Discovering the History of Psychiatry

DISCOVERING
THE HISTORY
OF PSYCHIATRY

Edited by

Mark S. Micale
Roy Porter

New York   Oxford
OXFORD UNIVERSITY PRESS
1994

Oxford University Press

Oxford   New York   Toronto
Delhi   Bombay   Calcutta   Madras   Karachi
Kuala Lumpur   Singapore   Hong Kong   Tokyo
Nairobi   Dar es Salaam   Cape Town
Melbourne   Auckland   Madrid

and associated companies in
Berlin   Ibadan

Published by Oxford University Press, Inc.,
200 Madison Avenue, New York, New York 10016

Oxford is a registered trademark of Oxford University Press

Library of Congress Cataloging-in-Publication Data
Discovering the history of psychiatry
edited by Mark S. Micale and Roy Porter
p. cm.   Includes bibliographical references and index.
ISBN 0-19-507739-3
1. Psychiatry—Historiography.
I. Micale, Mark S., 1957–   .
II. Porter, Roy, 1946–   .
[DNLM: 1. Psychiatry—history.   WM 11.1 D611 1994]
RC438.D58   1994
616.89′009—dc20   DNLM/DLC
for Library of Congress   93-12244

1 3 5 7 9 8 6 4 2

Printed in the United States of America
on acid-free paper

For

DR. ERIC T. CARLSON

Director

History of Psychiatry Section

Department of Psychiatry

The New York Hospital—Cornell Medical Center

1958–1992

Preface

The idea for this book originated in the fall of 1990, in a conversation between a British and an American historian over a Mexican meal in s'Hertogenbosch, the Netherlands. We were attending the First European Congress for the History of Psychiatry and Mental Health Care, sponsored by the Netherlands Institute of Mental Health, at which over 200 scholars from a dozen and a half countries gathered for the first time to share ideas about the history of the psychological sciences. It was a successful and exciting occasion, a fine expression of the new Europeanism. However, by the end of the conference, we were struck by the great diversity of styles of thinking and writing about the subjects under discussion. The question arose: Why do we have the psychiatric histories that we do? By the end of the meal, the solution seemed obvious: to assemble an international cast of eminent scholars, both psychiatrists and historians, and invite them to answer the question for us. The result is the present volume.

We would like to express our infinite gratitude to all the contributors. Not only did they too find the question intriguing; they proved willing rapidly to put pen to paper, often taking time from crowded schedules to address topics that were difficult and speculative. For close, critical, and constructive readings of our introductory essay, we acknowledge the assistance of Geoffrey Cocks, Gerald Grob, Anne Harrington, Nancy Tomes, Fernando Vidal, and Elisabeth Young-Bruehl. We also offer our deep thanks to Mr. Jeffrey House of Oxford University Press for his continual and enthusiastic support of an ambitious project.

Boston   M.S.M.
London   R.P.
February 1993

Contents

Contributors

DAVID F. ALLEN   M.A., M.Sc.,
   D.E.S.S.D.E.A.
Private Practice
Paris, France

JULIE V. BROWN   Ph.D.
Department of Sociology
University of North Carolina
Greensboro, North Carolina

GEOFFREY COCKS   Ph.D.
Department of History
Albion College
Albion, Michigan

NORMAN DAIN   Ph.D.
Department of History
Rutgers University
Newark, New Jersey

JOHN FORRESTER   Ph.D.
Department of the History and Philosophy
   of Science
Cambridge University
Cambridge, England

GERALD N. GROB   Ph.D.
Institute for Health, Health Care
   Policy, and Aging Research
Rutgers University
New Brunswick, New Jersey

PATRIZIA GUARNIERI   Ph.D.
Italian Center of Stanford University
   and Instituto degl'Innocenti
Florence, Italy

GARY GUTTING   Ph.D.
Department of Philosophy
University of Notre Dame
South Bend, Indiana

OTTO M. MARX   M.D.
West Chesterfield, New Hampshire

MARK S. MICALE   Ph.D. (Editor)
Department of History
Yale University
New Haven, Connecticut

GEORGE MORA   M.D.
Narragansett, Rhode Island

EDWARD T. MORMAN   M.S.L.S.,
   Ph.D.
Institute of the History of Medicine
The Johns Hopkins University
Baltimore, Maryland

KENNETH S. PIVER   M.A.
Enrolled in Medical School
The Johns Hopkins University
Baltimore, Maryland

ROY PORTER   Ph.D. (Editor)
Wellcome Institute for the History of
   Medicine
London, England

JACQUES POSTEL   M.D.
Centre Hospitalier Sainte-Anne
Paris, France

NANCY TOMES   Ph.D.
Department of History
State University of New York at Stony Brook
Stony Brook, New York

PATRICK VANDERMEERSCH   Ph.D.
Faculty of Theology
Groningen, The Netherlands

RICHARD E. VATZ   Ph.D.
Department of Communication
Towson State University
Baltimore, Maryland

FERNANDO VIDAL   Ph.D.
Faculté de Psychologie et des Sciences
   de l'Education
University of Geneva
Geneva, Switzerland

LEE S. WEINBERG   Ph.D., J.D.
Graduate School of Public
   and International Affairs
University of Pittsburgh
Pittsburgh, Pennsylvania

DORA B. WEINER   Ph.D.
Department of Medical Humanities
University of California, Los Angeles
Los Angeles, California

ELISABETH YOUNG-BRUEHL   Ph.D.
General Programs
Haverford College
Haverford, Pennsylvania

Discovering the History of Psychiatry

1

INTRODUCTION:
Reflections on Psychiatry and Its Histories[1]

ROY PORTER and MARK S. MICALE

History is a tale told about the past in the present for present purposes.
PAUL RICOEUR, "The Narrative Function," 1979

Among the most rapidly growing, controversy-ridden, and attention-attracting areas of history over the past generation has been the history of psychiatry. During the last three decades, debates have raged concerning the rise and fall of the asylum; the history of compulsory institutional confinement and deinstitutionalization; the origins, scientific validity, and therapeutic efficacy of Freudian theory; the merits of biological as opposed to psychodynamic models of the mind; the history of the insanity plea in the courts; the past uses of extreme physicalistic treatments for mental disability, such as frontal lobotomies and electroconvulsive therapy; and, most recently, the role played by psychiatry in the alleged processes of social and sexual control applied to women, workers, ethnic minorities, and gay people. The past thirty years have brought an outpouring of original scholarship—often passionate, partisan, and polemical—in all of these areas with no sign at present of slackening.

Strikingly, these controversies have by no means been confined to the world of medical practitioners and scholarly specialists. To the contrary, such disputes have displayed astonishing social, political, and cultural resonances. The historiography of psychiatry has decisively influenced thinking and writing in many neighboring fields of study, such as the history of medicine and science; women's studies; the history of law, crime, and deviance; the history of the professions; the history of sexuality; the history of the body; and cultural studies. A number of contributors to these literatures—most notably, the late Michel Foucault—are hailed less as commentators on a single branch of medical history than as social and cultural icons. Debates in Britain and the United States during the 1960s and 1970s concerning the institutional decarceration of mental patients were demonstrably linked to a body of scholarship exploring the nature, "discovery," and growth of the asylum in the nineteenth century. And a number of early, landmark texts in the women's movement, including Simone de Beauvoir's *The*

Second Sex, underscored the past functions of science and medicine generally, and psychiatry in particular, as intellectual justification for female subordination, while the first wave of scholarship by Anglo-American women's historians during the 1970s took nervous disorders in the Victorian middle-class woman as one of its subjects. In a somewhat similar way, the activities of Central European mental health care professionals during the Nazi era have emerged in the last ten years as a topic of intense and painful controversy in Germany. And the conditions for similar soul-searching interrogations about the past political usages of psychiatry in the former Soviet Union and eastern Europe have also now developed. The same issue is festering just under the surface of public discussion in Latin America.

The selective politicization of the history of psychiatry in recent years has been accompanied by the explosive growth of psychiatric history as an academic discipline. Scanning the field in its entirety today, we are perhaps most struck by the remarkable diversity of discourses about psychiatry's history. Cultural and social theorists; sociologists; historians of science and medicine; social, cultural, and intellectual historians; women's historians; and art and literary critics, as well as psychiatrists, neurologists, psychoanalysts, and clinical psychologists have all had, and are having, their say about psychiatry and its famous past. Not surprisingly, the histories of psychiatry that result—and it is a basic contention of this book that there are many separate *histories*—have varied enormously. Since the mid-twentieth century, something labeled ''the history of psychiatry'' by its authors has been diversely interpreted as the unilinear progress of humanitarianism and medical science; the gradual, centuries-long discovery of the unconscious psyche; the endless dialectical struggle between biologically and psychologically oriented theories and therapies of mind; the story of the emergence, formulation, and global diffusion of Freudian ideas; the continuing social and psychological mastering of unreason by an authoritarian bourgeois rationalism; a manipulation by male physicians of passive female patients; and an ancient but misconceived effort to medicalize mythical nonorganic illnesses. The list could easily be extended. Over the past thirty years, each of these historical visions has inspired—or, perhaps better, provoked—a revision, and each revision a counterrevision. We believe that in no branch of the history of science or medicine has there been less interpretive consensus. In few professions, inside or outside the sciences, has it been more difficult to demarcate the scholarly, historical enterprise from urgent, present-day debates. And perhaps no area of the humanities today attracts detailed and impassioned commentary from so wide a range of writers. This book is intended to explore the peculiar, complex, and powerful interplay between psychiatry, historiography, and social, cultural, and political ideology.

Like other human endeavors, the sciences—physical, biological, behavioral—develop their own histories as they evolve. They seek casts of ancestors, precursors, and founding fathers; they fashion pedigrees for themselves. Exemplary episodes are highlighted, along with occasional false steps and heroic breakthroughs, all pointing to moral lessons. Much like individuals creating an autobiography, a selective sense of past self, the sciences fashion for themselves idealized genealogies in which positive episodes are memorialized, taken as characteristic of the essence, while negative ones are forgotten.[2] To be sure, histories of scientific disciplines instruct, inform, and entertain. However, as recent scholarship has demonstrated, they serve other purposes, too. Disciplinary histories socialize scientific initiates into their endeavor by establishing a line of intellectual filiation between the great minds of the past and contemporary workers. With newly acquired bodies of knowledge, they may argue for the epistemological integrity, and therefore scientific credentials, of a discipline by tracing a suitable line of evolution. They may also assist in sharpening contested interdisciplinary or intra-disciplinary boundaries. Furthermore, in periods of paradigmatic conflict, science histories, by memorializing the proper lineage of figures, texts, and ideas, serve to legitimate particular theories and methodologies and to delegitimate others. More and more, they also operate to present a favorable image of the field not only internally but to the educated public, the media, and institutional sources of financial support.[3]

The history of psychiatry is no exception to the well-known phenomenon of "usable pasts."[4] However, a confluence of conditions has prodigiously complicated the construction of the psychiatric profession's collective memory. If today we inspect the major historical accounts of, say, biology or chemistry, or, within medical history, of surgery, dentistry, or anesthesiology, we find essential agreement on the subject matters, developmental themes, foundational figures, and transformational episodes that are central and constitutive of the discipline. The same cannot be claimed for histories of psychiatry. We venture to claim that, both empirically and interpretively, extant histories of psychiatry reveal a vastly greater degree of difference among themselves than historical accounts of any other discipline.

There are a number of likely reasons why this is so. Late twentieth-century psychiatry has come about not through the steady, unproblematic accumulation of ideas and practices through the centuries but sporadically, with long periods of advance, stagnation, and even regression. The sort of dramatic and decisive breakthroughs in understanding the nature and etiology of disease that have punctuated the history of organic medicine are few and far between for mental medicine. Other branches of medicine and science have, by and large, followed unilinear developments as they emerged from one or two "pre-scientific" forms into their modern incarnations—evolving, for instance, from alchemy to chemistry or astrology to astronomy. Comparatively speaking, the pathway of their disciplinary evolution (Thomas Kuhn's *The Structure of Scientific Revolutions* notwithstanding) has been clear, continuous, and cumulative; as a result, their histories are internally cohesive. The historical structure of psychiatry, however, is significantly different. Its disciplinary origins lie scattered in a multitude of areas of past activity and inquiry, including primitive medicine, mythology, hypnotism, theology, philosophy, law, anthropology, literature, and popular lay healing, all of which came together only in the late nineteenth century to form what we recognize today as the modern discipline of psychiatry. Furthermore, the subject matter of psychiatry itself has continually shifted. Poised precariously between the medical sciences and the human sciences, psychological medicine has routinely lost, gained, and then lost again its disciplinary territory as neighboring fields expanded and contracted.[5]

Perhaps most decisively, psychiatry boasts no stable and consensual theoretical vantage point from which to construct itself historically. From its earliest days, psychiatric medicine has been marked by the persistence of competing, if not bitterly opposing, schools. Most noticeably, the field since the eighteenth century has been convulsed by a deep, dichotomous debate between the somatic and mentalist philosophies of mind. The historiographical effects of this division have been great. From generation to generation, as the perceived cognitive content of the discipline has changed, the projected disciplinary past of psychiatry has changed with it. Moreover, for professional purposes, each generation of practitioners has written a history that highlights those past ideas and practices that anticipate its own formation and consigns to marginal status competing ideas and their heritages. In this process, individual figures and texts—indeed, entire historical periods and bodies of knowledge—have at times been omitted from the historical record. With an intensely subjective subject matter, complex multidisciplinary origins, an insecure and shifting epistemological base, porous disciplinary boundaries, and a sectarian and dialectical dynamic of development, it has thus far proved impossible to produce anything like an enduring, comprehensive, authoritative history of psychiatry.[6]

Notwithstanding these complications, there has been no dearth of attempts to write such a history. By the second quarter of the twentieth century, psychiatric practitioners were sufficiently self-confident about their speciality to produce the first full-scale narrative histories of the field. Early attempts by members of the profession to represent themselves historically assumed the form of what today is most commonly termed "Whig" historiography.[7] Works in this genre, which proliferated during the 1930s, 1940s, and 1950s, were indicatively titled *Men Against Madness, Man Above Humanity, From Medicine Man to Freud,* and *One Hundred Years and More of Conquests.*[8] Easily the most widely read work in this mold was *A History of Medical Psychology,* which appeared in 1941 and was authored by the Russian emigré psychoanalyst Gregory Zilboorg.[9] Whig narratives were presentist, progressivist, and tenaciously internalist. They typically presented a dual historical movement, from cruelty and barbarism to organized, institutional humanitarianism, and from ignorance, religion, and superstition to modern medical science. They often consisted of dramatically juxtaposed dark ages, enlightenments, and revolutions that heralded the way to the present.

We might cite one influential capsule statement of a historical vision of this kind. "The story in its broad outlines is familiar and dramatic," wrote Sir Aubrey Lewis, the distinguished senior psychiatrist of the Maudsley Hospital, in 1967.

> After the tortures and judicial murders of the Middle Ages and the Renaissance, which confounded demoniacal possession with delusion and frenzy, and smelt out witchcraft in the maunderings of demented old women, there were the cruelties and degradation of the madhouses of the seventeenth and eighteenth centuries, in which authority used chains and whips as its instruments. Humanitarian effort put an end to the abuses. Pinel in France, Chiarugi in Italy, Tuke in England inaugurated an era of kindness and medical care which prepared the way for a rational, humane approach to the mastery of mental illness. In the nineteenth century the pathology of insanity was investigated, its clinical forms described and classified, its kinship with physical disease and the psychoneuroses recognized. Treatment was undertaken in university hospitals, out-patient clinics multiplied, and social aspects [of psychiatric illness] were given increasing attention. By the end of the century the way had been opened for the ideas of such men as Kraepelin, Freud, Charcot and Janet, following in the paths of Kahlbaum and Griesinger, Conolly and Maudsley. In the twentieth century psychopathology has been elucidated, and psychological treatment given ever widening scope and sanction. Revolutionary changes have occurred in physical methods of treatment, the regime in mental hospitals has been further liberalized, and the varieties of care articulated into one another, individualized, and made elements in a continuous therapeutic process that extends well into the general community, beginning with the phase of onset, *Stadium incrementi,* and proceeding to the ultimate phase of rehabilitation and social resettlement.

"This," concluded Lewis, "is the conventional picture, one of progress and enlightenment . . . [and] it is not far out."[10] Zilboorg, too, summed up this view nicely in the epilogue of his *History of Medical Psychology*. His book closes with the inspired generalization that "[t]he history of psychiatry is essentially the history of humanism . . . Every time the spirit of humanism has arisen, a new contribution to psychiatry has been made."[11]

Latter-day critics of historical Whiggism have not failed to point out still other features of the scholarship in this camp. Traditional psychiatric historiography, it has been observed, was based on The Great Man, Hall-of-Fame approach. In its methodology, it was purely intellectual-historical, paying scant attention to the social, cultural, economic, and professional dimensions of the subject. It offered little original historical research, being limited to the best known printed texts of major theorists, which were more often than not cited reverently rather than read or researched. Moreover, Whig histories, in the standard view, are highly "presentist," evaluating past ideas and practices solely according to contemporary medical beliefs and standards. Finally, early psychiatric history writing, it has been alleged, functioned in effect as a kind of hallowed self-historiography. It consisted of uncritical "in-house" historical accounts written by psychiatrists, about psychiatrists, and for psychiatrists.

Not surprisingly, the historiographical optimism of the midcentury period, which corresponded with the height of the professional prestige of psychiatry in Europe and North America, eventually provoked The Great Revision. Clustered at the beginning of the 1960s, and foreshadowing the larger cultural radicalism of the new decade, came four key texts: Erving Goffman's *Asylums*, R. D. Laing's *The Divided Self*, Thomas Szasz's *The Myth of Mental Illness*, and Michel Foucault's *Histoire de la folie*.[12] Despite major differences in intellectual style and origin, these books offered similar historical perspectives on their subject. All of them questioned official assurances of the fundamental benignity of the psychiatric enterprise as well as the assumption that more psychiatry means better psychiatry. Laing, working in Britain, averred that schizophrenia, and by extension all mental illness, was not an illness but a diagnostic designation arbitrarily fixed by society and confirmed by psychiatrists. Goffman, an American sociologist much moved by Bruno Bettelheim's writings on concentration camps, portrayed the modern-day mental hospital as a "total" institution that degraded people and effectively created mad behavior. And Szasz began from the premise that institutional psychiatry is an unsupportable enterprise because it is based on a notion of mental illness that is itself fictitious. Accordingly, Szasz viewed the history of "compulsory psychiatry" as a gigantic error, if not a gigantic evil, and, rather in the manner of an atheistic reading of the annals of the Vatican, twisted the *idées reçues* of the Whig history of psychiatry on their head. In his view, the entire history of psychiatry is the obdurate and pitiless defense of a fantasy.

In a somewhat comparable manner, Foucault's *Madness and Civilization* proved such a bombshell because it utterly overturned conventional liberal and meliorist assumptions.[13] Foucault contended that the growth of institutional psychiatry was not a source of progress but a technique of alienation, not reason restored but rather madness expropriated, a new mode of unreason. In a quasi-Nietzschean transvaluative gesture, Foucault transformed the pantheonic heroes of the Whig accounts into villains. Thus, in the famous final chapter of his study, the Tuke family at the York Retreat in the 1770s and 1780s and Philippe Pinel at the Bicêtre hospital in the 1790s did not, after all, free the mad in traditionally celebrated liberations but only forged for them more sinister inner chains—the "gigantic moral imprisonment" of the insane asylum.[14] By the end of the 1960s, then, the ideas of Goffman, Laing, Szasz, and Foucault had combined with French and German Marxist psychologies, British anti-psychoanalytic sentiment, critical feminist theory, and the mental patients' liberation movement in a comprehensive attack on modern mental health institutions and practices. A powerful "anti-psychiatry" movement was under way.[15]

In turn, the 1970s brought a series of ambitious historical studies that applied the heady but general schemes of anti-psychiatry to particular countries. While the authors of the Whig literature had been self-appointed physician-historians, the new critical revisionists were either disaffected psychotherapists or radical sociologists and social historians from the universities.[16] Klaus Doerner's *Bürger und Irre*, David Rothman's *The Discovery of the Asylum*, Robert Castel's *L'Ordre psychiatrique*, and Andrew Scull's *Museums of Madness* brought the ideas of Laing, Foucault, Goffman, and Szasz, respectively, to German, American, French, and British psychiatry history of the nineteenth century.[17] Doerner, Rothman, Castel, and Scull eschewed the traditional genres of biography and the general longitudinal narrative in favor of a study of institutions. Relentlessly revisionist in interpretation, their books supplied sociologically literate historical analyses of psychiatry that stressed the covert social and moral normalizing function of the discipline. They also highlighted the deep functional similarities among modern institutions, such as asylums, prisons, factories, and schools.[18] In this process, the revisionist *Kritikers* of the 1970s, it has often been maintained, fatally challenged what they perceived as the shallow and idealizing historiography of previous generations and unveiled Whig medical history as the ideology of medical progress that it was. Not least of all, the new generation of commentators introduced professional scholarly standards into the historiography of psychiatry both by drawing on a much wider base of empirical evidence and by introducing into the field the ideal of objective and systematic analysis.[19]

All of this, we say, is well known. It may be well known, but in our view the account offered up to now in this introductory chapter, while assuredly containing an element of validity, is also highly tendentious and accurate at best only in parts. The debunking revisionism of the past generation has been impressive for its critical intellectual energy, and the dramatic, "historiclastic" interpretations it has advanced are responsible in no small measure for arousing widespread scholarly interest in a previously specialized and rather antiquarian area of study. Nevertheless, the way in which recent scholars in this tradition present their work, as well as their placement of that work in the historiographical field, cannot, we believe, be accepted at face value. In particular, the impression is forming that Whiggism today exists primarily in the ideological imagination of the latter-day revisionist historian who continues to find the concept an indispensable ideological straw man against which to define his or her own self-consciously radical interpretations.[20]

For one thing, The Great Revision of the last three decades pits "amateur" physician-cum-historians writing a naive and self-serving internalist intellectual history of psychiatry against "professional" historians producing a more methodologically sophisticated, empirically substantial, and sociologically oriented scholarship.[21] But an unbiased examination reveals this idea as a simple misreading of the historiographical record and suggests that such a value-laden professional polarization is, to a great degree, fictional. For example, the first major history of American psychiatry, often cited today for its putative Whiggishness, was Albert Deutsch's *The Mentally Ill in America*, published in 1937. But Deutsch, as we learn from George Mora's essay in this volume, was neither a physician nor a historian but a self-taught public servant in the New York State mental hygiene movement whose work was manifestly reformist in design. In addition, Deutsch's book draws heavily on virgin primary source materials, such as reports from mental hospitals, court proceedings, and local, state, and federal legislation.[22] Similarly, as Edward Morman indicates in his chapter in this volume, it was George Rosen, with doctorates in medicine and sociology, who learned the lessons of the functionalist social sciences of the 1950s and 1960s and went on to pioneer the concept of "the historical sociology of mental illness" contemporaneously with the writings of Goffman, Laing, Foucault, and Szasz.[23] Likewise, the second part of this book explores the work of five individuals—Richard Hunter, Ida Macalpine, George Rosen, Henri Ellenberger, and Jean Starobinski—who arguably are among the most powerful and original historical interpreters of psychiatry in our century. Yet all five were trained medically, and two of them—Hunter and Ellenberger—practiced institutional psychiatry daily throughout their professional lifetimes. Three of these figures—Hunter, Macalpine, and Ellenberger—were substantially distanced from, if not bitterly alienated by, many of the therapeutic practices of their time.

For another thing, it is difficult to dismiss the physician-historian as an amateur when the category includes such authors as Hunter, Macalpine, and Ellenberger, who immersed themselves to a profound depth in previously unknown source materials. An exemplary historical study of the asylum, quite unWhiggish, which integrated medical and sociological perspectives, was Hunter and Macalpine's *Psychiatry for the Poor, 1851: Colney Hatch Asylum, Friern Hospital 1973: A Medical and Social History* (1974). The finest study that we possess to date of private madhouse facilities in any country during any period remains *The Trade in Lunacy*, by William Parry-Jones, a physician. And, more recently, the most intelligent and comprehensive history of a psychodiagnostic category in the scholarly literature thus far has been provided by Stanley Jackson, a Yale professor of clinical psychiatry.[24] Also pertinent is the reaction of psychiatrist-historians to the remarks lodged against their work during the past twenty years. Confronted with the withering criticisms of sociologists and social historians, some doctors fled the field in horror or anger while others reacted uncomprehendingly.[25] Other authors accepted the criticisms, responded constructively, and, after a period of silence, are now returning with work of high caliber.[26] Moreover, some psychiatric practitioners of late have gone on the offensive and raised the specter of a historiography of psychiatry with the psychiatry left out.[27] Nor by any means have all "prefatory histories" of psychiatry been uncritical and Whiggish.[28]

Moreover, the past division of interpretive labor within the historiography of psychiatry has been far less neat than some have contended. Two of the four major so-called anti-psychiatric theorists—Szasz and Laing—hailed from the psychiatric community itself. The first critical questioning of the "heroic" image of one of the traditional originators of modern psychiatry appeared from the pen of a well-established medical historian two decades before the rise of historical anti-psychiatry.[29] In France, the first critical analysis of the founding myth of Pinel was produced by the French psychiatrist Gladys Swain, while the bulk of scholarship on the history of mental medicine in that country today, much of it informed by the precedents of anti-psychiatry, is written by physicians. Analogously, the best-informed historical critic of the anti-psychiatry movement in North America comes not from the defensive or conservative wing of the medical profession but within liberal historical studies.[30] Still further, the *guerre des savants* waged in the United States during the 1970s and 1980s over the origin and nature of the asylum opposed to one another not scientists and humanists but social historians within the universities.[31]

In addition, on close and honest inspection, the actual content of psychiatric history recounted in traditional textbooks, biographies, institutional histories, and the like proves to be more complex, nuanced, and ambiguous, and less complacent, progressivist, and filiopietistic, than many historians of the 1970s and 1980s wanted it to be and confidently declared it to be. Indeed, some so-called Whig treatments have taken a critical and rather gloomy view of their profession. Daniel Hack Tuke's *Chapters on the History of the Insane in the British Isles* (1882) is rather instructive. Near the close of that work, Tuke includes a paean to psychiatric progress written by Dr. Stokes, superintendent of the Mount Hope Retreat in Baltimore. But Tuke declines to endorse Stokes' vision. The history of psychiatry did not plot the path of progress:

> If the success of the treatment of insanity bore any considerable proportion to the number of the remedies which have been brought forward, it would be my easy and agreeable duty to record the triumphs of medicine in the distressing malady which they are employed to combat. But this, unhappily, is not the case.

Tuke proceeds to list some dozen worthless remedies that had come into and gone out of fashion during the previous half-century.[32]

Or, nearer to the present, juxtapose to the long, celebratory statement of Aubrey Lewis above the following prefatory lament from the 1960s by Hunter and Macalpine, the two leading British historians of psychiatry at the time:

> [In psychiatry], there is not even an objective method of describing or communicating clinical findings without subjective interpretation and no exact and uniform terminology which conveys precisely the same to all. In consequence there is wide divergence of diagnosis, even of diagnoses, a steady flow of new terms and an ever-changing nomenclature, as well as a surfeit of hypotheses which tend to be presented as fact. Furthermore, etiology remains speculative, pathogenesis largely obscure, classifications predominantly symptomatic and hence arbitrary and possibly ephemeral; physical treatments are empirical and subject to fashion, and psychotherapies still only in their infancy and doctrinaire.

The authors conclude that "rather than a chronicle of feats, facts, and discoveries, the history of psychiatry presents a record of perennial problems, recurrent ideas, disputes and treatments, trailing in the wake of medicine and exhibiting paradoxically—as medicine did of old—a mixture of as many false facts as false theories."[33] This passage was written in 1963, four years after the passage by Lewis, and by two historians who were physicians. Among the functions of this volume, then, are to reopen serious and unprejudiced scrutiny of older "in-house" psychiatric histories, to establish the extent and the richness of pre-Foucault historical writing about psychiatry, and to break down the artificial, value-laden bifurcation between medical and nonmedical scholarship.

Perhaps most relevant for present purposes, social revisionist analyses of the past generation may be critiqued on many of the same grounds that the revisionists themselves used with such effect against Whig psychiatric historiography. If social-historical revisionism alleges that practitioners' history has been shaped to serve the self-interested purposes of the medical profession, where does this leave the demystifying recensions written by the critics and radicals? "Labels such as 'presentism' have been attached to the historical studies of psychiatrists, but it is the revisionists themselves who often apply late twentieth-century value judgments to the activities of doctors, relatives, administrators, or politicians in the totally different conditions of the past," two recent skeptical readers have snapped.[34] Plainly, it is essential in this matter to have recourse to the principle of intellectual symmetry. Accepting that historians of the 1970s and 1980s had the right and duty to deconstruct past psychiatrists' histories of psychiatry, exposing their biases and ulterior motives, the histories constructed by such critics must equally be exposed to equivalent styles of analysis.[35]

In truth, to be outside psychiatry and to write about it historically has by no means ensured objectivity and disinterest. In fact, it is becoming apparent in retrospect that the challenging scholarship of the past three decades has been no less rooted in social, political, and professional circumstances than the literature it sought to displace. Graduate schooled during the tumultuous 1960s, the major authors in the revisionist tradition were steeped in the romantic anti-statism and anti-institutionalism of that decade. Consequently, much historiography in this category was intended as part of an attempt to reform present-day policy. It was with considerable aptness that Peter Sedgwick, the British historian of the anti-psychiatry movement, referred to "an anti-history of psychiatry."[36] What is more, the most militant historical anti-psychiatrists sought not just to reform but to *épater la psychiatrie*. In other words, The Great Revision, viewed in *its* historical context, may be seen as part and parcel of the larger, libertarian, countercultural interrogation of the basic institutional structures of power in modern capitalist society of the 1960s in which its practitioners shared the belief that their work as historians was contributing, however indirectly, to the forthcoming social transformation.

We suspect radically oriented social historians of psychiatry from the 1960s, 1970s, and 1980s are aware of their ideological orientation and would most likely acknowledge their (often laudable) political goals. However, by all indications, they are far less conscious of the myriad ways in which their political agendas served to select their subject matters, to shape their methodologies, to texture their interpretations, and to predetermine their conclusions. The literature of social revisionism has focused on the institutional aspects of psychiatry, and the blackest episodes of institutional history at that—the great confinement of the seventeenth century, cases of arbitrary confinement, instances of therapeutic excesses, the failures of decarceration in the twentieth century. It has centered its narratives on subjects that lend themselves to social, political, and economic (rather than scientific or clinical) analyses. In addition, its demystifications of Whig idealizations have often only generated "heroic" neo-Marxist and Foucauldian remystifications.[37] The historical picture it provides as a whole has not been free of ideology so much as counterideological. Lastly, the work done in this tradition has been no less self-promoting professionally than what preceded it. The highly charged division between amateur and professional historians, the programmatically externalist conceptualization of the discipline, and the methodologies appropriate to such a conceptualization that were announced loudly in the 1970s were all calculated to privilege the explanatory authority of the social historian and the social scientist over and above the physician. What are called Whig histories were written by, about, and for psychiatrists, we have said. But no less so, sixties, seventies, and eighties social revisionists, too, have written for members of their own guild—for ideologically like-minded, nonmedical intellectuals in the academy. As one of us writes below, "It is clear that to understand the history of psychiatry written by practitioners, it is a prerequisite to examine their own psychiatric commitments. It is equally clear that to understand the history of psychiatry written by historians, it is first necessary to examine the commitments of the historian."[38]

Our purpose in this line of analysis, we want to state clearly, is not to attack recent revisionist literature as such, nor to judge the comparative worth of the "Whig" and "revisionist" approaches. (Both groups had excesses and accomplishments and both labels no doubt are in part reductionistic.) Nor is our goal to apportion blame for the controversialism of the field. Our point, rather, is that the two main traditions of commentary about the history of psychiatry in the past half-century have been equally lacking in self-reflexivity and, for reasons that are not as dissimilar as members of either camp would care to acknowledge, both have been substantially politicized. For the first group, writing about psychiatry's past has typically functioned as the historical branch of current-day psychiatric practice. For the second, it has operated as the historical branch of the contemporary anti-psychiatry movement. What is perhaps most notable in all of this is that there has been so little serious self-examination by modern historians of madness of the many nonintellectual factors undergirding their enterprise. This want of reflective, philosophical discussion about the foundations and principles of writing about psychiatric history strikes us as surprising, disappointing, and even shocking. Psychiatry as a profession emphasizes the value and virtue of self-awareness, and in its medical practices often employs a developmental mode of inquiry; nevertheless, it has remained resolutely unintrospective about the methodological and ideological conditions under which it writes about its own past.

The silence on these matters is all the more peculiar in light of the past decade's extensive and sophisticated discussion concerning different conceptual, methodological, and epistemological strategies for writing the history of science generally. Should the history of science follow an "internalist" approach, stressing the cognitive development of natural knowledge, or an "externalist" approach, focusing on the social, economic, political, and professional determinants of scientific theory and practice? Should it offer an intellectual history or a social and cultural history? Should it be relativistic or progressivist? Presentist or contextualist?[39] Although less probingly, these same matters have been addressed by historians of medicine,[40] and several significant attempts have been made to achieve a critical and self-aware historiography of the behavioral sciences.[41] More broadly still, the issue of the nature, status, and validity of historical knowledge and historical language in general has been eagerly disputed within poststructuralist and deconstructionist theories.[42] It is striking, however, that so few of these issues have been raised within the history of psychiatry. As one of us has observed elsewhere, it appears that as historians of psychiatry we have been so preoccupied during the past generation with placing ourselves in the great ideological controversies animating the field that we have had little time to examine the methodological, epistemological, and ideological underpinnings of the discipline.[43]

One may or may not approve of the ongoing ideologization of the history of psychiatry, but the fact remains that these have been the defining conditions under which a good portion of it has been written. In all of this there has been much recrimination but little serious reflection about the varieties of the history of psychiatry that are, or should be, on offer, and the reasons why psychiatry has been interpreted in certain ways. Hence, in the editors' opinion, the need for this volume as the first systematic appraisal of the formation of successive and rival representations of the history of insanity.[44] As the history of psychiatry itself gropes toward the status of a mature and independent discipline of study, we believe that it is timely, and intellectually exciting, to have a work that invites the reader to peer into the mind, and the soul, of the historiography of psychiatry. In this volume, therefore, we offer a collection of essays that examines—collectively and comparatively, critically but constructively—the major psychohistoriographies of the century.

Of particular interest, we believe, is the constructedness of psychiatric histories or, put differently, the intense interpretability of psychiatry's past. To explore this phenomenon properly, we believe that it is necessary to conceptualize history writing as itself a historical act. It has been the goal of the editors and the contributors, therefore, to reconstruct the array of local issues and circumstances—of a personal, professional, institutional, scientific, cultural, intellectual, social, and political nature—which together have formed the culture and the sociology of history writing out of which the most important authors, texts, and analytical models in the field have emerged. To this end, we have posed recurrently to ourselves a number of questions: What is the range of relations that practicing psychiatrists have had to both their discipline's history and its historiography? In what ways has psychiatric historiography over the years operated as a form of internal, disciplinary self-presentation for professional psychological medicine? What are the hidden linkages between psychiatric history writing and contemporary social and political contexts that have often scripted subjects and ideas into historical writing about psychiatry, and how have these agendas operated? How has psychological theory and psychiatric practice affected the writing of psychiatric history? And, conversely, how has psychiatric historiography influenced theory and practice?

Finally, and rather more speculatively, we have attempted with this book to place our subject in a broad cultural setting. Over the past two decades, traditional hospital psychiatry has declined decisively in power and prestige. However, in a pattern that has not been sufficiently noted, the decrease in the institutional authority of psychological medicine has been accompanied by its seemingly endless intellectual extension. All around us today, we observe the influence and expansion of psychology-as-worldview. We live in pervasively secular societies in which people are preoccupied as never before with the self and in which psychology, in its myriad manifestations, is seen as the most appropriate instrument for exploring that self and the best means for ministering to its ills. We turn to the psychosciences to run our private relationships, to raise our children, to try our criminals, to interpret our works of art, to improve our sex lives, to tell us why we are unhappy, depressed, anxious, or fatigued.[45] Over the past few generations, an immense professional structure has developed to cater to our elaborate and expanding psychological needs. Hundreds of thousands of individuals in an increasing diversity of professional forms, including psychiatrists, psychoanalysts, clinical psychologists, psychotherapists, social workers, psychiatric nurses, marriage and family therapists, sexologists, guidance counselors, and lay therapists of all sorts administer our "advanced psychiatric society."[46] Millions of people each year receive psychotherapy in a multitude of forms, and we ingest tons of psychochemicals to alter our moods.[47] Furthermore, the number of populations conceptualized psychiatrically and the scope of behaviors diagnosed medically continue to multiply in an apparently endless process.[48]

Plainly, the "psychological revolution" that has taken place around us represents much more than the expansion of a single medical subspeciality. Rather, we suspect that it constitutes one of the major cultural transformations of the twentieth century. On the broadest level, then, we have attempted with this volume to work toward a kind of meta-historiographical perspective on the history of psychiatry by reflecting on past and present commentaries about psychiatry as forms of collective, cultural self-definition: How has the rush of critical writing about psychiatry and its history in recent decades been part of a larger disillusionment with scientific and medical knowledge in a modern, alienating technocratic world? In what ways may the literature of psychiatric historiography be read as a part of the cultural and intellectual history of the twentieth century? And, in this most psychological of centuries, how have we sought to understand ourselves and our society through the historical representation of psychiatric knowledge and practice?

The essays in this book seek to explore these questions, among others, in as many different domains of debate as possible. The authors come from the medical sciences, the social sciences, and the humanities. They issue from a variety of national and disciplinary backgrounds. Some of them are established, prominent figures who have lived through and participated in these controversies while others are young, promising scholars just entering the field. The book includes articles on individual historians and schools of historiography, on nineteenth- and twentieth-century topics, and on a spectrum of psychological systems and practices. Furthermore, we have attempted to construct a volume that moves beyond the traditional focus of English-language scholarship on the Anglo-Saxon world.[49] Throughout the book, we have eschewed an overtly ideological approach, instead encouraging contributors to develop a historicizing methodology. As the editors, we have made no effort whatsoever to adjudicate among different, even directly antagonistic, interpretations. To repeat: It is not our goal in these pages to defend, debunk, or deride particular historical readings of psychiatry but to study them, insofar as possible, from a critical, comparative, cultural perspective. It is our hope that readers will find the simple juxtaposition of essays to be suggestive and illuminating and that together they will serve to answer the question: Why do we have the histories of psychiatry that we do?

The twenty chapters that make up the balance of this book fall within five, large, thematically interconnected sections. Part I, "Early Developments," surveys two major interpretive traditions of historical writing about psychiatry that formed before the second half of the twentieth century.

In "The Beginning of Psychiatric Historiography in Nineteenth-Century Germany," Otto Marx establishes that the first historical commentary about psychiatry appeared in the German-speaking countries during the second quarter of the nineteenth century. Marx links this early appearance to the combined presence in Germany during the 1800s of philosophical historicism and positivist scholarship, which spawned the first "scientific" schools of historical studies, including medical and science histories. Marx reconstructs a rich but little-known sequence of texts by German-language asylum physicians and medical historians that appeared during the period 1820–1920.[50] In the process, he demonstrates that from its earliest years, psychiatric history writing was intimately caught up with the methodological and theoretical commitments of its authors. As already noted, the history of this subject has been marked by a deep dialectical clash between organic and psychogenic visions of the mind. This mind-body duality, Marx finds, was directly mirrored in the historiography of nineteenth-century Germany. During the 1820s, 1830s, and 1840s, psychiatrists and historians who wrote as *Psychiker* conceptualized the philosophical issue of relations between body, mind, and soul as the central theme of psychiatric theorizing and accordingly hailed the achievements of the so-called Romantic school of J. C. A. Heinroth, J. C. Reil, K. W. Ideler, Justinus Kerner, Friedrich Schelling, Novalis, C. W. M. Jacobi, and Alexander Haindorf. During the second half of the century, however, *Somatiker* dismissed the metaphysical psychiatry of the previous generation as the expression of a contemptible prescientific stage in the development of the discipline. In a series of historical introductions to psychiatric textbooks and chapters on psychiatry in general medical histories from 1850 to 1920, Marx shows, German writers traced the historical precedents of contemporary, anatomically and physiologically oriented psychiatry back to Gall's phrenological work earlier in the century, and farther still, to the Hippocratic treatise on epilepsy. At the same time, they presented Romantic psychiatry as an undifferentiated background of mystical nonsense from which contemporary psychiatric medicine had struggled to free itself in order to achieve its truly modern, scientific form.[51]

In a similar vein, George Mora in "Early American Historians of Psychiatry, 1910–1960" analyzes the varied writings of the first three generations of psychiatric historians in the United States. Some of Mora's most instructive observations concern Gregory Zilboorg, Franz Alexander, and Sheldon Selesnick. As David Werman has determined, Zilboorg's *A History of Medical Psychology* (1941) and Alexander and Selesnick's *History of Psychiatry* (1966) provided the standard version of psychiatric history for two generations of medical students in the United States.[52] Both works, Mora points out, are structured around a kind of Freudian historical teleology. Zilboorg and Alexander were charismatic emigré psychoanalysts, practicing respectively in New York City and Chicago, who wrote during the American psychoanalytic hegemony of the middle decades of the century. In their influential accounts, Mora shows, Freud gets interpreted as the central event in the history of the psychological sciences. Selected elements in the history of psychiatry are either criticized or eulogized according to their degree of anticipation of or divergence from the psychoanalytic model of mind. Analogously, the major figures of twentieth-century psychiatry are divided into categories of disciples or dissidents, based on their place in the schismatic history of the psychoanalytic movement. Texts in the Zilboorgian tradition, Mora finds further, have tended to expend considerable effort locating "prefigurations" of Freudian concepts, particularly the ideas of unconscious mental activity, psychogenesis, and psychosexuality. Conversely, those historical figures who produced competing nonpsychoanalytic psychodynamic theories, such as Pierre Janet, and contemporaneous nondynamic schools of psychology, like behavioralism and reflexology, are dealt with through systematic misrepresentation or even nonrepresentation. Mora's chapter illustrates ways in which history writing may serve to commemorate and consolidate the teachings of a dominant psychological paradigm while simultaneously discrediting its rivals.[53]

Part II, "Five Major Voices," concentrates on the *oeuvres* of five brilliant authors whose intellectual vision of the history of psychiatry was particularly original and whose writings have influenced—at times altered—the course of thinking and writing about the subject. In Chapter 4, Roy Porter dissects the wide-ranging writings of Ida Macalpine and Richard Hunter, the mother-and-son team that dominated British history of psychiatry from the mid-1950s. Prolific writers, their early publications display attempts to apply orthodox Freudian categories to historical cases. In time, however, they renounced Freudian categories, and, in the last ten years of their careers as historians, they abandoned psychogenic approaches completely and examined the historical record from a convinced organic viewpoint, a change that evidently reflected shifts in their psychiatric practice and in the wider climate of psychiatry. Along the way, Porter highlights the magnificent bibliographical labors of Hunter and Macalpine, who brought to scholarly attention dozens of unknown texts and whose unrivaled library of holdings in the history of psychiatry, The Hunter/Macalpine Collection, is now available for general use at Cambridge University.

In Chapter 5, Edward T. Morman discusses the American physician George Rosen. Best known for his writings on the history of public health and general medical history, Rosen in the latter half of his career produced some two dozen essays on the history of psychiatry. Rosen's primary methodological innovation in these papers, Morman indicates, was the notion of the "historical sociology of mental illness." While previous historians primarily conceived of psychiatry's past in intellectual terms, as a drama of ideas taking place in printed texts, Rosen focused intensely on social definitions of, attitudes toward, and determinants of, mental illness. In particular, he analyzed to great effect a series of historical episodes of mass psychopathology from ancient Greek times to the present. While not denying the sort of biological factors that Hunter and Macalpine emphasized, Rosen brought to attention the sociocultural contexts indispensable for understanding irrational behaviors, which he interpreted as expressions of deep structural stresses and anxieties in society. Morman explores the range of influences operating on Rosen's approach to psychiatric history, including a trade-unionist family background; ethnic, immigrant, working-class origins; a nondogmatic reading of Marxian political and economic theory; and exposure (as a graduate student at Columbia University) to the Mannheimian and Mertonian sociologies of knowledge. Morman closes by reflecting on the ways in which Rosen's work of the 1950s and 1960s anticipated the later project of the social history of psychiatry.

In Chapter 6, Mark S. Micale discusses a selection of themes in the historical writings of Henri F. Ellenberger, the Swiss author of *The Discovery of the Unconscious*. As Micale indicates, Ellenberger's magisterial study represents both a reaction against and an elaboration of the Freudian teleological model found in Zilboorg, Alexander, and Ernest Jones. Schooled broadly in French Catholic and Swiss Protestant settings, Ellenberger knew well that the tradition of theorizing about unconscious mental activity was very much larger than Freud. In his book, as well as in some thirty historical essays, he massively contextualized Freud's work by granting equal coverage to Pierre Janet, Alfred Adler, and Carl Jung (Freud's primary psychodynamic competitors) and by detailing the work of preceding physicians, philosophers, novelists, theologians, hypnotists, spiritists, and lay therapists who developed insights into the unconscious mind. At the same time, Micale proposes, Ellenberger was a product of "the age of the pure dynamic psychiatries" and, like the more orthodox Freud historians of his time, he centered his conceptualization of psychiatric history on the notion of the Unconscious as an autonomous unitary entity and its cumulative discovery over hundreds of years and across many fields of inquiry.[54]

Fernando Vidal concludes Part II with a contemplation of the elegant and evocative writings of Jean Starobinski. Less known in the United States, Starobinski is among the most renowned academic intellectuals in Europe today, a masterful essayist, literary critic, and cultural historian. Virtually unique among commentators in the field, he has been able, throughout his lifetime, to bridge very productively the divide between the two cultures of science and the humanities. Beginning with his medical dissertation in 1960, which dealt with the history of treatments of melancholia from ancient times to 1900, Starobinski's writings include much material pertinent to the history of psychiatry. Running sinuously through Starobinski's lifework, Vidal finds, is an evolving fascination with the historical experiences of melancholia and nostalgia, with the history of psychiatric semantics, with the expression of psychological sensibility in fiction and autobiography, with the relations between psychoanalytic theory and imaginative literature, and with the interaction of body sensation and self-consciousness. At the center of Starobinski's work, according to Vidal's reading, lies a concern with the complex and shifting connections between individual subjective experience, objective psychological concepts, and artistic style. Other critics and historians have ably studied the history of psychiatric ideas, therapies, and institutions. Thus far, Starobinski is arguably the only cultural historian of psychiatry of first rank.

Part III of this book, "The Psychoanalytic Strain," takes as its subject the sprawling, century-long corpus of commentary on Sigmund Freud. It comprises three complementary essays by Elisabeth Young-Bruehl, John Forrester, and Kenneth Piver. From the vantage point of the last decade in the century it seems clear that the single most important event in the intellectual history of the psychological sciences of the twentieth century has been the emergence and diffusion of psychoanalysis. The psychological revolution, however remote and diffuse its latter-day manifestations, was unquestionably set in motion by Freud's work. As Piver indicates, it is no coincidence that Philip Rieff's well-known concept of "Psychological Man" was cast in the form of a reading of Freud. Piver's essay, "Philip Rieff: The Critic of Psychoanalysis as Cultural Theorist," offers a close and sensitive reading of the evolution of this concept through forty years of Rieff's writings, on the eve of the publication of a major new work by that author.[55]

Over the past twenty years, the appeal and authority of doctrinal psychoanalytic theory and therapy have greatly declined. Nevertheless, the cultural influence of Freud remains immense, almost ubiquitous. Despite the contention of some critics today, Freudian psychodynamic themes and insights have not so much been discarded by contemporary psychiatry as integrated selectively into new theoretical syntheses while psychoanalysis itself, both theoretically and professionally, has diversified, bringing within its orbit many new ideas and practitioners.[56] Nearly every major critical current of thought in the last fifty years has passed through Freudianism. And psychoanalytic ideas and methodologies continue to operate in one branch of the humanities and behavioral sciences after another. Similarly, the psychobabble of ego, id, and superego, narcissism, sublimation, introversion, sibling rivalry, defense mechanism, and death wish pervades popular speech. Despite the progressive de-Freudianization of American psychiatry, Freud's place as one of the supreme makers of the twentieth-century mind, alongside Darwin, Marx, and Einstein, remains secure.[57]

By now, the historical literature about Freud consists of thousands of publications.[58] With his basic theories in place, and the psychoanalytic movement underway but beset by the defections of Jung and Adler, Freud wrote *On the History of the Psychoanalytic Movement* in 1914. His *Autobiographical Study* followed a decade later.[59] The attempt to create a suitable historical past for Freud and his movement began with Freud himself and in an explicitly polemical context. As Forrester observes, however, these two texts were only the beginning of a "writing and re-writing of the history of psychoanalysis" that has taken place over the last seventy-five years. Each defection of an individual from Freud's teachings, and each change in orientation of mainstream psychoanalytic theory, Forrester indicates, elicited a rewriting of the historical record while these rewritings at times doubled back and initiated conceptual reworkings of the theory.

Forrester outlines the great differences between the French and American historical visions of Freud. In "A History of Freud Biographies," Young-Bruehl explores the generational dialectic of Freud studies. To a remarkable degree, Young-Bruehl demonstrates, the successive waves of writing about Freud have been polemically interconnected. From the 1920s to the 1960s, nearly all historical commentary about Freud was produced either by psychoanalytic converts, who sought confirmation of their beliefs by commemorating the life and work of its founder, or by heretics, who desired to discredit psychoanalysis in favor of an alternative psychological school. A tendency emerged across the century, Young-Bruehl perceives further, to construe psychoanalytic history biographically—that is, as the story of its founder's own life. During the first thirty years after Freud's death in 1939, his friends, followers, and family members provided biographical accounts of him, translated and edited authoritatively his collected psychological writings, published volumes of his correspondence, recorded personal memories of him, and reflected eloquently on the moral significance of his thought. In what has come to be called traditional psychoanalytic historiography, two figures were especially important. During the 1950s Ernest Jones, the British psychoanalyst and Freud's most loyal follower, produced his three-volume *The Life and Work of Sigmund Freud*, which sought definitively to record Freud's biography.[60] And Kurt Eissler, a distinguished psychoanalyst trained in the best Central European tradition and the director of the Sigmund Freud Archives, for many years operated as the self-appointed guardian of the Freud heritage. With remarkably little criticism from historians of psychiatry, the traditional historiography of psychoanalysis prevailed throughout the 1940s, 1950s, and 1960s.[61]

Beginning in the 1970s, however, the disciples-and-dissenters historiography of the preceding fifty years gave way to a new, programmatically revisionist school of history writing about Freud. In contrast to earlier "official" accounts produced by psychoanalytic practitioners, the last twenty years has brought a ferocious critique of Freud and his work, which at this point constitutes a veritable counterliterature to the earlier writing.[62] The new critical literature about Freud has largely been generated by writers outside of psychiatric medicine—by clinical psychologists, intellectual and cultural historians, social historians, historians of science, women's historians, literary critics, freelance scholars, and angry ex-analysands. The assault on Freud in our time has been waged on at least five major fronts—biographical, clinical, epistemological, feminist, and linguistic—and shows no sign of slackening. In the forties, fifties, and sixties, Freud was the object of uncritical and repetitive hero worship. In the past fifteen years, he has been accused of being a poor clinician;[63] a therapeutic danger and fraud;[64] an episte-

mological failure;[65] a resentful, malicious, and authoritarian group leader;[66] the orga-
nizer of a declining or dead medical movement;[67] an intellectual conspirator of capitalism;[68] a leading figure in the Western misogynist tradition;[69] a polymorphous neurotic
who projected his own psychopathology into his psychological system;[70] the destroyer
of modern American psychiatry;[71] a subverter of the Western humanities;[72] an intellectual coward;[73] a failed and plagiarizing cryptobiologist;[74] a hateful, all-around fake;[75]
and an incestuous, murderous, masturbating, and abortionizing cocaine addict.[76] This
list could very easily be extended. "Freud bashing" has become an industry in its own
right.[77] In addition, a smaller group of Young Turks within this category has criticized
frontally what they perceive as the secrecy and censorship of the Freud establishment
and its attempt over the decades to create, control, and "correct" the image of Freud
for posterity.[78]

To outsiders, the literature on Freud, with its endless sectarian squabbles and personal antagonisms, may seem tiresome. But its flow remains so large and unstanched,
its points of national and disciplinary origins so diverse, and its tone so engaged, impassioned, at times irrational, as to suggest another reading. Earlier historians, by definition,
acknowledged their intellectual kinship to Freud. But we are disposed to believe that
the *nouvelle vague* anti-Freudians, some of whom have displayed lifelong critical
engagements with their subject, are no less implicated in the Freudian century than the
predecessors against whom they define themselves so sharply. As we approach the
centenary of the *Studies on Hysteria* (1895), and therefore arguably the centenary of
the birth of psychoanalysis, we are beginning to be able to perceive that the history of
Freud interpretation as a whole constitutes an important and intriguing chapter in twentieth-century cultural and intellectual history. From the self-representations of Freud,
to the officially sanctioned Jones biography, to the moderate revisionism of Henri Ellenberger, to the brilliant, brooding ruminations of Rieff, to the harsh, if not hostile, clinical,
feminist, epistemological, hermeneutical, and psychobiographical critiques of today,
the avalanche of writing about Freud may be interpreted as an ongoing attempt to
determine the meaning of Freud for our time. Freud has been written about from every
conceivable point of view. He has aroused reactions ranging from adoration to disgust,
from the idolatrous to the murderous. Each national culture has absorbed him differently. As we approach the end of the 1900s, he appears to be the single most inter-
pretable figure in twentieth-century culture. The literature on him as a whole may be
seen (if we may use the phrase) as an expression of the collective working-through of
Freud by the twentieth-century Freudians.[79]

Part IV, the largest section of the book, "Historical Themes and Topics," offers a
series of essays on historical subjects of exceptional interest and controversy. In *"Les
mythes d'origine* in the History of Psychiatry," Patrick Vandermeersch examines comparatively a number of originary episodes in the traditional historiography of psychiatry
that have served a didactic, self-defining function for the profession. Vandermeersch
explores less the historical veracity of these myths than the reasons for their creation
and invocation at particular times. Frequently, he concludes, such mythic stories have
served to confirm the scientific character of psychiatry, to memorialize the triumph of
medicine over what was perceived as religious obscurantism and philosophical mysticism, and to project psychiatry's origins into the remote, "pre-scientific" past.[80]

Illustrating Vandermeersch's general study is Dora Weiner's *"Le geste de Pinel*:
The History of a Psychiatric Myth." Historians of science have observed that founder

myths have played a prominent part in the professional and ideological evolution of the sciences.[81] Weiner, the leading Pinel scholar in the English-speaking world today,[82] takes as her topic the formation of the premier *mythe d'origine* in psychiatric history, the legendary image of Pinel as liberator of the insane. Pinel's gesture, Weiner carefully points out, was noble in its way; but historical research, rather than hagiographical repetition, reveals that Pinel freed only a small percentage of his hospital patients; moreover, he often replaced the shackles with other forms of mechanical restraint, and his actions reflected less personal innovations than a manifestation of a late Enlightenment *Zeitgeist*, which found expression simultaneously at other hospital sites in Europe. The widespread overemphasis on the heroism of this single gesture, Weiner asserts, has obscured Pinel's very substantial and systematic contributions in other areas to modern psychiatric thought and practice. In a close analysis, Weiner proceeds to outline the construction of the myth of Pinel as chainbreaker. Building on the recent work of French scholars, she demonstrates that the historical story was first formed and circulated in the 1820s and 1830s by Pinel's eldest son, Dr. Scipion Pinel, and by Pinel's students, including the alienist J. E. D. Esquirol.[83] Then, throughout the nineteenth century, Pinel's alleged emancipatory gesture was perceived by the French to carry a clear revolutionary charge and was employed for political purposes. The conservative, clerical right rejected Pinel as dangerous, whereas successive republican regimes, in search of heroic figures from the secular professions, immortalized him.[84] Here, then, we find an instance in which history writing was employed at once to express familial piety and to foster a particular political ideology.

Patrizia Guarnieri's "The History of Psychiatry in Italy" next introduces us to the lively, if little-known, literature of Italian psychiatric history. Guarnieri highlights the ways in which psychiatric historiography has been, and continues to be, pressed into the service of cultural nationalism. In Italy, for example, Guarnieri notes that there existed little interest in writing psychiatric history until the immediate postunification era, when a group of scholars began arguing for the eighteenth-century Italian precursors of Pinel, such as Antonio Valsalva and Vincenzo Chiarugi. Fifty years later, during the fascist years of the 1920s, historians again clamored for national recognition by insisting on the Graeco-Roman, and hence Italian, origins of all modern European psychiatry. Despite these efforts, the Italian contribution to the history of the discipline did not make it into mainstream historiography. Chiarugi has only recently been brought to the attention of medical historians outside of Italy—and this due to the tireless efforts of an Italian-American historian.[85] Ironically, current scholarship suggests that the actual institutional beginnings of Western psychiatry lie not in late Enlightenment France, England, or Italy but in sixteenth-century Spain, where Catholic asylums were founded in Valencia (1409), Saragossa (1425), Seville (1436), Toledo (1436), Valladolid (1489), and Madrid (1546). A periodical literature exists on the subject;[86] yet this fact has failed to gain recognition in British, French, or German historiographies, which have perhaps been reluctant to trace their discipline to church-run establishments during the period of the Inquisition. More recently, Guarnieri explains, Italian psychiatric historiography has been tied to national events in a different way. Today, the study of the history of psychiatry in Italy, where it is a rapidly growing field of interest, was directly inspired by the boisterous anti-psychiatric campaign of Enrico Basaglia during the early 1970s and the drastic changes in state medical policy introduced as a result of Basaglia's actions.

In a similar way, Gerald Grob demonstrates that aspects of Anglo-American psychiatric historiography have been acutely shaped by controversies within contemporary public health policy. The most obvious instance of this is the remarkable interest over the past thirty years in asylum history. The post–World War II era witnessed an enormous growth in state-run psychiatric institutions in both Europe and North America. By the 1960s and 1970s, however, the combination of dissatisfaction with traditional institutional mechanisms within mainstream psychiatry, the advent of drug therapies, the efforts of the mental patients' liberation movement, and anti-psychiatric critiques led, in Britain and the United States, to a process of deinstitutionalization, or the transferring of large numbers of mental patients from state facilities to so-called community health care centers. Almost inevitably, writing about the history of asylums in these countries during this period was deeply colored by the politics of psychiatric hospital closure. The discrediting of psychiatry's key institution within the context of changing mental health policies went hand in hand with its discrediting within psychiatric history: The processes were parallel and interactive. The fiercest debate within Anglo-American psychiatric historiography since the early 1970s—a debate that has been tracked in many other areas of study—focused on the nature, origin, and evolution of the asylum. This historical controversy has been charged with contemporary significance, as each historical study seemed to defend or delegitimize the mental hospital as an institutional form.[87] Indicatively, at one time or another, most of the *dramatis personae* in the debate took time from their historical labors to address directly the public debate on decarceration swirling around them.[88] In Chapter 14, "The History of the Asylum Revisited: Personal Reflections," Gerald Grob, one of the most prominent participants in the controversy, combines historiographical and autobiographical perspectives to review the development of his own thinking about the history of American institutional psychiatry and to place his evolving work in the heady political and historical debates of the sixties and seventies.

Grob's essay is followed by Geoffrey Cocks's responsible study of one of the most dramatic developments anywhere in the psychiatric historiography of the last decade. It has now been established that during the Third Reich many German psychiatrists working at mental hospitals conspired in euthanizing thousands of persons deemed chronically psychotic and in conducting extensive, often sadistic, eugenic experimentation on many more. Germany boasts a rich tradition of writing on the history of psychiatry. Nevertheless, as Cocks discusses in "German Psychiatry, Psychotherapy, and Psychoanalysis during the Nazi Period: Historiographical Reflections," virtually none of the historical accounts produced by German authors until the late 1970s acknowledged this episode. For a generation following the Second World War, German psychiatry remained officially oblivious to this portion of its past; some historians still believe it is best to pass over this shameful period in silence or to dismiss it as a lamentable aberration. Cocks speculates on the psychological functions of the collective repression of the past and raises the issue of the insidious and morally ambiguous ways in which modern professions may opportunistically serve political regimes.

Since 1980, however, Cocks goes on to show, a burst of publications has appeared concerning the activities of German and Austrian psychiatrists, psychotherapists, psychoanalysts, and mental health care workers under National Socialism. Tellingly, this literature has not been produced by the mainstream medical establishment. The first programmatic call for an examination of the subject was sounded by Klaus Doerner, the leading German social revisionist historian of psychiatry from the 1970s, who is deeply read in critical Marxist theory and Continental anti-psychiatry.[89] Likewise, the first study of German institutional psychotherapy during the 1930s and 1940s came from a foreign scholar.[90] Most impressively, the story of the extermination of mental patients is being exposed today in unflinching detail by German medical students and young psychoanalysts in the form of monographs, essay collections, conferences, exhibitions, and collections of documents.[91] These young authors are reconstructing the story of "Nazi psychiatry"; but they are also addressing, often angrily, the unwillingness of their teachers' generation—at times, of their teachers—to confront a shared professional heritage. Clearly, this literature is part of the collective soul-searching of a new generation of Germans about their national past.[92] With the reunification of the country in 1990, and the end of the political abuse of psychiatry in former Communist East Germany, Cocks comments in closing, German psychiatric historians now have a second painful past to discover, write, and work through.

As with the contribution by Cocks, Julie Brown's essay reminds us again that some of the darkest chapters in psychiatric history have occurred in our own century. In Soviet Russian history from the late 1920s until the late 1980s, we have, without a doubt, the most overt politicization of psychiatry in the twentieth century. For obvious reasons, the numbers remain highly imprecise; but scholars today agree that during these decades hundreds, perhaps thousands, of political dissenters in the Soviet Union were declared insane and interned involuntarily in institutions designated as mental hospitals. At times, these political cases were subjected to the Orwellian use of psychopharmacological techniques to "reeducate" individuals politically. The number of forced, arbitrary, and often prolonged internments for social misconduct is believed to have been much higher. The image of the psychiatric gulag is among the most striking of our time.[93] In Chapter 16, "Heroes and Non-Heroes: Recurring Themes in the Historiography of Russian-Soviet Psychiatry," Brown examines the historical literature of psychiatry coming out of Russia during the crucial years around the Bolshevik Revolution of 1917. History writing about psychiatry, she discovers, first became ideologized at that time. Increasingly during the 1920s, the new Communist government expressed an official preference for the history of materialist over psychodynamic psychologies and for commemorating the past achievements of the Moscow psychiatric community over that of individuals outside the new Communist capital.[94] Following her historical analysis, Brown poses the question: What will the historiography of psychiatry in post-Communist Russia look like? With the world-historical dissolution of the USSR and its Communist satellite states, it has suddenly become possible for both Russian and foreign scholars to write the history of psychiatry in these countries "as it really happened."[95] Psychological theories and schools that were previously suppressed, and that bring new historical perspectives, may experience revivals. Furthermore, it seems likely that some sort of intensely "revisionist," "anti-psychiatric" reaction will develop in the former Soviet Union as Russian scholars, with their new freedom, begin to study aggressively the full history of the Soviet state and its oppressive institutions.[96] Another problematic past is being confronted.

"Critics of Psychiatry" is the fifth and final part of the book. Because psychiatry remains, as Hunter and Macalpine observed, more embroiled with aspects of its past than other branches of science or medicine, it has often proved possible to cast critiques of current-day practice in historical terms. Among the major "anti-psychiatry" movements of the 1960s and 1970s, only the British critique lacked a substantial historical dimension. However, as Guarnieri rightly reminds us, "[t]here has not been only one anti-psychiatry, just as there has not been only one psychiatry."[97] Therefore, the essays gathered loosely under this final heading explore five major critics of, or bodies of critical theory about, psychiatry that appeared during the last half century.

Richard Vatz and Lee Weinberg provide a rigorous and well-informed defense of the work of Thomas Szasz, whose *The Myth of Mental Illness* (1961), they observe, was an event in itself in the historiography of psychiatry.[98] Vatz and Weinberg employ Thomas Kuhn's concept of a revolutionary paradigmatic critique of normal science to account for the challenge represented by Szaszian ideas to the theoretical and clinical premises of modern scientific psychiatry. The authors also highlight the strong historical component in Szasz's thought. In many of his writings, Szasz has offered fundamental rereadings of exemplary episodes and topics in the history of mental medicine, such as the role of doctors in the European witch-hunts, the medical practices of Benjamin Rush, the eighteenth- and nineteenth-century medical literature on masturbatory insanity, and past scientific writing about homosexuality. A timeline appended to Szasz's *The Manufacture of Madness* (1970) enumerates with ironic commentary the landmark dates of the triumphalist Whig version of psychiatric history.[99]

Dovetailing nicely with Vatz and Weinberg's discussion of Szasz is Gary Gutting's chapter, "Michel Foucault's *Phänomenologie des Krankengeistes*." Gutting explores the distinctive Foucauldian concept of "a history of reason and unreason." He furnishes an up-to-date review of the spirited (and apparently unceasing) debate surrounding Foucault's *Histoire de la folie* of 1961. This book has easily been the single most influential text of psychiatric historiography in the second half of the century. Gutting provides a defense of the Frenchman's powerful but unconventional vision of history in the face of recent Anglo-American empirical criticism. In his analysis, he emphasizes the differences in explanatory styles between Foucault and most of his critics, and he underscores the importance of Foucault's early intellectual encounters with Kantian idealist philosophy and the phenomenological psychiatry of Ludwig Binswanger in comprehending these differences.[100]

With Nancy Tomes's "Feminist Histories of Psychiatry," we learn that a body of powerful contemporary critical social theory may force a wholesale reconceptualization of inherited historiographical traditions.[101] As Tomes indicates, women as historical subjects and gender as an analytical category were wholly absent from historical psychiatric narratives before 1965. Over the past thirty years, however, feminist scholarship has systematically laid bare the deep masculinist assumptions of much past psychological theory and psychiatric practice and in the process has challenged yet another feature of traditional Whig history writing. As Tomes demonstrates, the development of the historical literature on psychiatry and women has mirrored the overall intellectual history of women's studies as well as the women's movement generally. Within the academy, feminist psychiatric historiography has joined in turns with radical "anti-psychiatric" sociology, with the "new social history" of the 1960s and 1970s, with psychoanalytic studies, and, most recently, with feminist deconstructive literary criticism. As the field of women's studies has gained institutional recognition and intellectual respect, feminist historical scholarship on psychiatry has become increasingly sophisticated and is marked today, both empirically and interpretively, by rich internal diversity, even dissent. Over the last decade, no subfield of psychiatric historiography has expanded more energetically. Tomes provides a very full account of the burgeoning British and North American historical literatures, which have clustered around several research areas: the representation of women in psychological texts, women in the institutionalized hospital world, women and the doctor-patient relationship, famous past female patients, the representation of women in psychoanalytic theory, literary representations of women and madness, women and historical psychopathology, early female psychiatrists and psychoanalysts, and the role of gendered language in medical science. Most recently, feminist-informed psychiatric historians in the United States, reflecting the new critical multiculturalism of the 1990s, have been enlarging their purview beyond the experience of white, middle-class, heterosexual women. Furthermore, the historical exploration of other populations that have been similarly misrepresented by psychiatry is beginning to be explored following the feminist model.[102]

Employing very different styles of exposition, the final two essays in *Discovering the History of Psychiatry* investigate the anti-psychiatry movements of France and the United States.[103] In a dense and fascinating study, Jacques Postel and David Allen reconstruct the clinical, theoretical, philosophical, political, and cultural foundations of French anti-psychiatry. In the process, they provide a tour through a labyrinthine world of ideas and texts and introduce us to a raft of figures—P. C. Racamier, H. Heyward, R. Gentis, G. Césari, C. Delacampagne, G. Jervis, J. Oury, C. Koupernik—that most likely will be unfamiliar to English-language readers. During its heyday in the late 1960s and early 1970s, Postel and Allen show, French anti-psychiatric agitation appeared as part of the proliferation of left-wing ideologies that swarmed around the Vietnam War and the 1968 student riots in Paris. However, the intellectual prehistory of the movement is, in fact, long and intricate. A decisive impulse came from the importation from Britain of the writings of R. D. Laing, David Cooper, and Aaron Esterson in a series of influential translations during the sixties and seventies. Within the history of French ideas in the post–World War II era, neo-Hegelianism, Marxian humanism, Sartre's existential Marxism, Eugène Minkowski's phenomenological psychiatry, and the teachings of Jacques Lacan and Michel Foucault contributed as well. Furthermore, behind the French Left of the 1950s lay strong and unresolved wartime experiences that created a profound moral and social distrust of incarcerative "total" institutions. More distantly still, the shifting aggregation of ideas and events that was French anti-psychiatry, Postel and Allen demonstrate, can be traced back to a tradition of anti-Kraepelinian and anti-Bleulerian opposition and a critique of the classic schizophrenia concept from the early years of the twentieth century. In closing, Postel and Allen reflect on the ways in which anti-psychiatry used, wrote, and eventually made psychiatric history, as well as on the current status of the movement.

Finally, Norman Dain investigates North American anti-psychiatry, which reveals highly interesting similarities to, and divergences from, its principal Continental counterparts. Like Postel and Allen, Dain casts his historical net very widely. He finds that anti-psychiatric sentiment in the United States has an extensive and more or less continuous history since the end of the eighteenth century. Opposition to psychiatry has at times come from religious leaders, lay healers, jurists, neurologists, clinical psychologists, social workers, and ex-patients, as well as from disaffected psychiatrists. It has been associated alternatively with the political Left and the Right and has been based on a remarkable spectrum of arguments. Like Postel and Allen, Dain sketches the long-range history of ideas, attitudes, and activities that came together during the 1960s to form the first nationally and internationally organized anti-psychiatric "movement." With the exception of organized ex-patient activism, every element of the anti-psychiatry of the second half of the twentieth century, he affirms, has antecedents in earlier times, although anti-psychiatry writers at that time tended to be ignorant of the historical background of their own work. Whereas Postel and Allen emphasize the intellectual history of French anti-psychiatry, Dain reconstructs the complex of local social and political factors that produced past and present anti-psychiatries in America. Two forces—continual economic constraints on the care of the mentally disabled and the chronic recalcitrance of many forms of mental disease itself—appear most persistently in his mildly tragic historical portrait. Dain closes this exceptionally well-informed survey, and the book as a whole, with a consideration of the most recent writings in the United States against psychiatry, which respond to the conditions of the post-Freudian biological psychiatry of the early 1990s.

In summation, the essays in this volume establish that a great many factors have gone into the interpretation of the history of psychiatry. Psychiatric history writing may inform, instruct, and entertain. It may reflect the intellectual personality, the cultural background, or the emotional temperament of the historian. It may be informed by internal disciplinary dimensions of a clinical, theoretical, or professional nature. And it may be shaped externally by contemporary social movements or political exigencies. It may also embody cultural structures and processes of a deeper and longer-term nature. Psychiatric historiography has served purposes that are antiquarian, pedagogical, justificatory, and ideological. We hope that the understanding and the exploration of all these forces and functions, as well as many others, will be stimulated by this collection of original and far-ranging essays.

From what we have written thus far, it should be clear that we view all history writing as perspectival, the expression of a particular historical environment. The present book, and its introduction, are assuredly no exception to this rule. In 1970, two American authors—a child psychiatrist and a government archivist and historian—first opened up the possibility of a more critical historiography of the mental sciences, which they attempted to explore in an international symposium.[104] For all of its promise, this effort was obscured by the emergence of a passionate, generation-long, dialectical argument about basic ideological issues within psychiatric history. The 1990s, we believe, bring a propitious confluence of circumstances for reviving this project and for moving from thesis and antithesis to historiographical synthesis. Over the past two decades, a large body of historical writing about psychiatry has accumulated, which proffers sharply conflicting interpretations. By consensus, the critical ideological currents that challenged psychiatry during the third quarter of this century have, after achieving selected successes, now waned. A quantity of sophisticated scholarship concerning the methodology and epistemology of other branches of the history of science has come into being. Contemporary Western psychiatry is experiencing a "paradigm shift" as it progressively deprivileges psychodynamic psychologies and embraces new, more biologically oriented theories and therapies. And the history of psychiatry as a field of professional study, with its own practitioners, periodicals, organizations, and international congresses, is itself expanding rapidly. Lastly, developments in the world at large strongly suggest that the ideological universe of the past two generations, which in subtle ways structured much of our thinking throughout this period, has been fundamentally altered. As the anti-psychiatry movement passes, as Freud studies enter their second century, as psychiatric history writing achieves independent disciplinary status, and as we enter a new ''postideological'' age, the time seems ripe for a renewed discussion of this subject. We hope that this volume will at once capture and encourage this distinctive moment in the historical development of the field.

It should also be evident from what has been said, and from the chapters that follow, that historical debate about the history of psychiatry has displayed not a panorama of serene scholarship but a stormy sea of rhetoric and at times even abuse. The field today remains in enormous flux. Psychiatry is a deeply controversial aspect of our modern, secular world of knowledge. It raises questions about the very nature of the Self, about the relations of body and mind, about our emotions and our sexuality, about the individual and the expert, about the nature of disease and illness, about the status and limits of applied science, and about compulsion and state power. We do not expect in the foreseeable future that the history of psychiatry will reflect a consensus. It is not for consensus that this book is calling. Within both psychiatric medicine and historical studies, the conditions giving rise to its diversity and divisions remain very much in place. Rather, this volume, we suspect, reflects in the final analysis the supremely postmodernist preoccupation with self-awareness. In all of our combined professional reading, there is one book we have failed to find, and that book is titled *The History of Psychiatry: An Interpretation*. We know of no study of the subject from any period or in any language that contains an acknowledgment, much less ample discussion, of its own methodological, epistemological, and ideological assumptions. Thus far, scholars have told us a great many tales about the past, in the present, for present purposes. Future histories of psychiatry may be no fewer; but they will, we hope, be more self-aware.

Notes

1. Our title alludes to three earlier commentaries that we hope to extend: George Mora and Jeanne L. Brand (eds.), *Psychiatry and Its History: Methodological Problems in Research* (Springfield, Illinois: Charles C Thomas, 1970); Sir Martin Roth, ''Psychiatry and Its Critics,'' *British Journal of Psychiatry*, cxxii (1973), 374–402; and Andrew Scull, ''Psychiatry and Its Historians,'' *History of Psychiatry*, ii (1991), 239–250.

2. In the history of science and medicine, many celebrated texts open with significant historical fanfare. A distinguished instance of such an overview that shaped historical interpretation for many decades is the overture to Charles Lyell's *Principles of Geology* (1830–33). For an evaluation of the ideological aims of Lyell's narrative, see Roy Porter, ''Charles Lyell and the Principles of the History of Geology,'' *The British Journal for the History of Science*, ix (1976), 91–103.

3. Wolf Lepenies, ''Wissenschaftsgeschichte und Disziplingeschichte,'' *Geschichte und Gesellschaft*, iv (1978), 437–451; Loren Graham, Wolf Lepenies, and Peter Weingart (eds.), *Functions and Uses of Disciplinary Histories* (Dordrecht/Boston/Lancaster: D. Reidel, 1983); and R. C. Olby, G. N. Cantor, J. R. R. Christie, and J. J. S. Hodge (eds.), *Companion to the History of Modern Science* (London: Routledge, 1990), sections of which are organized disciplinarily.

4. For the general philosophy of usable pasts, and the broader notion of the usefulness of custom, tradition, and history, see Peter Burke, *The Renaissance Sense of the Past* (New York:

St. Martin's Press, 1970); and Eric Hobsbawm and Terence Ranger (eds.), *The Invention of Tradition* (Cambridge: Cambridge University Press, 1983).

5. The classic discussion of this last point is Charles Rosenberg's "The Crisis of Psychiatric Legitimacy: Reflections on Psychiatry, Medicine, and Public Policy" in G. Kriegman et al. (eds.), *American Psychiatry: Past, Present, and Future* (Charlottesville: University Press of Virginia, 1975), 135–148.

6. What the British historians of psychiatry Ida Macalpine and Richard Hunter observed sagely in 1963 remains true today: "There can be as yet no definitive history of the subject since psychiatry is still too little differentiated from its past, and accordingly each age must interpret it from its own vantage point and temper and in relation to the contemporary medical scene" (Richard Hunter and Ida Macalpine, *Three Hundred Years of Psychiatry 1535–1860* [London: Oxford University Press, 1963], ix). Whether a "definitive" history of psychiatry can be written without the unification of the psychological sciences themselves—or, conversely, whether the profession can ever stabilize itself without a consensual history—are questions worthy of speculation.

7. The classic discussion is Herbert Butterfield's *The Whig Interpretation of History* (London: Bell, 1931). On the concept in science history, refer to C. B. Wilde, "Whig History" in W. F. Bynum, E. J. Browne, and Roy Porter (eds.), *Dictionary of the History of Science* (Princeton: Princeton University Press, 1981), 445–446; and A. R. Hall, "On Whiggism," *History of Science*, xxi (1983), 45–59.

8. Lowell S. Selling, *Men Against Madness* (New York: Greenberg, 1940); Walter Bromberg, *Man Above Humanity: A History of Psychotherapy* (Philadelphia: Lippincott, 1954); and Jan Ehrenwald, *From Medicine Man to Freud: A History of Psychotherapy* (New York: Dell, 1957). *Cento e più anni di conquiste* was the title proposed by Enrico Morselli in 1920 for a history of psychiatry. For other works in the Whig tradition, see René Semelaigne, *Les pionniers de la psychiatrie française avant et après Pinel*, 2 vols. (Paris: J. B. Baillière, 1930–32); J. R. Whitwell, *Historical Notes on Psychiatry* (London: Lewis, 1936); Walter Bromberg, *The Mind of Man: The Story of Man's Conquest of Mental Illness* (New York: Harper, 1937); John K. Winkler and Walter Bromberg, *Mind Explorers* (New York: Reynal & Hitchcock, 1939); Nolan D. C. Lewis, *A Short History of Psychiatric Achievements* (New York: Norton, 1941); John K. Hall et al. (eds.), *One Hundred Years of American Psychiatry* (New York: Columbia University Press, 1944); Johannes Heinrich Schulz, *Psychotherapie. Leben und Werk grosser Aerzte* (Stuttgart: Hippokrates-Verlag Marquardt, 1952); A. M. Sackler (ed.), *The Great Physiodynamic Therapies in Psychiatry* (New York: 1956); and Franz G. Alexander and Sheldon T. Selesnick, *The History of Psychiatry: An Evaluation of Psychiatric Thought and Practice from Prehistoric Times to the Present* (New York: Harper & Row, 1966). The Whig view was also promulgated in many historical prefaces to psychiatric texts during the midcentury period.

9. Gregory Zilboorg, in collaboration with George W. Henry, *A History of Medical Psychology* (New York: Norton, 1941).

10. Sir Aubrey Lewis, *The State of Psychiatry* (London: Routledge & Kegan Paul, 1967), 3.

11. Zilboorg, *History of Medical Psychology*, 524–525.

12. R. D. Laing, *The Divided Self: A Study of Sanity and Madness* (London: Tavistock, 1960); Erving Goffman, *Asylums: Essays on the Social Situation of Mental Patients and Other Inmates* (Garden City, New York: Anchor, 1961); Thomas Szasz, *The Myth of Mental Illness: Foundations of a Theory of Personal Conduct* (New York: Hoeber-Harper, 1961); Michael Foucault, *Histoire de la folie à l'âge classique* (Paris: Plon, 1961).

13. Foucault, *Madness and Civilization: A History of Insanity in the Age of Reason* (New York: Random House, 1965).

14. Historiographically, Foucault's chapter may be seen as a response to René Semelaigne's *Aliénistes et philanthropes: Les Pinels et les Tukes* (Paris: Steinheil, 1912).

15. The term was first used by David Cooper in *Psychiatry and Anti-Psychiatry* (London:

Granada/Paladin, 1970). For a review of the compendious literature in this camp, consult K. Portland Frank's *The Anti-Psychiatry Bibliography and Resources Guide*, 2nd ed. (Vancouver, British Columbia: Press Gang, 1979).

16. For a useful cautionary note about the need to discriminate among social revisionisms within psychiatric historiography, see Andrew Scull, *Social Order/Social Disorder: Anglo-American Psychiatry in Historical Perspective* (Berkeley: University of California Press, 1990), ch. 2.

17. Klaus Doerner, *Bürger und Irre. Zur Sozialgeschichte und Wissenschaftssoziologie der Psychiatrie* (Frankfurt am Main: Europänische Verlagsanstalt, 1969); trans. *Madmen and the Bourgeoisie: A Social History of Insanity and Psychiatry* (Oxford: Basil Blackwell, 1981); David Rothman, *The Discovery of the Asylum: Social Order and Disorder in the New Republic* (Boston: Little, Brown, 1971); Robert Castel, *L'Ordre psychiatrique: L'Age d'or de l'aliénisme* (Paris: Minuit, 1976); trans. *The Regulation of Madness: Origins of Incarceration in France* (Berkeley: University of California Press, 1988); Andrew Scull, *Museums of Madness: The Social Organization of Insanity in Nineteenth-Century England* (London: Allen Lane, 1979).

18. In addition to the books of Doerner, Castel, Rothman, and Scull, literature in the social revisionist category includes Thomas Scheff, *Being Mentally Ill: A Sociological Theory* (Chicago: Aldine Press, 1966); David Ingleby (ed.), *Critical Psychiatry: The Politics of Mental Health* (Harmondsworth: Penguin, 1981); Ingleby, "The Social Construction of Mental Illness" in P. Wright and A. Treacher (eds.), *The Problem of Medical Knowledge* (Edinburgh: Edinburgh University Press, 1982), 123–143; Joan Busfield, *Managing Madness: Changing Ideas and Practice* (London: Hutchinson, 1986); and David Rothman, "Social Control: The Uses and Abuses of the Concept in the History of Incarceration" and Robert Castel, "Moral Treatment: Mental Therapy and Social Control in the Nineteenth Century," both in Stanley Cohen and Andrew Scull (eds.), *Social Control and the State: Historical and Comparative Essays* (New York: St. Martin's Press, 1981).

19. For intelligent and influential articulations of these evaluations, see the combative historiographical introduction to Andrew Scull, *Social Order/Mental Disorder*, ch. 1, as well as idem, "The Social History of Psychiatry in the Victorian Era" in Scull (ed.), *Madhouses, Mad-Doctors, and Madmen: The Social History of Psychiatry in the Victorian Era* (London: Athlone Press, 1981), 5–32; and idem, "Psychiatry and Its Historians," *History of Psychiatry*, 239–250.

20. For some skeptical general reflections on the adjective "Whiggish" as an all-purpose epithet in contemporary academic writing, see Ernst Mayr, "When Is Historiography Whiggish?" *Journal of the History of Ideas*, li (1990), 301–309.

21. "Until the last two decades, psychiatric history has been written primarily by amateur historians, and a peculiar group of amateurs at that—psychiatrists themselves." "The resulting distortions have seriously compromised the scholarly usefulness of the accounts offered—creating versions of the past that serve (in ways generally obscured from their authors) to legitimate the profession's present-day activities; or that represent a harmless form of antiquarianism but largely fail to satisfy the elementary canons of good historiography" (Scull, "Psychiatry and Its Historians," 239).

22. See George Mora, "Early American Historians of Psychiatry, 1910–1960," this volume.

23. Edward Morman, "George Rosen and the History of Mental Illness," this volume. See also Walter Bromberg, "Some Social Aspects of the History of Psychiatry," *Bulletin of the History of Medicine*, xi (1942), 117–132.

24. Richard Hunter and Ida Macalpine, *Psychiatry for the Poor, 1851. Colney Hatch Asylum, Friern Hospital 1973: A Medical and Social History* (London: Dawsons, 1974); William Llewellyn Parry-Jones, *The Trade in Lunacy: A Study of Private Madhouses in England in the Eighteenth and Nineteenth Centuries* (London: Routledge & Kegan Paul, 1971); Stanley W. Jackson, *Melancholia and Depression: From Hippocratic Times to Modern Times* (New Haven: Yale University Press, 1986).

25. Henri Baruk, "L'Oeuvre de Pinel et Esquirol devant 'l'anti-psychiatrie,' " *Académie nationale de médecine* (9 March 1971), 205–215.

26. See, for instance, German E. Berrios and Hugh Freeman, *150 Years of British Psychiatry, 1841–1991* (London: Gaskell, 1991), which consists of twenty-eight essays, mostly by clinicians.

27. Ibid., introduction; and G. Daumezon, "Légitimité de l'intérêt pour l'histoire de la psychiatrie," *L'Information psychiatrique*, xlv (1980), 637–653. Our reference to a "history of psychiatry with the psychiatry left out" alludes to the controversial editorial note, "Medical History without Medicine," which appeared in the *Journal of the History of Medicine and Allied Sciences*, xxv (1980), 5–7.

28. For a fine exception, consider W. F. Bynum, "Psychiatry in Its Historical Context" in M. Shepherd and O. L. Zangwill (eds.), *Handbook of Psychiatry, i: General Psychopathology* (Cambridge: Cambridge University Press, 1983), 11–38. See as well Henri F. Ellenberger, "Histoire de la psychiatrie" in R. Duguay et al. (eds.), *Précis pratique de psychiatrie* (Montreal: Chenelière and Stanké, 1981), 1–12; and George Mora, "Historical and Theoretical Trends in Psychiatry" in Harold I. Kaplan, Alfred M. Freedman, and Benjamin J. Sadock (eds.), *Comprehensive Textbook of Psychiatry*, 3rd ed. (Baltimore: Williams & Wilkins, 1980), i: 4–98.

29. Richard Shryock, "The Psychiatry of Benjamin Rush," *American Journal of Psychiatry*, x (1941), 429–432. See also idem, "The Medical Reputation of Benjamin Rush," *Bulletin of the History of Medicine*, xlv (1971), 507–552.

30. Norman Dain, "Critics and Dissenters: Reflections on 'Anti-Psychiatry' in the United States," *Journal of the History of the Behavioral Sciences*, xxv (1989), 3–25; and idem, "Psychiatry and Anti-Psychiatry in the United States," this volume.

31. The chief disputants in this debate included David Rothman, Gerald Grob, Norman Dain, Jacques Quen, and Andrew Scull. See the introduction to this volume, p. 21, as well as Grob, "The Rise of the Asylum Revisited: Personal Reflections," this volume.

32. Daniel Hack Tuke, *Chapters on the History of the Insane in the British Isles* (London: Kegan Paul, Trench & Co., 1882), 484–485.

33. Richard Hunter and Ida Macalpine, *Three Hundred Years of Psychiatry: 1535–1860* (London: Oxford University Press, 1963), vii.

34. Berrios and Freeman, *150 Years of British Psychiatry*, introduction, ix.

35. Especially valuable here is the insistence of the so-called Edinburgh School of the historical sociology of science upon "explanatory symmetry" in treating different, allegedly scientific as well as non-, pre-, or pseudoscientific thought systems. The same explanatory structures, members of this school argue persuasively, must direct our accounts of what perhaps seem to us true or at least progressive and successful beliefs as govern the interpretation of those that appear irrational or which fell by the wayside. See especially David Bloor, *Knowledge and Social Imagery* (London: Routledge & Kegan Paul, 1976); Barry Barnes, *Interests and the Growth of Knowledge* (London: Routledge & Kegan Paul, 1977); and Harry M. Collins, *Changing Order: Replication and Induction in Scientific Practice* (Beverly Hills: Sage, 1985).

36. Peter Sedgwick, "Michel Foucault: The Anti-History of Psychiatry," *Psychological Medicine*, xi (1981), 235–248.

37. On these countermyths, Martin Roth and Jerome Kroll, *The Reality of Mental Illness* (Cambridge: Cambridge University Press, 1986) levies some trenchant criticisms. See especially 26–29.

38. Roy Porter, "Ida Macalpine and Richard Hunter: History between Psychoanalysis and Psychiatry," this volume, p. 90.

39. From a large literature, see Arnold Thackray, "Science: Has Its Present Past a Future?" in Roger H. Stuewer (ed.), *Historical and Philosophical Perspectives of Science* (Minneapolis: University of Minnesota Press, 1970), 112–133; Imre Lakatos, "History of Science and Its Rational Reconstructions" in Yehuka Elkana (ed.), *The Interaction between Science and Philosophy* (Atlantic Highlands, New Jersey: Humanities Press, 1974), 195–241; Barry Barnes, "'Internal'

Versus 'External' Factors in the History of Science'' in Barnes (ed.), *Scientific Knowledge and Sociological Theory* (London: Routledge & Kegan Paul, 1974), ch. 5; Pietro Corsi, "History of Science, History of Philosophy, and History of Theology'' in Pietro Corsi and Paul Weindling (eds.), *Information Sources in the History of Science and Medicine* (London: Butterworth, 1983), 3–28; Charles Rosenberg, "Science in American Society: A Generation of Historical Debate,'' *Isis*, lxxiv (1983), 356–367; H. Kragh, *An Introduction to the Historiography of Science* (Cambridge: Cambridge University Press, 1987); Steven Shapin, "Social Uses of Science'' in George S. Rousseau and Roy Porter (eds.), *The Ferment of Knowledge: Perspectives on Scholarship of Eighteenth Century Science* (Cambridge: Cambridge University Press, 1980), 93–142; idem, "History of Science and Its Sociological Reconstructions,'' *History of Science*, xx (1982), 157–211; idem, "Discipline and Bounding: The History and Sociology of Science as Seen Through the Externalism-Internalism Debate,'' *History of Science*, xxx (1992), 333–369; "Ideology in the Life Sciences,'' International symposium held at Harvard University, Department of Science, 19–21 April 1989.

40. J. Woodward, "Towards a Social History of Medicine'' in J. Woodward and D. Richards (eds.), *Health Care and Popular Medicine in England: Essays in the Social History of Medicine* (London: Croom Helm; New York: Holmes and Meier, 1977), 15–55; Karl N. Figlio, "The Historiography of Scientific Medicine: An Invitation to the Human Sciences,'' *Comparative Studies in Society and History*, xlx (1977), 262–286; Lloyd Stevenson (ed.), *A Celebration of Medical History: The Fiftieth Anniversary of the Johns Hopkins Institute of the History of Medicine and the Welch Medical Library* (Baltimore: Johns Hopkins University Press, 1982); Charles Webster, "The Historiography of Medicine'' in Pietro Corsi and Paul Weindling, *Information Sources in the History of Science and Medicine*, 29–43; Gert H. Brieger, "History of Medicine'' in Paul T. Durbin (ed.), *A Guide to the Culture of Science, Technology and Medicine* (New York: Free Press, 1980), 121–194; idem, "Medical Historiography'' in W. F. Bynum and Roy Porter (eds.), *Companion Encyclopedia of the History of Medicine* (London: Routledge, 1993), 24–44; Peter W. G. Wright and A. Treacher (eds.), *The Problem of Medical Knowledge* (Edinburgh: Edinburgh University Press, 1982); John Harley Warner, "Science in Medicine,'' *Osiris*, second series, i (1985), 37–58.

41. George W. Stocking, Jr., "On the Limits of 'Presentism' and 'Historicism' in the Historiography of the Behavioral Sciences,'' *Journal of the History of the Behavioral Sciences*, i (1965), 211–218; W. R. Woodward, "Toward a Critical Historiography of Psychology'' in Josef Brozek and Ludwig H. Pongratz (eds.), *Historiography of Modern Psychology: Aims, Resources, Approaches* (Toronto: C. J. Hogrefe, 1980), 29–67; B. N. Kelly, "Inventing Psychology's Past: E. G. Boring's Historiography in Relation to the Psychology of His Time,'' *Journal of Mind and Behavior*, ii (1981), 229–241B; U. Geuter, "The Uses of History for the Shaping of a Field: Observations on German Psychology'' in Graham et al., *Functions and Uses of Disciplinary Histories*, 191–228; Kurt Danziger, "Towards a Conceptual Framework for a Critical History of Psychology'' in Helio Carpintero and J. M. Peiro (eds.), *Psychology in Its Historical Context* (Valencia: Monografias de la Revista de Historia de la Psicologia, Universidad de Valencia, 1984), 99–107; idem, *Constructing the Subject: Historical Origins of Psychological Research* (Cambridge: Cambridge University Press, 1990); and Roger Smith, "Does the History of Psychology Have a Subject?'' *History of the Human Sciences*, i (1988), 147–177.

42. On some of the implications of these debates for the historiography of science, see Richard J. Bernstein, *Beyond Objectivism and Relativism: Science, Hermeneutics, and Praxis* (Philadelphia: University of Pennsylvania Press, 1983).

43. Mark S. Micale, "Hysteria and Its Historiography—The Future Perspective,'' *History of Psychiatry*, i (1990), [33–124], 37.

44. Several earlier efforts pointed in this direction and provide the foundation on which the present volume builds: George Mora, "The Historiography of Psychiatry and Its Development: A Re-Evaluation,'' *Journal of the History of the Behavioral Sciences*, i (1965), 43–52; Klaus

Doerner, "Criteria for a Historiography of Psychiatry" in Doerner, *Madmen and the Bourgeoisie* (1969), appendix, 292–300; Mora and Brand, *Psychiatry and Its History* (1970); and Otto M. Marx, "What is the History of Psychiatry?" *American Journal of Orthopsychiatry*, xl (1970), 593–605. Also, implicit in some recent psychiatric historiography has been a more sophisticated, self-aware approach. See, for example, the three dozen essays in W. F. Bynum, Roy Porter, and Michael Shepherd (eds.), *The Anatomy of Madness: Essays in the History of Psychiatry*, 3 vols. (London: Tavistock, 1985; 1985; 1988) as well as Nancy Tomes, "The Anatomy of Madness: New Directions in the History of Psychiatry," *Social Studies of Science*, xvii (1987), 358–370.

45. The classic formulation of this development remains Philip Rieff's notion of "the emergence of Psychological Man" in *Freud: The Mind of the Moralist* (Garden City, New York: Doubleday, 1959), ch. 10.

46. Robert Castel, Françoise Castel, and Anne Lovell, *La société psychiatrique avancée* (Paris: Grasset, 1979).

47. On the psychologization of self and society, see Arnold A. Rogow, *The Psychiatrists* (New York: G. P. Putnam, 1970); Martin L. Gross, *The Psychological Society: A Critical Analysis of Psychiatry, Psychotherapy, Psychoanalysis, and the Psychological Revolution* (New York: Simon & Schuster, 1978); Jonas Robitscher, *The Powers of Psychiatry* (Boston: Houghton Mifflin, 1980); Robert Castel, Françoise Castel, and Anne Lovell, *The Psychiatric Society* (New York: Columbia University Press, 1982); and Nikolas Rose, *Governing the Soul: The Shaping of the Private Self* (London: Routledge, 1990).

48. In the fourth edition of the *Diagnostic and Statistical Manual of Mental Disorders*, poised for publication shortly, over twenty new diagnostic categories will be introduced. The diagnostic areas of most rapid growth will be depressive disorders, eating disorders, sleep disorders, personality disorders, and dissociative disorders. See Allen J. Frances et al., "An A to Z Guide to DSM-IV Conundrums," *Journal of Abnormal Psychology*, c (1991), 407–412; and Erica E. Goode, "Sick, or Just Quirky?: Psychiatrists are Labelling More Human Behaviors Abnormal," *U.S. News and World Report*, cxii, 10 February 1992, 49–50.

49. Nevertheless, we cannot claim comprehensive coverage, and a number of significant topics, due to limitations of space, have not been included. The book does not, for instance, consider the French tradition of psychiatric historiography before the 1960s (Semelaigne, Sérieux, Laignel-Lavastine, Vinchon, Pélicier, etc.), the rich Swiss or Spanish contributions to the field, or the anti-psychiatric ideas of Laing or Basaglia. Similarly, we have not included articles on the history of somatic psychiatry. This is due largely to the fact that biological psychiatry, while ascendant in psychiatric medicine today, is too new to have generated a significant body of historical commentary about itself, a fact that is almost certain to change with time.

50. See also Ernest Harms, "The Early Historians of Psychiatry," *American Journal of Psychiatry*, cxiii (1957), 749–752.

51. For more on this topic, consult Marx, "What Is Psychiatry?" 593–605, esp. 594–597 as well as Henri Baruk, "Quelques réflexions sur l'historie de la psychiatrie," *Histoire des sciences médicales*, xviii (1984), 205–207.

52. David S. Werman, "The Teaching of the History of Psychiatry," *Archives of General Psychiatry*, xxvi (1972), 287–289.

53. For other Freudocentric histories from the midcentury era, see Lewis, *A Short History of Psychiatric Achievement* (1941); Ehrenwald, *From Medicine Man to Freud* (1957); Bromberg, *The Mind of Man* (1959); Jerome M. Schneck, *A History of Psychiatry* (Springfield, Illinois: Charles C Thomas, 1960); and Dieter Wyss, *Depth Psychology: A Critical History* (London: Allen & Unwin, 1966; German ed., 1961).

54. See also *Beyond the Unconscious: Selected Essays by Henri F. Ellenberger in the History of Psychiatry*, edited and introduced by Mark S. Micale (Princeton: Princeton University Press, 1993).

55. Philip Rieff, *Sacred Order/Social Order: Image Entries to the Aesthetics of Authority*, 3 vols. (Chicago: University of Chicago Press, forthcoming).

56. These points are brought out clearly in J. S. Maxmen, *The New Psychiatry* (New York: Morrow, 1985).

57. On the global cultural and intellectual diffusion of psychoanalytic ideas, the most comprehensive source thus far is Roland Jaccard (ed.), *Histoire de la psychanalyse*, 2 vols. (Paris: Hachette, 1982). On "cultures of psychoanalysis," see Edith Kurzweil, *The Freudians: A Comparative Perspective* (New Haven: Yale University Press, 1989); Steven Marcus, *Freud and the Culture of Psychoanalysis* (London: Allen & Unwin, 1984); and Forrester, "'A Whole Climate of Opinion': Rewriting the History of Psychoanalysis," this volume. For statistical analyses showing Freud to be the most heavily cited European or North American author in the major arts, humanities, and social sciences citation indexes, see Allan Megill, "The Reception of Foucault by Historians," *Journal of the History of Ideas*, xlviii (1987), [117–141], 121, n. 13 and 139.

58. There is no comprehensive catalogue of the secondary literature on Freud. However, for a lively and wide-ranging tour through the major writings, see the extended bibliographical essay in Peter Gay's *Freud: A Life for Our Time* (New York: Norton, 1988), 741–779.

59. Freud, *On the History of the Psychoanalytic Movement* (1914), in *The Standard Edition of the Complete Psychological Works of Sigmund Freud*, translated from the German and under the editorship of James Strachey, with Anna Freud, Alix Strachey, and Alan Tyson (London: Hogarth, 1957), xiv, 7–66; idem, *An Autobiographical Study* (1925), *Standard Edition*, xx, 7–70.

60. Ernest Jones, *The Life and Work of Sigmund Freud*, 3 vols. (New York: Basic, 1953–1957).

61. To the best of our knowledge, the only explicit general challenge to Jones's canonical history during this period by a historian of psychiatry was Ernest Harms's *Origins of Modern Psychiatry* (Springfield, Illinois: Charles C Thomas, 1967), ch. 24.

62. For some perceptive observations about the distinction between "traditional" and "revisionist" historiographies of Freud, and about Freud studies generally today, see John Kerr's epilogue to Toby Gelfand and John Kerr (eds.), *Freud and the History of Psychoanalysis* (Hillsdale, New Jersey: Analytic Press, 1992), 357–383.

63. Adolf Grünbaum, "Epistemological Liabilities of the Clinical Appraisal of Psychoanalytic Theory," *Noûs*, xiv (1979), 307–385; idem, "The Role of the Case Study Method in the Foundations of Psychoanalysis," *Canadian Journal of Philosophy*, xviii (1988), 623–658; Anthony Clare, "Freud's Cases: The Clinical Basis of Psychoanalysis" in Bynum, Porter, and Shepherd, *Anatomy of Madness*, i: 271–288; Frank J. Sulloway, "Reassessing Freud's Case Histories: The Social Construction of Psychoanalysis," *Isis*, lxxxii (1991), 245–275.

64. Maurice Natenberg, *Freudian Psycho-Antics: Fact and Fraud in Psychoanalysis* (Chicago: Regent House, 1953); François Roustang, *Psychoanalysis Never Lets Go* (Baltimore: Johns Hopkins University Press, 1980); Daniel Goleman, "As a Therapist, Freud Fell Short, Scholars Find," *New York Times* (Science Times section), 6 March 1990, C1, C12; Paul Taylor, "Freud Undergoes Analysis and Is Found Inadequate," *The Globe and Mail* (Toronto), 13 October 1990. See also H. M. Lohmann (ed.), *Die Psychoanalyse auf der Couch* (Frankfurt: Fischer, 1984).

65. Adolf Grünbaum, *The Foundations of Psychoanalysis: A Philosophical Critique* (Berkeley: University of California Press, 1984); Frank J. Sulloway, "Grünbaum on Freud: Flawed Methodologist or Serendipitous Scientist?" *Free Inquiry* (Fall, 1985), 23–27. See also Paul Kline, *Fact and Fantasy in Freudian Theory* (London: Methuen, 1972); Seymour Fisher and Roger P. Greenberg, *The Scientific Credibility of Freud's Theories and Therapy* (New York: Basic, 1977); Fisher and Greenberg (eds.), *The Scientific Evaluation of Freud's Theories and Therapy* (New York: Basic, 1978); and Marshall Edelson, *Hypothesis and Evidence in Psychoanalysis* (Chicago: University of Chicago Press, 1984).

66. Paul Roazen, *Freud and His Followers* (New York: Knopf, 1975); idem, *Encountering Freud: The Politics and Histories of Psychoanalysis* (New Brunswick, New Jersey: Transaction Publishers, 1990); Robert Castel, *Le psychanalysme: L'Ordre psychanalytique et le pouvoir* (Paris: Union générale d'Éditions, 1976); François Roustang, *Dire Mastery: Discipleship from Freud to Lacan* (Baltimore: Johns Hopkins University Press, 1982); Russell Jacoby, *The Repression of Psychoanalysis: Otto Fenichel and the Political Freudians* (New York: Basic, 1983); E. Gellner, *The Psychoanalytic Movement: Or, the Coming of Unreason* (London: Paladin, 1985); J. N. Isbister, *Freud: An Introduction to His Life and Work* (New York: Blackwell, 1985); Stephen Frosh, *The Politics of Psychoanalysis* (New Haven: Yale University Press, 1987); and Phyllis Grosskurth, *The Secret Ring: Freud's Inner Circle and the Politics of Psychoanalysis* (London: J. Cape, 1991).

67. H. J. Eysenck, *The Decline and Fall of the Freudian Empire* (Harmondsworth: Viking, 1985); J. Reppen (ed.), *Beyond Freud* (Hillsdale, New Jersey: Analytic Press, 1985).

68. Gilles Deleuze and Félix Guattari, *Anti-Oedipus: Capitalism and Schizophrenia* (New York: Viking, 1977; French ed., 1972).

69. From many titles, see Monique Schneider, *De l'exorcisme à la psychanalyse: Le féminin expurgé* (Paris: Retz, 1979); Renat Schleisier, *Konstrucktionen der Weiblichkeit bei Sigmund Freud* (Frankfurt: Europeanishe Verlagsamtatt, 1981); Jane Gallop, *The Daughter's Seduction: Feminism and Psychoanalysis* (London: Macmillan, 1982); Charles Bernheimer and Claire Kahane (eds.), *In Dora's Case: Freud—Feminism—Hysteria* (New York: Columbia University Press, 1985); and Catherine Clément, *The Weary Sons of Freud* [1978] (New York: Verso, 1987).

70. Marie Balmary, *Psychoanalyzing Psychoanalysis: Freud and the Hidden Fault of the Father* (Baltimore: Johns Hopkins University Press, 1982); Jean A. Harris and Jay E. Harris, *The One-Eyed Doctor Sigismund Freud: Psychological Origins of Freud's Works* (New York: Aronson, 1984); and Bernheimer and Kahane, *In Dora's Case*, especially the essays by Toril Moi and Suzanne Gearhart.

71. E. Fuller Torrey, *Freudian Fraud: The Malignant Effect of Freud's Theory on American Thought and Culture* (New York: HarperCollins, 1992).

72. Jacques Barzun, *Clio and the Doctors: Psycho-History, Quanto-History & History* (Chicago: University of Chicago Press, 1974); David E. Stannard, *Shrinking History: On Freud and the Failure of Psychohistory* (New York: Oxford University Press, 1980); Torrey, *Freudian Fraud* (1992).

73. Jeffrey Moussaieff Masson, *The Assault on Truth: Freud's Suppression of the Seduction Theory* (New York: Farrar, Straus, and Giroux, 1984).

74. Frank J. Sulloway, *Freud, Biologist of the Mind: Beyond the Psychoanalytic Legend* (New York: Basic, 1979); idem, "Freud and Biology: The Hidden Legacy" in W. R. Woodward and M. B. Ash (eds.), *The Problematic Science* (New York: Praeger, 1982), 198–227.

75. Frederick Crews, "Analysis Terminable," *Commentary* (July 1980), 25–34; idem, "The Freudian Way of Knowledge," *New Criterion* (June 1984), 7–25; idem, "The Future of an Illusion," *New Republic* (January 1985), 28–33; and idem, "Beyond Sulloway's *Freud*: Psychoanalysis Minus the Myth of the Hero," all available in Crews, *Skeptical Engagements* (New York: Oxford University Press, 1986), 18–111.

76. Peter J. Swales, "Freud, His Teacher, and the Birth of Psychoanalysis" in Paul Stepansky (ed.), *Freud: Appraisals and Reappraisals* (Hillsdale, New Jersey: Analytic Press, 1986), i, 3–82; idem, "Freud, Minna Bernays and the Conquest of Rome: New Light on the Origins of Psychoanalysis," *The New American Review*, i (1982), 1–23; idem, "Freud, Fliess, and Fratricide: The Role of Fliess in Freud's Conception of Paranoia" in Laurence Spurling (ed.), *Sigmund Freud: Critical Assessments* (London: Routledge, 1989), i: *Freud and the Origins of Psychoanalysis*, 302–330; idem, "Freud, Cocaine and Sexual Chemistry: The Role of Cocaine in Freud's Conception of the Libido" in Spurling, *Freud: Critical Assessments*, i, 273–301; and idem, "Freud, Martha Bernays and the Language of Flowers: Masturbation, Cocaine, and the Inflation

of Fantasy" (privately printed, 1983). On the final charge, see also E. M. Thornton, *Freud and Cocaine: The Freudian Fallacy* (London: Blond & Briggs, 1983).

77. At the same time, other scholars, unabashed, have continued to write in traditional historiographical molds. See, for instance, Peter Gay, *Freud: A Life for Our Time* (New York: Norton, 1988); Elisabeth Young-Bruehl, *Anna Freud: A Biography* (New York: Summit, 1988); and Sigmund Freud, *A Phylogenetic Fantasy: Overview of the Transference Neuroses*, edited with an essay by Ilse Grubrich-Simitis (Cambridge: Harvard University Press, 1987).

78. Paul Roazen, "The Legend of Freud," *Virginia Quarterly Review*, xlvii (1971), 33–45; Sulloway, *Freud: Beyond the Psychoanalytic Legend*, especially Part Three; and idem, "Reassessing Freud's Case Histories," *Isis*, especially 246–251. See also George Weisz, "Scientists and Sectarians: The Case of Psychoanalysis," *Journal of the History of the Behavioral Sciences* xi (1975), 350–364.

79. As Young-Bruehl notes, there are indications that recent writing on Freud is achieving a new level of critical and cultural self-consciousness. In addition to Young-Bruehl, "A History of Freud Biographies," this volume, see N. Rand and M. Torok, "The History of Psychoanalysis: History Reads Theory," *Critical Inquiry*, xiii (1987), 504–509; Arnold I. Davidson, "How to Do the History of Psychoanalysis: A Reading of Freud's *Three Essays on the Theory of Sexuality*" in Françoise Meltzer (ed.), *The Trial(s) of Psychoanalysis* (Chicago: University of Chicago Press, 1988), 39–64; and John E. Toews, "Historicizing Psychoanalysis: Freud in His Time and for Our Time," *Journal of Modern History*, xliii (1991), 504–554.

80. See also Vandermeersch, "The Victory of Psychiatry over Demonology: The Origins of the Nineteenth-Century Myth," *History of Psychiatry*, ii (1991), 351–363.

81. L. S. Jacyna, "Images of John Hunter in the Nineteenth Century," *History of Science*, xxi (1983), 85–108; George Weisz, "The Posthumous Laennec: Creating a Modern Medical Hero, 1826–1870," *Bulletin of the History of Medicine*, lxi (1987), 541–562; Bernadette Bensaude-Vincent, "A Founder Myth in the History of Sciences?—The Lavoisier Case" in Graham, *Functions and Uses of Disciplinary Histories*, 53–78.

82. Dora B. Weiner, *The Citizen-Patient in Revolutionary and Imperial Paris* (Baltimore: John Hopkins University Press, 1993), ch. 9.

83. See also Gladys Swain, *Le sujet de la folie: Naissance de la psychiatrie* (Toulouse: Privat, 1977), Pt. 3, "Les chaines qu'on enlève"; and Jacques Postel, "Philippe Pinel et le mythe fondateur de la psychiatrie française," *Psychanalyse à l'Université*, iv (1979), 197–244.

84. Historiographically, the image of Pinel as absolute liberator was then transmitted from *Philippe Pinel et son oeuvre au point de vue de la médecine mentale* (1888) by René Semelaigne (who turns out to have been Pinel's great nephew!), to Zilboorg's *A History of Medical Psychology*, and from there to generations of English-language readers up to the present.

85. George Mora, "Vincenzo Chiarugi (1759–1820). His Contribution to Psychiatry," *Bulletin of the Isaac Ray Medical Library*, ii (1954), 50–104; idem, "Italy" in John G. Howells (ed.), *World History of Psychiatry* (New York: Brunner/Mazel, 1975), 39–89; idem, introduction to Vincenzo Chiarugi, *On Insanity and Its Classification (1793–94)* (Canton, Massachusetts: Science History Publications, 1987), xiii–cxli.

86. Peter Bassoe, "Spain as the Cradle of Psychiatry," *American Journal of Psychiatry*, ci (1945), 731–738; Ajparo S. Chamberlain, "Early Mental Hospitals in Spain," *American Journal of Psychiatry*, cxxiii (1966–1967), 143–149; Ruben D. Rumbaut, "The First Psychiatric Hospital of the Western World," *American Journal of Psychiatry*, cxxviii (1972), 1305–1309; Raquel Alvarez, "The History of Psychiatry in Spain," *History of Psychiatry*, ii (1991), 303–306.

87. The major statements in chronological order were Gerald N. Grob, *The State and the Mentally Ill: A History of Worcester State Hospital in Massachusetts* (Chapel Hill: University of North Carolina Press, 1966); David J. Rothman, *The Discovery of the Asylum: Social Order and Disorder in the New Republic* (Boston: Little, Brown, 1971); Grob, *Mental Institutions in*

America: Social Policy to 1875 (New York: Free Press, 1973); Jacques Quen, "David Rothman's *Discovery of the Asylum*," *Journal of Psychiatry and the Law*, ii (1974), 105–120; Andrew Scull, "Madness and Segregative Control: The Rise of the Insane Asylum," *Social Problems*, xxiv (1977), 338–351; idem, *Museums of Madness* (1979); Grob, "Rediscovering the Asylum: The Unhistorical History of the Mental Hospital" in Morris Vogel and Charles E. Rosenberg (eds.), *The Therapeutic Revolution: Essays in the Social History of American Medicine* (Philadelphia: University of Pennsylvania Press, 1979), 135–157; Rothman, *Conscience and Convenience: The Asylum and Its Alternatives in Progressive America* (Boston: Little, Brown, 1980); Kathleen Jones, "Scull's Dilemma," *British Journal of Psychiatry*, cvli (1982), 221–226; and Grob, *Mental Illness and American Society, 1875–1940* (Princeton: Princeton University Press, 1983).

Twenty-five years after its inception, the controversy continues. Recent publications include Grob, *From Asylum to Community: Mental Health Policy in Modern America* (Princeton: Princeton University Press, 1991), especially chs. 4 and 10; Scull, "Humanitarianism or Control? Some Observations on the Historiography of Anglo-American Psychiatry" and "The Discovery of the Asylum Revisited" in *Social Order/Mental Disorder*, chs. 2 and 5; Rothman, *Discovery of the Asylum*, rev. ed (Boston: Little, Brown, 1990), introduction to the 1990 edition, viii–xliv; Grob, "Marxian Analysis and Mental Illness," *History of Psychiatry*, i (1990), 223–232; Scull, *The Most Solitary Affliction: Madness and Society in Britain, 1700–1900* (New Haven: Yale University Press, 1993), introduction; and Grob, "The History of the Asylum Revisited: Personal Reflections," this volume.

88. Andrew Scull, "The Decarceration of the Mentally Ill: A Critical View," *Politics and Society*, vi (1976), 173–212; idem, "Deinstitutionalization and the Rights of the Deviant," *Journal of Social Issues*, xxxvii (1981), 6–20; idem, "Whose Dilemma? The Crisis of the Mental Health Services," *British Journal of Psychiatry*, cxlii (1983), 98; idem, *Decarceration: Community Treatment and the Deviant—A Radical View*, 2nd ed. (Oxford: Polity Press, 1984); Kathleen Jones, *Mental Hospitals at Work* (London: Routledge & Kegan Paul, 1962); idem, "Deinstitutionalization in Context," *Milbank Memorial Fund Quarterly*, lvii (1979), 552–569; idem, "Scull's Dilemma" (1982); Gerald Grob, "Doing Well and Getting Worse: The Dilemma of Social Policy," *Michigan Law Review*, lxxvii (1979), 761–783.

89. Klaus Doerner, "Nationalsozialismus und Lebensvernichtung," *Vierteljahreshefte für Zeitgeschichte*, xv (1967), 121–152. Among Doerner's later publications on the topic, see his searching analysis, *Tödliches Mitleid* (Gütersloh: J. van Hoddis, 1988).

90. Geoffrey Cocks, "Psyche and Swastika: *Neue deutsche Seelenheilkunde, 1933–1945*," (Ph.D. diss., University of California, Los Angeles, 1975). See also idem, *Psychotherapy in the Third Reich: The Göring Institute* (New York: Oxford University Press, 1985); and idem, "The Professionalization of Psychotherapy in Germany, 1928–1949" in Geoffrey Cocks and Konrad H. Jarausch (eds.), *German Professions, 1800–1950* (New York: Oxford University Press, 1990), 308–328.

91. Hans-Martin Lohmann (ed.), *Psychoanalyse und Nationalsozialismus. Beiträge zur Bearbeitung eines unbewältigten Traumas* (Frankfurt: Fischer Verlag, 1984); Ulfried Geuter, *Die Professionalisierung der deutschen Psychologie im Nationalsozialismus*, 2nd ed. (Frankfurt, Suhrkamp, 1988); trans. *The Professionalization of Psychology in Nazi Germany* (Cambridge: Cambridge University Press, 1992); Regine Lockot, *Erinnern und Durcharbeiten. Zur Geschichte der Psychoanalyse und Psychotherapie im Nationalsozialismus* (Frankfurt: Fischer Verlag, 1985).

92. Nor is Germany the only nation now confronting its wartime psychiatric history. See the recent, remarkable volume by Max Lafont entitled *L'Extermination douce* (Nantes: Areppi, 1987), which relates the story of some 40,000 inmates of French mental hospitals who were allowed to starve to death under the Vichy regime.

93. Sidney Bloch and Peter Reddaway, *Psychiatric Terror: How Soviet Psychiatry Is Used to Suppress Dissent* (New York: Basic, 1977); idem, *Soviet Psychiatric Abuse: The Shadow over*

World Psychiatry (London: V. Gollancz, 1984); David Joravsky, *Russian Psychology: A Critical History* (Oxford: Basil Blackwell, 1989), ch. 15.

94. See also Martin Miller, "Freudian Theory under Bolshevik Rule: The Theoretical Controversy during the 1920s," *Slavic Review*, xliv (1983), 625–646; Hans Lobner and Vladimir Levitin, "A Short History of Freudism: Notes on the History of Psychoanalysis in the U.S.S.R.," *Sigmund Freud House Bulletin*, ii (1978), 5–30; and Joravsky, *Russian Psychology*, Part III.

95. This story, incidentally, need not be a tale of horrors. For example, the fledgling psychoanalytic movements that flourished in a number of Russian cities and in Budapest during the 1920s have a history that can now be written properly.

96. The history of state-sponsored psychiatric terrorism in other countries is beginning to be told, too. Most prominently, see Léon Grinberg, "La mémoire accuse: Des psychanalystes sous les régimes totalitaires," *Revue internationale d'histoire de psychanalyse*, v (1992), 445–472; and Nancy Caro Hollander, "Psychanalyse et terreur d'état en Argentine," *Revue internationale d'histoire de psychanalyse*, v (1992), 473–507.

97. Guarnieri, "The History of Psychiatry in Italy," this volume.

98. See as well Richard E. Vatz and Lee S. Weinberg (eds.), *Thomas Szasz: Primary Values and Major Contentions* (Buffalo, New York: Prometheus, 1983), which includes a complete bibliography of Szasz's publications, pp. 237–253.

99. Szasz, *The Manufacture of Madness*, appendix, 293–321.

100. See also Gutting, *Michel Foucault's Archaeology of Scientific Reason* (Cambridge: Cambridge University Press, 1989), ch. 2.

101. Also see Tomes's earlier survey, "Historical Perspectives on Women and Mental Illness" in Rima Apple (ed.), *Women, Health, and Medicine in America: A Historical Handbook* (New York: Garland, 1990), 143–171.

102. Ronald Bayer, *Homosexuality and American Psychiatry: The Politics of Diagnosis* (Princeton: Princeton University Press, 1987); Roland Littlewood and Maurice Lipsedge (eds.), *Aliens and Alienists: Ethnic Minorities and Psychiatry*, 2nd ed. (London: Unwin Hyman, 1989).

103. Virtually all authors in this section acknowledge the semantic inadequacies and ambiguities of the term *anti-psychiatry*. They employ the term with reservation to denote a loose and shifting collection of critical ideas, attitudes, and theories about psychiatric theory and practice that culminated in the 1960s and 1970s.

104. Mora and Brand, *Psychiatry and Its History* (1970).

I

EARLY DEVELOPMENTS

2

The Beginning of Psychiatric Historiography in Nineteenth-Century Germany

OTTO M. MARX

Traditionally medicine had its share of patients with mental derangement or behavioral disorder, and medical texts included the careful description of these symptoms and their treatment. While in some patients these disturbances preceded the onset of other recognizable physical symptoms, were concomitant with them or subsided with recovery, in still others the mental symptoms or disordered behavior remained. In yet another group of patients mental symptoms or disordered behavior was all that a physician could discern. The situation was further complicated by the fact that there was much overlap among these groups of patients, and that relatively few patients with mental symptoms only came to the attention of physicians. After all a physician was called only when there was grave concern for a sick person and when the physician's services could be afforded. When the physician was consulted no radically different measures of treatment were prescribed, since medical theory provided guidelines for the treatment of all diseases. In the majority of cases, mental, emotional, or behavioral changes were concomitants of many diseases, and there was no need for a special literature to address these secondary changes, or complications. People who developed mental or behavioral changes without other discernible signs of illness were not necessarily candidates for medical attention; even today we are still uncertain whether all instances of disturbed behavior represent an illness. In such cases, as in all others, the economics of the patient's situation played an important role, and physicians were ready to interpret a variety of complaints as medical problems when the patient could afford their services.

In late eighteenth-century Western Europe, this situation changed dramatically, and mental illness of all social classes became the subject of medical attention and the concern of governments. While the reasons for this are still widely debated by historians of psychiatry, the physicians' interest and writings on the subject began with literary efforts based on experience with upper- and middle-class private patients in Britain. But urbanization did not support only private practice; it also brought with it an ever-growing proletariat that lived under the most horrific conditions in the slums. Madness was clearly a concomitant of violence, hunger, and disease. Both private patients and the proletariat thus played a role in the development of what came to be known as psychiatry, which, at the time, was viewed as but another example of the fruits of the Enlightenment. Even if more recently historians of psychiatry have played down the significance of Enlightenment thought or philosophy, all those who were then engaged in improving the lot of the mentally ill, whether as physicians or reformers or as representatives of government, did so in the name of the Enlightenment or, more specifically, its values of reason, science, and philanthropy. Yet there were significant differences in what was meant by these ideals when they were promoted by authors from different countries.

Although most German rulers saw themselves as men of the Enlightenment and protagonists of the new philosophy, they had no intention of giving up their autocratic rule or of abolishing the privileges of the aristocracy. Moreover, each had his own ideas and standards, making it difficult to generalize about the conglomerate of states, duchies, principalities, and cities that made up Germany—except, perhaps, in regard to one institution—the university.

With the Enlightenment, many German rulers increased their support for or founded their own universities as proof of their personal cultural status, and in competition with each other. The professors at these—mostly very small—universities had no better way to show their gratitude and further their professional status than to publish learned works dedicated to their king or his minister of education and to compete with the professors serving other rulers. In medicine one professor often represented several specialities, and since hospital facilities were limited, the publication of a book was the preferred way of establishing expertise in a specialty. Erudite and polyglot, they read voraciously and were quick to review, criticize, or elaborate on the European literature and the clinical or experimental findings of their foreign colleagues. For most of the first half of the nineteenth century their own universities had, at best, small clinical facilities and lacked the funds for laboratories and experimentation.

At the turn of the century, the direction British and French medicine took with its emphasis on observation, statistics, and natural science seemed to lead toward materialism, a philosophy abhorrent not only to the German rulers who paid the professors' salaries but to the professors themselves as devout Christians. That their positions were not secure is evident from the experience of the philosopher J. G. Fichte, who was forced to leave Jena in the 1790s and F. J. Gall who was prohibited from lecturing in Vienna in 1801. Both were accused of materialism. It was safer to speak of sciences, *Wissenschaften*, as including the humanities (*Geisteswissenschaften*) and to consider the natural sciences (*Naturwissenschaften*) as merely complementary to them. In this situation, when the fear of revolution and danger of materialism conflicted with the ideals of the Enlightenment and the *Sturm und Drang* that had taken hold of people's imagination, F. Schelling's philosophy of nature seemed to offer a perfect solution. Schelling proposed a revolution limited to the individual's soul. Man could gain his freedom without political change. Man and nature were to be unified and the dichotomy between mind and matter, science and philosophy, subject and object was to disappear. In this context German psychiatric literature had its beginnings, and its focus on the philosophical issues of the relations between body and mind and soul is readily understood.

While German efforts in the care of the mentally ill and a psychiatry based on hospital experience came late in relation to those in England and France, psychiatric historiography seems to have begun in Germany as part of this psychiatric literature. Psychiatric historiography began in Germany with the self-conscious efforts of J. C. A. Heinroth (1773–1843). The very first professor of mental therapy (*Professor der Psychischen Heilkunde*) at Leipzig, Heinroth thought to initiate a new period in the history of the theory and treatment of mental disturbances, or as he preferred to put it in the *Theorie und Technik der Seelenstörungen*.[1] To that end he wrote a two-volume psychiatric text, a guide for the training of physicians in psychiatry, a *History and Critique of the Mysticism of All Known People and Times*, a two-volume text on *Mental Health*, and a book titled *Instruction in Appropriate Self-treatment in the Early Stages of Mental Diseases*, and much more.[2] Heinroth's lengthy history of psychiatry has a number of noteworthy aspects, which we can only highlight within the constraints of this chapter. Heinroth ascribes different mental illnesses to humanity at different stages of civilization. Uncontrolled affect, rage, and revenge characterized the age of heroes; later, with the rise of different kinds of religions, ecstasy, fantasy, and reveries could lead to mental disturbances of another sort; melancholy and madness (*Wahnsinn*) came only at the final stage of higher civilization. Heinroth laments the absence of a true theory and art of mental medicine or medicine of the mind, at the time of Hippocrates. After Hippocrates, only a few medical authors wrote on mental therapy. As a whole, the medicine of the antique world was steeped in a misguided somatic orientation.[3] Heinroth passes over the "barbarism" with which mental illness was conceptualized and treated in the Middle Ages and has only contempt for the aberrant superstitions of Jews, Christians, and heathens, which ruled the thinking of that time.

The preliminary phase of mental medicine came between the fifteenth and the eighteenth centuries, and closed with Hermann Boerhaave (1668–1738). The freer spirit of the eighteenth century allowed for a better separation of old opinions from new observations and supernatural belief. National schools of psychiatry developed in Italy, France, England, and Germany. Heinroth's detailed analyses of the psychiatric authors of the generations immediately preceding him are most astute. His greatest praise goes to the English for their superior intuitive approach to practice, although he finds that their institutions are not necessarily better. In Germany he sees J. C. Reil (1759–1813) as the originator of a medicine of the mind (*psychische Medicin*) and considers Ernst Horn's (1774–1848) psychiatry to represent the final summit of the empiric approach to mental disorder.

Clearly Heinroth did not share Reil's opposition to physicians specialized in a medicine of the mind (*psychische Medicin*) and did not find much use for the term *Psychiaterie*, which Reil had coined in 1808. Heinroth's own *rational* point of view was to begin a new era in psychiatry. He took leave of empiricism, confident that at worst "new error leads to newer, higher truth."[4] Having read our way through the lengthy history of *mental medicine* presented by Heinroth, we now realize that he sees over 2,000 years of history merely as preliminary to his own work, with which the real medicine of the mind was to begin.

Heinroth's audacious formulation of psychiatric history as a preamble to his own literary contributions—his experience in practice remains unknown but was certainly not extensive—was countered eighteen years later by a younger contemporary, J. B. Friedreich (1796–1862). Heinroth's most vociferous opponent and a self-declared somaticist, Friedreich expressed his views on history in his *Critical Historical Presentation of the Theories on the Nature and the Seat of Mental Diseases*.[5] For Friedreich,

Heinroth's new mental medicine was an abomination and a throwback to the religious mysticism Heinroth had condemned in his history but which his opponents saw Heinroth blatantly perpetuating in his own work. Like Heinroth, Friedreich was one of the early German authors who wrote extensively in order to establish a personal reputation in psychiatry on the basis of philosophical-theoretical elaborations. For both Heinroth and Friedreich their historical efforts were intended to substantiate their points of view regarding the nature of mental illness.

A third author of this genre and period had a different aim in mind when he wrote a *General History of Medical Science*, subtitled *A Basis for Lectures and Self-instruction*.[6] Johann Michael Leupoldt, professor of medical sciences at Erlangen (1794–1874), had written the book in the absence of a suitable text for the course of lectures on medical history he was required to teach.[7] Seeing himself as a mediator between the extreme positions represented by Heinroth and Friedreich, Leupoldt remains even-handed in his praise and criticisms of different schools. Basic to Leupoldt's history is the notion that humanity and nature have developed according to the same God-given organic plan. When the human "spirit" embarked on its search for the causes of health, disease, and healing, this search also had to follow the very same plan of development. Unless one recognizes this basic universal plan of all development, the history of medical science remains a dead aggregate of data and becomes an additional burden to our memory. If historical study is to become useful, its findings must be applied to contemporary practice.[8]

Leupoldt's discussion of the most recent history of medicine opens with a section on "Brown's System and other Irritability and Contrastimulation Theories," followed by a section on "Theoretical and Practical Efforts with regard to so-called Animal Magnetism."[9] For Leupoldt these efforts are related to the mysticism of the fifteenth and sixteenth centuries, but not to the new field of psychiatry that is the subject of a brief section later on. Significantly the section titled *"Psychiatrie"*[10] follows one on the revision of medicine by philosophy of nature (*Naturphilosophische Bearbeitung der Medicin*). This term was not used by Heinroth nor by Friedreich in the titles of their histories.

Leupoldt links the increased frequency and variety of diseases that primarily express themselves by the way of mental disturbances, to the "impetuously progressive" development of the "nerves and spirits" (*Nerven und Geistesentwicklung*) of mankind in Europe: Revolutions and wars are not the causes of the increased incidence of mental diseases, as Pinel and others had suggested earlier. Revolutions and the increase in mental illness were both products of an exuberance of the human spirit in recent times. Thus they were related, but not causally. Since every author had his own unique theoretical assumptions, recent German psychiatric literature was of no help in practice. Although the newly opened mental hospitals flourished, as had leprosaria in the distant past, Leupoldt questioned their usefulness. They had abandoned J. G. Langermann's pedagogical principles and Philippe Pinel's management much too quickly in favor of chemical remedies and the mechanical measures of J. M. Cox and E. Horn (1774–1848).[11]

Speaking on the history of psychiatry seven years later, Leupoldt abandoned his cautious and circumspect stance and presented the development of psychiatry as the final phase in the evolution of medicine.[12] From its bases in the body and in the mind, the psychiatric conceptualizations envisioned by Leupoldt would reach the level of the spirit hovering above them. But since man relates to God at the spiritual level, science would unite at this level with religious belief and thereby reach its highest level of fulfillment. The "marriage" between science and religion would bring about the greatest revolution in history. Once again medicine would follow a great leader like Galen, for medicine like all sciences was subject to the "monarchic" principle. All the "little spirits" will join "One [*sic*] greatest" and become like him. Clearly Leupoldt, like other German Romantics then and since envisioned the millennium.[13] Surprisingly, Leupoldt's great vision of twenty-five hundred years of medical history culminating in a new psychosomatic, religious-ethical-scientific medicine, thanks to the development of psychiatry, had been elaborated by the youthful Heinrich Damerow at least three years earlier.

A leader of German psychiatry in later years, and the founding editor of the *German Psychiatric Journal* (*Allgemeine Zeitschrift für Psychiatrie*) in 1844, Heinrich Damerow had expounded these ideas in greater detail in his *Elements of the Near Future of Medicine Developed out of Past and Present.*[14] In this nearly 400-page "glimpse" of Heinrich Damerow, the boundaries between past, present, and future fell as well, and the theme of the superior, chosen Germans is most prominent. German philosophy and German psychology, German brain research and physiology provided the proper basis for the foundation of a superior German psychiatry.[15] For Damerow the "law" that the history of medicine followed the same principles as the natural history of the human race required the addition to medical science of a medicine of the soul, just as the addition of the soul to animal life had culminated in the development of humanity. In the visions of Damerow and Leupoldt the introduction of psychiatry into medical science would elevate medicine from a somatic, scientific endeavor to a psychosomatic, religious-scientific enterprise, thus relegating the earlier twenty-five hundred-year history of medical science to a preliminary evolutionary phase, just as Heinroth had done. Damerow's conviction of great things to come in the wake of the breakdown of old structures and concepts, the unification of opposites, and the disappearance of boundaries on the eve of the great revolution of the individual human mind, places his and Leupoldt's thoughts within Schelling's *Philosophy of Nature* and in the early nineteenth-century Romantic era of German medicine and psychiatry. When this messianic vision of all striving for the common good of a superior and healthy Germany under the guidance of an omniscient leader was realized a century later, the systematic murder of psychiatric patients in Germany and her territories was part of this utopia.

With the failure of the revolution of 1848, Romantic aspirations lost their fervor. In psychiatry the confrontation with large numbers of institutionalized patients called for a more realistic assessment of what could be done and a more critical view of the philosophical flights of imagination of German psychiatric authors. Although Romantic ideas persisted in psychiatry and in the history of psychiatry, more sober voices were heard in the 1840s. The excesses of the Romantic influence were increasingly seen as a heavy burden that had prevented German medicine and perhaps even psychiatry from catching up with the rapid progress evident in England and France with their emphasis on empiric fact and an unequivocal commitment to a materialistic natural science.

Ernst Freiherr von Feuchtersleben (1806–1845), renowned poet, author of the popular *Dietetics of the Soul*, and dean of the Medical Faculty of Vienna, claimed that he favored fact over speculation in his medicine. But when it came to psychiatry he recognized that there was little fact in that specialty. In his lecture course on *Medical Psychology*, generally considered the first lecture series on psychiatry at the University of Vienna, he retained a deeply philosophical perspective with which he hoped to overcome the body-mind dichotomy. To that end he combined the scientific perspective with the philosophical in the hope of providing an approach that would accommodate the different points of view. Since Feuchtersleben believed that the dictum "the history of science is the science itself" also applied to this "totally new field,"[16] the volume of over 400 pages opens with a nearly sixty-page history. There was no difference between science and philosophy in this respect, for to the extent to which psychiatry is philosophical, historical knowledge is essential as well, Feuchtersleben wrote, and proposed to present, a history of psychiatry that included the general characteristics of every age, the state of mental health and its mental diseases, and the history of science at the time.

Clearly Feuchtersleben's definitions of science and of philosophy differed from those of the reader of his work today. Throughout history, Feuchtersleben finds no new modes of thought but a repetition of the four positions first elucidated in antiquity by Plato, Aristotle, the Epicureans, and the Stoics. In nineteenth-century psychiatry these are represented, with some modifications, by J. C. A. Heinroth, J. C. Hoffbauer, A. Combe and M. Jacobi, and F. Groos. Finally "three semi-philosophical half medical" phenomena would also have to be integrated into the history of psychiatry: animal magnetism, craniology, and physiognomy. The shadow that fell over medieval Europe did not lead to a preponderance of mental diseases, as Leupoldt had asserted, but the Crusades could be best understood as a form of epidemic mental illness such as dance mania. Paracelsus represented the culmination of the mystical school. He should be seen as standing at the end of an age, not at the beginning of a new one.[17] Feuchtersleben concluded that expertise in medical psychology was essential for all physicians, since in common parlance a good physician was referred to as a "psychological doctor." But a physician could never limit himself to psychology, since regardless of his specialty he must be able to treat somatically as well.[18]

None of the academic authors mentioned so far was a professor of psychiatry,[19] and not all psychiatric works at that period contained historical chapters. Two of the most important, the mature work of M. Jacobi, *On Mania*, of 1844, and young W. Griesinger's text of 1845, did not.[20] But at midcentury, we find a number of scholarly historical articles by practicing psychiatrists of remarkable quality based on primary sources in the *General Psychiatric Journal*. The purpose of at least one of these historical case studies was to establish whether the treatment of the mentally ill had improved at all with the arrival of psychiatry.[21] For all the ink that had been spilt on the subject of psychiatry, most physicians would have agreed with Damerow's assessment, that midnineteenth century psychiatry was keenly aware of how much it did not know.

Among historians of medicine of the mid-1840s we can differentiate between the old and the new just as in psychiatry we had differentiated between Jacobi representing the old and Griesinger the new, although their work appeared within one year of each other. Emil Isensee's (1807–1845) nearly 2,000-page *History of Medicine* represents the old, and is a remarkable accomplishment for a thirty-seven-year-old man.[22] For the section on the history of psychiatry, which adds up to over 100 pages, Isensee made frequent use of Heinroth's and Friedreich's work, but added extensive sections on the literature and institutions of the most recent twenty years. Isensee implies that Luther,

Paracelsus, and van Helmont were themselves mad. Once again we are told that Stahl, Langermann, and Pinel picked up where Aretaeus and Caelius Aurelianus had left off. For the most recent period, a very thoughtful section on German psychiatric journals— the first ones in the world; another on forensic psychiatry; one on geography and statistics; and a final section on Heinrich Damerow are quite unique.[23] Strangely, nsee agrees with Heinroth on the importance of Ernst Horn, and dwells on Horn's horrifying treatment methods—as depicted by Sandmann—without any sign of revulsion.[24]

Heinrich Haeser's *History of Medicine and Diseases of People*, which first appeared in 1845, devoted only 9 out of nearly 900 pages to psychiatry. But then Haeser believed that "in historiography as in natural science and law the most exactly possible determination of the state of facts must precede any judgement" and he found that "the incontrovertible effect of philosophy on medical practice was not as great as had been usually assumed."[25] Nearly forty years later, in the third edition of his text, now expanded to three heavy volumes, Haeser presents the development of psychiatry going through the same stages as pathology: a purely theoretical beginning in the animism of G. E. Stahl, a descriptive phase in the work of P. Pinel and J. E. D. Esquirol, a pathological anatomical phase in the work of C. Spurzheim, and a contemporary physiological stage with W. Griesinger, in which the somatic and mental spheres were equally emphasized. According to Haeser, greatest credit for humane treatment went to the English. Despite Pinel's efforts in France, the Code Napoleon still dealt with the *insensées ou furiaux* mad or raging people on one and the same line with *animaux malfaisans ou feroces*, i.e. dangerous or ferocious animals.[26]

Whereas Haeser and his predecessors had written for the medical profession, August Hirsch produced a volume on the *History of the Medical Sciences in Germany* in a series dedicated to the edification of the history of sciences in Germany, directed at all educated classes.[27] Despite the purpose of the series, the author maintains a well-balanced critical point of view. He notes that theoretical efforts such as Stahl's did little for psychiatry, which received its first meaningful impulses from the foundation of hospitals dedicated to the treatment of the mentally ill in England. Hirsch believed that only after the establishment of mental hospitals was it possible to approach psychiatry scientifically.[28]

Not everyone agreed with the new medical science and its perspective on the past. Over thirty years after his first historical effort, J. M. Leupoldt authored yet another volume, *The History of Medicine According to its Objective and Subjective Aspects*. Leupoldt thought that the perspective from which older works were written was no longer tenable and that newer contributors paid too much homage to contemporary opinion. History of medicine should be written as a part of the history of culture, a point with which Carl Wunderlich (see below) was in full agreement. Medical history must combine the objective side, that is, the history of health and diseases, with the subjective side, that is, the physicians' knowledge, practice, their literature, institutions, and lives. Finally the relations to the natural sciences, philosophy, religion, and God's will must be integrated by the active historian willing to speculate. It did not seem speculative to Leupoldt, when he wrote that the appearance of Christianity was *the* turning point in history. The section on magnetism is quite separate from that on psychiatry as is "Gall's phrenology."[29] Leupoldt thought that psychiatry should work against the physical one-sidedness of medicine, he credited Paracelsus for bringing the spirit into medicine, and he praised Pargeter for emphasizing the appropriate personal relations with the patient.[30] But Leupoldt no longer espoused his extravagant goals for psychiatry of three decades earlier, and his depiction of current psychiatry did not meet the criteria he set himself in the introduction.

Carl A. Wunderlich's *Medical History*—lectures given in 1858—deserves mention, because the author was the most prominent leader of the new physiological medicine with its allegiance to natural scientific principles and basic sciences. For Wunderlich there was no value in philosophy of nature. Its influence on medicine was disastrous, moreover "the evaporation of all basis in fact as it existed in the school of philosophy of nature certainly promoted the three fraudulent movements" (*Schwindelrichtungen*) of animal magnetism, cranioscopy, and homeopathy, which, unlike the philosophy of nature, "greedily tried to take hold of the public".[31] Transcendental problems were for Wunderlich on the *other* side of medicine's border. "Although committed to science as never before, the medicine of today is aware of its social and human purpose, and the future does not lie in onesided physical or chemical examination, neurology or research of blood or cell, a more subtle or exact diagnosis, or in new principles of therapy." The future of medicine is unpredictable. "It was," Wunderlich wrote, "to seek and find truth wherever and whatever truth may be, and by what way it could be found."[32] Psychiatry did not warrant a special section.

The young Leupoldt, Isensee, Haeser, Wunderlich, and the older Leupoldt cannot easily be placed on one scale of historiography, whether progressive or regressive, nor is it clear what, if any, influence they had on each other. Despite significant changes in Leupoldt's beliefs he maintained more of his overall philosophical perspective and remained less concerned with rigorous method. In the new volume of 1863, Leupoldt gave up some of the self-conscious evenhandedness of his volume of 1825 in which he had apposed Alexander of Hohenlohe's attempt to heal through prayer and blessing (1812) to the most recent psychiatric developments.

Before returning to histories of psychiatry proper it is well to look at a standard medical historical text from the end of the nineteenth century to discover what was happening in medical historiography and its depiction of the history of psychiatry. In 1897 Julius L. Pagel noted in his preface to the first edition of his *Introduction to the History of Medicine* that a rigorously correct presentation of the literature and practice of medicine of the second half of the nineteenth century would require the cooperation of several specialists of the twentieth century.[33] The task was beyond any one individual. Yet in the revised version of Pagel's text of 1915, edited by K. Sudhoff, psychiatry is presented as a purely somatic discipline founded by Pinel who recognized that his patients were suffering from ailments of the brain (*Gehirnleiden*), physical diseases like all others. Yet after Pinel it was still "a long way" until this was generally accepted. That "all coercion must fall" and that "treatment must proceed along somatic points of view as with all diseases" was "finally found and recognized to be the only correct way."[34]

From the meager statements by the historians of medicine, one could not have guessed that the most extensive preliminary work on the history of psychiatry had been completed long since by Heinrich Laehr (1820–1905), the director of his own private hospital, the *Schweizerhof*, in Zehlendorf, a suburb of Berlin. He became known as a leader when he assumed the editorship of the *General Psychiatric Journal (Allgemeine Zeitschrift)* from H. Damerow in 1858, and successfully aborted Wilhelm Griesinger's attempt to take over the journal and the Psychiatric Association in the 1860s. Laehr conducted the most extensive search of past psychiatric literature. First came the *Days to Remember in Psychiatry and Its Accessory Sciences in all Countries* in 1885, followed by the *Literature of Psychiatry, Neurology and Psychology in the Eighteenth Century*. Its first edition of 1892 listing 1,250 authors and 1,728 titles, increased to 4,085 authors and 14,578 titles in the second edition only two years later.[35] In 1900 the nearly 2,500-page *Literature of Psychiatry, Neurology and Psychology 1459–1799* followed. As Laehr wrote in 1899, in the preface to this last work, he had hoped to write a history based on primary sources, but the preliminary work alone had taken up all his time.[36] He recognized that psychiatry depended on knowledge of all parts of the organism but primarily on neurology and psychology, which he had therefore included.

The increasing importance of psychiatry was established by the statistics for the second half of the century: The population of Germany had increased by ten percent, the number of institutions had doubled, and the number of physicians and patients at institutions had both increased by a factor of nearly seven.[37] But their history was of little interest to most psychiatrists, and Laehr had noted that errors had already crept into historical accounts of this "youngest branch of medicine."[38] Toward the end of the century, Laehr observed that most German psychiatrists did not know that animal experimentation, castration for mental deficiency, therapeutic use of electricity, autopsies, measurement of mental processes, and studies of the brain were performed, and that male hysteria was known in the eighteenth century, which had also been called the "century of the nervous constitution."[39]

More importantly, the psychiatrists were now officials in the new united German Reich, whose power, military might, and industry placed it among the great powers with imperial ambitions. Science and medicine received the support of government and industry. From that perspective, reminders of the early nineteenth century and suggestions of continuity were not welcome. In the twentieth century, the early decades of the nineteenth, when Romanticism flourished, were just a brief regression in an altogether progressive history that had been only once before interrupted—by the Middle Ages.

Having completed this preliminary account of German historiography in the nineteenth century, I can offer but a glimpse of what happened subsequently, limiting myself to some comments on a few examples of German historiographic literature.[40] The great history of psychiatry that Laehr envisaged and for which he had completed the preliminary work was never written. The heyday of German nationalism was over when World War I was lost. Emil Kraepelin (1856–1926), the internationally recognized undisputed leader of German psychiatry, himself a fervent nationalist who contributed significantly to the preeminence of German psychiatry, wrote a brief *One Hundred Years of Psychiatry* and saw to it that Theodor Kirchhoff would edit a collection of biographies under the title *Deutsche Irrenärzte*.[41] How little historiography subsequently changed is evident from a comparison of these biographies with the collection of biographies edited by Kurt Kolle after the Second World War.[42] Both are typical biographies of, by, and for physicians. At the same time, Erwin Ackerknecht produced his brief but ever useful *Short History of Psychiatry*.[43] Written from a Whiggish perspective it gives just the most essential information. The antithesis to Ackerknecht is the voluminous *Madness—a History of Occidental Psychopathology* by W. Leibbrand and A. Wettley, which combines the presentation of extraordinary literary detail with careful philosophical analysis.[44]

The first break in the medical tradition of psychiatric historiography came only in

1969 with Klaus Doerner's *Madmen and the Bourgeoisie. A Social History and Sociology of Psychiatric Science.*[45] The patients, society, and politics, and the realities of psychiatric practice and institutions were now given their rightful place in the history of psychiatry. The physicians were finally placed in context but not absolved of their responsibilities. As a member of the post–World War II generation Doerner attempted to deal with the terrible burden of his professional inheritance: the systematic mass murder of patients by German psychiatrists of his teachers' generation.

A less-known work by H. G. Güse and N. Schmacke sought the historical background of that tragedy in a study of *Psychiatry between Bourgeois Revolution and Fascism.*[46] They were first to reverse the hallowed tradition of a progressive development from Griesinger to Kraepelin. Kraepelin's work, heretofore considered the acme of German clinical psychiatric science, was shown to be a thinly disguised ideology that subsequently permitted the complete destruction of the human bond between psychiatrist and patient during the Third Reich. Finally, with B. Pauleickhoff's *Image of Man through Changing Times, a History of Ideas of Psychiatry and Clinical Psychology* we return once again to the more traditional narrow perspective with its focus on the philosophical analysis of psychiatric theory and ignoring the practice that is psychiatric reality.[47]

Finally, among recent bibliographies, G. Fichtner's *Index to Current Work in the History of Medicine* and his *Indices of Dissertations* as well as U. Benzenhöfer's *Bibliography of German Psychiatric Historiography (1975–1989)*[48] deserve mention.

Notes

1. J. C. A. Heinroth, *Lehrbuch der Störungen des Seelenlebens* (Leipzig: Vogel, 1818). vol. 1. "Kritische Geschichte der Theorie und Technik der Seelenstörungen," 64–170. I translate the word *psychisch* with mental; see my paper on J. C. A. Heinroth: "A Reevaluation of the Mentalists in Early Nineteenth Century German Psychiatry," *American Journal of Psychiatry*, 121 (1965), 752–760.

2. J. C. A. Heinroth, *Anweisungen für angehende Irrenärzte zu richtiger Behandlung ihrer Kranken* (Leipzig: Vogel, 1825); J. C. A. Heinroth, *Geschichte und Kritik des Mysticismus aller bekannten Völker und Zeiten* (Leipzig: Hartmann, 1830); J. C. A. Heinroth, *Lehrbuch der Seelengesundheitskunde* (Leipzig: Vogel, 1823); J. C. A. Heinroth, *Unterricht in zweckmässiger Selbstbehandlung bei beginnenden Seelenkrankheiten* (Leipzig: Vogel, 1834). See also L. Cauwenbergh, "J. Chr. A. Heinroth (1773–1843): Psychiatrist of the German Romantic Era," *History of Psychiatry*, 2 (1991), 365–384, and O. Marx, "German Romantic Psychiatry," Part 1, *History of Psychiatry*, 1 (1990), 351–381. Heinroth, J. C. *Textbook of Disturbances of Mental Life*. trans. and Introduction by G. Mora. (Baltimore: Johns Hopkins, 1975), 2 vols.

3. J. C. A. Heinroth, *Lehrbuch*, vol. 1, 96. Heinroth speaks in most of his writings of a *psychische Medicin* and a *psychischer Arzt* meaning a physician of the mind using mental treatment methods. It is a more complicated situation, however. Please see my paper, "German Romantic Psychiatry," Part 1.

4. Heinroth, *Lehrbuch*, p. 170. J. C. Reil, professor of medicine at Halle, had authored the *Rhapsodien über die Anwendung der psychischen Curmethode auf Geisteszerrüttungen* (Halle: Enke, 1803), and in 1808 proposed the term *Psychiaterie* to refer to all mental interventions by physicians directed toward the therapy of any illness. Reil specifically objected to a special mental medicine. "Ueber den Begriff der Medicin und ihren Verzweigungen, besonders in Beziehung auf die Berichtigung der Topik der Psychiaterie," *Beyträge zur Beförderung einer Kurmethode*

derung einer Kurmethode I (1808), 161–279. See also O. Marx, "German Romantic Psychiatry, Part 1, *History of Psychiatry*, 1, 351–381.

5. *Historisch Kritische Darstellung der Theorien über das Wesen und den Sitz der psychischen Krankheiten* (Leipzig: Wigand, 1836). See also K. C. Kirkby, Classic Text No. 8, *History of Psychiatry*, 2 (1991), 457–469 for an introduction to this book and a translation of pages 7–22 of the book.

6. Johann Michael Leupoldt, *Allgemeine Geschichte der Heilkunde. eine Grundlage zu Vorlesungen und zum Selbstunterricht* (Erlangen: Palm & Enke, 1825).

7. Ibid., III–IV, X. Leupoldt provides an eight-page bibliography (pp. 7–15) of medical history texts of which only two are nineteenth-century German: Kurt Sprengel, *Versuch einer pragmatischen Geschichte der Arzneikunde*, first published in Halle in 1792, 3rd ed. 1823; and Aug. Fr. Hecker, *Die Heilkunde auf ihren Wegen zur Gewissheit, oder die Theorien, Systeme und Heilsmethoden der Aerzte seit Hippokrates bis auf unsere Zeiten* (Erfurt, 1802, rev. ed. 1805).

8. Leupoldt, *Gesch. Heilk.*, V–VI. He goes on to say that only with this overall concept of development does the spirit of peace (*Frieden*) come to live, but perhaps he meant freedom (*Freiheit*)? Without applicability to the present, history remains barren!

9. Ibid., 260–266, "Theoretische und praktische Bemühungen in Betreff des sog. [*sic*] thierischen Magnetismus."

10. Ibid., "Psychiatrie," 273–279.

11. Ernst Horn, professor in Brunswick, later in Wittenberg, Erlangen, and Berlin. First to teach psychiatry in Berlin.

12. J. M. Leupoldt, *Ueber den Entwicklungsgang der Psychiatrie* (Erlangen: Heyder, 1833).

13. Ibid., 46–48.

14. Heinrich Damerow, *Die Elemente der nächsten Zukunft der Medizin entwickelt aus der Vergangenheit und Gegenwart. Ein Blick* (Berlin: Reimer, 1829). Damerow was also the first director of the Halle mental hospital and worked in the Prussian Ministry for many years. In the introduction he notes that he had promised himself not to publish his ideas before age thirty.

15. Ibid. Madness was presented to medicine as bait to open her eyes for her higher a evolution (p.277). Although Brownian Theory came from England it "metamorphosed" to a higher level in Germany. Pinel was first to work on madness, "its study threw deeper roots" in Germany. "Germany became the home for the soul which medicine was to educate" (p. 278). Also pp. 279ff, 293, 305.

16. E. Freiherr von Feuchtersleben, *Lehrbuch der ärztlichen Seelenkunde* (Wien: Gerold, 1845), 5. Translated into English by the Sydenham Society much sooner than usual because of its importance: *The Principles of Medical Psychology*, trans. H. E. Lloyd, revised and edited by G. G. Babington (London: 1847). Though they are absent from the title, Feuchtersleben uses the terms *Psychiatrik* and *Psychiater* freely in his text. His *Dietetics of the Soul* was republished for over a century.

17. Feuchtersleben, *Lehrbuch*, 30, 39, 45, 59.

18. Ibid., 72. To the question of whether treating independent mental conditions by education, teaching, etc., is the business of the physician, Feuchtersleben replied with an unequivocal no; in the present state of the world where moral influences are entrusted to parents and teachers, the physician must deal with somatic illnesses, since only those are considered diseases in the nonfigurative sense.

19. Including Heinroth, whose chair was not filled after his death; it was over forty years before Leipzig had a professor of psychiatry. Griesinger's professorial title did not specify psychiatry.

20. W. Griesinger, *Pathologie und Therapie der psychischen Krankheiten*, 4th ed. (Braunschweig: Wreden, 1876). Although Griesinger also taught medical history at Tübingen, he did not add a history chapter even after the first edition of 1845. M. Jacobi, *Die Hauptformen der*

Seelenstoerungen in ihren Beziehungen zur Heilkunde. Vol. 1 *Die Tobsucht.* (Leipzig: Weidmann, 1844).

21. The list offered here is just a random partial selection: Friedrich Bird, "Geschichte der Seelenstörungen Johanna's von Castilien; ein Beitrag zur Geschichte der Psychiatrie im 15. und 16. Jahrhundert," *Allgemeine Zeitschrift für Psychiatrie,* 5 (1848), 151–162; Friedrich Bird, "Geschichte der Geisteskrankheit Carls VI. Königs von Frankreich in den Jahren 1392 bis 1422 und Geschichte des abnormen geistigen Zustandes Carls IX. Königs von Frankreich, besonders nach Bartholomäus 1572," *Allgemeine Zeitschrift für Psychiatrie,* 5 (1848), 569–579; Willers Jessen, "Ueber die Convulsionen unter den Jansenisten in Paris," *Allgemeine Zeitschrift für Psychiatrie,* 7 (1850), 430–473; Friedrich Bird, "Zur Geschichte der Psychiatrie", *Allgemeine Zeitschrift für Psychiatrie,* 7 (1850), 45–62; Friedrich Bird, "Beiträge zur Geschichte der Psychiatrie," *Allgemeine Zeitschrift für Psychiatrie,* 8 (1851), 17–27; P. B. Bergrath, "Zur Geschichte der Geistesstörungen des Herzogs Wilhelm des Reichen und seines Sohnes Johann Wilhelm von Jülich-Cleve-Berg," *Allgemeine Zeitschrift für Psychiatrie,* 10 (1853), 249–280; Wilhelm Jessen, "Ueber die Fanatiker von Languedoc 1688–1780," *Allgemeine Zeitschrift für Psychiatrie,* 11 (1854), 173–197, 448–461.

22. Emil Isensee, (1807–1845), *Geschichte der Medicin, Chirurgie, Geburtshilfe, Staatsarzneikunde, Pharmazie u.a. Naturwissenschaften,* 6th book: *Neuere und neueste Geschichte der öffentlichen und allgemeinen Medizinal-Angelegenheiten,* (bound with 5th book) (Berlin: Nauck, 1844). An amazing work of nearly 2,000 pages, with an extensive literature, literature reviews, and an index of over 130 pages. Clearly an incredible compilation, Isensee maintains a very personal, sometimes chatty style, mixing data with anecdotes, opinions, and bits of information.

23. Isensee, "Zur Geschichte der Psychiatrie", 1211–1313.

24. Since Horn did not publish these methods in detail he quotes from his pupil Sandmann, *Nonnulla de quibusdam remediis ad animi morbos curandos summa cum fructu adhibendis* (Berlin: 1817). (*On Therapeutics of Treatable Mental Diseases, Especially on their Successful Application.*)

25. Heinrich Haeser, *Lehrbuch der Geschichte der Medicin und der Volkskrankheiten* (Jena: Mauke, 1845), VII, X. According to Haeser, psychiatry began with Pinel whose "beautiful and noble gestures" found nowhere as much "enthusiastic approval" as in Germany. Langermann and Reil are the initiators of psychiatry in Germany. Reil intimately connected this branch of pathology with physiology. Psychiatry needed a psychological basis. This must come from neurology, which preoccupied with nerve activity has not been giving mental life the necessary attention (pp. 775–776). Haeser refers to J. B. Friedrich, *Versuch einer Literaturgeschichte der Pathologie und Therapie der psychischen Krankheiten* (Würzburg: 1830); U. Trelat, *Recherches historiques sur la folie* (Paris: 1839), and Choulant, *Bibl. hist. Med.*

26. Haeser, *Lehrbuch,* vol. 2, 3rd ed. (Jena: Fischer, 1881), 1027–1040. In three volumes, with a total of nearly 3,000 pages, 14 deal with psychiatry.

27. Ibid., 1028, 1036. Haeser notes that "among the 'cerebrists' following Spurzheim, some extremists even consider hysteria a disease of the brain." He quotes the *Code penal* (1804), art. 574 on p. 1029. Haeser also makes reference to C. W. Ideler, *Langermann und Stahl als Begründer der Seelenheilkunde dargestellt* (Berlin: 1835). But he only partially subscribes to Ideler's thesis. Even that is surprising, given Haeser's criteria for historiography and the fact that the whole book is mostly based on Ideler's personal feelings of indebtedness to Langermann.

28. August Hirsch, *Geschichte der medicinischen Wissenschaften in Deutschland,* vol. 22 in *Geschichte der Wissenschaften in Deutschland—Neuere Zeit* (München & Leipzig: Oldenbourg, 1893) edit.: Historische Kommission der Königlichen Akademie der Wissenschaften auf Veranlassung des Königs von Bayern. In the preface Hirsch explains that he expanded the task to include the international background. August Hirsch was the editor of the invaluable *Biographisches Lexikon der hervorragenden Ärzte aller Zeiten und Völker,* first published in 1883.

More recent editions were published in 1929 and 1962 by Verlag Urban und Schwarzenberg (München & Berlin).

29. Leupoldt, J. M., *Die Geschichte der Medicin nach ihrer objectiven und subjectiven Seite* (Berlin: Hirschwald, 1863). See pp. IV, 1, 6, 8. For the section on magnetism see pp. 422–433; on psychiatry see pp. 618–647; on phrenology see p. 581.

30. Ibid., 619, 623.

31. C. A. Wunderlich, *Geschichte der Medicin* (Stuttgart: Ebner & Seubert, 1859).

32. Ibid., 364, 366.

33. K. Sudhoff, (ed.), *J. P. Pagels Einführung in die Geschichte der Medizin* (Berlin: Karger, 1915), preface, 536, 537.

34. Hirsch, *Gesch.*, 626. "Mental institutions which did not serve the segregation of the patients, but their treatment" and the publication of their findings and autopsies, p. 628.

35. Heinrich Laehr, *Gedenktage der Psychiatrie und ihrer Hülfsdisciplinen in allen Ländern*, rev. 4th and enlarged ed. (Berlin: Reimer, 1893) (1st ed., 1885); H. Laehr, *Die Literatur der Psychiatrie, Neurologie und Psychologie im XVIII. Jahrhundert*, 1st ed. of 1892 dedicated to the fiftieth anniversary of the Illenau in Achern, and the 2nd ed. to the fiftieth anniversary of Nietleben near Halle (Berlin: Reimer, 1895).

36. H. Laehr, *Die Literatur der Psychiatrie, Neurologie und Psychologie 1459–1699*, vol. I (1459–1699), vol. II-1 and II-2 (1700–1799) with vol. III (an author and subject index) (Berlin: Reimer, 1990). See preface p. VII.

37. Ibid., vol. I, preface:

Germany	Inhabitants	Institutions	Physicians	Patients
1852	47,100,000	134	110	11,622
1898	52,300,000	262	741	74,087

38. Laehr, *Gedenktage*, preface to 1st ed. (1885). He expected that these errors would reproduce themselves and increase.

39. Laehr, *Literatur, 18. Jahrhundert* (1895), preface. Laehr also wrote: *Die Heil- und Pflegeanstalten für Psychisch-Kranke des deutschen Sprachgebietes im Jahr 1890* (Berlin: Reimer, 1891) and again with M. Lewald, under the same title but "im Jahr 1898," (Berlin: Reimer, 1899).

40. I am all the more ready to do so since Klaus Doerner, *Bürger und Irre* (Frankfurt: Europ. Verlagsanstalt, 1969), contains a section on *Criteria of Psychiatric Historiography* (pp. 381–388) in which Dörner criticizes selected twentieth-century histories of psychiatry.

41. Emil, Kraepelin, *Hundert Jahre Psychiatrie* (Berlin: 1918), first appeared in *Zschr. f. ger. Neurol. & Psychiat.*, 38 (1918), 173ff. Kraepelin tries to dissociate psychiatry in the second half of the nineteenth century from the first and attributed the error of the early part to Romanticism and lack of clinical experience. Theodor Kirchhoff, *Deutsche Irrenärzte. Einzelbilder ihres Lebens und Wirkens* (Berlin: Springer, vol. 1 1921; vol. 2 1924). Still a useful, quick reference for individual psychiatrists usually written from a favorable personal perspective. Earlier, Kirchhoff had written an *Outline of a History of German Care of the Mentally Ill. Grundriß einer Geschichte der deutschen Irrenpflege* (Berlin: Hirschwald, 1890), 182 pages of text. The slender volume deals primarily with the ways in which the mentally ill were cared for before the nineteenth century and by psychiatrists during the early decades of the nineteenth century with their emphasis on coercion, restraint, evacuation, shock, and horror.

42. Kurt Kolle, *Große Nervenärzte, vol. 1 1956, vol. 2 1959, vol. 3 1963 (Stuttgart: Thieme)*.

43. Erwin Ackernecht, *Kurze Geschichte der Psychiatrie*, 3rd improved ed. (Stuttgart: Enke, 1985). Unfortunately the English translation is of an earlier edition and compares unfavorably with this last, much improved one.

44. W. Leibbrand, and A. Wettley, *Der Wahnsinn. Geschichte der abendlägndischen Psycho-*

pathologie, vol. II/12 in Orbis Academicus, *Probleme der Wissenschaft in Dokumenten und Darstellungen* (Freiburg: Alber, 1961). Leibbrand's *Romantische Medizin* (Hamburg: Goverts, 1937) proves that honest expression of ideas in conflict with Nazi doctrine was possible at the height of Nazi power.

45. Klaus Dörner, *Bürger und Irre. Zur Sozialgeschichte und Wissenschaftssoziologie der Psychiatrie* (Frankfurt: Europ. Verlagsanstalt, 1969); *Madmen and the Bourgeoise*, J. Neugroschel & J. Steinberg trans. (Oxford, Blackwell, 1981).

46. H. G. Güse, and N. Schmacke, *Psychiatrie zwischen Revolution und Faschismus* (Kronberg: Athenäum, 1976).

47. B. Pauleickhoff, *Das Menschenbild im Wandel der Zeit. Ideengeschichte der Psychiatrie und der Klinischen Psychologie*, (Hürtgenwald: Pressler, vol. 1–4, 1983–1989). *Partnerschaft im Wandel der Zeit*, 1st suppl. vol. 1989. Zeit und Sein, 2nd suppl. vol. 1990.

48. G. Fichtner, Tübingen Institut Geschichte der Medizin: *Index wissenschaftshistorischer Dissertationen (IWD). Verzeichnis abgeschlossener Dissertationen auf dem Gebiet der Geschichte der Medizin, der Pharmazie, der Naturwissenschaften und der Technik*, Nr. 1: 1970–1980, (Tübingen: 1981); *Index wissenschaftshistorischer Dissertationen (IWD/LWD). Verzeichnis abgeschlossener und in Bearbeitung befindlicher Dissertationen auf dem Gebiet der Geschichte der Medizin, der Pharmazie, der Naturwissenschaften und der Technik*, Nr. 3: 1987–1992; *Laufende Wissenschaftshistorische Dissertationen (LWD). Verzeichnis in Bearbeitung befindlicher Dissertationen auf dem Gebiet der Geschichte der Medizin, der Pharmazie, der Naturwissenschaften und der Technik*, Nr. 1 (Tübingen: 1981); U. Benzenhöfer, *Bibliographie der zwischen 1975 und 1989 erschienen Schriften zur Geschichte der Psychiatrie im deutschsprachigen Raum* (Tecklenburg: Burgverlag, 1992) (Hannoversche Abhandlungen zur Geschichte der Medizin und der Naturwissenschaften, edited by. W. U. Eckart). See also Dietrich Langen, (ed.), *Bibliographie deutschsprachiger Veröffentlichungen über Hypnose, autogenes Training und andere Versenkungsmethoden (1890–1969)*, 1st ed. 1974.

3

Early American Historians of Psychiatry: 1910–1960[1]

GEORGE MORA

The first scholarly writing in the United States on the history of psychiatry appeared well after that in the major Western and Central European countries. In the New World, the long, cumulative cultural traditions of classical antiquity, the Middle Ages, and the Renaissance were lacking. By and large, throughout the nineteenth century, intellectual and scientific inquiry remained at a level far below Europe's. As a consequence, nine-teenth-century American asylum physicians displayed almost no interest in the history of the care of the mentally ill. There is no evidence in the publications or private libraries of American alienists during this period of the historical writings of figures such as Philippe Pinel, J. E. D. Esquirol, J. C. A. Heinroth, and E. Feuchtersleben. Even the British literature on the history of psychiatry, such as Daniel Hack Tuke's *Insanity in Ancient and Modern Life* (1878), which was available to American doctors in view of the common language, elicited little resonance in psychiatric circles. To be sure, some of the earliest representatives of American psychiatry (particularly Pliny Earle) spent time in European centers and visited old and well-known facilities for the mentally ill, such as the famous colony of Gheel in Belgium. But their reports about these travels focused on current practical approaches to the mentally ill rather than on historical background. A perusal of the volumes of the *American Journal of Insanity* indicates that the overriding emphasis was on institutional and clinical matters.[2] Similarly, the pioneering historical monographs by nineteenth-century German psychiatrists that Otto Marx discussed in the preceding essay in this volume seem to have remained unknown in America until the advent of the twentieth century.

Precursory Figures

Henry Mills Hurd and Smith Ely Jelliffe

Soon after the turn of the last century, a small number of publications pertinent to the history of psychiatry began to appear in the United States. The methodology employed in these early writings left much to be desired, and in content they consisted essentially of chronicles of events or short biographies of individual doctors or lay reformers that in comparison with psychiatric historiography today were devoid of analytical depth.

The most significant of these early writers was Henry Mills Hurd, a little-known figure who, undeservedly, is generally omitted from accounts of psychiatric history writing. Hurd was born in Michigan in 1843 and after graduating from the medical school of the University of Michigan in 1866 served for eleven years as superintendent of the Eastern Michigan Asylum in Pontiac, Michigan.[3] In 1889, he assumed the position of superintendent of the Johns Hopkins Hospitals in Baltimore, Maryland, which was then staffed by such eminent physicians as William Osler (general medicine), William Halstead (general surgery), Howard Kelly (gynecology), and William Welch (pathology). In 1890, Hurd launched *The Johns Hopkins Hospital Bulletin*, which was soon ranked one of the leading American medical journals. Hurd's new publication regularly included historical papers.

In 1910, the American Medico-Psychological Association, subsequently renamed the American Psychiatric Association, established a committee of well-known psychiatrists, operating under Hurd's chairmanship, to prepare a comprehensive history of the institutional care of the insane in the United States and Canada. Hurd's committee worked tirelessly, and the final product, consisting of four massive volumes for a total of 2,296 pages, was published by The Johns Hopkins Press in 1916–17. The first volume of the set, written singly by Hurd, provided a comprehensive overview of the development of the care of the mentally ill in North America, with particular emphasis on the events that occurred in state institutions and on legal issues relevant to mental illness. Hurd's volume, mainly a compendium of factual material, is now overlooked; yet, in the early 1970s, it was reprinted and still serves as a valuable source of information.[4]

A second significant precursor of American psychiatric historiography was the early psychoanalyst Smith Ely Jelliffe. Born in 1866 in New York City, Jelliffe studied civil engineering at Brooklyn Collegiate and Polytechnic Institute and then enrolled at the College of Physicians and Surgeons of Columbia University where he received his medical degree in 1889.[5] Shortly thereafter he spent a year in Europe, mostly as a postgraduate trainee in the great medical centers of Vienna, Berlin, and Paris. From these foreign experiences, Jelliffe acquired proficiency in French and German, a large amount of knowledge of psychiatry and culture in general, and a cosmopolitan attitude that made him rather unique among contemporary American neurologists and psychiatrists.

Back in the United States, Jelliffe developed a strong interest in botany and pharmacology. In 1896, he had spent a summer as a physician at the Binghamton State Hospital, where he became acquainted with William Alanson White (1870–1937), by whom he was influenced professionally toward the fields of neurology and psychiatry. Indeed, the two men remained friends and collaborators for several decades. Eventually Jelliffe became an assistant in neurology at the Vanderbilt Clinic of Columbia University and the outpatient department of the Presbyterian Hospital. Later, he engaged extensively in medical journalism, which resulted in his appointment as editor of the weekly *Medical News* in 1900. In addition, he served as associate editor of the *Journal of Nervous and Mental Disease*, which he later purchased in 1901 and which under his leadership succeeded in introducing European medical literature to many Americans.

By 1906, Jelliffe had decided to devote himself to neurology, psychiatry, and psychoanalysis. He undertook a series of study trips to Europe where he became acquainted with scores of well-known clinicians, among whom were Kraepelin, Dubois, Freud, Jung, Maeder, Bernheim, Déjerine, Janet, Babinski, Ziehen, and Oppenheim. In 1907, along with White, he founded the *Nervous and Mental Diseases Monograph Series*, whose first issue published White's influential *Outline of Psychiatry*, followed by a series of important publications (mostly in translation) by Jung, Freud, Brill, Maeder, Rank, Kraepelin, and others. During a period as professor in the medical school of Fordham University (1907–1913), Jelliffe invited Jung to speak there in 1911. He also became involved with the Post-Graduate Medical School in New York and the Neurological Institute, in addition to carrying on a substantial medical practice and being active in the American Neurological Association.

In 1913, Jelliffe and White launched the *Psychoanalytic Review*, the first periodical in the English language open to all currents of the emerging psychoanalytic movement. In 1915, again jointly with White, he published his massive handbook, *Diseases of the Nervous System: A Textbook of Neurology and Psychiatry*, which was well received and went through many editions. Increasingly influenced by Freud, Jelliffe two years later published *The Technique of Psychoanalysis*; for many years, he was also active in the New York Psychoanalytic Society.

In the light of such an active and productive career, Jelliffe's contributions to the history of psychiatry are modest. In the bibliography of his writings amounting to hundreds of items, only a few publications are of specifically historical interest, although historical materials are scattered throughout many of his works. These mainly take the forms of historical surveys of psychopathological concepts, among which stands out a valuable, detailed study of the manic-depressive syndrome.[6] Again, although these papers may not meet the standards of the historical monographs of our own time, they are written in a lively style, which serves to make the topics interesting, especially to clinicians with little historical background.

In addition to these writings, Jelliffe produced a series of translations of European, mostly German, sources from the nineteenth century that dealt with the history of psychiatry, particularly ancient Greek and Roman psychological medicine. This series of sixteen papers, which run to approximately 300 pages, appeared consecutively in the journal *Alienist and Neurologist* (1880–1920) between 1910 and 1917.[7] Because of the unavailability of such a journal in most libraries, these papers have, by and large, remained unknown, even to psychiatric historians. Moreover, being a mixture of translations (at times, abridged) and commentary, they impress at times as repetitious and poorly organized. Nonetheless, Jelliffe's sequence of articles are quite interesting and, taken together, they offer a comprehensive view of mental illness and its treatment in classical times.

Albert Deutsch (1905–1961)

Beginning with the 1930s, American psychiatric historiography entered a period of greater confidence, maturity, and accomplishment. The second quarter of the century, in fact, gave rise to three major historians of psychiatry whose work I will consider in turn. They are Albert Deutsch, Gregory Zilboorg, and Walther Riese. Interestingly, two of the three figures were intellectual emigrés who drew upon their distinctive European cultural heritages in making their careers in the New World. Each of the three came from different personal, national, and disciplinary backgrounds, and each as a result developed a distinctive vision of psychiatric history.

Albert Deutsch was born to a Jewish family that emigrated from Latvia in 1905 to a depressed area of New York City's Lower East Side. Being the fourth of nine brothers and sisters may have contributed to Deutsch's gregarious and jovial personality, which was apparently not affected by the enucleation of his right eye at the age of five as a result of an accident. Coming from a poor family, he was unable to attend college and during his teens performed menial jobs. This did not prevent young Deutsch from making extensive use of public libraries in New York, where his thirst for learning was satisfied through voracious reading, mainly of history books and biographies.

In his twenties, while doing research for publishing firms, Deutsch happened across a cache of old documents concerning the history of the New York State Department of Welfare. Many of these documents were pertinent to the mentally ill, who in the past had fallen under the domain of public assistance. Progressively, Deutsch became absorbed in the history of this subject. Very likely, his personal humble origins and his familiarity with the environment of the poor made him receptive to the lot of the destitute mentally ill as recorded in these obscure materials.

In 1934, Deutsch, aged 29, submitted to the National Foundation for Mental Hygiene a proposal to research and write a history of the care of the mentally ill in the United States. Impressively, Deutsch's proposal was approved and funded—for a total of $5,000! He worked intensely for the next two years, as an independent scholar surveying virtual *terra incognita* and deeply immersed in all manner of primary sources. In 1937, Deutsch published *The Mentally Ill in America*, a 530-page book that covered the entire development of the care of the mentally ill from colonial times to the present.[8] With this work, the 32-year-old Deutsch emerged as a pioneer in the social and intellectual history of psychiatry and the most substantial historian of American psychiatry up to that time.

Following publication of his monograph, Deutsch worked modestly for a few years as Research Associate for the New York State Department of Welfare. In 1941, he coauthored with David Schneider *The History of Public Welfare in New York State, 1867–1940*. Three years later, he contributed to the volume commemorating the centennial of the American Psychiatric Association two detailed chapters dealing with the history of the mental hygiene movement and with military psychiatry during the American Civil War.[9] During the 1940s and 1950s, he published miscellaneous writings about contemporary psychiatry and public health. In these writings, Deutsch did not hesitate to criticize harshly the psychiatric programs carried on in Veterans Administration hospitals or to publicize abuses and shortcomings in other psychiatric institutions and organizations, risking at times being cited for contempt of Congress. In 1945 and 1946, he received special citations for his exposés of Veterans Administration hospitals and mental hospitals by the American Newspaper Guild's Heywood Brown Award Committee. In 1947, the New York Newspaper Guild honored him as "the most distinguished and effective humanitarian crusading in American journalism." In 1953, he was presented with the Adolf Meyer Memorial Award in Mental Hygiene, and in 1958 he was elected Honorary Fellow of the American Psychiatric Association.[10]

Eventually, Deutsch published much of this material in a book entitled *The Shame of the States* (1948).[11] This was followed by *Our Rejected Children* (1950) and *The*

Trouble with Cops (1955). In 1956, under a grant from the National Association for Mental Health, he initiated a project to survey comprehensively current mental health research in the United States. He visited several research centers and gathered a great deal of material. In view of the size of the project, in 1958 and 1959 he was awarded additional funds by the National Institute of Mental Health. Unfortunately, this important endeavor could not be completed due to his sudden death from a heart attack while attending an international research conference in England sponsored by the World Federation for Mental Health in 1961. Deutsch was only 55 years of age.

As a psychiatric historian, Deutsch's *magnum opus* remains *The Mentally Ill in America*, which, since its appearance in 1937, has been widely recognized as a landmark in American psychiatric historiography. Deutsch's book represents the first attempt at a synthetic overview of the history of care of the mentally ill in the United States. Moreover, to my knowledge, no comprehensive narrative had been written of this subject up to that point, even in the Western and Central European nations, where historical studies on psychiatry continued to take the form of textbook prefaces, biographical compendia, and bibliographical compilations.

In retrospect, two main innovative features of Deutsch's book stand out. First, methodologically *The Mentally Ill in America* is based largely on a careful and critical assessment of primary sources, such as reports from mental hospitals, official local, state, and federal legislation, court proceedings, little-known documents, and so forth. Second, structurally Deutsch's book provides a set of thematic subdivisions and a scheme of periodization for the history of mentally health care in the United States that has virtually been accepted by all later historians. This schematization includes the colonial period, early pioneers (with strong emphasis on Benjamin Rush as "the father of American psychiatry"), the rise of moral treatment, a period of retrogression, the development of a network of state institutions (largely through the efforts of Dorothea Dix), the controversies concerning restraint and the etiology of mental illness in the midnineteenth century, and finally the emergence of the mental hygiene movement and of the modern ideology of psychiatry in the early twentieth century.

Several other aspects of Deutsch's reading of psychiatric history are also noteworthy. As his title indicates, Deutsch largely limits his treatment to the American arena with occasional but fairly superficial considerations of the pertinent European background. By far, he pays the closest attention to developments in New England and the mid-Atlantic states. Throughout the book, and particularly in the early chapters, he conceptualizes the history of psychiatry almost entirely as the story of humanitarianism, marked by alternating periods of progress and regress, optimism and disillusionment. He grants Benjamin Rush a full and thoughtful chapter of his own, presenting him as the founding figure of American psychiatry. The following chapter, "The Rise of the Moral Treatment," provides a dramatic and classically "Whiggish" account of the work of Pinel and the Tukes (much as Michel Foucault would later reinterpret in the final chapter of his *Madness and Civilization*). However, after a rapid review of their work, Deutsch added tellingly that "[i]f Pinel and Tuke had never lived, it is quite possible that the same reforms would have been achieved by others about the same time"—a clear anticipation of the argument for the *Zeitgeist* as opposed to the Great Man theory of history.[12]

In two interlocking chapters entitled "Retrogression" and "The Cult of Curability," Deutsch explores in intelligent detail the complex of social, financial, clinical, institutional, and therapeutic reasons for the national failure of the moral treatment within American mental hospitals by the midnineteenth-century period. He does an excellent job of reconstructing the emergence, consolidation, and bureaucratization of the system of state care for the mentally ill, laying emphasis on the autonomy of states under the American system and the consequent differences among their psychiatric policies. Like Rush, Dorothea Dix receives an enthusiastic and extensive chapter of her own. Deutsch also devotes considerable space to expositions of individual key texts, such as Isaac Ray's *Treatise on the Medical Jurisprudence of Insanity* (1837), Thomas Kirkbride's *On the Construction and Organization of Hospitals for the Insane* (1854), and Clifford Beers, *A Mind that Found Itself* (1908). He provides as well a novel discussion of the impact of the Civil War on the course of American psychiatry. Spurred by the large numbers of neurological casualties from the Civil War, private "nerve specialists," such as Spitzka, Hammond, and Mitchell, appeared during the 1870s and 1880s to compete professionally with the medical authority of institutional alienists.

Yet another significant feature of *The Mentally Ill in America* is Deutsch's copious coverage of twentieth-century psychiatry up to the late 1930s. Deutsch's heroes from this period are Clifford Beers (who was still alive in 1937 when Deutsch published his book) and Adolf Meyer. Deutsch's historical study of American psychiatry culminates in the mental hygiene movement of the 1920s. Deutsch also discusses many other early twentieth-century developments, including the involvement of psychiatry during World War I, the emergence of the field of social work and of the child guidance movement, and the impact of mental hygiene on industry and criminology. He pays close attention as well to the First International Congress on Mental Hygiene held in Washington, D.C., in 1930, with the participation of fifty countries, an event that he sees as representing the official international recognition of American psychiatry. Finally, Deutsch includes in the closing sections of his book separate chapters on two interesting ancillary aspects of psychiatry—the history of treatment of the mentally deficient and the history of legal psychiatry in America.

Deutsch's book assuredly is not without its faults. As a young autodidact, Deutsch lacked even a minimum of professional training in either psychiatry or history. As a result, his knowledge of psychiatric historiography was scanty. Along similar lines, by and large, he overlooked in his historical presentation the strictly psychiatric aspects of the care of the mentally ill. Indicatively, he lavishes attention on Benjamin Rush's practical approach to the mentally ill and his humanitarian concern for many other causes while ignoring Rush's textbook, *Medical Inquiries and Observations upon the Diseases of the Mind* (1812). In the same way, he hardly mentions Wilhelm Griesinger's famous handbook of psychiatry, which had a great impact in Anglo-Saxon countries. There are other important omissions, too. For some reason, Deutsch ignores the phrenological movement, which was taken quite seriously by American psychiatrists in the first half of the nineteenth century. He also overlooks entirely George Beard's description of neurasthenia, the first indigenously American contribution to psychopathology. And likewise, he leaves out the theory of degeneration, which exerted great influence during the second half of the nineteenth century. Interestingly, Freud and the coming of psychoanalytic psychotherapeutics does not figure in Deutsch's book at all.[13]

Nonetheless, in my judgment, these shortcomings are more than offset by the positive aspects of Deutsch's book. As a young man not trained medically or historically (indeed, not even a college graduate), Deutsch's accomplishment was extraordinary, fully justifying the esteem in which he has subsequently been held by historians and psychiatrists. In fairness, Deutsch was less interested in the intellectual history of psychology and psychiatry than in the history of mental health care, and he properly entitled his book *The Mentally Ill in America*. Within this category, Deutsch explored virtually uncharted territory to produce a unique history of the mentally ill in his own country that, half a century after its appearance, is still very valuable and appreciated in many quarters. To this day, no single, book-length study of the subject has replaced it.

In his historical account, Deutsch clearly paid particular attention to the care—often the neglect, if not cruelty—that was given to the mentally ill belonging to the lower classes of society. Underlying his well-documented description of methods of care, developments of mental hospitals, and periods of progress and retrogression was his deep and sincere empathic understanding of the experience of the poor. As mentioned earlier, Deutsch's personal low-income background seems to have sensitized him to this dimension of psychiatry's past; indeed, he maintained a direct interest in the underprivileged throughout his life. Perhaps reflecting his own professional status, Deutsch also expressed in his historical writings a particular admiration for, and perhaps unconscious identification with, the contributions of laymen—most notably Dorothea Dix and Clifford Beers—who devoted their lives to alleviating the lot of the mentally ill. In fact, of the major heroic figures in his study, only two—Rush and Meyer—hailed from professional medical backgrounds. (This, we will see shortly, contrasted sharply with the orientation of other contemporaneous historians.) Retrospectively, a perusal of his work in its totality suggests that Albert Deutsch was primarily a social historian, a journalist-reformer, and, in a certain sense, a maverick.[14]

Gregory Zilboorg (1891–1959)

Gregory Zilboorg is one of the most interesting and charismatic figures in the history of twentieth-century American psychiatry. Zilboorg (whom I had the personal pleasure of knowing quite well) was born in 1891 in Kiev, Ukraine. He graduated from the medical school of the University of St. Petersburg in 1916 and then attended the Psychoneurological Institute in that city where he studied under Vladimir Bekhterev. Bekhterev is generally known today as the founder of the school of "psychoreflexology," according to which, human behavior, including the highest mental activities, is purely the result of "associative reflexes." This fact is interesting in light of Zilboorg's later strong psychodynamic allegiance and his intense opposition, in both his clinical and historical writings, to materialist psychologies. Moreover, Bekhterev had trained with some of the greatest medical scientists of the nineteenth century, so that, through him, Zilboorg was exposed to the teachings of Flechsig, Du Bois-Reymond, Meynert, Westphal, Charcot, and Wundt. In this way, the young Zilboorg became educated in the main psychiatric, psychological, and neurological schools of thought from Western and Central Europe as well as from Russia of the late nineteenth and early twentieth centuries.

During the early stages of the Russian Revolution in 1917, Zilboorg experienced a short period of personal involvement in politics. In fact, he served for several weeks as Secretary to the Minister of Labor in the Provisional Government of Kerensky. However, following the Bolshevik coup of 1917, he was forced to flee Russia surreptitiously, which he accomplished by walking out of the country to Finland. In 1919, he came to the United States. In America, Zilboorg supported himself at first by lecturing, writing, and translating from the Russian works for the theater, and contributing to the journal *Drama*. Among his translations is a rendition of the early anti-utopian political novel, *We* by E. I. Zamiatin, which is still read widely today.

Zilboorg learned upon his arrival in the United States that his Russian medical degree was not recognized in this country. Therefore he took additional training at the medical school of Columbia University and obtained a second medical degree from that institution in 1926. For the next five years, Zilboorg served on the staff of the Bloomingdale Hospital (now the Westchester Division of New York Hospital) in White Plains, New York. During that period, he also passed a year in Germany (1929–1930) at the Berlin Psychoanalytic Institute.

By 1930, he made the decision to devote himself professionally to psychoanalysis. From 1931 onward, he engaged in private psychoanalytic practice in New York City. In time, he became one of the most sought-after analysts in New York, who counted among his analysands numerous celebrated social and cultural personalities. In the early thirties, he translated from the German two important psychoanalytic texts, *The Criminal, the Judge and the Public* by Franz Alexander and H. Staub and the *Outline of Psychoanalysis* by Otto Fenichel. Among Zilboorg's original contributions to clinical matters are several papers on postpartum psychosis, on suicide, and on what he called "ambulatory schizophrenia," approximately corresponding to present-day "borderline personality."

It is unfortunate that Zilboorg did not write an autobiography. It remains uncertain how he first developed an interest in psychiatric history. Clearly, however, such an interest goes back at least to the early 1930s. In 1935, Zilboorg's first historical book, *The Medical Man and the Witch During the Renaissance*, appeared. This work consists of the Noguchi Lectures delivered at the Institute of the History of Medicine of Johns Hopkins University, then headed by Henry Sigerist.[15] In 1941, his major historical work, *A History of Medical Psychology*, was published.[16] In 1944, on the occasion of the one hundredth anniversary of the American Psychiatric Association, he coedited the important volume, *One Hundred Years of American Psychiatry, 1844–1944* (the same volume to which Deutsch contributed), for which he wrote the lengthy historical chapter "Legal Aspects of Psychiatry."[17] Zilboorg again expressed his longstanding interest in legal psychiatry in 1954 with *The Psychology of the Criminal Act and Punishment*, a series of lectures delivered at Yale University.[18]

By the early 1950s, Zilboorg had become strongly involved in religious matters as related to psychiatry. Born to Orthodox Jewish parents, he became progressively attracted to Christianity, resulting in his official joining of the Roman Catholic Church in 1954. His two books from this period—*Mind, Medicine and Man* (1943), a collection of essays on aspects of psychoanalysis, and *Sigmund Freud: His Exploration of the Mind and Man* (1951), a short, encomiastic monograph[19]—reflect his increasing involvement in philosophical and religious matters in relation to psychoanalysis. These later publications in the main fall outside the arena of the history of psychiatry.

Within the field of psychoanalysis, Zilboorg took active part in the American psychoanalytic movement, as charter member since 1931 of the New York Psychoanalytic Institute and cofounder in 1932 of the *Psychoanalytic Quarterly*. A training analyst for many years, he held academic positions in various medical schools, mainly at the College of Medicine of the State University of New York and at the New York Medical

College. He also became a much sought-after speaker, able to attract large audiences on many occasions, most notably as Gimbel Lecturer at the University of California in 1947 and as the first academic lecturer at the annual convention of the American Psychiatric Association in 1952.

A forceful and multitalented personality, a linguist, a scholar, and an indefatigable traveler at home in North America as well as in several European countries, Zilboorg was also an expert photographer, an outstanding bibliophile, and an excellent cook. Perhaps as a reaction against the collectivism of the Communist regime, he became a champion of individualism, for which he found identification in some of the outstanding Renaissance medical personalities, notably Vives, Weyer, and Paracelsus. A man both greatly admired and resented by contemporaries because of his tremendous ability to love (as evidenced by the warmth he conveyed to his family and friends) as well as for his uncompromising attitude in some circumstances, he appeared to many of his contemporaries, as Franz Alexander once put it, "a master of the written and spoken word" and "great actor," able to exercise a magnetic influence on his audience. In any case, Zilboorg "was anything but a representative of the stereotype of the psychoanalyst. . . . [He was] individualistic, nonconformist, philosophically inclined, [and] deeply rooted in nineteenth-century culture."[20] At a deeper level, according to Francis Braceland, Zilboorg elicited "admiration, usually unexpressed; antipathy, usually openly expressed; envy, disguised; and occasionally loyalty and affection."[21] Finally, characteristic of Zilboorg was his personal lifelong journey from outward public interests (politics and drama), to psychological and social themes (psychoanalysis, criminology, and psychiatric history), to private moral and religious issues. He died in New York City in 1959 at age 68.

As with Deutsch, Zilboorg's significance for psychiatric historiography centers around a single scholarly text, *A History of Medical Psychology* (1941). It is interesting that Zilboorg opted in his title for the term *medical psychology*, rather than the more common *psychiatry*, a term that he believed was older and more comprehensive. In the foreword to the book, he observes that he has used two main bodies of sources. He has read widely in printed medical texts in the history of psychiatry in several languages. And (unlike Hurd, Jelliffe, and Deutsch) he has utilized the existing works of European psychiatric historiography. In particular, he is familiar with the major nineteenth-century writings of Friedreich, Lélut, Trélat, and D. H. Tuke. He draws heavily throughout the book on the extensive biographical volumes about French psychiatrists by René Semelaigne and about German psychiatrists by Theodore Kirchhoff. Furthermore, he makes use of the only full-scale narrative history of psychiatry then available in any language, *Istoriya psikhiatrii* [*History of Psychiatry*] by the Russian Yuriy V. Kannabikh, which was available to Zilboorg because of his Russian background.[22]

The History of Medical Psychology deals almost entirely with European matters. As for the history of psychiatry in the United States, Zilboorg stated that "a special history of American psychiatry should be written," followed later by the statement that "the story of American psychiatry still awaits its historian."[23] This statement in 1941 is hard to understand, as Deutsch's *The Mentally Ill in America* had appeared only four years earlier; and Zilboorg was undoubtedly aware of its existence, as he refers to it twice, but only as marginal notes.[24] As mentioned previously, perhaps the best way to understand Zilboorg's disregard for Deutsch's book is that Deutsch was not a physician, and therefore, in Zilboorg's eyes, not the appropciate person to write authoritatively about *medical* psychology. Indeed, Zilboorg's lack of interest, even contempt, for the nonmedical contributions to the history of psychiatry is strikingly in contrast with Deutsch's view.

Following a prologue, the second and third chapters of Zilboorg's book concern primitive and oriental medicine, and ancient Greek and Roman culture and psychology. His discussion of shamanism consists of a succinct and rather traditional synthesis of ideas from the anthropological, historical, and philosophical presentations of the time. As for the Greeks, Zilboorg emphasizes exclusively their rationalistic approach to life, culture, and madness, with disregard of the opposite aspect, the Dionysiac (brought forward originally by Nietzsche). Consequently, hardly any mention is made of the therapeutic approach used in the Asclepian temples or of the cathartic effect of the tragedy. Zilboorg's discussions of mental illness by classical medical authors (Asclepiades, Celsus, Aretaeus, Soranus, Caelius Aurelianus) are detailed and comprehensive. In line with traditional thinking at the time, he views Galen's role in regard to mental illness as rather minimal. Also notable from the early chapters of the book onward is Zilboorg's willingness unproblematically to label as mentally ill individuals in the past endowed with unusual psychological traits—from the Hebrew prophets, to the Phytian and Delphic oracles, to Socrates' demon. Indeed, the retrospective diagnosis of past behaviors from premedical times occurs often in the book.

Chapters four and five of Zilboorg's study deal with the Middle Ages and the Renaissance. The very titles of the chapters—''The Great Decline'' and ''The Restless Surrender to Demonology''—reveal the author's interpretive approach. In these chapters, Zilboorg adheres to the nineteenth-century positivistic view of the Middle Ages as a period of great, unbroken obscurantism and superstition.[25] As expected, he treats St. Augustine's work prominently, although he makes no mention of the influence of Augustine's personal struggle to master his own sexuality on his theological views. The presentation of the most important medieval authors and beliefs constitutes a good part of these chapters, which terminate with the initial outbreak of witch-hunting. Zilboorg contends in this section, without documentation, that there occurred during this period an immense, almost epidemical, increase in the number of mentally ill persons across Europe, many of whom were persecuted as cases of witchcraft.[26]

The sixth and seventh chapters of *The History of Medical Psychology* are by far the strongest in the book and, in my view, Zilboorg's most original contribution to psychiatric history generally. Zilboorg here brings to prominence a trio of medical humanists—Johann Weyer, Luis Vives, and Cornelius Agrippa—whose work in the field of psychiatry was previously unknown or undervalued but who represent in Zilboorg's estimation figures of the first rank. The great achievement of these men rested in their rational opposition to the witch-hunting mania of the time and their advancement of a naturalistic, rather than demonological, model of madness. Zilboorg lays particular stress on Weyer's compendious study *De Praestigiis Daemonum* of 1563, which he reviews in detail.

As might be expected, Zilboorg's emphasis is on the emergence of a psychiatric conceptualization of the witch-mania in sixteenth- and seventeenth-century Europe. He centers his discussion on the state of mind of the women accused of witchcraft and on the sadistic attitude of the men representing the law, both ecclesiastic and secular. A number of points in Zilboorg's handling of the subject have subsequently been singled out by historians and sociologists as controversial: the assertion that most of the alleged witches were mentally ill; the statement that, on the basis of the behavior presented by these women, Sprenger and Kraemer's *Malleus Maleficarum* "at times may well be considered a handbook of sexual psychopathies"; and the assertion that the *Malleus Maleficarum* "described literally every type of neurosis or psychosis which we find today in our daily psychiatric work."[27] These are strong statements, perhaps understandable in the 1930s, when the historiography on demonology was just beginning and little attention was paid to local social and cultural aspects of Renaissance witchcraft. The evident presentist shortcomings of these chapters, however, should not in my opinion distract us from recognizing the importance of Zilboorg's virtual rediscovery of Weyer's masterpiece. Indeed, the presentation of Weyer and his book was the culmination of Zilboorg's study of Weyer, which traces back to his *The Medical Man and the Witch During the Renaissance*. Throughout his narrative, Zilboorg shows a considerable preoccupation with points of origins and founding figures in the prehistory of psychiatry. Of Weyer, he comments that he "stands out as the true founder of modern psychiatry and a true revolutionary genius in the science of man";[28] hence, the title of the chapter, "The First Psychiatric Revolution."

In this same long and important chapter, Zilboorg also includes a delightful, fifteen-page presentation of the work of the Spanish-born Luis Vives (1492–1540), who spent most of his life in Bruges, Flanders. Although well known among scholars of the Renaissance for his progressive views on education and his program of relief for the poor, the handicapped, and the mentally ill, Vives's work on psychology had been overlooked. Zilboorg offers a careful assessment of Vives's views on human emotional life in his last book, *De anima et vita* (*On Soul and Life*, 1538), pointing to his precursory role in modern dynamic psychology, especially in regard to the importance of free associations and the concept of the unconscious. Similar discussions of Paracelsus and Agrippa follow. In particular, he reviews the conglomeration of philosophical, mystical, and medical concepts in Paracelsus's difficult tract, *The Diseases That Deprive Man of Reason* (1567), a text that Zilboorg had translated from German into English.[29]

"The Age of Reconstruction," the eighth chapter of Zilboorg's book, extends to nearly 100 pages. It covers a great variety of figures and surveys a succession of concepts, events, and classificatory systems of mental illness from the seventeenth and eighteenth centuries. In contrast to the originality of his discussion of the Renaissance, this chapter essentially synthesizes secondary sources. Although during that period the new methodologies of experimental sciences had an impact on the entire field of medicine, especially in regard to anatomy and physiology, Zilboorg shows that psychopathology continued to be influenced by old-fashioned, unproved beliefs. Even more important, the practical approach to treatment of the mentally ill continued to be characterized by neglect and cruelty, resulting in an increased gap between such an attitude and the progressive advancement in the understanding of man and society leading to the European Enlightenment.

In view of the complexity of this period, Zilboorg's analysis is, on the whole, adequate and well informed. He does an excellent job of reviewing the most significant new clinical descriptions of psychopathological symptoms and syndromes from that period. He also notes the emerging interest in psychology during these centuries by a number of philosophers, such as Hobbes, Malebranche, Locke, Condillac, Spinoza, and, later, Kant. However, the actual importance of this development to mental illness he considers negligible, and he emphasizes the wide disparity in views of psychopathology between philosophers and physicians during the early modern period. He states next that two attempts to deal with the mind in a more systematic way also emerged during the eighteenth century: on the psychological side, Stahl's theory of vitalism and, on the organic side, Gall's system of phrenology, both of which boasted considerable followings. Characteristically, Zilboorg praised highly Stahl's views as anticipating modern psychodynamic concepts while barely mentioning Gall's contributions to neurology and to the influence of phrenology on the later notions of cerebral localizations. These historical assessments assuredly reflect Zilboorg's own psychiatric theoretical allegiances. Interesting in retrospect is the fact that the new system of care (or, rather, confinement) of the mentally ill in the French "Hôpital Général" beginning in the midseventeenth century is overlooked entirely.

Considerable space is also devoted in this chapter to Pinel's reform of the treatment of the mentally ill. In contrast to Deutsch, Zilboorg says comparatively little about Pinel's famous physical liberation of the insane. Rather, he stresses Pinel's medical credentials and argues that it was Pinel's achievement to open up an appropriately medical path to the understanding of the mentally ill. To convey the importance of Pinel's work, Zilboorg usefully includes a translation of Pinel's full introduction to the *Traité médico-philosophique*, which was thus far unavailable in English. Yet, in spite of this, he does not interpret Pinel's innovation as constituting one of the great "revolutions" in psychiatric history—as did Weyer before him and Freud after. Zilboorg grants hardly any space to the early history of the moral treatment brought forward at the same time as Pinel at the York Retreat under the guidance of William Tuke and his descendants.[30] Again, this is most likely because the Tukes were laymen rather than physicians. In general, Zilboorg's coverage of British contributions to the history of psychiatry, with the exception of Conolly's work and the "no-restraint" controversy, is very scanty throughout.

In the ninth chapter, "The Discovery of Neuroses," Zilboorg offers a detailed and accurate exposition of the work of Franz Anton Mesmer and his followers. He discusses the work on hypnotism and the unconscious of a string of figures working loosely within the Mesmeric tradition, including Puységur, Elliotson, Braid (who coined the word "hypnotism"), Charcot and his pupils, Liébeault, Bernheim, and Janet. In his discussion of Pierre Janet (who was still alive in 1941), Zilboorg includes the one statement in the book critical of Freud, where he observes that Janet was not treated fairly by Freud in Freud's autobiography.[31]

In "The Era of Systems," another 100-page chapter, Zilboorg presents an abundance of information about psychiatry in the nineteenth century. He reviews a series of newly identified clinical syndromes, from Bayle's general paralysis onward. He examines the emergence of national trends and "schools" of psychiatry in France, England, and Germany. And he relates the appearance of the first psychiatric societies and journals. He even includes some remarks on the beginnings of psychiatric historiography. A large section of this chapter is devoted to the great nineteenth-century controversy within German psychiatry between the "somatologists" and the "psychologists." "The somatologists won the battle, and in the middle of the century German psychiatry asserted the supremacy of the brain over any other structure and proceeded systematically to produce a psychiatry without a psychology."[32] It is clear to which school Zilboorg gives his preference. He devotes space to a discussion of Griesinger's textbook, although he fails to recognize its historical or theoretical importance, wondering why the work went through so many editions. He discusses the ideas of Heinroth, Haindorf, Groos, Ideler, and Feuchtersleben, for example, in considerably greater detail than was typical at the time. He concludes with a concise account of Emil Kraepelin's work, whose many good points he acknowledges, but with the conclusion that "the system of Kraepelin appears to have become a thing of the past as it announced its own birth in 1896."[33] This again seems a statement influenced by a psychoanalytic disregard for psychiatric symptoms and classifications.

The final chapter of Zilboorg's history, "The Second Psychiatric Revolution," is surprisingly short in light of all that precedes it. In thirty pages, it covers the entire span of the modern psychodynamic schools. The chapter opens with a discussion of the intellectual and artistic trends that preannounced the importance of the Freudian unconscious. This is followed by a quick review of Freud's most notable theoretical accomplishments. Zilboorg then rather grandly advances an interpretation of Freud that subsumes him under the long and noble tradition of Western humanism. The point particularly stressed is that Freud, by digging fearlessly into the unconscious and by openly acknowledging the importance of sexuality, did not hesitate to accept what is intrinsic to the humanity of man. In Zilboorg's reading, Freud is "the last representative of the Renaissance and the humanism which wanted man free" and "the first humanist in clinical psychology."[34] In conspicuous contrast, he grants Carl Jung and Alfred Adler only two paragraphs of coverage. Moreover, he severely criticizes contemporaneous, nondynamic medical psychologies, such as the experimental and laboratory study of personality, leading to the dehumanizing (and therefore anti-humanistic) excesses of behavioralism and reflexology. This latter theory, which remained associated in Zilboorg's mind with his old teacher Bekhterev and with Pavlov, represented a theoretical parallel, he believed, to the degrading and all-leveling philosophy of communism that was then officially entrenched in Soviet Russia. Zilboorg expresses the antithesis between the two trends in the strongest terms. The chapter concludes with a brief consideration of a number of early twentieth-century American Freudians, such as Jelliffe and Brill. Whereas Deutsch envisions the mental hygiene movement as the culminant event in the history of psychiatry, to Zilboorg this event is represented by Freudian psychoanalysis and its successful transplantation in the United States.

Zilboorg's book ends with a spirited and idealized epilogue. Here, Zilboorg gives an English translation from the French of a long letter addressed to him by René Semelaigne in which, inevitably, Pinel's reform of the treatment of the mentally ill is eulogized. Philanthropism and humanitarianism have opened the path to a better understanding of the mentally ill; but only "the Freudian revolution . . . was the first practical step in the history of medical psychology toward the foundation of a psychiatry which would be a medical discipline."[35] This section includes a final paean to the triad of Weyer, Pinel, and Freud, the major Zilboorgian heroes, who have in common a courageous, rationalizing approach to the understanding of mental disease in the face of societal ignorance and opposition. This leads to the parting paragraph of the book. It reads:

> The whole course of the history of medical psychology is punctuated by the medical man's struggle to rise above the prejudices of all ages in order to identify himself with the psychological realities of his patients. Every time such an identification was achieved the medical man became a psychiatrist. The history of psychiatry is essentially the history of humanism. Every time humanism has diminished or degenerated into mere philanthropic sentimentality, psychiatry has entered a new ebb.

Every time the spirit of humanism has arisen, a new contribution to psychiatry has been made.[36]

Just over half a century after its appearance, Gregory Zilboorg's *A History of Medical Psychology* is, by consensus, outdated. Its concentration on single personalities has been replaced by a new concern with social, political, economic, and cultural determinants, while the analytical focus has switched from heroic individuals to the common person. However, historiographically, Zilboorg's book has been immensely important. Along with Erwin Ackerknecht's *A Short History of Psychiatry* (1959), *A History of Medical Psychology* has probably been read more widely over the past five decades than any other general history of the subject in any language. In its chronological sweep and lively, attractive style of writing, the book remains highly readable. In retrospect, the salient interpretive features of Zilboorg's reading of psychiatric history are (1) an emphasis on the progressive medicalization of the care of the insane; (2) a marked preference for professional medical approaches to madness (rather than those of religion, philosophy, academic psychology, or lay reform); (3) a preoccupation with bringing out the many scattered anticipations of Freud's ideas in earlier centuries; and (4) the assimilation of the history of psychiatry to the great Western tradition of humanism, spanning from the ancient Greeks, to the geniuses of the Renaissance, to Sigmund Freud. In biographical context, these interpretations take on added meaning. Zilboorg wrote as a psychoanalytic physician, trained in the broad intellectual and cultural traditions of Central Europe, who emigrated to the United States during the beginning of the golden age of psychoanalysis in this country. In more ways than one, he wrote a history of psychiatry for a generation of readers who shared this distinctive background.

Walther Riese (1890–1976)

German-born and educated, Walther Riese, who passed the first half of his career in Germany and France and the later half in the United States, is one of the most undervalued historians of psychiatry in this century. Riese wrote alternately in German, French, and English. And his elegant, erudite, and highly intelligent books and essays range over a great many subjects. Riese is one of the very few commentators on psychiatric history who was also a first-rate practicing medical scientist. He is also one of the few who wrote about the history of dynamic psychiatry as a professional neuroscientist.

Riese had such a long and multifarious career, spanning six productive decades, that only certain highlights can be mentioned here. Born in Germany in 1890, Riese received his medical degree from the University of Königsberg, Germany, in 1914. After training in neurology, he did private practice and research in this field in Frankfurt from 1917 to 1933 at the well-known Hospital for Brain Injured Soldiers, where he was greatly influenced by Kurt Goldstein's "Gestalt" approach and Constantin von Monakow's empirical novel approach to neurology. From 1933 to 1936, Riese, a Rockefeller Fellow, conducted research at the Neuropsychiatric Clinic of the Medical School of Lyon, France. From 1937 to 1940, he headed the research program at the National Center of Scientific Research, Department of Physiology, Sorbonne, and at the National Museum of National History in Paris. In 1941, again as a Rockefeller

Fellow, Riese for political reasons moved to the United States and for the remainder of his life held various positions at the Medical College of Virginia in Richmond, first as research associate at the Neuropsychiatric Clinic, and then as associate professor of neurology, psychiatry, and the history of medicine. In his later years, he was appointed emeritus professor at Johann Wolfgang Goethe University in Frankfurt, Germany. Riese died in 1976, at the age of 86. His wife of many years, Hertha Riese, a child psychiatrist, died shortly thereafter.

In total, Riese was the author of no fewer than 277 articles and 15 books. His writings encompass neurology, neuroanatomy, comparative neurology, neuropathology, medical psychology (including forensic psychology, pathology, and psychiatry), the history of medicine, and the philosophy of medicine.[37] It is little wonder that no one thus far has taken up the challenge of writing a biography of him. Riese did not produce a single, comprehensive study of psychiatric history, along the lines of Deutsch, Zilboorg, or Ellenberger. However, upon close reading, his wide-ranging essays and monographs reveal a clear thematic and stylistic unity. I will limit this discussion to a consideration of four themes, or areas of interest, that appear recurrently in his work. These subjects are psychiatry and antiquity; Enlightenment psychological theory, with an emphasis on the seventeenth-century theory of the passions; the work of Pinel; and the historical origins of psychoanalysis. In addition, I will briefly consider a single, important excursion of Riese's into the field of psychobiography.

Raised with a classical German education, Riese had a fine working knowledge of the major ancient Greek and Roman medical writers. Although he tended to trace many modern concepts of mental illness to Hippocratic sources, it is in regard to Galen that his work in psychiatry was most original. In spite of his immense output, Galen was generally considered as having shown little interest in mental disorders. (Zilboorg's cursory handling of his work was typical.) However, in 1963, Riese published an English translation, along with an extensive, interpretive introduction, of two little-known treatises by Galen combined in one volume under the title *On the Passions and Errors of the Soul*.[38]

Although his life coincided with the emerging Judeo-Christian movement, Galen, we learn in Riese's introduction, remained refractory to the new moral and psychological messages intrinsic to Christianity. Influenced by Platonic, Aristotelian, Stoic, and Epicurean doctrines, the Galenic understanding of the human passions, rooted in the biological constitution of man (the Hippocratic *crasis*), remained essentially rationalistic and pedagogic. Galen's text is replete with concrete examples of achieving the mastery of the two instinctual drives, i.e., the irascible and the concupiscible. Yet, regardless of his rationalistic orientation, Riese emphasizes, Galen throughout his lifetime was attracted by the mysterious beliefs and techniques affecting the emotional life of the individual and the therapeutic implications of these beliefs. This is perhaps, Riese speculates, because Galen was born in Pergamon, Asia Minor, the seat of a famous asclepeion (i.e., a temple devoted to Asclepius and geared to the treatment of many illnesses). Riese highlights many passages of Galen's text that remain pertinent to contemporary psychotherapy. What interests Riese were the many psychological insights and formulations implicit in Galenic moral theory. In a previous publication, *La pensée morale en médecine*, he had stressed that "what is generally lacking in the ethics of the ancients is the element of 'conflict' and 'strength.' "[39] True, the Galenic view of the passions as diseases of the soul can be traced back to the Stoic school. But, rather than being conceived from a static perspective, the passions should be actively perceived as useful in a curative capacity. This, Riese points out, is what Descartes argued centuries later in his famous treatise *Passions of the Soul*, especially as concerns the positive aspect of "delay" in dealing with violent passions.

A second theme investigated very perceptively by Riese concerns the period of Enlightenment rationalism in the history of psychiatry. Riese's major contribution in this area is the small but remarkable volume, published in 1965, entitled *La théorie des passions à la lumière de la pensée médicale du XVIIe siècle*.[40] Despite its importance for seventeenth- and eighteenth-century theorizing about human nature, the subject of Riese's book had been largely passed over in historical, including medical-historical, scholarship. Riese was intrigued by the changing valuations of the passions through different times and cultures. In line with the Stoic submission of passions to reason and the Christian devaluation of passions as leading to sin, hardly anyone perceived the positive value of passions from the Middle Ages, to the Counter-Reformation, to the succeeding rationalistic philosophy. Yet, the passions, crucial to the understanding of mental illness, became paramount in Western culture during the Romantic period of the late eighteenth and early nineteenth centuries, the same period that witnessed the birth of modern psychiatry.

In his historical study of the passions, Riese reconstructs a sequence of seventeenth century texts—some well known but most quite obscure—which theorized at length about the origins, nature, meaning, and manipulation of the human emotions. In the first chapter, Riese stresses the inability of Descartes to conceptualize the passions as a means of overcoming the dichotomy between body and mind (through his famous localization of the soul in the pineal gland). At the same time, Riese underscores the implications of Descartes' "instrumental use of passions" in his *Passions de l'âme* (1649) and in his well-known letters to Princess Elizabeth of Bohemia. The same problematic relation between reason and passions, Riese notes next, is evident in the writings of the physician Louis de la Forge, who, following Malebranche, assumed a divine intervention between body and mind. Riese then shows that Cureau de la Chambre, a court physician of Louis XIV and the author of *L'art de connaître les hommes* (1660), offered a symptomatological description of the passions, a discussion of their nature and classification, an analysis of the altered anatomical and physiological mechanisms they could elicit, and speculations on their causes. Underlying these topics is Cureau de la Chambre's position vis-a-vis Descartes' dualism and Stahl's animism, leading to a typically Baroque emphasis on movement and the transition from the basic etymology of passions from "passive" to "active."

Following this, Riese analyzes Spinoza's monism, which he discusses in detail as anticipating modern dynamic psychology. The passions were seen by Spinoza not as movement but rather as "thought" on the basis of the psycho-physical parallelism that, according to Riese, characterizes much nineteenth-century biological and neurological thinking from Claude Bernard to Hughlings Jackson. Riese's slender volume terminates with a discussion of the often republished book *De l'usage des passions* (1641) by the French priest François Senault in which the manipulation of the passions is openly advocated in the context of Christian principles. Riese notes in conclusion that all of these writers tended to consider the passions from the objective, external perspective, independent of the subjective, inner perception of the individual. In essence, Riese's book brings forward the full range of medical and philosophical interpretations of the passions during the "Age of Reason," from their complete submission to the imperatives of reason to their systematic spiritual and psychological use. The book is both a study of the intellectual prehistory of modern psychiatry and a chapter in Enlightenment intellectual history. In my opinion, it is one of the best and subtlest of Riese's works pertinent to psychiatry, not least of all because it displays the author's fine psychological insights and his underlying artistic disposition. The volume requires more than one reading to capture the nuances of the texts under review and the analyses of them. Undoubtedly, Riese preferred to write it in French to be close, in the spirit as well as in the letter, to the thoughts of the authors he considers.

Riese also maintained a longstanding interest in the work of Pinel as evidenced by various papers as well as a monograph published in 1969. Riese's interest in Pinel was somewhat revisionist in nature. What stands out clearly is the contrast between his sober and deep analysis of Pinel's complete medical work as opposed to the hagiographic account of Pinel's dramatic presentation of his reform of the treatment of the mentally ill standardly found in other accounts up to this time. Hence, the disappointment of some readers when unexpectedly encountering a scholarly and technical inquiry into the essence of Pinel's thought as mentioned in the subtitle of the book, *The Legacy of Philippe Pinel. An Inquiry into Thought on Mental Alienation.*[41]

In "The Importance of Pinel," the introduction to the book, Riese argues for a view of Pinel primarily as a "medical philosopher" in the late eighteenth-century sense of the term, as someone who, according to the definition of the *Dictionnaire de l'Académie Française* in 1762, is "a person who devotes himself to the study of science and who tries to derive effects from their causes and their principles."[42] Riese emphasizes Pinel's theory of the passions as both pathogenic and therapeutic. He attempts to place Pinel in the moral and intellectual setting of his time. And he lays considerable emphasis on the importance of Hippocratic medicine for understanding Pinel's teachings, particularly for the Frenchman's observation of the course of a disease over time in the individual patient. Similarly, he analyzes Pinel's continual attempts to achieve a rational classification of mental symptoms; in the process, he discusses in depth Pinel's *Nosographie philosophique ou méthode de l'analyse appliquée à la médecine* (1798), which is much less known to psychiatrists today than his treatise on insanity.

In commentary upon his English translation of the introduction to the first edition of Pinel's *Traité médico-philosophique sur l'aliénation mentale ou la manie* (1801), Riese underscores Pinel's reliance on both ancient medical writers and modern French moralists (Montaigne, La Rochefoucault, Rousseau), the influence of eighteenth-century British reformers (Crichton and Haslam), and the crucial importance of the lay hospital superintendent Pussin in the formation of Pinel's ideas.[43] Elsewhere, Riese explores the meanings of the term *moral treatment* in Pinel's time, and he observes that Pinel continued to advocate the exercise of both authority and leniency in dealing with patients. He accentuates Pinel's efforts to achieve an individualized understanding of each patient's case as one of his most significant innovations.[44] As Riese puts it in his monograph: "No matter whether he approached the subject as a natural historian, a clinician, a diagnostician, a therapist, or a superintendent, he always approached the mentally ill disturbed individual in his own terms."[45] In stressing these matters, Riese certainly did not intend to minimize Pinel's pioneering humanitarian efforts but simply to play down the widespread overdramatization of the gesture of freeing the mentally ill from their chains. In its insistent emphasis on the conceptual, rather than humanitarian, aspects of

Pinel's medical thought, Riese's book, which has largely been ignored in psychiatric historiography, should receive careful attention; it anticipates several key points advanced recently by the best French and American scholars in their reassessment of Pinel's work.[46]

Finally, there is Riese's work on the historical foundations of psychoanalysis. Material pertinent to this subject is scattered throughout many of his scholarly writings. It is likely that Riese contemplated a comprehensive study of this subject, which unfortunately he was never able to accomplish. However, as a preview of what might have been, in 1957 he delivered a major address on "The Pre-Freudian Origins of Psychoanalysis" at the founding meeting of the Academy of Psychoanalysis in Chicago. The speech was later enlarged into a substantial essay that attempts a synoptic overview of the intellectual antecedents of psychoanalytic theory.[47] In this context, Riese explores the intricate historical backgrounds to the Freudian categories of catharsis, the unconscious, repression, the psychogenesis of symptoms, the interpretation of dreams, the instincts, regression, and the neurosis concept. This is unquestionably a masterful presentation, indicating, aside from the author's philosophical and medico-historical background, a thorough knowledge of Freud's writings. Riese's long essay represents one of the very few attempts in the 1950s, at a time when Ernest Jones's three-volume biography was widely regarded as the definitive view of Freud's intellectual biography, to reconstruct what is today known as "the historical Freud."[48]

As an addendum, I would also like to cite Riese's interest in psychobiography. This manifested itself most notably in his fascination with the case of the painter Van Gogh. In *Vincent van Gogh in der Krankheit* (1926), as well as in other later publications, Riese speculates that Van Gogh suffered from "episodic twilight states." However, the search for diagnostic clarification in this case, he believed, was secondary "to the problem of the relationship of the disease to the artistic productivity and certainly to the ultimate maturation of his style."[49] The essence of Van Gogh's psychodynamics, Riese suggests, consisted in the conflict between his striving for the essential and absolute and his need for the love of others, a conflict that can be traced to a struggle to achieve his unique style before and after the outbreak of psychosis.

In my view, what stands out most strongly in Walter Riese's history writing about psychiatry is the contrast between the high quality of his thinking and writing and the almost complete lack of professional recognition Riese has received, both in North America and in Europe. Most likely, Riese's multidisciplinary background, embracing neurology, medical history, philosophy, and psychiatry, made it possible for him to do work at a level achievable by only a few. Yet, his very polymorphous orientation, as well as the shifting circumstances of his career, presented assets and liabilities. Riese wrote in a rather dense, scholarly style, assuming a certain degree of knowledge and sophistication in his audience, with the result that many readers dismissed him as too elaborate and difficult to follow. In addition, despite the thirty-five years of his activity in the United States, Riese's *forma mentis* remained very formal and European. He continued to publish in French and occasionally in German. To my knowledge, he never became involved in any aspect of American culture. Furthermore, probably because of his comparatively senior age (he arrived in this country at the age of 51), Riese remained at the fringe of American academic life, and consequently his work became known only to a limited and specialized audience. Also, he never identified himself closely with any particular school of thought and therefore did not enjoy stable professional support. Finally, in contrast to Deutsch, Zilboorg, or Ellenberger (with whom he shared some of the same traits),[50] Riese failed to produce a single, synthetic work; rather, his writings remain scattered in many books and journals, both European and American, and are far from being easily accessible.

In essence, we should accept Riese as a unique example of a scientist, humanist, and scholar, equally comfortable in the ancient, the rationalistic, the Romantic, the positivistic, and the contemporary traditions. Although his work lacked the sort of external unity that at least superficially allows for the production of a *magnum opus*, it reveals upon careful reading an internal, thematic, and stylistic unity. To a large degree, Riese was a philosopher of medicine, always preferring broad concepts to detailed, empirical analyses. As such, it is not unnatural that his work has remained somewhat alien to the prevailing American pragmatic mentality. It is greatly to be hoped that this essay may contribute to a renewed attention to his writings.

Additional Developments

Bromberg, Alexander, Ackerknecht, Schneck

Albert Deutsch, Gregory Zilboorg, and Walther Riese have by no means been the only historians of psychiatry operating in North America up to the 1960s. A number of other scholars have also addressed the field, including writing general histories. In my view, however, these authors, while they may have produced titles that are relatively well known, appear in retrospect less original interpretively than Deutsch, Zilboorg, and Riese, and therefore are less significant for this volume. For this reason, as well as due to limitations of space, I would like to acknowledge these authors and texts but to review their work rather summarily.

Walter Bromberg (1900–) has had a long career as a practicing psychiatrist spanning a good part of our century. As he relates in his autobiographical account, *Psychiatry Between the Wars, 1918–1945*, Bromberg grew up in a Jewish environment in New York City, received a medical degree from the Long Island Medical College, and obtained postgraduate training in various centers of that metropolis.[51] He then devoted a great deal of his clinical work to legal psychiatric activities (on which he wrote extensively) in New York City and from 1946 onward mostly in California. In spite of exposure to psychoanalytic training in the late thirties, he maintained a rather eclectic attitude in his psychiatric thinking and practice.

Bromberg states that he was attracted specifically to the history of psychotherapy as a result of a request made to him by a publisher to write "a brief book on the differences between Freud, Jung, and Adler." The outcome of this proposal was *The Mind of Man*, which appeared in 1937. Since that date, he has continued to bring the same book up to date, first under the title *Man Above Humanity: A History of Psychotherapy* (1954) and later in a shorter version as *From Shaman to Psychotherapy: A History of the Treatment of Mental Illness* (1975).[52] Of the various versions of this book (which are essentially the same, although appearing under different names, thus leading to some misunderstanding), *Man Above Humanity* is the most extensive and well known, in part because it was issued in paperback edition. My comments will focus on this book.

A number of features of *Mind Above Humanity* may be noted. Generally speaking, Bromberg makes clear that he has been less interested in the history of psychiatry per se than in history as a long prologue to present-day psychiatry. Although he has not elaborated on his methodology, he relies almost entirely on secondary sources in English, mostly published in the United States. In the introductory chapter, Bromberg advances a kind of Comtian evolutionary perspective according to which the development of psychiatry divides into five stages: the polytheistic religion of the Greeks; the monotheism of the Judeo-Christian tradition; humanitarianism based on religion in the Middle Ages; humanitarianism based on individual consciousness in the Renaissance; and the confluence of humanitarianism and social changes from the Enlightenment onward.

Succeeding chapters relate the stories of important and dramatic events, such as Pinel's work at the Bicêtre hospital, in which historical developments are discussed only in terms of the individual physician.[53] As a result, Bromberg's account reads rather episodically, with individuals as isolated phenomena, operating outside of larger intellectual, political, religious, and economic contexts. These attributes of the book, it must be acknowledged, are typical of what today is known as the Whig historiography of psychiatry. Moreover, many important subjects are intermingled rather ahistorically. For instance, Bromberg deals with the beginning of hospital treatment of the mentally ill in Europe and in the United States on the same page, irrespective of the substantial differences between the two continents. He discusses the history of Bethlehem Hospital in London and the Williamsburg Hospital in Virginia in the same paragraph.[54] At times, the chronology of events is loose and the historical data are of questionable accuracy, as, for example, when he presents Paracelsus as part of medieval faith healing.[55] Bromberg's account of Renaissance witchcraft is rather eccentric and is based in part on the controversial works by the English priest Montague Summers, who in the twentieth century believed in the reality of witchcraft!

All of this, however, should not detract from appreciating the good qualities of Bromberg's book. In particular, and in contrast to the preceding work of Zilboorg and the succeeding text of Alexander and Selesnick, *Man Above Humanity* presents the history of psychiatry not stricly in the context of the psychoanalytic school, but of the overall eclectic view of contemporary psychiatry. While this may be taken for granted today, it was an innovative and somewhat daring approach in 1954, when psychiatry in the United States was heavily dominated by psychoanalysis.

Franz Alexander (1891–1964) requires little introduction as he is well known as one of the main exponents of the psychoanalytic movement in the United States. Born in Budapest, and after studying medicine at the University of Göttingen, Alexander became the first student to graduate from the Berlin Institute for Psychoanalysis, which was founded by Karl Abraham in 1910. Following this formative ten-year period at the Berlin Psychoanalytic Institute (1920–1930), which corresponded with the era of the Weimar Republic, Alexander (in spite of Freud's personal warnings) accepted the challenge to move to the United States. The success of Alexander's early books, dealing with psychoanalytic ego psychology and forensic psychiatry, contributed to his appointment in 1931 as professor of psychoanalysis at the University of Chicago, the first official academic recognition of this new field anywhere in the world. Soon thereafter, Alexander founded and then led for twenty-five years the Chicago Institute for Psychoanalysis. In 1956, he became the director of a new Psychiatric Research Department at the Mount Sinai Hospital in Los Angeles, where he attempted to investigate critically the psychotherapeutic relationship between patient and analyst. In the field of psychiatric medicine, Alexander is particularly recognized for original contributions to the dynamics and treatment of psychosomatic disorders, for the introduction of a new short-term method of psychotherapy, and for his organization of an excellent postgraduate training program at the Chicago Institute for Psychoanalysis. Among psychoanalysts-cum-historians-of-psychiatry, he is among the most accomplished.

The History of Psychiatry: An Evaluation of Psychiatric Thought and Practice from Prehistoric Times to the Present, written by Alexander with the assistance of his former student Sheldon Selesnick, appeared in 1966.[56] Alexander, who died in 1964, just as the manuscript was nearing completion, had been working on the book, we learn in the preface, since 1959. The history of Alexander and Selesnick in effect constitutes an introduction to the work of Freud, his followers, his dissenters, and of modern psychiatric psychodynamism generally. In a word, it gives us the history of psychiatry as a long and elaborate prehistory to psychoanalysis. The first third of the book deals with the full evolution of psychiatry from ancient times to the late nineteenth century. The second third, "The Freudian Age," tells the story of Freud's work and the history of the psychoanalytic movement. In this section, the work of Adler, Jung, and Rank are relegated to a chapter entitled "The Dissenters," while a brief but accusatory appendix discusses Jung's alleged complicity with the Nazis.[57] Pierre Janet's psychological system is granted all of two paragraphs.[58] The final third of the book canvasses the latest developments in Western psychiatry and as such is not historical.

Without entering into a detailed exposition, several main points stand out in the Alexander and Selesnick volume. There is hardly any evidence of originality of interpretation and the material presented is mainly taken from previously published books, in particular Zilboorg's *History of Medical Psychology*.[59] There is a pervasive pattern in the book to stress concepts and events considered as anticipations of twentieth-century psychodynamic tenets. Readers continually hear that psychoanalytic concepts have been hinted at or somehow prefigured in the past, thus providing additional confirmation of their validity. In short, the volume suffers from what is today termed a presentist bias of stressing events in the past that support present-day notions irrespective of their cultural and historical frames of reference. Viewed in historiographical context, this approach is probably understandable; the book was composed in the late fifties and early sixties, at a time when the various psychoanalytic schools had reached their highest degree of acceptance but on the eves of the first so-called anti-psychiatric historical writings and of the "new social history."

By and large Alexander and Selesnick's book offers an overview of psychiatric developments that still retains some use for clinicians today. However, in the light of current-day methodological critiques of presentism and contemporary critical reassessments of Freud's work and the psychoanalytic perspective, the underlying approach of the book—tracing back throughout history authors and concepts forerunning Freud's tenets—is outdated and objectionable. Nonetheless, the book by Alexander and Selesnick, like Zilboorg's, circulated widely during the fifteen years following its appearance and, in particular, was used extensively in teaching psychiatric history to American medical students. Their *History of Psychiatry* may be viewed as the last narrative, historiographical expression of the heroic age of American psychoanalysis.

Around 1960, two other longitudinal intellectual histories of psychiatry appeared in

America. Both works are under 200 pages in length. The methodology and orientation of these works are quite different. The first, *A Short History of Psychiatry*, is actually a translation from German of a monograph originally published in 1957 by the distinguished German medical historian Erwin Ackerknecht.[60] Ackerknecht was born and passed the second half of his career in Germany and Switzerland. However, I make brief mention of him here because from 1945 to 1957 he lived and worked in the United States, first in New York City and then as professor of the history of medicine at the University of Wisconsin in Madison, Wisconsin. Ackerknecht's history is very well informed and extremely compact. It emphasizes throughout the historical working out of the dialectic between somatic and psychological models of the mind. In notable contrast to the volumes by Zilboorg and Alexander, Ackerknecht's conspectus is comparatively uninterested in the story of Freud and the psychoanalytic movement and may even be faulted for devoting too little attention to the historical significance of this subject. It is unfortunate that the much-revised third edition of this book has never been translated into English.[61]

The second book from this period, *A History of Psychiatry*, was authored by Jerome Schneck (1920–), a psychiatrist practicing in New York City who has been particularly involved in treatment by hypnosis.[62] As stated in his preface, Schneck bases his historical study on the works of previous medical and psychiatric historians, mainly through books and papers published in English, mostly in American journals. By and large, the material presented is accurate and the chapters are well balanced. However, there are various factual omissions, idiosyncrasies of interpretation, and chronological confusions. Galen's notion of spirits, for instance, is overlooked. Inexplicably, Sprenger's and Kraemer's *Malleus Maleficarum* (published in 1486) is discussed in the chapter on the seventeenth century. And there is no discussion whatsoever of moral treatment. In spite of these facts and of a lack of originality, the book is a fairly solid survey of the history of psychiatry as seen by a clinician and may still serve as a useful and unpretentious overview of psychiatric developments.

In addition to Bromberg, Alexander, Ackerknecht, and Schneck, two American medical historians also contributed significantly to historical studies during the period under consideration. George Rosen (1910–1977), a physician and social scientist who taught public health at Columbia University and, later in his career, the history of medicine at Yale University, is remembered for his superb studies on social attitudes toward the mentally ill and the cultural dimensions of psychopathology.[63] Rosen's work as a psychiatric historian is analyzed in another essay in this collection.[64] Second, Ilza Veith, a pupil of the well-known Swiss-American medical historian Henry Sigerist (who founded and led for many years the Institute of the History of Medicine at Johns Hopkins University), taught at the University of Chicago and then at the University of California in San Francisco. Veith, who was the first individual to receive a Ph.D. in medical history in the United States, wrote numerous articles on psychiatric history, including Far Eastern psychiatry. She also produced a monograph on the history of hysteria, which for many years remained the best comprehensive study of that centuries-old puzzling syndrome.[65]

Naturally, aside from these scholars, many others contributed studies of historical significance about psychiatry during the first sixty years of the century. These works have taken the form of monographs on psychiatric pioneers and innovators,[66] chronicles of psychiatric institutions,[67] surveys of the history of psychotherapy and of organic therapies,[68] histories of the psychoanalytic movement and its various schools,[69] auto-biographical reports,[70] presentations of the mental illness of persons from the past,[71] narratives of movements presaging modern psychiatry,[72] discussions of psychiatric developments in other countries,[73] and studies on various other aspects of American psychiatry.[74] Most of these writings have been written by clinicians (mainly psychiatrists, occasionally psychologists, seldom by historians) and reflect the methodological limitations of their authors. In contrast to them, the works by medical historians are impressive for their level of scholarship and methodological sophistication. In addition, many other scholars—John Burnham, Eric Carlson, Norman Dain, Iago Galdston, Gerald Grob, Stanley Jackson, and Jacques Quen, to mention only a sampling—have made, and are making, important contributions to psychiatric historiography in the United States.[75]

Finally, it should be observed that the historiography of psychiatry made impressive professional and organizational gains in the United States during the 1950s and early 1960s. This is apparent by the republication of a large number of psychiatric classics;[76] by the beginning of a highly successful, pioneering effort to introduce the teaching of the history of psychiatry into select postgraduate medical programs, most notably at the New York Hospital-Cornell Medical Center in New York City;[77] by the launching, as an offspring of the latter center, of the *Journal of the History of the Behavioral Sciences* in 1965, which has printed a large amount of scholarship in the history of psychiatry; and by the establishment of a committee on historical matters at the American Psychiatric Association. Last, but certainly not least, mention should be made of the program in the history of medicine at the National Library of Medicine and the National Institutes of Health near Washington D. C., which for the past several decades—mainly through Jeanne Brand's dedication—has offered financial support for many projects, undertaken by both American and foreign scholars, concerning the history of psychiatry.[78] In assaying the state of psychiatric historiography in this country up until the 1960s, these developments too should be taken into consideration.

Conclusion

The Demedicalization of American Psychiatric Historiography

This assessment of some authors' contributions to the history of psychiatry brings us chronologically to the middle of the 1960s, a logical point of termination for this essay. Beginning in the mid-1960s, psychiatry began rapidly to undergo substantial practical, professional, and ideological changes connected with the almost simultaneous new emphases on community psychiatry on the one hand and on psychopharmacology on the other. Equally important for our purposes was the sudden rise of "anti-psychiatry," stemming in part from the overall movement of the sixties counterculture. These changes initiated a fundamentally new type of psychiatric history writing, one that, directly or indirectly, has often responded critically to the scholarly literature that preceded it. A number of these subsequent historiographical developments are dealt with in other chapters of this volume.

In conclusion, the historiography of psychiatry in the United States, in contrast with Europe, emerged quite late, only at the end of the 1930s and beginning of the 1940s.

Unlike German nineteenth-century historiography, the American historical literature between 1910 and 1960 does not fall into a single historiographical tradition or two. The most dominant perspective informing psychiatric historiography during this fifty-year period was the psychoanalytic; yet, as the writings of Deutsch, Riese, and Ackerknecht reveal, the influence of Freud on history writing was by no means exclusive. Indeed, reviewing it as a whole, we are struck by the considerable interpretive diversity and intellectual individuality of the work under review. The particular vision of psychiatry's past that these scholars developed often reflected directly their personal, cultural, professional, and theoretical identities. In contrast to the commonly held view that history writing during this period constitutes a desert of Whiggish writing, American psychiatric historiography before the 1960s is rich, interesting, informative, and multifarious.

With the exception of Albert Deutsch, all of the scholars considered in this essay were trained professionally either in medicine or the history of medicine. Within the medical field, however, their specialities varied considerably, from the establishment psychoanalysis of Alexander to the research neuroscience of Riese. It is also striking to observe that a majority of individuals writing psychiatric history in America during these years had Central European backgrounds. Several—Zilboorg, Riese, Alexander, Ackerknecht, and Veith—were in fact emigré intellectuals. Like the cultural and intellectual life of the country as a whole during the twentieth century, American psychiatric historiography owes much to the great migration of Central European intellectuals to the United States during the 1930s and 1940s.

Since the close of this period, there has occurred a surging interest in the history of psychiatry, particularly its institutional and psychodynamic aspects; however, this has taken place largely on the part of academic historians and social scientists, resulting in a large number of studies supported by a much improved methodology. The era of the amateur physician-historian, the self-taught humanitarian, and the scholarly humanist, as well as that of the all-encompassing narrative, historical survey, appears to be gone forever. Nonetheless, as I have attempted to show in these pages, the early generations of workers in this country, with their manifold strengths and limitations, continue today to serve as a valuable model of historical inquiry by a few exceptional individuals into the perennial mysteries of the human mind.

Notes

1. I wish to express my gratitude to Mark Micale for his editorial assistance in the preparation of this essay.

2. W. R. Dunton, "The American Journal of Psychiatry, 1844–1944" in C. B. Farrar (ed.), *American Journal of Psychiatry, 1844–1944*, Centennial Anniversary Issue (Philadelphia, 1944), 45–60.

3. For biographical information, consult T. S. Cullen, *Henry Mills Hurd* (Baltimore: The Johns Hopkins Press, 1920).

4. Henry Mills Hurd (ed.), *The Institutional Care of the Insane in the United States and Canada*, 4 vols. (Baltimore: The Johns Hopkins Press, 1916–1917; reprint, New York: Arno, 1973).

5. For biographical information on Jelliffe, consult John C. Burnham, *Jelliffe: American Psychoanalyst and Physician & His Correspondence with Sigmund Freud and C. G. Jung*, edited

by William McGuire (Chicago: University of Chicago Press, 1983); and N. D. C. Lewis, "Smith Ely Jelliffe, 1866–1945" in F. Alexander, S. Eisenstein, and M. Grotjahn (eds.), *Psychoanalytic Pioneers* (New York: Basic, 1966), 224–234.

6. S. E. Jelliffe, "Dementia Praecox: An Historical Summary," *New York Medical Journal*, xci (1910), 521–530; and idem, "Some Historical Phases of the Manic-Depressive Synthesis," *Journal of Nervous and Mental Disease*, lxxiii (1931), 353–374, 499–521. See also "Psychiatry of Our Colonial Fathers," *Archives of Neurology and Psychiatry*, cxxiv (1930), 667–681.

7. S. E. Jelliffe, "Notes on the History of Psychiatry," *The Alienist and Neurologist*, xxxi (1910), 80–89; xxxii (1910), 141–155, 297–314, 478–490, 649–668; xxxiii (1912), 69–90, 307–322; xxxiv (1913), 26–37, 235–248; xxxvi (1915), 365–371; xxxxvii (1916), 35–51, 159–183, 287–312, 331–346; xxxviii (1917), 41–56, 147–159.

8. Albert Deutsch, *The Mentally Ill in America. A History of Their Care and Treatment from Colonial Times* (Garden City, New York: Doubleday, 1937). A second edition of the book, slightly enlarged, was published under the same title in 1949 by Columbia University Press.

9. Albert Deutsch, "The History of Mental Hygiene," and "Military Psychiatry: The Civil War, 1861–1865" in J. K. Hall (ed.), *One Hundred Years of American Psychiatry* (New York: Columbia University Press, 1944), 325–366, 367–384.

10. On his later psychiatric reformism, see M. E. Kenworth, "Albert Deutsch (1905–1961)," *American Journal of Psychiatry*, cxviii (1962), 1064–1068; and Jeanne L. Brand, "Albert Deutsch: The Historian as Social Reformer," *Journal of the History of Medicine and Allied Sciences*, xviii (1963), 149–157.

11. Albert Deutsch, *The Shame of the States* (New York: Harcourt, Brace, 1948).

12. Deutsch, *The Mentally Ill in America*, 94.

13. It may be with these absences in mind that Gregory Zilboorg, several years after the appearance of Deutsch's book, commented that the history of American psychiatry remained to be written.

14. See again Brand, "Albert Deutsch: The Historian as Social Reformer," (1963).

15. Gregory Zilboorg, *The Medical Man and the Witch During the Renaissance* (The Noguchi Lectures) (Baltimore: The Johns Hopkins Press, 1935; reprint, New York: Cooper Square Publishers, 1969).

16. Gregory Zilboorg, in collaboration with George W. Henry, *A History of Medical Psychology* (New York: Norton, 1941; paperback ed., New York: Norton, 1967; Spanish trans., Buenos Aires: Hachette, 1945; Italian trans., Milano: Feltrinelli, 1963). In the hardback edition, Zilboorg's book includes at the end additional chapters about the history of organic diseases and mental hospitals written by George Henry.

17. Zilboorg, "Legal Aspects of Psychiatry" in *One Hundred Years of American Psychiatry*, edited by J. K. Hall with the assistance of Gregory Zilboorg and Henry Alden Bunker (New York: Columbia University Press, 1944), 507–584.

18. Zilboorg, *The Psychology of the Criminal Act and Punishment* (New York: Harcourt, Brace, 1954).

19. Zilboorg, *Mind, Medicine and Man* (New York: Harcourt, Brace, 1943); idem, *Sigmund Freud: His Exploration of the Mind of Man* (New York: Scribner, 1951).

20. Franz Alexander, "Gregory Zilboorg," *Journal of the American Psychoanalytic Association*, viii (1960), 380–381.

21. Francis J. Braceland, "In Memoriam—Gregory Zilboorg," *American Journal of Psychiatry*, xvi (1960), 671–672.

22. Zilboorg, *History of Medical Psychology*, 12.

23. Ibid., 14, 411.

24. Ibid., 382, 387.

25. For more on this topic, see Patrick Vandermeersch's " '*Les mythes d'origine*' in the History of Psychiatry" in this volume.

26. H. Institoris (i.e., Kraemer) and J. Sprenger, *Malleus Maleficarum* (*Hammer for Witches*), originally published in Strasbourg in 1486 and reprinted many times. English Trans. by Montague Summers (London: Rodker, 1928; repr. New York: Dover, 1971). Quotation from Zilboorg, *History of Medical Psychology*, 109, 133, 144.

27. Zilboorg, *The Medical Man and the Witch*, 50.

28. Zilboorg, *History of Medical Psychology*, 226.

29. Paracelsus, "The Diseases That Deprive Man of His Reason," tr. by Gregory Zilboorg, in H. E. Sigerist (ed.), *Four Treatises of Theophrastus von Hohenheim Called Paracelsus* (Baltimore: The Johns Hopkins Press, 1941), 127–212.

30. Ibid., 317, 407.

31. Ibid., 377.

32. Ibid., 434–435.

33. Ibid., 455.

34. Ibid., 494, 500. See also Zilboorg's later statement, *Sigmund Freud, His Exploration of the Mind of Man* (New York: Scribner, 1951).

35. Zilboorg, *History of Medical Psychology*, 523.

36. Zilboorg, *History of Medical Psychology*, 524–525.

37. See the commemorative volume of essays, Hertha Riese (ed.), *Historical Explorations in Medicine and Psychiatry* (New York: Springer, 1978), which includes a bibliography of Riese's major writings, pp. 228–232.

38. Galen, *On the Passions and Errors of the Soul*, edited by Walther Riese, translated from the Latin by P. W. Harkins (Columbus: Ohio State University Press, 1963).

39. Walther Riese, *La pensée morale en médecine* (Paris: Presses Universitaires de France, 1954), 121.

40. Walther Riese, *La théorie des passions à la lumière de la pensée médicale du dix-septième siècle*, supplement to *Confinia Psychiatrica*, viii (Basel: Karger, 1965).

41. Walther Riese, *The Legacy of Philippe Pinel. An Inquiry into Thought on Mental Alienation* (New York: Springer, 1969).

42. Ibid., 3.

43. Philippe Pinel, *Traité médico-philosophique sur l'aliénation mentale ou la manie* (Paris: Richard, Caille et Ravier, 1801; photostatic edition, Paris: Circle du Livre Précieux, 1965), Introduction, v–lvi.

44. Walther Riese, "Philippe Pinel (1745–1826). His Views on Human Nature and Disease. His Medical Thought," *Journal of Nervous and Mental Disease*, cxiv (1951), 313–323; idem, "Le raisonnement expérimental dans l'oeuvre de Pinel," *L'évolution psychiatrique*, xxxi (1966), 407–413; idem, "La méthode analytique de Condillac et ses rapports avec l'oeuvre de Philippe Pinel," *Revue philosophique*, lxxiv (1968), 321–336; idem, "Les sources hippocratiques de l'oeuvre de Philippe Pinel," *Société Moreau de Tours, Annales de Thérapeutique Psychiatrique*, iv (1969), 130–148; idem, "L'idée de la maladie dans l'oeuvre de Philippe Pinel," *Episteme*, vi (1972), 247–251.

45. Riese, *The Legacy of Philippe Pinel*, 153.

46. See in this regard Dora Weiner's essay in this volume, "'*Le geste de Pinel*': The History of a Psychiatric Myth."

47. Walther Riese, "The Pre-Freudian Origins of Psychoanalysis" in Jules Masserman (ed.), *Science and Psychoanalysis* (New York: Grune & Stratton, 1958), i, 29–72.

48. See also Walther Riese, "The Impact of Nineteenth-Century Thought on Psychiatry," *International Record of Medicine*, clxxiii (1960), 7–19; idem, "Changing Concepts of Cerebral Localizations," *Clio Medica*, ii (1967), 182–230; and idem, "Phenomenology and Existentialism in Psychiatry. An Historical Analysis," *Journal of Nervous and Mental Diseases*, cxxxii (1961), 469–484.

49. Walter Riese, *Vincent van Gogh in der Krankheit. Ein Beitrag zum Problem der Bezie-

hung zwischen Kunstwerk und Krankheit (Munich: Bergmann, 1926), 199. See also idem, ''The Disease of Vincent van Gogh, Its Significance in the Life and Work of an Artist,'' *Ciba Symposia*, vi (1948), 198–205.

50. See Mark S. Micale, ''Henri F. Ellenberger: The History of Psychiatry as the History of the Unconscious,'' in this volume.

51. Walter Bromberg, *Psychiatry Between the Wars, 1918–1945. A Recollection* (Westport, Connecticut: Greenwood Press, 1982).

52. Walter Bromberg, *The Mind of Man* (New York: Harper & Brothers, 1937); idem, *Man Above Humanity. A History of Psychotherapy* (Philadelphia: Lippincott, 1954; reissued in paperback edition under the title, *The Mind of Man: A History of Psychotherapy and Psychoanalysis* (New York: Harper & Brothers, 1959); idem, *From Shaman to Psychotherapist: A History of the Treatment of Mental Illness* (Chicago: Regnery, 1975). Bromberg also contributed a popularized history of psychiatry in the nineteenth and early twentieth centuries, which appeared as J. Winkler and Walter Bromberg, *Mind Explorers* (New York: Reynald & Hitchcock, 1939).

53. Bromberg, *Man Above Humanity*, 82–85.

54. Ibid., 97, 77.

55. Ibid., 35.

56. Franz Alexander and Sheldon T. Selesnick, *The History of Psychiatry: An Evaluation of Psychiatric Thought and Practice from Prehistoric Times to the Present* (New York: Harper & Row, 1966).

57. Ibid., 226–252; Appendix B, 407–409.

58. Ibid., 173.

59. The relationship between Zilboorg and Alexander is complicated. During the period in which he was enrolled at the Berlin Psychoanalytic Institute (1929–1930), Zilboorg was Alexander's analysand. In 1931, the year in which Alexander moved to the United States, the English translation, by Zilboorg, of Alexander and Staub's *The Criminal, The Judge and the Public* appeared. Three and a half decades later, Alexander published his *History of Psychiatry*, which was strongly, although not always openly, indebted to *A History of Medical Psychology*.

60. Erwin Ackerknecht, *A Short History of Psychiatry* [1957], Eng. trans. Sullamith Wolff (New York: Hafner, 1959).

61. Ackerknecht, *Kurze Geschichte der Psychiatrie*, 3rd rev. ed. (Stuttgart: Enke, 1985).

62. Jerome Schneck, *A History of Psychiatry* (Springfield, Illinois: Charles C Thomas, 1960).

63. George Rosen, *Madness in Society. Chapters in the Historical Sociology of Mental Illness* (Chicago: University of Chicago Press, 1968).

64. Edward T. Morman, ''George Rosen and the History of Mental Illness,'' this volume. See also my earlier article, ''Three American Historians of Psychiatry: Albert Deutsch, Gregory Zilboorg, George Rosen'' in Edwin R. Wallace and Lucius C. Pressley (eds.), *Essays in the History of Psychiatry*, Supplementary Volume to the *Psychiatric Forum* (Columbia, South Carolina: William S. Hall Psychiatric Institute, 1980), 1–21.

65. Ilza Veith, *Hysteria: The History of a Disease* (Chicago: University of Chicago Press, 1965).

66. A. R. Burr, *Weir Mitchell, His Life and Letters* (New York: Duffield, 1929); B. Evans, *The Psychiatry of Robert Burton* (New York: Columbia University Press, 1944); E. Bond, *Dr. Kirkbride and His Mental Hospital* (Philadelphia: Lippincott, 1947); Bond, *Thomas Salmon: Psychiatrist* (New York: Norton, 1950); H. Marshall, *Dorothea Dix: Forgotten Samaritan* (Chapel Hill, North Carolina: University of North Carolina Press, 1937); F. Gay, *The Open Mind: Elmer Ernest Southard, 1876–1920* (Chicago: Normandie House, 1938); Ernst Earnest, *Silas Weir Mitchell, Novelist and Physician* (Philadelphia: University of Pennsylvania Press, 1950); N. Goodman, *Benjamin Rush: Physician and Citizen, 1746–1813* (Philadelphia: University of Pennsylvania Press, 1934); E. Harms, *Origins of Modern Psychiatry* (Springfield, Illinois: Charles C Thomas, 1967) (a collection of papers published in the 1950s); Iago Galdston (ed.), *Historic*

Derivations of Modern Psychiatry (New York: McGraw-Hill, 1967). (Dr. Galdston was also the author of several valuable papers on the history of psychiatry.)

67. *Centennial Papers, Saint Elizabeths Hospital, 1855–1955* (Baltimore: Waverly Press, 1956); W. Russell, *The New York Hospital: A History of the Psychiatric Services, 1771–1936* (New York: Columbia University Press, 1945; reprint, New York: Arno, 1973).

68. Jan Ehrenwald, *From Medicine Man to Freud: A History of Psychotherapy* (New York: Dell, 1957); A. M. Sackler et al. (eds.), *The Great Physiodynamic Therapies in Psychiatry* (New York: Hoeber-Harper, 1956); Nolan D. C. Lewis, *A Short History of Psychiatric Achievements* (New York: Norton, 1941).

69. C. Oberndorf, *A History of Psychoanalysis in America* (New York: Grune & Stratton, 1953).

70. W. A. White, *The Autobiography of a Purpose* (Garden City, New York: Doubleday, 1938).

71. M. Guttmacher, *America's Last King: An Interpretation of the Madness of George III* (New York: Scribner, 1941); E. Hitschmann, *Great Men: Psychoanalytic Studies* (New York: International Universities Press, 1956).

72. "Mesmerism," *Ciba Symposia*, ix (1948), 826–856 (articles by E. Ackerknecht, I. Galdston, G. Rosen); J. Davies, *Phrenology, Fad and Science* (New Haven: Yale University Press, 1955).

73. J. Wortis, *Soviet Psychiatry* (Baltimore: Williams & Wilkins, 1950).

74. W. L. Cross (ed.), *Twenty-five Years After. Sidelights on the Mental Hygiene Movement and Its Founder* (Garden City, New York: Doubleday, 1934); A. E. Fink, *Causes of Crime. Biological Theories in the United States, 1800–1915* (Philadelphia: University of Pennsylvania Press, 1938; reprint, New York: Barnes, 1962); H. Mannheim (ed.), *Pioneers in Criminology* (Chicago: Quadrangle, 1960); J. S. Bockhoven, *Moral Treatment in American Psychiatry* (New York: Springer, 1963).

75. [Editors' Note: Dr. Mora modestly excludes himself from this discussion of American historians of psychiatry during the period 1910–1960. For a review of his many scholarly contributions to the field, readers are directed to "Knowing Members of the Advisory Board: George Mora," *History of Psychiatry*, iii (1992), 271–278.]

76. For a list of republished psychiatric classics, see D. Blain and M. Barton (eds.), *The History of American Psychiatry: A Teaching and Research Guide* (Washington, D. C.: American Psychiatric Association, 1979), ch. 14.

77. On this training and research center, see Eric T. Carlson and M. M. Simpson, "A Program on the History of Psychiatry and the Behavioral Sciences at Cornell University Medical College," *Journal of the History of Behavioral Sciences*, iii (1967), 370–372.

78. As an example of the federal support of scholarship by non-Americans, consider the case of Henri Ellenberger. During the early 1960s, Ellenberger received from NIH a three-year grant that permitted him to research and write *The Discovery of the Unconscious*.

II

FIVE MAJOR VOICES

4

Ida Macalpine and Richard Hunter: History between Psychoanalysis and Psychiatry

ROY PORTER

Collaborative writing in the history of psychiatry is not unknown—one thinks of Franz G. Alexander and Sheldon T. Selesnick's *The History of Psychiatry: An Evaluation of Psychiatric Thought and Practice from Prehistoric Times to the Present* (1967), discussed by George Mora in the preceding chapter; but Ida Macalpine and Richard Hunter constitute easily the most productive collaboration and certainly the only mother-and-son team. Psychobiographical questions of a Freudian hue are naturally raised by this scholarly liaison and its prolific progeny, which I shall not attempt to resolve in this paper.[1] Nevertheless, any understanding of the changing interpretative framework adopted in their work must hinge upon biographical elements, and so it may be useful here to sketch their careers.[2]

Ida Macalpine was born Ida Wertheimer in Nuremberg on 19 June 1899. In 1918 she began her medical studies at Erlangen, later studying at Freiburg, Munich, and Berlin. She interrupted her medical studies in 1921 to marry, but returned to medicine while her two children were still young and graduated MD at Erlangen in 1925. She then practiced in Berlin, working with children, and holding a part-time appointment in the Pestalozzi Froebel House. Her MD thesis was published and there followed a monograph, coauthored with her brother, on the problem of "surplus" women and the expected decline in the birthrate after the losses of the First World War.

Seeing the shadow of coming events, she left Germany in 1933, migrating to London with her two young sons. In 1934, she became registered with the Scottish triple diploma and settled in London in practice. She later remarried, and during the war and for some years afterward lived in Lancashire, spending part of her time helping in short-staffed mental hospitals. In 1948, she returned to London and was appointed assistant psychiatrist in the dermatology department of St. Bartholomew's Hospital; she engaged in active psychiatric practice. It was at this time that she developed her interest in the history of medicine, particularly the history of psychiatry. Observations of mental symptoms made by early physicians, she believed, might often still be valid; and that study of the development of psychiatric thought might thus provide clues to the solution of modern psychiatric mysteries. From the 1950s she published widely in psychiatry, and, generally in collaboration with her son Richard, in the history of psychiatry. She died in 1974.

Her son, Richard Alfred Hunter, was born in Nuremberg on 11 November 1923. Brought to London in 1933, he was educated at St. Paul's School and St. Bartholomew's Hospital, where he graduated MB in 1946. Between house posts, he served as a captain in the RAMC, and eventually joined the staff of the National Hospital, Queen Square, becoming physician in psychological medicine in 1960. Three years later, he received an appointment at Friern, the large North London psychiatric hospital.

In 1953, Hunter gained his membership in the Royal College of Physicians and was elected a fellow in 1972. He served as president of the sections of psychiatry and of history of medicine of the Royal Society of Medicine and was visiting Trent Lecturer at Duke University, North Carolina, and Sloan Professor at the Menninger Foundation, Topeka, Kansas. On his mother's death in 1974, his lifestyle changed completely. He married in his fifties, had three children, and moved out of London. He also ceased to publish in the history of psychiatry. He died in 1983. For the moment, the point of significance I wish to note for their *historical* writings—I will say nothing about their contributions to psychiatry proper—is that all their major writings were coauthored, but that it is possible to discern a major shift in the nature of the collaboration.

In the first half of the twentieth century, it would be fair to say, the British psychiatric community displayed little scholarly interest in the history of their discipline.[3] Against this backdrop of general indifference, the *oeuvre* of Macalpine and Hunter is quite astonishing. Despite being in active medical practice, they produced in their spare time three fundamental historical books. *Three Hundred Years of Psychiatry: 1535–1860* (1963)[4] is a stunningly complete and scholarly anthology of psychiatric texts; *George III and the Mad Business* (1969)[5] remains easily the best-documented case history we possess; and *Psychiatry for the Poor, 1851. Colney Hatch Asylum, Friern Hospital 1973: A Medical and Social History* (1974)[6] set new standards in exploring the history of a single asylum from its foundation to the present. They also found time to set up and edit the "Dawson" series of psychiatric reprints—they were the sole contributors. This series once more made readily available classic texts such as those of William Battie, Samuel Tuke, and John Conolly, with the added bonus of superb new scholarly introductions. They also brought out in that series the first English translation of the *Memoirs* of Daniel Schreber.[7] On top of this, they produced (singly, jointly, and with others) numerous papers on varied topics in the history of psychiatry,[8] bearing ample evidence of primary, archival research and enviable bio-bibliographical erudition. Their vast private library, which includes many hitherto unexploited items, has been preserved intact and is now housed in Cambridge University Library.[9] Aside from the sheer range and quantity of their output, numerous aspects of their work helped raise the history of psychiatry in Britain to a higher plane. Four may be singled out. First, they emphasized that the investigation and treatment of mental disturbance are not merely modern developments, but have long histories. The use of "schizophrenia" in the title of *Schizophrenia 1677* (their study of the seventeenth-century painter, Christoph Haizmann) and "psychiatry" in *Three Hundred Years of Psychiatry* is arguably tendentious, and historians may be bothered by the authors' Whiggish, and, perhaps, psychiatrically imperialistic implications. Nevertheless, Macalpine and Hunter's insistence that the history of British psychiatry did not begin with the York Retreat, or with John Conolly or Henry Maudsley, opened up fresh vistas on the past. For the first time, the wealth of writings about the mind and its disorders produced in Tudor, Stuart, and Georgian times became objects of serious scholarly scrutiny. Not least, their emphasis upon continuity and tradition did much to enrich perceptions of the historical record.[10]

Putting this in a slightly different way, my second point is that Macalpine and Hunter decisively broke with Great Man, heroic approaches to the history of psychiatry. No doubt they studied such generals of psychiatry as Freud and Conolly; but they were also passionately concerned with the rank-and-file, with minor private asylum-keepers, and the hundreds of obscure "divines, philosophers, philanthropists, lawyers [and] men of letters,"[11] who, over the centuries, expressed their views on the disturbed and their treatment, and whose often obscure and forgotten labors finally found immortality through a page or two of extracts, introduced by a brief biographical sketch, in *Three Hundred Years of Psychiatry*. For the first time, the history of British psychiatry ceased to be a grand tour from capital to capital—Bright, Burton, Battie, Burrows, Bucknill, and so forth—and became an exploration of a highly complex, well-populated, and deeply contested terrain.[12]

Third, in so doing, and despite the fact that they were both medically qualified, Macalpine and Hunter did not restrict their interests and sympathies to their professional predecessors. They were interested in the York Retreat, founded by the Quaker tea-merchant, William Tuke—an institution that emphasized the inefficacy of medicine for relieving the insane; they edited the writings of mentally disturbed individuals like Christoph Haizmann and Daniel Schreber; and they also researched the early Victorian patients' rights activist, John Perceval.[13] Nonmedical writers on the mad, for instance, Sir Thomas More, are copiously represented in *Three Hundred Years of Psychiatry*.[14]

Fourth, Macalpine and Hunter deserve credit as sticklers for scholarship. They unearthed records and resources hitherto overlooked or hardly used: for example, the late eighteenth-century County Register for patients in private lunatic asylums.[15] They argued for the importance of preserving, and working from, manuscript sources, demonstrating from their own researches how archives, especially those housed in English County Record Offices, could alone provide the key to a much richer picture than heretofore available.[16] Their history of Colney Hatch Asylum was exemplarily based upon intimate knowledge of Governors' Minutes and many other unpublished materials.

How did Macalpine and Hunter construe the history of psychiatry? It is often implied nowadays that, for all their strengths, they committed the sin of Whiggery. They looked at the past, it is alleged, with hindsight, anachronistically applying modern psychiatric labels and searching for "precursors" and "anticipations" of later views.[17] To a fair degree, this was their practice, indeed, avowedly so: They were certainly concerned with assessing "achievements" not merely on their own terms but in respect of the long-term development of what they saw as psychiatry. Certainly, theirs was an approach that emphasized continuity, and they saw no great epistemological ruptures in the evolution of psychiatric thought. They pointed to links in the historical chain—John Locke looked forward to William Battie and Thomas Arnold; Alexander Crichton and John Conolly drew upon Battie and Locke, and so forth—and they documented those links. "Many contemporary attitudes to 'mental' illness can be traced back to 16th and 17th century authors and institutions," Hunter argued:[18]

Bedlam, the prototype mental hospital, sheltered the socially incompetent or disruptive who were excluded from society. Robert Burton's *Anatomy of melancholy*, 1621, provided chapter and verse for the popular romantic or psychopathological approach. The biological approach which sought to correlate mental symptoms with brain lesions was pioneered in Professor Thomas Willis's *De anima brutorum* 1672. The Reverend Doctor Timothie Bright's *Treatise of melancholie*, 1586, suggested physical causes to be treated by appropriate medicines with simultaneous relief through the mind. Medicine's first professional mad-doctor and teacher of psychiatry, William Battie, in his *Treatise on madness*, 1758, made the distinction between "original" and "consequential" madness, that is between what are nowadays called functional psychoses, a term which tends to be equated with psychological, and organic psychoses caused by obvious disease of the brain. Neurotic or nervous disorders were described by George Cheyne in *The English Malady*, 1733.

They were thus unabashed about a certain "presentism," applying modern categories to earlier figures (*vide* the challenging usage of the term "schizophrenia" in the very title: *Schizophrenia 1677*). But if the essence of Whig history lies in the habit of making anachronistic *value* judgments about the past in the light of the present, Macalpine and Hunter come off well. Their scholarship is fully contextualized, remarkably unjudgmental, and extraordinarily free of psychiatric triumphalism.

This is not to deny that their works drew attention to elements of psychiatric progress. In their history of Colney Hatch Asylum, they cited instances of asylum patients from earlier centuries, once routinely (mis)diagnosed as cases of "melancholia" or depression, who could confidently nowadays be identified as having been stricken with neurological disorders like parkinsonism. "Early parkinsonism," they commented,

> is still of all extrapyramidal syndromes the most likely to be missed because psychomotor impoverishment and anergy are judged by their mental component and labelled endogenous depression. Photographs of many patients called melancholic in the old casebooks of Colney Hatch show unmistakable signs of parkinsonism. Their hang-head posture and what appeared as painful facial expression were interpreted as a feeling state, or the abnormal play of facial muscles as responding to inner voices or hallucinations. Bowed head, furrowed brow, fixed gaze, bent arms, rigid posture, and trembling hands made patients appear—and doubtless feel—anxious and sad. This is why in former times catatonia was called picturesquely *melancholia attonita* because patients appeared thunder-struck in a posture.[19]

The art of diagnosis had improved, and etiologies were better understood. According to Hunter and Macalpine, the humanistic "moral therapies" of earlier generations, and the Freudian psychodynamics that stepped into their shoes, made the mistake of interpreting in terms of emotional and behavioral disorders cases later clinicians could confidently ascribe to neuropathy. They noted, for instance, that the blepharospasm, or blinking tic characteristic of encephalitic parkinsonism, commonly found in mental hospitals in the interwar years, and numerous other facial tics and spasms, used to be called "mannerisms" and were read as signs of abnormal emotional disturbance or evidence of hallucination. These could today be satisfactorily reascribed as motoneuron problems.

Yet Macalpine and Hunter were far from spinning simplistic stories of psychiatric progress. In part, scholarly scruples kept them from that solecism. But their caution may also be related to the fact that their own situations within British psychiatry were rather maverick, unestablishmentarian, embattled, and in flux. A German refugee, Ida Macalpine never received ready admission into the metropolitan psychiatric citadel: It was only on her deathbed that she was admitted to the fellowship of the Royal College of Physicians.[20] Her institutional employment was in a dermatological department. Richard Hunter certainly rose up the ladder, but he trenchantly adopted some unfashionable poses, and fiercely dissented from many of the sacred cows of modern psychiatry. As a consultant at Friern Hospital, he was violently opposed to the psychosurgery and the shock treatments then practiced, seeing them as higher quackery. At a time when new psychotropic drugs were being hailed as panaceas for mental illness, he regarded them with deep suspicion. A brash and abrasive man who did not suffer fools gladly, he was equally hostile to the growing use in the 1960s of psychiatric social workers. Their therapeutics he regarded as bogus; only the medically qualified should be permitted to treat the disturbed. Yet while considering mental disorder to be organic in its etiology, Hunter insisted that these origins were largely unknown; hence radical surgical and pharmacological interventions were unjustifiable. Though believing passionately in the ideal of asylum as sanctuary, he judged that overcrowding, understaffing, and underfunding had, in actuality, turned psychiatric hospitals into a sham. Holding complex, unfashionable, and dissenting views like these, it is no surprise that Macalpine and Hunter did not subscribe to any simplistic Whig view of history that construed the present as the pinnacle of the past.

Indeed, psychiatry appeared to have lost its way. Freudian psychoanalysis had turned into a dogma. Its relationship to psychiatry was unsatisfactory. And whereas general medicine had made rapid and certain progress, the treatment of mental illness lagged behind: "Despite all that is said and written psychiatry does not possess a body of exact and established knowledge on which all can agree comparable with medicine."[21] By contrast with medicine, psychiatry was hardly a success story:

> Rather than a chronicle of feats, facts and discoveries, the history of psychiatry presents a record of perennial problems, recurrent ideas, disputes and treatments, trailing in the wake of medicine and exhibiting paradoxically—as medicine did of old—a mixture of as many false facts as false theories. How far psychiatry is still behind medicine is shown not only by the survival of therapeutic principles long since discarded from the parent science as for instance treatment by shock, but also by the persistence of schools of psychiatry, not to mention psychology or psychotherapy, the like of which vanished from the medical scene one hundred years ago with the scientific developments of the nineteenth century. This is why the historical study of psychiatry, again unlike that of medicine, is inseparable from that appreciation of its current problems and uncertainties which only the practical pursuit of it can give.[22]

To make these points is not, of course, to deny that Macalpine and Hunter read the past from a promontory of the present, or that they held strong convictions about the reality of mental illness and its historical manifestations, and about the proper role of psychiatry.[23] It is, rather, to insist that these convictions were complex: In addition to vindicating the general enterprise of psychiatry, they were fighting intraprofessional battles within the discipline, and doing so partly through emphasizing the problems and paradoxes of psychiatry in the past. Moreover, their views seem to have undergone a dramatic shift, which can only be sketched here.[24]

In the immediate postwar years, Ida Macalpine's outlook was primarily Freudian. In her early 1950s publications, she emphasized the "unconscious factors" involved in, and the psychosomatic roots of, skin disorders, boldly and confidently interpreting their stigmata in the light of Freudian theories of the unconscious and of neurotic conversion.[25] To mar

k the centenary of Freud's birth in 1956, Macalpine delivered a glowing "Tribute to Freud": He was, she declared, the Harvey of the mind. In collaboration with her son, then at the beginning of his career, she published at that time reverential Freudian accounts of transference.[26] Their first jointly written historical paper constitutes a piece of Freudian psychohistorical sleuthing so orthodox and insistent in its Oedipal themes that today it reads almost as a parody of the genre. Arguing that the composer Rossini manifested an "incestuous fixation on his mother," they offered an Oedipal interpretation of a late set of piano pieces, ostensibly about a train journey, interpreting the program and titles of the items as the "son's unconscious phantasy of the primal scene."[27]

During the 1950s, the orientation and allegiances of Macalpine and Hunter as investigators of the psyche were moving from a position sympathetic to Freud toward the more Kleinian or object-relations stance then fashionable in London, and at the same time they were growing more troubled by the unsatisfactory relations between psychoanalysis and psychiatry, and between psychiatry and medicine.[28] These themes come across loud and clear in their two major historical ventures in the midfifties, their 1955 translation, the first in English, of Daniel Schreber's *Memoirs of My Nervous Illness*,[29] and, a year later, their *Psychiatric Study of An Illustrated Autobiographical Record of Demonical Possession*, that is, the writings and paintings of the seventeenth-century Bavarian demoniac, Christoph Haizmann.[30] Both Schreber and Haizmann had already been metaphorically set on the couch by Freud, who contended that each presented a case of paranoia, deriving from a suppressed homosexual desire for the father.[31] Seemingly distancing themselves from Macalpine's earlier Freudian loyalties, Macalpine and Hunter argue in both instances that Freud's interpretation cannot be supported in the light of the texts and of other empirical evidence. They imply that Freud was guilty of projecting from his own personal case onto Haizmann; and they contend for the importance to both Haizmann and Schreber of "archaic, pregenital," pre-Oedipal longings involving gender-identity uncertainty and male fantasies of being female and producing babies. Today, Hunter and Macalpine's readings may seem almost as forced and dated as Freud's. Back in the 1950s, however, it was probably a bold act to offer rival psychohistorical readings of cases that (Schreber in particular) had long remained exemplary for Freudian orthodoxy.

From the mid-1950s, Macalpine and Hunter's psychiatric orientation underwent a sea change. Sensing that psychiatry was treading water while general medicine zoomed forward, they became convinced that symptoms they had hitherto viewed psychopathologically could be explained in the light of advances in somatic medicine and neuropsychiatry.[32] They certainly ceased to write psychohistory: Indeed, they were soon to denounce its follies.

Their *magnum opus, Three Hundred Years of Psychiatry* (1963), is completely different from these psychobiographical projects. Early in the book, Hunter and Macalpine nailed their colors to the mast, asserting their faith in the organic basis of most psychiatric disorders. They suggested in their notes and commentaries that it was possible retrospectively to diagnose many patients from earlier centuries as suffering from identifiable organic conditions (for example, tabes dorsalis, tertiary syphilis, or Parkinson's disease); and they proffered superficial histories of the development of modern understanding of the somatic basis of, and treatment for, such disorders.[33]

In *Three Hundred Years of Psychiatry*, the message is emphatic but it is discreetly stated. Their next major work, *George III and the Mad Business* (1969), grounded upon meticulous research into unpublished manuscript materials, carried a dynamite charge. It ridiculed psychodynamic interpretations of the king's supposed madness as wild and speculative, and hammered the psychohistorians with all the zeal of new converts.[34] Macalpine and Hunter claimed that George III could confidently be retrospectively diagnosed as having suffered from an inherited metabolic disorder, porphyria, which produces delirium and other epiphenomenal secondary psychiatric symptoms. Freudian delvings into the king's psyche—the idea that he went "mad" (J. H. Plumb had written of a "total flight from reality") because he was sexually frustrated and displayed an overanxious personality—were thus otiose, because he was suffering from an inborn error of metabolism. Such readings were, in any case, flimsy and fatuous. Equally silly was the idea that George had been "cured" by the Reverend Dr. Francis Willis, or any other doctor touting forms of primitive psychotherapy.[35] Neither medicines nor moral therapy had made much difference, or *could* have made much difference to the royal complaint. George had enjoyed a natural, spontaneous remission, and he suffered later relapses. *George III and the Mad Business* was clearly offered by its authors as the final triumph of scholarship and science over fantasy and system-building. Commenting on psychohistorical interpretations, they wrote:

> To such absurdities may historic figures be reduced when the mutterings of a delirious mind temporarily disordered by an intoxicated brain are mistaken for the expressions of psychological complexes. The royal malady was not insanity, not mania, nor manic-depressive psychosis. The psychiatric symptoms were but one manifestation of a physical disease, the bodily symptoms and signs of which were overshadowed by the mental because of the imperfect state of medical knowledge and the unique position of the patient.[36]

Much the same applies to *Psychiatry for the Poor, 1851. Colney Hatch Asylum, Friern Hospital 1973: A Medical and Social History* (1974). This is a meticulous institutional history of the hospital at which Hunter served as a consultant. It does not, it goes without saying, embrace the anti-psychiatric currents that were then rejecting the mental hospital as necessarily an abomination. Neither, however, does it provide a defense of, or apologia for, the Victorian asylum as it actually was. It shows that, from the first, Colney Hatch was starved of staff and resources. Magistrates treated lunacy as an administrative and economic, not a medical, problem. Preoccupied with administrative order, superintendents neglected caring and curing. The verdict is that Colney Hatch was a noble ideal that, in reality, consistently failed its patients.[37]

But the book also fires a polemic. The authors deployed patient records to demonstrate the reality of mental illness rooted in authentic lesions of the brain and the nervous system, and metabolic disturbance. Historical evidence was adduced to confute psychogenetic theories past (moral therapy) and present (psychoanalysis), and to support a medical model of insanity. "There are conflicting opinions about psychiatry and even among psychiatrists there is hardly a body of knowledge on which all agree," they wrote, yet:

> the historian of the contemporary scene must work from a viewpoint. Ours is that psychiatry is foremost a branch of medicine and subject to its discipline. We do not accept that mental illness is somehow different from physical as terms like neurosis, psychosis and their subdivisions imply. Patients suffer from mental symptoms which like bodily symptoms are caused by disease. It is the psychiatrist's task to identify its seat and nature by the methods of modern investigative and laboratory medicine. This diagnostic approach makes psychiatry at the present time one of the most exciting and rewarding areas of medicine. Patients are still sent to psychiatrists for treatment but go to physicians for diagnosis. Effective treatment can only follow on discovery of causes. Neurology which split off from psychiatry in the asylum's first decade established itself as a science when it became anatomical. Today enough is known of the brain to place psychiatry on the same footing.[38]

Thus the curative aspirations of the asylum were mistaken. At best, the asylum received oblique justification thanks to its potential to serve as a kind of giant laboratory for the close observation of the behavioral symptoms of what in the end proved to be largely neurological afflictions.[39]

Thus the reading of psychiatric history offered by Macalpine and Hunter changed dramatically in the course of twenty years. "Evidence is now accumulating," Hunter emphasized in 1971:

> that when mental patients are investigated by modern methods, mental symptoms are found to be epiphenomena which depend on type, rate of onset, localization and severity of the underlying disease process—and this may be one of as many as modern medicine has discovered. Under these circumstances, the abnormal mental state, however attractive, becomes a manifestation of the disease, equivalent to any other sign of disordered bodily function. It ceases to be mistaken for the disease itself. It follows also that its psychosocial ramifications, however tortuously they are traced out, do not lead to the cause of the illness and therefore do not make a diagnosis, any more than fever did. Furthermore, normal personality may be regarded as suspended during the time of illness. This is not to say that social consequences are not important, nor to deny that professional sympathising or psychotherapy may not be helpful in enabling patients to adjust. But the onus of being ill is entirely lifted off the patient who is the victim not of his mind but of his brain.[40]

It might be tempting to see in this turnabout a case of the female psychiatrist, trained in the Central Europe of the mature Freud, initially dominating the partnership with her theories of psychogenesis, but being mastered intellectually in due course by her son, who adopted the more medico-scientific outlook—the "psychiatric gaze"—required of the mental hospital consultant.[41] This switch might also, more broadly, be said to register the greater confidence in psychological medicine developing in the Anglo-American world from the late 1950s. The rewriting of history thus corresponded to new directions in psychiatry itself. Whichever, it is clear that to understand the history of psychiatry written by practitioners, it is a prerequisite to examine their own psychiatric commitments. It is equally clear that to understand the history of psychiatry written by historians, it is first necessary to examine the commitments of the historians.

Notes

1. I shall not attempt that task for two reasons. First, I do not feel professionally qualified, historically or psychiatrically. Second, I do not know enough intimate personal details of their lives, singly or together. A full-length biography of the pair would be highly desirable. I would like to take the opportunity here of thanking many individuals who have volunteered their reminiscences, particularly of Richard Hunter.

2. My sources are chiefly published obituary notices: see above all, for Ida Macalpine, *British Medical Journal*, 25 May 1974, 449; and, for Richard Hunter, *Lancet*, 2 January 1982; *The Times*, 1 December 1981; *British Medical Journal*, 12 December 1981; and Henry Rollin, "Richard Hunter, MD (1923–81)," *Cambridge Review*, civ (1983), 71–74.

3. See Roy Porter, "History of Psychiatry in the U.K.," *History of Psychiatry*, ii (1991), 271–280.

4. Richard Hunter and Ida Macalpine, *Three Hundred Years of Psychiatry: 1535–1860* (London: Oxford University Press, 1963).

5. Ida Macalpine and Richard Hunter, *George III and the Mad Business* (London: Allen Lane, 1969). The book forms the basis for Alan Bennett's play, "The Madness of George the Third," produced in 1991 at the National Theatre in London. Ida Macalpine was a character in that play.

6. Richard Hunter and Ida Macalpine, *Psychiatry for the Poor, 1851. Colney Hatch Asylum, Friern Hospital 1973: A Medical and Social History* (London: Dawsons, 1974).

7. For the Dawsons series, Ida Macalpine and Richard Hunter produced the following editions: *Memoirs of My Nervous Illness, by Daniel Paul Schreber* (London: Dawsons, 1955); idem, *Schizophrenia 1677: A Psychiatric Study of An Illustrated Autobiographical Record of Demonical Possession* (London: Dawsons, 1956); William Battie, *A Treatise on Madness, and John Monro, Remarks on Dr. Battie's Treatise on Madness* (London: Dawsons, 1962); John Conolly, *An Inquiry Concerning the Indications of Insanity, with Suggestions for the Better Protection and Care of the Insane* (London: Dawsons, 1964); John Conolly, *The Construction and Government of Lunatic Asylums and Hospitals for the Insane* (London: Dawsons, 1968); John Conolly, *The Treatment of the Insane Without Mechanical Restraint* (Folkestone: Dawsons, 1973); Samuel Tuke, *Description of the Retreat, an Institution near York for Insane Persons of the Society of Friends* (London: Dawsons, 1964). I stand in some awe of their entrepreneurial success in persuading a publisher to undertake these reprints. W. F. Bynum and I revived this series of reprints with Routledge in the late 1980s, but Routledge rapidly abandoned it as not sufficiently profitable.

8. See, for instance, R. A. Hunter and Ida Macalpine, "William Battie, M.D., F.R.S.; Pioneer Psychiatrist," *Practitioner*, clxxiv (1955), 208–215; R. A. Hunter and H. P. Greenberg, "Sir William Gull and Psychiatry," *Guy's Hospital Reports*, cv (1956), 361–375; Richard Hunter and Ida Macalpine, "The Reverend William Pargeter, M. A., M. D. (1760–1810), Psychiatrist," *St. Bartholomew's Hospital Journal*, lx (1956), 52–60; Richard Hunter, "A Brief Review of the Use of Electricity in Psychiatry," *British Journal of Physical Medicine*, n.s. xx (1957), 99–100; R. A. Hunter, Ida Macalpine, "William Harvey: His Neurological and Psychiatric Observations," *Journal of the History of Medicine and Allied Sciences*, xii (1957), 126–139; (October 1957), 512–515; R. Hunter and Ida Macalpine, "John Haslam: His Will and His Daughter," *Medical History*, vi (1962), 22–26; R. Hunter and Ida Macalpine, "Samuel Tuke's First Publication on the Treatment of Patients at The Retreat, 1811," *British Journal of Psychiatry*, cxi (1965), 769–772; R. Hunter and Ida Macalpine, "The Reverend John Ashbourne (c. 1611–61) and the Origins of the Private Madhouse System," *British Medical Journal*, ii (1972), 513–515.

9. Hunter and Macalpine's card catalogue is available in the Cambridge University Library.

10. Hunter and Macalpine's *Three Hundred Years of Psychiatry: 1535–1860* is especially remarkable for recovering long-forgotten figures from the seventeenth and eighteenth centuries. Ironically, the work's coverage becomes thinner the nearer it approaches its terminal date.

11. Ibid., viii.

12. E.g., Richard Hunter and J. B. Wood, "Nathaniel Cotton, M.D., Poet and Physician," *King's College Hospital Gazette*, xxxvi (1957), 120. See also R. Hunter, "Some Lessons from the History of Psychiatry (Abstr)," *Society for the Social History of Medicine Bulletin*, 5 (1971), 11–12.

13. Richard Hunter and Ida Macalpine, "John Thomas Perceval (1803–1876): Patient and Reformer," *Medical History*, vi (1961), 391–395.

14. Richard Hunter and Ida Macalpine, *Three Hundred Years of Psychiatry: 1535–1860*, p. 5 for Sir Thomas More.

15. Richard A. Hunter, Ida Macalpine, L. M. Payne, "The County Register of Houses for the Reception of Lunatics, 1798–1812," *Journal of Mental Science*, cii (1956), 856–863.

16. Richard Hunter, "Some Notes on the Importance of Manuscript Records for Psychiatric History," *Archives*, iv (1959), 9–11 (where Hunter states, regarding manuscript materials, "if the information contained in them is added up a picture emerges very different from the one generally accepted"); R. Hunter and Ida Macalpine, "Manuscript Evidence for William Nisbet's Authorship of a Picture of . . . The Royal College of Physicians of London, 1817 Retitled Authentic Memoirs . . . of the Most Eminent Physicians and Surgeons of Great Britain, 1818 and 1822," *Medical History*, vi (1962), 187–189.

17. For Whiggery, see Herbert Butterfield, *The Whig Interpretation of History* (London: Bell, 1931); A. R. Hall, "On Whiggism," *History of Science*, xxi (1983), 45–59.

18. R. Hunter, "Some Lessons from the History of Psychiatry (Abstr)," *Society for the Social History of Medicine Bulletin*, v (1971), 11–12. See also Hunter and Macalpine, *Three Hundred Years of Psychiatry: 1535–1860*, 236, 402, 559. Their contrast of the "progressive" Battie to the backward-looking Monro is incisively dissected in Akihito Suzuki, "Mind and Its Disease in Enlightenment British Medicine" (Ph.D. thesis, University of London, 1992).

19. Richard Hunter and Ida Macalpine, *Psychiatry for the Poor*, 222.

20. Research into the professional politics of postwar medicine is a desideratum. See for some glimpses John G. Howells, "The Establishment of the Royal College of Psychiatrists" in German Berrios and Hugh Freeman (eds.), *150 Years of British Psychiatry, 1841–1991* (London: Gaskell, 1991), 117–36.

21. Richard Hunter and Ida Macalpine, *Three Hundred Years of Psychiatry: 1535–1860*, viii.

22. Ibid., viii–ix.

23. It is interesting that Macalpine and Hunter never felt the need to polemicize against antipsychiatry.

24. Proper evaluation of the significance of shifts in their positions, and the respective roles played by Macalpine and by Hunter in them, would repay much closer analysis.

25. Ida Macalpine, "A Case of 'De-conversion,' " *International Journal of Psycho-Analysis*, xxx (1949), 57–58; Ida Macalpine, "The Development of the Transference," *Psychoanalytic Quarterly*, xix (1950), 501–539; R. M. B. MacKenna and Ida Macalpine, "Application of Psychology to Dermatology," *Lancet*, cclx (1951), 65–68; Ida Macalpine, "Psychosomatic Symptom Formation," *Lancet*, 1 (1952), 278–282; Ida Macalpine, "Psychiatric Observations on Facial Dermatoses," *British Journal of Dermatology*, lxv (1953), 177–182; Ida Macalpine, "Pruritus Ani; a Psychiatric Study," *Psychosomatic Medicine*, xv (1953), 498–508; Ida Macalpine, "Present Status of Psychosomatic Medicine," *American Journal of Psychotherapy*, viii (1954), 454–465.

26. Ida Macalpine, "Tribute to Freud," *Journal of the History of Medicine and Allied Sciences*, xi (1956), 247–260 (for Harvey, see p. 259); Ida Macalpine and R. A. Hunter, "The Importance of the Concept of Transference for Present-day Theories of Mental Diseases," *Acta Psychotherapeutica, Psychosomatica et Orthopaedagogica*, iii (1955), 237–243; Richard A. Hunter and Ida Macalpine, "Follow-up Study of a Case Treated in 1910 by 'The Freud Psychoanalytic Method,' " *British Journal of Medical Psychology*, xxvi (1953), 64–67; Ida Macal-

pine, "Syphilophobia; a Psychiatric Study," *British Journal of Venereal Diseases*, 33 (1957), 92–99.

27. "The various pieces in their original order are headed as follows:

The Devilish Whistle
The Sweet Melody of the Brake
The Terrible Derailment
First Wounded Man
Second Wounded Man
Funeral Ode
Amen

These titles may be taken as a thinly disguised symbolic presentation of an only son's unconscious phantasy of the primal scene." Ida Macalpine and Richard A. Hunter, "Rossini: Piano Pieces for the Primal Scene," *American Imago*, ix (1952), 213–219. Of course, the paper invites speculation about the significance of the authorial mother-son relationship for the orientation of their work.

28. Richard Hunter and Ida Macalpine, *Schizophrenia 1677: A Psychiatric Study of an Illustrated Autobiographical Record of Demonical Possession* (London: Dawsons, 1956); the introduction is a fascinating attempt to "take stock." See also Ida Macalpine and Richard A. Hunter, "Observations on the Psychoanalytic Theory of Psychosis: Freud's 'A Neurosis of Demoniacal Possession in the Seventeenth Century,' " *British Journal of Medical Psychology*, xxvii (1954), 175–192.

29. Ida Macalpine and Richard Hunter, *Memoirs of My Nervous Illness, by Daniel Paul Schreber* (London: Dawsons, 1955); see also their "The Schreber Case; a Contribution to Schizophrenia, Hypochondria, and Psychosomatic Symptom-formation," *Psychoanalytic Quarterly*, xxii (1953), 328–371.

30. See Richard Hunter and Ida Macalpine, *Schizophrenia 1677*, 42f.

31. For further discussion of Schreber, see the introduction by Samuel M. Weber to the reissue of Ida Macalpine and Richard Hunter, *Memoirs of My Nervous Illness, by Daniel Paul Schreber*, and, above all Han Israëls, *Schreber, Father and Son* (Amsterdam: Han Israëls, 1991).

32. One wonders, of course, about the respective contributions here of mother and son. It would seem as though the young Hunter, abreast of recent neurological developments, must have been instrumental in converting his mother.

33. See Richard Hunter and Ida Macalpine, *Three Hundred Years of Psychiatry*, 196, 197, 614, 268, 861. The subject index lists modern psychiatric categories like schizophrenia, referring back to cases and writings from earlier centuries.

34. In book form it was Ida Macalpine and Richard Hunter, *George III and the Mad Business*; it was attended by the following articles: Ida Macalpine and R. Hunter, "A Clinical Reassessment of the 'Insanity' of George III and Some of Its Historical Implications," *Bulletin of the Institure of Historical Research*, xl (1967), 166–185; Ida Macalpine, R. Hunter, and C. Rimington, "Porphyria in the Royal Houses of Stuart, Hanover, and Prussia: A Follow-up Study of George III's Illness (And Subsequent Correspondence)," *British Medical Journal*, 1 (1968), 7–18, 178, 311–313, 443–444; 509–510, 705–706, 841–842; 2 (1968), 118–119, 243–244, 430–431; Ida Macalpine and R. Hunter, "Some Effects of the Royal Malady on the Development of Psychiatry," *History of Medicine (London)*, October (1968), 15–16, 21–22; Ida Macalpine and R. Hunter, "George III's Illness and its Impact on Psychiatry," *Proceedings of the Royal Society of Medicine*, lxi (1968), 1017–1026; G. Dean and Ida Macalpine, "Porphyria and King George III," *Scientific American*, ccxxi (1969), 8–9; Ida Macalpine and R. Hunter, "Porphyria and King George III," *Scientific American*, ccxxi (1969), 38–48. The irony, of course, is that the mode of psychohistory attacked in *George III and the Mad Business* has much in common with the historical interpretation that Macalpine and Hunter had themselves been touting some fifteen years earlier.

35. See Ida Macalpine and Richard Hunter, *George III and the Mad Business.*

36. Ida Macalpine and R. Hunter, "George III's Illness and its Impact on Psychiatry," *Proceedings of the Royal Society of Medicine,* lxi (1968), 1017–1026. Debate of course rages among historians today as to the validity of psychohistory. See, *inter alia,* Peter Gay, *Freud for Historians* (New York: Oxford University Press, 1985); Peter Loewenberg, *Decoding the Past: The Psychohistorical Approach* (New York: Knopf, 1983); Lloyd DeMause, *The New Psychohistory* (New York: Psychohistory Press, 1975); David E. Stannard, *Shrinking History: On Freud and the Failure of Psychohistory* (New York: Oxford University Press, 1980); and, in this volume, Elisabeth Young-Bruehl, "A History of Freud Biographies."

37. Richard Hunter and Ida Macalpine, *Psychiatry for the Poor,* 12.

38. Ibid., 11f.

39. Ibid., 223f.

40. R. Hunter, "Some Lessons from the History of Psychiatry (Abstr)," *Society for the Social History of Medicine Bulletin,* 5 (1971), 11–12.

41. Hunter engaged in clinical research. See, for instance, Richard A. Hunter, "Confusional Psychosis with Residual Organic Cerebral Impairment Following Isoniazid Therapy," *Lancet,* 2 (1952), 960–962; R. A. Hunter and W. H. Merivale, "A Case Illustrating Some Effects of Barbiturates on the Glucose Tolerance Test," *Guy's Hospital Reports,* ciii (4) (1954), 375–380; Richard A. Hunter, H. P. Greenberg, "Barbiturate Addiction Simulating Spontaneous Hyperinsulinism," *Lancet,* 2 (1954), 58–62; W.H.H. Merivale and Richard A. Hunter, "Abnormal Glucose-tolerance Tests in Patients Treated with Sedative Drugs," *Lancet,* 2 (1954), 939–942; Richard Hunter, Muriel Jones, B.A.L. Hurn, et al., "Impaired Glucose Tolerance: A Late Effect of Insulin Shock Treatment," *British Medical Journal,* 1 (1970), 465–468; R. Hunter, J. Smith, T. Thomson, A. D. Dayan, "Hemiparkinsonism with Infarction of the Ipsilateral Substantia Nigra," *Neuropathology and Applied Neurobiology,* 4 (1978), 297–301.

5

George Rosen and the History of Mental Illness[1]

EDWARD T. MORMAN

Between 1936 and the end of his life, George Rosen published almost three dozen articles on subjects relating to the history of psychiatry.[2] His concentrated work in this area, however, dates only from the late 1950s, by which time he was already among the United States' leading historians of medicine. Rosen was not particularly concerned with psychiatry as a body of theory, an aspect of medical practice, or a professional specialty; nor was the development of mental health services a central focus of his research. He was drawn, rather, to the history of irrational behavior, the etiology of mental illness, and the evolution of attitudes toward the mentally ill. His one essay on Sigmund Freud was very much a diversion, and his discussion of somatic factors in mental disease resolved itself into a means of dealing with some evident counterinstances to his argument that mental illness is culturally generated.

Why did Rosen turn to psychiatry after decades of work in other areas of the history of health care? While George Mora has suggested that Rosen's sociological interest in mental illness was "only natural . . . in the light of his tremendous grasp of people and ideas,"[3] it should be possible to construct a more historically grounded explanation. Looking for clues elsewhere in Rosen's writings and in the cultural and institutional environments in which he lived, we can identify several factors that together help explain this development.

First is Rosen's personal regard for associates working in psychiatric history. Rosen came to know Albert Deutsch and Gregory Zilboorg in the late 1930s, as he was getting involved in the New York City medical history scene. Both Deutsch and Zilboorg were moderate leftists who, with Rosen, looked to Henry Sigerist of Johns Hopkins for leadership and inspiration.[4] Deutsch, primarily a journalist, may have exemplified for Rosen the historian who helps change the present world by demonstrating the relevance of the past; and Zilboorg, a highly cultured physician-historian of the sort Rosen admired, produced work on Renaissance witchcraft posing questions that Rosen tried to answer decades later.[5]

A more practical source of Rosen's interest in mental health was his position on the faculty of the Columbia University School of Public Health and Administrative Medicine at a time when all such institutions in the United States were confronting the

problems of community mental health. In December 1959, Columbia hosted a conference, financed by the National Institute of Mental Health (NIMH) and sponsored by
the Association of Schools of Public Health, on mental health teaching in public health
schools. To the report that came out of this meeting, Rosen contributed a chapter that
assessed trends in psychiatric social work, public health nursing, child guidance, general
psychiatry, public health education, and the social sciences.[6] Within this seventy-five-
page essay is the substance of a well-reasoned, historically sophisticated, short article;
but it is clear from its sloppy structure and tedious style that Rosen was not engaged
by the policy questions at hand. He was, however, very much interested in related
sociological and historical issues.

The concept of community mental health was rooted in the mental hygiene movement of the 1910s and given new life as a result of the experiences of military psychiatrists during the Second World War.[7] In the immediate postwar period, William C.
Menninger specifically advocated an activist ''social psychiatry'' based on ''commu-
nity-caused sources of emotional stress.''[8] The founding of the NIMH in 1946 presup-
posed a community orientation,[9] and leaders of the social psychiatry movement
regarded an expanded community orientation to be the natural next step in the development of psychiatry. As a founding editor of the *International Journal of Social Psychiatry* wrote in its first issue:

> Social psychiatry is concerned not only with facts of prevalence and incidence. It
> searches more deeply into the possible significance of social and cultural factors in
> the etiology and dynamics of mental disorder. . . . Social psychiatry is etiological
> in its aim, but its point of attack is the whole social framework of contemporary
> living.[10]

Having participated in the social medicine upsurge of the late forties,[11] Rosen was
bound to pay attention to a parallel movement within psychiatry; and he initially
approached the history of mental illness in order to understand the origins of social
psychiatry.[12] Rosen's turn to psychiatric history in the late 1950s was a continuation of
his earlier work on the history of public health and social medicine. With momentum
provided by social psychiatry and community mental health, Rosen hoped to use the
history of mental illness as a means to understand the cultural origins of irrational
behavior. He would thereby demystify or ''naturalize'' madness and irrationality by
making them normal components of any society, which predictably wax and wane in
response to other cultural factors.

George Rosen was born in Brooklyn on June 23, 1910.[13] His parents were immigrant
Jews who spoke Yiddish at home; and it was not until he entered the New York City
public schools that he himself learned English. His father, a presser in a laundry, was
an ardent trade unionist who sometimes took him to union functions. As an undergraduate at the College of the City of New York, Rosen devoted himself to schoolwork, a
paying job, and his voracious extracurricular reading. After completing the premedical
course, however, he found himself the victim of the anti-Semitic admissions policies
prevailing at American medical colleges. He chose then to go to Berlin, where he joined
several dozen other young American men (all Jews except for one African American)
who had gone abroad for the type of high-quality medical education denied them at

home. Much about Weimar Germany impressed Rosen, especially the national health insurance system; and he never confused the crimes of the Nazis with the general legacy of German culture.[14] While in Germany he married Beate Caspari, a fellow medical student and the daughter of a successful Berlin Jewish physician who suffered greatly after the Nazis came to power.

In the fall of 1933, Rosen's advisor, Paul Diepgen, urged him to contact Henry Sigerist for advice on choosing a topic for his MD thesis. Sigerist responded warmly to Rosen's inquiry; and once Rosen completed the thesis, both Sigerist and Diepgen praised it highly.[15] Rosen left Berlin in May 1935 to start an internship in Brooklyn, and soon began submitting articles to Sigerist's *Bulletin of the History of Medicine*. Rosen and Sigerist shared common interests in social history and the organization of medical care, and over the next several years they developed a warm student-teacher relationship.[16] Between 1936 and 1947, Rosen published no fewer than twenty articles in the *Bulletin*.

While continuing his work in medical history, Rosen completed his internship and opened a medical practice, but he quickly found that he was not suited for clinical work. To relieve the resulting financial strain, he took a part-time job in the tuberculosis service of the New York City Department of Health. Meanwhile, Sigerist found him work with the publisher Alfred A. Knopf as a translator and with the Ciba-Geigy drug firm as editor of their new magazine, *Ciba Symposia*. It was relatively easy for Sigerist to find lucrative part-time work for a protégé as capable as Rosen; but it was impossible for him to help Rosen with what he desperately wanted—an academic post in medical history.

Rosen was intent on getting out of private practice and improving his chances of finding a university position. In the fall of 1939, he began graduate work in sociology at Columbia, developing close ties with several prominent faculty members, including Robert K. Merton and Robert Lynd. He closed his office to become a full-time health officer for the New York City Department of Health in 1942; and in 1944 he completed his Ph.D.[17] He joined the army in the spring of 1943 and spent the following two years working in Washington, D. C., making frequent visits to nearby Baltimore to see Sigerist. Toward the end of the war, he eagerly awaited his return to civilian life so he could devote his free time to the prestigious task of editing the newly founded *Journal of the History of Medicine and Allied Sciences*.

After his discharge in April 1946, Rosen returned to the New York City Department of Health and continued writing medical history articles and editing the new journal for no pay. The following winter, he had renewed hopes of an academic position in history of medicine when he learned of Sigerist's plans to retire from Hopkins; but he soon realized that he was not likely to succeed his mentor. The most honest appraisal of his chances was provided by his friend Erwin Ackerknecht, who warned him of anti-Semitism at Hopkins.[18] In addition, the administration and trustees of Hopkins were dissatisfied with Sigerist's vocal advocacy of socialized medicine and friendliness toward the Soviet Union. Closely associated with Sigerist, Rosen was regarded with suspicion even though his opinions about the USSR were quite different.

With the Hopkins job closed to him and no other positions likely to open in history of medicine, Rosen continued his historical scholarship while earning his living in public health. In 1949, he became director of health education for New York City; and in 1950 he left city government for the Health Insurance Plan of Greater New York (HIP), a pioneering prepaid group medical practice regarded by some as a small-scale model for a national health system.[19] In 1951, Rosen took a part-time public health faculty position at Columbia, which was made full-time when he was appointed editor of the *American Journal of Public Health* in 1957. This allowed him to leave HIP and concentrate on his scholarship and editorial duties. Finally, in 1969, he acceded to the chair of history of medicine at Yale. Rosen died in Oxford in August 1977, while touring Great Britain on his way to an international history of science conference in Edinburgh.

The best of Rosen's contributions to the history of medicine and psychiatry, the ones with which he was most engaged, are those in which he makes good use of what he learned as a graduate student at Columbia and as an insatiable reader of sociology and political philosophy while a medical student. Once he had mastered the German language, Rosen immersed himself in the traditions of German intellectual culture, including Hegelian philosophy and other strains of German idealism. Rosen's youthful writings particularly reflect the prominent influence of the Marxist works he had read in Germany. In one early work Rosen stressed that diseases are not immutable entities and are intelligible only within their biological *and* social contexts, and he suggested that history of medicine had been deficient in viewing the patient as "only an accident in the history of the disease."[20] He claimed to have learned from Marx and Engels that human beings were "central actors on the stage of history"; and until the very end of his career he protested against a "biologism" in history that devalued human action in relationship to disease and other natural forces.[21]

While examining sources for his medical school thesis, Rosen had come upon John Elliotson, an early supporter of mesmerism in England, and was inspired almost immediately to prepare a short sketch of him for publication in Sigerist's *Bulletin*.[22] This piece of juvenilia was little more than a rehashing of secondary sources spiced with several long quotations; but Rosen kept it in mind and ten years later reshaped much of the same material into an article on the use of hypnotism in surgery.[23] In this piece he brought Elliotson to life as a medical innovator and social reformer, a complex but consistent historical actor, whose atheism and philosophical materialism were closely tied to his belief in an animal magnetic fluid.[24] Rosen's early work also included two short references to "sexual abnormalities" in a 1940 issue of *Ciba Symposia*,[25] in which he claimed that only because contemporary Western society provided no place for homosexuals did it therefore regard them as abnormal. While he did not question the reification of "homosexuality" as descriptive of a category of people, Rosen wanted to place the moral valuation of sexual preference clearly in a cultural context.

His works on mesmerism and sexuality provide indications of how the more mature Rosen would pursue the history of psychiatry, but none of his writings better represents the continuity between his early and later work than his 1952 article on conceptions of health in late eighteenth century North America.[26] Conceived as a chapter in his never-completed treatise on the history of social medicine, this article aimed to enlist Thomas Jefferson and Benjamin Rush among the precursors of the social medicine movement. In presenting Rush as a believer in the social causation of disease, Rosen pointed out that Rush associated good mental health with partisans of the revolution, and hypochondriasis with the Loyalists.[27]

Revolution, aborted revolution, and any sort of social disruption or dislocation remained constant in Rosen's writings on mental illness.[28] Having earlier invoked Rudolf Virchow as a physician conscious of the significance of social factors in disease causation,[29] Rosen called on him again in 1959, to explain that military defeats and suppressed revolutions may be the source of "psychic epidemics" of irrational behavior.[30] Virchow had been particularly concerned about the consequences of the failure of the German revolution of 1848, but Rosen extended the concept to include examples as far removed as the North American Indian Ghost Dance of the late nineteenth century, which was supposed to lend invulnerability in battle to a people on the verge of physical extermination. Rosen strongly believed that such "psychic epidemics" are not inexplicable occasions of group psychopathology. He considered them to be the result of stress and the product of social relations; and he wanted to study them as a means to criticize existing social circumstances.[31]

Rosen's discussions of mass psychopathology invariably turned to extreme forms of religious observance, and he was particularly fascinated by the radical Protestant sects of seventeenth-century England.[32] He became familiar with the English sectarians in the late 1930s, when he read Robert Merton's doctoral dissertation on Puritanism and science in England,[33] and pursued the topic himself while a student of Merton's at Columbia.[34] As a Jew, an atheist, and a critical admirer of Enlightenment rationalism, Rosen may have regarded fundamentalist Christianity as particularly hard to understand. On the other hand, he was a man of the Left, of proletarian origins, and had himself been the victim of religious prejudice—and seventeenth-century radical Protestantism was a revolutionary expression of the aspirations of the oppressed lower classes. Recognizing Mannheimian sociology of knowledge as a useful tool for understanding the beliefs of rational scientists,[35] Rosen also wanted to analyze the irrationality of religious sects like the Diggers, Levellers, and Fifth Monarchists, in order to find the ill-defined border between such beliefs and true mental illness.

As a case study in religious irrationality, Rosen took on the psychopathology of Renaissance witch-hunting,[36] emphasizing cultural values, such as misogyny and religious intolerance, in his explanation of the witch-craze. He clearly differentiated himself from the tradition in psychiatric historiography that accepted the idea that most of those accused of witchcraft were actually mad, and that hailed the development of this notion in the seventeenth century as a foundation of modern psychiatry.[37] Rosen thought that neither the victims nor the persecutors were necessarily insane, and that although a minority of both might have been mentally ill, most of the people involved in witch-hunting learned to participate because of fear. When he alluded to analogues in more recent times, he mentioned the Red Scare of 1919–20, but not the period that he had recently lived through. Though never directly victimized during what is known as the McCarthy period, Rosen knew enough people who had suffered to himself remain fearful.[38]

In discussing dance frenzies and revival movements,[39] Rosen stepped even further back from calling "psychic epidemics" instances of psychotic or psychopathological behavior. Citing several witnesses to the dancing mania of 1374, he was able to provide a vivid description of the participants—naked, holding hands or clapping, twitching, falling on the ground, describing visions, and foaming at the mouth[40]—and claimed that such behavior was easily explained:

> Obviously desires, beliefs, and rites were allied to satisfy moral demands and frustrated aspirations. To satisfy these needs, song and dance were employed to achieve a state of ritual trance or possession. In this situation it was possible to reduce emotional tensions and to achieve some degree of relief.[41]

The prophetic utterances and bizarre physical acts of religious extremists and millenarians from the Middle Ages to his own time "may be psychopathological in nature, but they also serve a social purpose as the means for generating superhuman efforts required to change conditions."[42] To the downtrodden, it makes sense to esteem what was despised by the society that has oppressed them.

Rosen also explored another connection between religion, ecstasy, and madness: the role of the prophet, shaman, or medicine man, especially among the ancient Hebrews. He may have been drawn to this because of his continuing identification as a Jew and his pride in his childhood religious training.[43] If he was not competent to make use of the primary documents of ancient Greek and Roman medicine, he was still able to display the potential breadth of his original scholarship by using the Hebrew Bible as a primary source. In addition, his friend Erwin Ackerknecht had grappled with the problem of the apparent madness of medicine men, and as editor of *Ciba Symposia* in the 1940s, Rosen had also become familiar with this issue.[44] Shamanism and prophetism interested him because of the evident connection between the ecstatic states achieved by individuals with specific religious functions and group phenomena such as revival meetings or witch-hunting. Rosen specifically wanted to know why the Hebrew word for behaving like a prophet also meant to rave, and why, since biblical prophets were taken seriously and had an important role to play in affairs of state, they were viewed as akin to madmen. He insisted that the behavior of the prophets was functional, constructing an argument that associated the actions of the prophets with the needs of the secular powers.[45]

In his 1967 Benjamin Rush lecture before the American Psychiatric Association,[46] Rosen discussed the notion of an "age of anxiety," such as his own times, in which insecurity and uneasiness are dominant emotions. He saw connections between this calmer form of irrationality and more frenzied instances of mass psychopathology, in that those living during an oppressive or alienating moment in history might turn inward and seek comfort by resorting to the irrational. Alternatively, they might become revolutionaries. Building on an observation of Mannheim's, Rosen described how frustrated "revolutionary optimism and hope give way to resignation and quietism, apathy and despair,"[47] and that this can lead to "naked mass-frenzy and a despiritualized fury."[48]

In the context of the 1960s, Rosen also took on the youth revolt, another nonreligious irrational phenomenon that he regarded as needing a fuller sociocultural explanation.[49] Although sympathetic to the political outlook of the youth movement of the time, Rosen was put off by its irrationality and potential threat to the academic culture he valued.[50] To demonstrate how culture naturally generates counterculture just as it generates madness and irrationality, he presented four case studies from the Middle Ages through the 1910s, choosing examples he could criticize for self-indulgence, cynicism, and inward vision. His analysis of youth revolts finally resembled his approach to psychic epidemics. Both occur in societies in a state of disruption and both help people deal with insecurity and meaninglessness; and while there are some psychopaths among the participants in both, neither phenomenon should be regarded as an instance of collective mental illness. In discussing both irrational revolts of youth and psychic epidemics, Rosen implicitly left room for radical progressive political movements as nonirrational alternatives—which themselves can flourish only in the proper cultural climate.[51]

Fundamentally a philosophical materialist and a believer in scientific advance, Rosen did not want the lessons of his cultural approach to be that psychiatric illness could directly touch off physical disease or that there were never proximate somatic causes for at least some mental disorders. In his discussions of "nostalgia,"[52] a pathologized form of homesickness that rose and fell as a disease entity between the mid-seventeenth and late nineteenth centuries, Rosen uncharacteristically argued against some of the historical figures who were the subject of his essay—claiming that those who believed that melancholy could cause affections of the lungs had made a mistake. While he appreciated what he would have called the "sociological explanations" that contemporaries provided for the genesis and disappearance of the psychiatric disease, he wanted to make clear that microscopic pathogens and poor living conditions could have caused the associated pneumonia or tuberculosis regardless of whether a student or soldier far from home was feeling depressed.

An argument similar in feeling prevails in his discussion of general paresis, pellagra, and cretinism.[53] Taking psychiatrists of his own day to task for adopting an obscurantist attitude toward the cause of mental illness, he reminded them that progressive doctors of the nineteenth century recognized that paresis was merely a symptom of syphilis even before the Wassermann test or the identification of spirochetes in the brains of paretics. Rosen was fighting a battle against the notion that mental illness arose from problems of individual psychodynamics. The cause of mental illness—like the cause of physical illness—in a broad sense was always cultural; but this did not mean that a pathogen, a nutritional deficiency, or a hormonal imbalance might not activate individual cases.

Rosen concerned himself not only with the social and somatic basis of mental illness but also with the cultural values embodied in social attitudes toward those perceived to be mentally disordered. He wanted to know how a society determines where madness begins on the continuum of aberrant behavior, suggesting that the answer lay in the degree of that society's tolerance for eccentricity and whether that society is equipped with "social institutions which enable such deviant individuals to function in some acceptable manner."[54] He denied that the insane were necessarily treated more poorly in the past, and especially wanted to refute the notion that before the time of Pinel and Tuke, all mental patients were shackled or condemned to a wretched existence in inhumane institutions.[55]

In a series of essays dealing with attitudes toward madness from the ancient world through early modern times,[56] Rosen showed that the nonviolent insane were generally permitted to wander freely, and that at various moments those perceived to be mad were esteemed either because they achieved a state nearer the divine or because they symbolized the folly of all humanity when compared with God and His wisdom. Rosen recognized a shift in attitudes toward the insane that he associated with Protestantism and Absolutism. Like several other observers he correlated the disappearance of leper houses with the growth of institutions for the insane and noted that by the early seventeenth century, the image of the ship of fools was replaced by that of the madhouse.[57] Rosen saw a commonality in development among the madhouse, the hospital, and the workhouse, associated with a repression of idleness based on political and economic, as well as moral, concerns.[58] For Rosen, discussion of all subsequent developments in care for the mentally ill would have to be seen in the context of social control within capitalist society.

It is interesting that to underscore his points about the social etiology of mental illness and the social determination of what constitutes madness, Rosen pointed to the modern sociological observation that it is too easy to judge the behavior of a black person in America as paranoid if one misses the fact that he or she lives in a persecuting society.[59] "From this position, it is not far to the standpoint that all individual break-downs are actually indices of a sick society, that society or culture are actually the patient."[60] Rosen pursued the historical study of attitudes, because he believed that the basis for psychiatric practice was not aberrant activity in itself but rather the societal reaction to such behavior. The fact that there were people on the streets as mad as those in mental hospitals signified to him that there are many contingencies that determine who becomes a psychiatric patient. For Rosen, the methodological issue was the relationship between sociocultural deviance and psychological abnormality.[61]

In 1972 Rosen published an essay on Freud's medical training in an illustrated anthology celebrating Freud's life and work.[62] This essay bears no relationship to the rest of Rosen's work in the history of psychiatry, but it does reveal something of his self-image. Anticipating more recent work on Freud,[63] Rosen's thesis was that as a medical student and house officer Freud was well acculturated into the world of Viennese scientific medicine, with several years in the laboratory of physiologist Ernst Brücke followed by six months in the clinic of internist Hermann Nothnagel before moving on to psychiatry. Nothnagel, fifteen years Freud's senior and the image of the successful academic doctor, remained close to Freud for decades. Deeply involved in the development of clinical research laboratories in German-language area hospitals, he encouraged Freud to think that scientific clinicians worked in the same way as the physiologists whom Freud admired. Rosen suggested that Freud, after failing as a laboratory investigator, saw Nothnagel as an alternative exemplar of maintaining science in medicine, but remained ambivalent about and jealous of the older man, to whom he felt himself superior in talent.

Rosen's work on Freud was evidently inspired by something other than his interest in social psychiatry or his desire to understand the irrational. In the work area he maintained in his Manhattan apartment, Rosen kept a collection of odd objects—chess pieces, reproductions of Egyptian statuettes, and the like—a collection described by his daughter as reminiscent of what he saw in Freud's study during a visit to the Freud Museum in London.[64] In some ways, what Rosen saw in Freud was a reflection of himself and his own aspirations: a secular Jew, a cosmopolitan intellectual, trained in medical science but inclined to the humanities, with an uncertain relationship to a mentor who was key in his early career.[65]

Interested in the mentally ill and attitudes toward them, rather than psychiatric practice, George Rosen was part of what George Mora has described as the mainstream of American psychiatric historiography.[66] Despite the innovativeness of his scholarship, though, Rosen generally has been overlooked as a major contributor to the field. This may be the result of certain stylistic problems with his work; his often repetitive thirty-odd publications in the history of psychiatry could probably have been distilled down to five or six significant articles. And while he pursued an ambitious and methodologically sound research program, hoping to achieve historical specificity as he searched for socioeconomic correlates of behavior and attitudes, he had difficulty accomplishing what he set out to do. His conclusions often failed to make adequate use of his empirical evidence, and he never fully managed to provide detail to the program with which he began his work.

Moreover, while contemporary social historians of medicine and public health generally view Rosen's work in those areas to be fundamental, historians of psychiatry and mental illness typically look to other writers in the recent past in constructing their intellectual genealogies. In approaching what has been called "the great confinement," for example, Rosen independently devised an argument similar to that put forth by Michel Foucault on the relationship between absolutism, capitalism, and institutionalization; but because Foucault's literary-philosophical method developed a vogue during the 1970s and 1980s, Rosen's history was largely overlooked by a generation of potential followers. This is particularly unfortunate, because Rosen's use of a more traditional method of empirical historical research potentially provides a more solid foundation for the conclusions drawn by both men and their successors.

Working for most of his career at a school of public health, with a formal appointment that had nothing to do with history, in isolation from the communities of both academic historians and psychiatrists, and following a research program that flowed mainly out of his own work on the history of social medicine and the social causation of somatic illness, Rosen developed an approach to the history of psychiatry that implicitly questioned most earlier scholarship and adumbrated the findings of later scholars. He refused to glorify the "great men" of the past; he turned away from intellectual history, except insofar as it provided or fed upon the general cultural context; he sought out sources other than the best-known printed medical texts; and, though he was inclined to believe in human progress, he rejected the notion that history had necessarily led away from the irrational and in the direction of more humane attitudes to those judged to be mad.

The breadth of Rosen's gaze was astounding. He tried to comprehend social attitudes and the social determinants of irrationality and madness in cultures from all parts of the world, from all historical epochs, and from all levels of industrial-economic development. Rosen worked in a field that he called the historical sociology of mental illness, and that now would be described as the social history of psychiatry. For him this necessarily meant understanding what has come to be called "social constructionism"; but even in anticipating this development, Rosen avoided its most dangerous relativistic pitfalls.

Rosen's concern with war and revolution, and his interest in religious enthusiasm and convulsive epidemics as manifestations of broad social malaise point to a basic concern with moments when "the world seems out of joint."[67] By taking up the history of psychiatry, Rosen could express his own dissatisfaction with social and cultural conditions at the same time as he could justify his academic aspirations. Throughout his career as a successful bureaucrat and academic, he continually felt a personal anxiety, and by considering past and present "ages of anxiety" he was able to participate in the world by writing about it. He expressed basic truths of a radical worldview in connecting the personal to the social; but he made the emotional or religious response to social upheaval dominant. For Rosen the political response was less problematic intellectually, though it did not suit him temperamentally.

In a sense, Rosen was contributing to a project undertaken by Marx in *The German Ideology*, by Mannheim in developing *Wissenschaftsociologie*, and by Gramsci (with whose writings there is no evidence of Rosen's familiarity) in his attempts to understand hegemony. By approaching the irrational—whether in the form of insanity, religious enthusiasm, youth revolts, or even social attitudes—Rosen was trying to understand the dominant thought patterns of a particular era, and what in the material existence of members of a given society caused ideologies to arise and be perpetuated.

Rosen was always conscious and somewhat proud of being identifiable as a New Yorker of proletarian Jewish origin[68] who succeeded by hard work and intelligence despite the obstacles set against him. Very much rooted in Enlightenment thought, he dealt with his own irrational tendencies by confronting the social roots of irrationality. In one discussion of religious frenzy, he hinted at such a direct connection between his work and his life:

> These phenomena are irrational in that among those who exhibit such behavior emotion overrides reason, but this does not mean that they are inaccessible to rational analysis. How to explain these phenomena is to be answered on several levels, social, cultural and psychological . . . An important factor . . . is socio-cultural alienation which may be a consequence of repression on grounds of religion, race, ethnicity, class, or sex. Alienation develops where desires and aspirations of individuals and groups are blocked by the absence of suitable channels and means for expression and achievement, by deliberate policies of repression and segregation, and above all where fear, insecurity and a sense of powerlessness pervade the socio-psychological atmosphere.[69]

Rosen insisted that the boundary between eccentricity and the sort of erratic behavior that indicated madness was very movable and, without using the phrase, socially constructed. To prove his point, he provided much evidence on tolerance of odd behavior in a range of historical periods. He pointed out that madness could be esteemed in certain social settings, and that people could act extremely irrationally without being mad at all. Rosen had hoped to analyze the irrational and to "naturalize" it by explaining it in cultural terms. For Rosen, very self-consciously an intellectual descendant of eighteenth-century rationalism,[70] this was an important tactic for survival in a world that made him feel very uneasy.

Notes

1. I would like to acknowledge Mark Micale's assistance in getting a late draft of this essay in shape for publication and for helping me to understand Rosen's work within the context of more recent historiography of psychiatry.

2. The appended bibliography is a complete list of Rosen's work related to psychiatry. His *Madness in Society: Chapters in the Historical Sociology of Mental Illness* (Chicago: University of Chicago Press, 1968) is essentially a compilation of eight articles prepared originally for publication elsewhere, with two new chapters on madness in ancient times (portions of which were themselves reprinted in other publications). Rosen acknowledged that this book was put together hastily and that the material in it was not well integrated. He justified this on the grounds

that the book was intended as "the illustration of an approach" that he intended to develop further in another volume (Rosen to Otto Klineberg, 20 March 1969, George Rosen Papers, Yale University Archives Manuscript Group 862 [hereinafter GRP], addition of 28 August 1978).

3. Mora, "Three American Historians of Psychiatry: Albert Deutsch, Gregory Zilboorg, George Rosen" in Edwin R. Wallace IV and Lucius C. Pressley (eds.), *Essays in the History of Psychiatry: A Tenth Anniversary Supplementary Volume to the Psychiatric Forum* (Columbia, South Carolina: Wm. S. Hall Psychiatric Institute, 1980), 14.

4. From Baltimore, Sigerist helped organize the New York Society for Medical History, on whose executive committee in 1941 sat Rosen, Zilboorg, and Deutsch. Early in his career, Rosen also participated in the Kings County (Brooklyn) Medical Society's Section on History of Medicine, at one meeting of which he shared the podium with Iago Galdston, who spoke on a psychiatric topic. I am grateful to Milton Roemer for providing photocopies of several documents originating from the New York Society, and for a copy of his unpublished talk "George Rosen: Historian of Social Medicine," delivered at the American Public Health Association's memorial session in honor of Rosen, 2 November 1977, in which he discussed Sigerist's relationship with the New York Society. A flier advertising the program of the Kings County Society is in GRP, accession of March 1978, Box II.

5. See Deutsch, *The Mentally Ill in America* (New York: Doubleday, 1937), and Zilboorg, *The Medical Man and the Witch during the Renaissance* (Baltimore: Johns Hopkins Press, 1935). Zilboorg left to some "future historical sociologist" the responsibility of finding "a definite scientific explanation for the various forces that combined to make the idea of the witch such a tenaciously cruel and almost ineradicable concept in medicine" (p. 91). Rosen, a historian with a doctorate in sociology, may have considered himself the appropriate person to take up Zilboorg's challenge. Mora (1980, p. 19) notes, however, that Rosen, despite his tremendous knowledge of the literature, never cited Zilboorg on the witchcraft issue. Rosen believed Zilboorg to be wrong in viewing as mad those accused of witchcraft. Since he liked and respected Zilboorg, Rosen may have preferred not to attack him directly.

6. Rosen, "Historical Background" in *Mental Health Teaching in Schools of Public Health* (New York: Columbia University School of Public Health and Administrative Medicine, 1961), 1–75; reprinted as "Public Health and Mental Health: Converging Trends and Emerging Issues" in *Madness in Society*, 263–328).

7. Gerald Grob, *From Asylum to Community: Mental Health Policy in Modern America* (Princeton: Princeton University Press, 1991), 16–23.

8. Ibid., 20.

9. Ibid., 53.

10. Thomas A. C. Rennie, "Social Psychiatry—A Definition." *International Journal of Social Psychiatry*, i (1955), 10.

11. For more on the social medicine movement of the 1940s, see Dorothy Watkins (Porter), "What Was Social Medicine? A Historiography of the Concept (or, George Rosen Revisited)," *Bulletin of the Society for the Social History of Medicine*, no. 38 (1985), 47–51; Dorothy Porter and Roy Porter, "What Was Social Medicine? An Historiographical Essay," *Journal of Historical Sociology*, i (1989), 90–106; and Dorothy Porter, "Changing Disciplines: John Ryle and the Making of Social Medicine in Britain in the 1940s," *History of Science*, xxx (1992), 137–164.

12. Rosen, "Social Stress and Mental Disease from the 18th Century to the Present: Some Origins of Social Psychiatry," *Milbank Memorial Fund Quarterly*, xxxvii (1959), 5–32 (reprinted as "Some Origins of Social Psychiatry: Social Stress and Mental Disease from the Eighteenth Century to the Present" in *Madness in Society*, 172–184).

13. Unless otherwise noted, information on Rosen's life throughout this essay was abstracted from a series of interviews with relatives, friends, and associates of Rosen. I would especially like to acknowledge the cooperation of Dr. Beate Caspari-Rosen, Dr. Louis Schneider, Prof. Susan Koslow (aka Susan Rosen-Olejarz), Prof. Arnold Koslow, and Mr. Erich Meyerhoff. I

have discussed Rosen's life and career in greater depth in "George Rosen, Public Health and History" in George Rosen's *A History of Public Health*, reprint ed. (Baltimore: Johns Hopkins University Press, 1993).

14. See Rosen, "Medicine under Hitler," *Bulletin of the New York Academy of Medicine*, xxv (1949), 125–129.

15. Rosen later translated the thesis and published it as *The Reception of William Beaumont's Discovery in Europe* (New York: Schuman's, 1942).

16. The entire Rosen–Sigerist correspondence through June 1947 is preserved in the papers of the Institute of the History of Medicine at the Alan Mason Chesney Medical Archives of the Johns Hopkins Medical Institution (hereinafter IHMP). Unless otherwise noted, all discussion of Rosen's activities through 1947 is based on this correspondence.

17. His dissertation, *The Specialization of Medicine with Particular Reference to Ophthalmology* (New York: Froben Press, 1944), remains a standard work.

18. Ackerknecht to Rosen, 7 March 1947 (GRP, addition of 4 June 1979, Box II). Ackerknecht, who was not Jewish but had been a political refugee from Nazi Germany, admired Rosen's continuing self-identification as a Jew. See Ackerknecht, "George Rosen as I Knew Him," *Journal of the History of Medicine and Allied Sciences*, xxxiii (1978), 254–255.

19. See John Z. Bowers, "Remarks at George Rosen Memorial Service, 14 October 1977, Yale University," *Journal of the History of Medicine and Allied Sciences*, xxxiii (1978), 256. A good source on the early history of HIP is Louis L. Feldman, "Organization of a Medical Group Practice Prepayment Program in New York City" (New York: Health Insurance Plan of Greater New York, 1953), mimeographed.

20. Rosen, "Disease and Social Criticism: A Contribution to a Theory of Medical History," *Bulletin of the History of Medicine*, x (1941), 5–15.

21. See Rosen, "Some Pre-Suppositions of Marxian Socialism" (unpublished typescript [1942], GRP, addition of 15 June 1979, Box I); and Rosen, "The Biological Element in Human History," *Medical History*, i (1957), 150–159. In 1975, Rosen recommended to a publishing house that it reject a manuscript that proposed that biological factors determined much of human history. He wrote: "After all, the acts of empire builders . . . were not simply a matter of bio-chemical urges, but involved human thought and intentionality" (Rosen to Jeffrey House, 16 January 1975, GRP, addition of 28 August 1978, Box V).

22. Rosen, "John Elliotson—Physician and Hypnotist," *Bulletin of the History of Medicine*, iv (1936), 600–603.

23. Rosen, "Mesmerism and Surgery: A Strange Chapter in the History of Anesthesia," *Journal of the History of Medicine and Allied Sciences*, i (1946), 328–339.

24. A well-received recent study that places Elliotson and his interest in mesmerism and phrenology clearly within the broader context of early Victorian medical radicalism is Adrian J. Desmond, *The Politics of Evolution* (Chicago: University of Chicago Press, 1989).

25. [Rosen], "Some Ancient References to Sexual Abnormalities," *Ciba Symposia*, ii (1940), 492; and [Rosen] "Homosexuality in Primitive Societies," *Ciba Symposia*, ii (1940), 495.

26. Rosen, "Political Order and Human Health in Jeffersonian Thought," *Bulletin of the History of Medicine*, xxvi (1952), 32–44.

27. Ibid., 34.

28. See, for example, Rosen, "Social Stress and Mental Disease."

29. See, for example, Rosen, "What is Social Medicine? A Genetic Analysis of the Concept," *Bulletin of the History of Medicine*, xxi (1947), 674–733.

30. Rosen urged that Virchow's view "be seen in terms of a concept of an 'organic' historical process, clearly a concept with Hegelian overtones" ("Social Stress and Mental Disease," 14).

31. Rosen, "Psychopathology in the Social Process: II. Dance Frenzies, Demonic Possession,

Revival Movements and Similar So-called Psychic Epidemics: An Interpretation,'' *Bulletin of the History of Medicine*, xxxvi (1962), 13–44 (reprinted as ''Psychic Epidemics in Europe and the United States: Dance Frenzies, Demonic Possession, Revival Movements and Related Phenomena, Fourteenth to Twentieth Centuries'' in *Madness in Society*, 195–225).

32. See especially, Rosen, ''Enthusiasm: A Dark Lanthorn of the Spirit,'' *Bulletin of the History of Medicine*, xlii (1968), 393–421.

33. First published as ''Science, Technology & Society in Seventeenth-Century England,'' *Osiris*, iv (1938), 360–632. Rosen wrote to Sigerist as soon as he heard of Merton's dissertation to ask whether the Institute of the History of Medicine had a copy he could borrow (Rosen to Sigerist, 28 May 1938, IHMP).

34. See Rosen, ''Left-Wing Puritanism and Science,'' *Bulletin of the History of Medicine*, xv (1944), 375–380.

35. See, for example, Rosen, ''Social Aspects of Jacob Henle's Medical Thought,'' *Bulletin of the History of Medicine*, v (1937), 509–537.

36. Rosen, ''Psychopathology in the Social Process: I. A Study of the Persecution of Witches in Europe as a Contribution to the Understanding of Mass Delusions and Psychic Epidemics,'' *Journal of Health and Human Behavior*, i (1960), 200–211 (reprinted as ''Psychopathology in the Social Process'' in *Madness in Society*, 1–20). Unfortunately, it is impossible to discuss this article without reference to the likelihood that Rosen copied a portion of it almost directly from a 1959 essay by H. R. Trevor-Roper (see Trevor-Roper, ''Words'' *New York Review of Books*, 31 August 1972, p. 330). Rosen's plagiarism, here or elsewhere, is of a piece with what is frequently wrong with his writing. For over thirty years he produced prolifically in medical history for no pay while earning his living in medical practice and public health. His writing, therefore, often reflects a certain haste. He freely reused his own prose—and occasionally, without attribution, apparently used the prose of others. In this case we can suppose that he took almost verbatim notes, lost the citation, and later assumed the words were his own all along. Rosen's writing is sloppy in many ways. If—because his intentions were good and his object was greater enlightenment—he can be forgiven for some very clumsy prose, he can also be forgiven for very occasionally borrowing from other authors.

37. Gregory Zilboorg is generally regarded as the chief twentieth-century exponent of the view that a great advance occurred in the seventeenth century when physicians like Johann Weyer claimed that witches were mentally ill rather than possessed by Satan. See Zilboorg, *The Medical Man and the Witch*, and idem, *A History of Medical Psychology* (New York: Norton, 1941). This position, originally developed by nineteenth-century psychiatrists in search of a myth of origin, has been challenged since the middle 1970s, but with little reference to Rosen's anti-Zilboorgian contribution. See, for example, Thomas J. Schoeneman, ''The Role of Mental Illness in the European Witch Hunts of the Sixteenth and Seventeenth Centuries: An Assessment,'' *Journal of the History of the Behavioral Sciences*, xiii (1977), 337–351, which briefly mentions Rosen's work in two places (pp. 340, 354) and cites the 1968 *Madness in Society* rather than Rosen's original 1960 publication. Historians of psychiatry would also do well to look to nonspecialist European historians for broader cultural interpretations of witch-hunting. See, especially, H. R. Trevor-Roper, ''The European Witch-craze of the Sixteenth and Seventeenth Centuries'' in his *Religion, the Reformation, and Social Change, and Other Essays* (London: Macmillan, 1967), 90–192. The question of mental illness, witch-hunting, and the origins of psychiatry is taken up elsewhere in this volume by Patrick Vandermeersch.

38. Milton Roemer, for example, lamented to Rosen in 1953 that he had little chance of an academic position, because of his outspoken leftist position on health insurance (Roemer to Rosen, 10 June 1953, GRP, accession of 28 October 1978).

39. Rosen, ''Dance Frenzies.''

40. Ibid, 16.

41. Ibid, 19.

42. Rosen, "Social Change and Psychopathology in the Emotional Climate of Millennial Movements," *American Behavioral Scientist,* xvi (1972), 157.

43. In personal communications, Rosen's daughter, Susan Koslow (aka Susan Rosen-Olejarz), and his former son-in-law, Arnold Koslow, have described Rosen's pride in his ability to supervise a ritual Passover seder despite his lack of any religious belief.

44. Ackerknecht, "Psychopathology, Primitive Medicine and Primitive Culture," *Bulletin of the History of Medicine,* xiv (1944), 30–67. See also the April 1942 issue of *Ciba Symposia* (vol. 4, no. 1), whose theme was "Shamans and Medicine Men."

45. Rosen, *Madness in Society,* 57.

46. Rosen, "Emotion and Sensibility in Ages of Anxiety: A Comparative Historical Review," *American Journal of Psychiatry,* cxxiv (1967), 771–784.

47. Ibid., 775.

48. Karl Mannheim, *Ideology and Utopia* (New York: Harcourt, Brace & Co., 1936), 193, as quoted in "Emotion and Sensibility in Ages of Anxiety," 775.

49. "The Revolt of Youth: Some Historical Comparisons," *Yale Journal of Biology and Medicine,* xlii (1969), 86–98 (reprinted in J. Zubin and A. M. Freedman [eds.], *The Psychopathology of Adolescence* [New York: Grune & Stratton, 1970], 1–14).

50. Personal communication from Dr. Beate Caspari-Rosen.

51. Rosen, "Emotion and Sensibility," 781.

52. Rosen, "Percussion and Nostalgia," *Journal of the History of Medicine and Allied Sciences,* xxvii (1972), 447–450; Rosen, "Nostalgia: A 'Forgotten' Psychological Disorder," *Clio Medica,* x (1975), 28–51 (reprinted in *Psychological Medicine,* v [1975], 340–354).

53. Rosen, "Patterns of Discovery and Control of Mental Illness," *American Journal of Public Health,* i (1960), 855–866 (reprinted in *Madness in Society,* 247–262).

54. Rosen, *Madness in Society,* 102.

55. See Rosen, "Social Attitudes to Irrationality and Madness in 17th and 18th Century Europe," *Journal of the History of Medicine and Allied Sciences,* xviii (1963), 220–240 (reprinted as "Irrationality and Madness in Seventeenth and Eighteenth Century Europe" in *Madness in Society,* 151–171). In this essay, Rosen particularly criticized Zilboorg for regarding all of history to the end of the eighteenth century as characterized by incarceration of the mentally ill. A revisionist view similar to Rosen's has flourished since the mideighties, but with minimal reference to Rosen's contribution. See, for example, Roy Porter, *Mind-Forg'd Manacles: A History of Madness in England from the Restoration to the Regency* (London: Athlone, 1987), ch. 3; Patricia H. Allderidge, "Bedlam: Fact or Fantasy?" in W. F. Bynum, Roy Porter, and Michael Shepherd (eds.), *The Anatomy of Madness,* ii (London: Tavistock, 1985), 17–33; Allderidge, "Management and Mismanagement at Bedlam, 1547–1633" in Charles Webster (ed.), *Health, Medicine and Mortality in the Sixteenth Century* (Cambridge: Cambridge University Press, 1979); and Jonathan Andrews, "A History of Bethlem Hospital, c.1600–c.1750" (Ph.D. diss., University of London, 1990).

56. "Ancient Palestine and Neighboring Adjacent Areas" in *Madness in Society,* 21–70 (a portion of which appeared earlier as "Is Saul also among the Prophets?" *Gesnerus,* xxiii [1966], 132–146); "Greece and Rome" in *Madness in Society,* 71–136 (partially reprinted as "Some Notes on Greek and Roman Attitudes Toward the Mentally Ill" in Lloyd G. Stevenson and Robert P. Multhauf [eds.], *Medicine, Science and Culture: Historical Essays in Honor of Owsei Temkin* [Baltimore: Johns Hopkins Press, 1968], 17–24); "The Mentally Ill and the Community in Western and Central Europe during the Late Middle Ages and the Renaissance," *Journal of the History of Medicine and Allied Sciences,* xix (1964), 377–388 (reprinted as "Western and Central Europe During the Late Middle Ages and the Renaissance" in *Madness in Society,* 139–150); "Social Attitudes to Irrationality and Madness in 17th and 18th Century Europe," *Journal of the History of Medicine and Allied Sciences,* xviii (1963), 220–240 (reprinted as "Irrationality and Madness in Seventeenth and Eighteenth Century Europe" in *Madness in Society,* 151–171);

"Modes of Feeling and Intellectual Attitudes toward Medical Problems from the Late Fifteenth to the Seventeenth Centuries: Current Problems in the History of Medicine" in *Proceedings of the XIXth International Congress of the History of Medicine, Basel, 1964* (Basel: Karger, 1966), 142–154; "Cross-Cultural and Historical Approaches" in Paul H. Hoch and Joseph Zubin (eds.), *Psychopathology of Aging* (New York: Grune & Stratton, 1961), 1–20 (reprinted as "Psychopathology of Ageing: Cross-Cultural and Historical Approaches" in *Madness in Society*, 229–246); and "History in the Study of Suicide," *Psychological Medicine*, i (1971) *1*: 267–285 (reprinted as "History" in Seymour Perlin [ed.], *A Handbook for the Study of Suicide* [New York: Oxford University Press, 1975], 3–29).

57. "The Mentally Ill and the Community," 381. Rosen's cited sources on the relationship between leprosaria and insane asylums are F. R. Salter (ed.), *Some Early Tracts on Poor Relief* (London: Methuen, 1926), 16; and T. Kirchhoff, *Grundriss einer Geschichte der Deutschen Irrenpflege* (Berlin: Hirschwald, 1890), 93ff. Kirchhoff's book, in particular, was a major source for this entire article of Rosen's. Interestingly, Rosen makes no reference to Foucault—with whom the idea of madhouses taking the place of leper houses is most closely associated—here or anywhere else in his writings on mental illness.

58. "Social Attitudes to Irrationality and Madness," 227.

59. "Mental Disorder, Social Deviance and Culture Pattern: Some Methodological Issues in the Historical Study of Mental Illness" in George Mora and Jeanne L. Brand (eds.), *Psychiatry and Its History: Methodological Problems in Research* (Springfield, Illinois: Charles C Thomas, 1970), 174.

60. Ibid, 180.

61. "Symptoms of mental disorder begin as violations of social norms. . . ." Ibid., 175.

62. Rosen, "Freud and Medicine in Vienna" in Jonathan Miller (ed.), *Freud: The Man, His World, His Influence* (London: Weidenfeld and Nicolson, 1972), 22–39 (reprinted as "Freud and Medicine in Vienna: Some Scientific and Medical Sources of His Thought," *Psychological Medicine*, ii [1972], 332–344).

63. See, for example, Frank J. Sulloway, *Freud, Biologist of the Mind: Beyond the Psychoanalytic Legend* (New York: Basic, 1979).

64. Personal communication from Susan Koslow (aka Susan Rosen-Olejarz).

65. Rosen noted that Freud wrote about Nothnagel in 1924, twenty years after Nothnagel's death, minimizing the older man's influence ("Freud and Medicine in Vienna," 34). Curiously, in 1976, almost twenty years after Sigerist died, Rosen replied to an inquiry about Sigerist with some bitterness about the older man's unwillingness to devote himself to the task of creating more chairs of medical history in the United States. Rosen also denied that Sigerist had ever really understood sociology (Rosen to Fernando C. Vescia, 22 December 1976, GRP). On the other hand, according to Rosen's former son-in-law, Arnold Koslow, Rosen "always talked of Sigerist with adulation" (interview with Arnold Koslow, August 1991).

66. Mora (1980), 1.

67. "Emotion and Sensibility," 773.

68. Ackerknecht, "George Rosen as I Knew Him."

69. "Forms of Irrationality in the Eighteenth Century" in Harold E. Pagliaro (ed.), *Irrationalism in the Eighteenth-Century*, Studies in Eighteenth-Century Culture, vol. 2. (Cleveland: Press of Case Western Reserve University, 1972), 261–262.

70. The philosopher Arnold Koslow, Rosen's former son-in-law, reported in a personal communication that "he was like an eighteenth-century rationalist studying madness."

Addendum—George Rosen: Writings on the History of Mental Illness

1936 "John Elliotson—Physician and Hypnotist," *Bulletin of the History of Medicine*, iv, 600–603.

1940 "Some Ancient References to Sexual Abnormalities," *Ciba Symposia*, ii, 492.
"Homosexuality in Primitive Societies," *Ciba Symposia*, ii, 495.

1946 "Mesmerism and Surgery: A Strange Chapter in the History of Anesthesia," *Journal of the History of Medicine and Allied Sciences*, i, 328–339.

1948 "From Mesmerism to Hypnotism," *Ciba Symposia*, ix, 838–844.

1952 "Political Order and Human Health in Jeffersonian Thought," *Bulletin of the History of Medicine*, xxvi, 32–44.

1953 "History of Medical Hypnosis" in Jerome C. Schneck (ed.), *Hypnosis in Modern Medicine* (Springfield, Illinois: Charles C Thomas), 3–27.

1959 "Social Stress and Mental Disease from the 18th Century to the Present: Some Origins of Social Psychiatry," *Milbank Memorial Fund Quarterly*, xxxvii, 5–32. (Reprinted as "Some Origins of Social Psychiatry: Social Stress and Mental Disease from the Eighteenth Century to the Present" in *Madness in Society* [1968], 172–184.)

1960 "Psychopathology in the Social Process: I. A Study of the Persecution of Witches in Europe as a Contribution to the Understanding of Mass Delusions and Psychic Epidemics," *Journal of Health and Human Behavior*, i, 200–211. (Reprinted as "Psychopathology in the Social Process" in *Madness in Society* [1968], 1–20.)
"Patterns of Discovery and Control of Mental Illness, *American Journal of Public Health*," 1, 855–866. (Reprinted in *Madness in Society* [1968], 247–262.)

1961 "Cross-Cultural and Historical Approaches" in P. H. Hoch and J. Zubin (eds.), *Psychopathology of Aging* (New York: Grune & Stratton), 1–20. (Reprinted as "Psychopathology of Ageing: Cross-Cultural and Historical Approaches" in *Madness in Society* [1968] 229–246.
"Discussion of Alexander H. Leighton: Cultures as a Causative of Mental Disorder," *Milbank Memorial Fund Quarterly*, xxxix, 471–485.
"Public Health and Mental Health: Converging Trends and Emerging Issues; Historical Background" in *Mental Health Teaching in Schools of Public Health* (New York: Columbia University School of Public Health and Administrative Medicine), 1–75. (Reprinted in *Madness in Society* [1968], 263–328.)

1962 "Psychopathology in the Social Process: II. Dance Frenzies, Demonic Possession, Revival Movements and Similar So-Called Psychic Epidemics: An Interpretation," *Bulletin of the History of Medicine*, xxxvi, 13–44. (Reprinted as "Psychic Epidemics in Europe and the United States: Dance Frenzies, Demonic Possession, Revival Movements and Related Phenomena, Fourteenth to Twentieth Centuries" in *Madness in Society* [1968], 195–225.)

1963 "Social Attitudes to Irrationality and Madness in 17th and 18th Century Europe," *Journal of the History of Medicine and Allied Sciences*, xviii, 220–240. (Reprinted as "Irrationality and Madness in Seventeenth and Eighteenth Century Europe" in *Madness in Society* [1968], 151–171.)

1964 "The Mentally Ill and the Community in Western and Central Europe during the Late Middle Ages and the Renaissance," *Journal of the History of Medicine and Allied Sciences*, xix, 377–388. (Reprinted as "Western and Central Europe During the Late Middle Ages and the Renaissance" in *Madness in Society* [1968], 139–150.)

1966 "Modes of Feeling and Intellectual Attitudes toward Medical Problems from the Late Fifteenth to the Seventeenth Centuries: Current Problems in the History of Medicine" in *Proceedings of the XIXth International Congress of the History of Medicine, Basel, 1964* (Basel: Karger), 142–154.

"Is Saul Also among the Prophets?" *Gesnerus*, xxiii, 132–146. (Reprinted as pp. 21–34 of "Ancient Palestine and Neighboring Adjacent Areas" in *Madness in Society* [1968]).

1967 "People, Disease, and Emotion: Some Newer Problems for Research in Medical History," *Bulletin of the History of Medicine*, xli, 5–23.

"Emotion and Sensibility in Ages of Anxiety: A Comparative Historical Review," *American Journal of Psychiatry*, cxxiv, 771–784.

1968 *Madness in Society: Chapters in the Historical Sociology of Mental Illness* (London: Routledge & Kegan Paul; Chicago: University of Chicago Press). Spanish translation, 1974.

"Some Notes on Greek and Roman Attitudes Toward the Mentally Ill" in Lloyd G. Stevenson and Robert P. Multhauf (eds.), *Medicine, Science and Culture: Historical Essays in Honor of Owsei Temkin* (Baltimore: Johns Hopkins Press, 1968), 17–24. "This paper . . . forms part of a chapter . . . in *Madness in Society* (i.e., pp. 83–90)."

"Enthusiasm: A Dark Lanthorn of the Spirit," *Bulletin of the History of Medicine*, xlii, 393–421.

"Benjamin Rush" in *International Encyclopedia of the Social Sciences*, xiii (New York: Free Press), 588–589.

1969 "The Revolt of Youth: Some Historical Comparisons," *Yale Journal of Biology and Medicine*, xlii, 86–98. (Reprinted in J. Zubin and A. M. Freedman [eds.], *The Psychopathology of Adolescence* [New York: Grune & Stratton, 1970], 1–14.)

1970 "Mental Disorder, Social Deviance and Culture Pattern: Some Methodological Issues in the Historical Study of Mental Illness" in George Mora and Jeanne L. Brand (eds.), *Psychiatry and Its History: Methodological Problems in Research*. Springfield, Illinois: Charles C Thomas), 172–194.

1971 "Auenbrugger on Suicide" in Hans-Heinz Eulner et al. (eds.), *Medizingeschichte in unserer Zeit* (Stuttgart: Enke), 294–299.

"History in the Study of Suicide," *Psychological Medicine*, i, 267–285. (Reprinted as "History" in Seymour Perlin [ed.], *A Handbook for the Study of Suicide* [New York: Oxford University Press, 1975], 3–29.)

1972 "Forms of Irrationality in the Eighteenth Century" in Harold E. Pagliaro (ed.), *Irrationalism in the Eighteenth Century* (Cleveland: Press of Case Western Reserve University), 255–288. (Studies in Eighteenth Century Culture, ii.)

"Editorial: Psyche and History," *Psychological Medicine*, ii, 205–207.

"Freud and Medicine in Vienna: Some Scientific and Medical Sources of His Thought," *Psychological Medicine*, ii, 332–344. (Reprinted as "Freud and Medicine in Vienna" in Jonathan Miller [ed.], *Freud: The Man, His World, His Influence* [London: Weidenfeld and Nicolson], 22–39.)

"Percussion and Nostalgia," *Journal of the History of Medicine and Allied Sciences*, xxvii, 447–450.

"Social Change and Psychopathology in the Emotional Climate of Millennial Movements," *American Behavioral Scientist*, xvi, 153–167.

1975 "Nostalgia: a 'Forgotten' Psychological Disorder," *Clio Medica*, x, 28–51. (Reprinted in *Psychological Medicine*, v [1975], 340–354.)

1976 "Benjamin Rush on Health and the American Revolution," *American Journal of Public Health*, lxvi, 397–398.

6

Henri F. Ellenberger: The History of Psychiatry as the History of the Unconscious

MARK S. MICALE

The French-Canadian medical historian Henri F. Ellenberger is best remembered today as the author of *The Discovery of the Unconscious*, published in 1970.[1] A brilliant, encyclopedic study of psychological theory and therapeutics from primitive times to the middle of the twentieth century, Ellenberger's book was widely regarded upon publication as a major, masterly work. Twenty years later, it remains simply indispensable to research in many areas of the history of psychology, psychiatry, and psychoanalysis.

In addition to *The Discovery of the Unconscious*, Ellenberger across a span of some thirty years has produced many shorter writings in psychiatric history. His first piece of historical scholarship, which is all but impossible to locate today, was a short but factually dense and highly interesting monograph on the history of psychiatry in Switzerland.[2] Furthermore, before the appearance of *The Discovery of the Unconscious*, Ellenberger had published approximately twenty articles on historical subjects, and since 1970 has written fifteen additional essays of a historical nature.[3] Many of these shorter pieces exhibit the same outstanding qualities found in the book, including the isolation of new or ignored subject matters and the mining of rich, previously untapped, primary source materials. With all of Ellenberger's writings, the chronological emphasis is on the nineteenth and twentieth centuries, the methodological concentration is on the clinical, cultural, and intellectual aspects of the psychological sciences, and the geographical focus is on the Central and Western European experiences.

Upon initial publication, *The Discovery of the Unconscious* was widely reviewed and very well received. The book was acknowledged early on as a minor classic in the field—as one reviewer commented, it established Ellenberger at once as "the premier historian of 'dynamic psychiatry' "[4]—and within five years the volume had been translated into Spanish, Italian, German, French, and Japanese. Curiously, however, since the early 1970's Ellenberger has been largely invisible, both personally and professionally. There appear to be a number of reasons for this: Lacking a position within the academy, Ellenberger found it difficult to secure a format for the professional sponsorship of his additional scholarly work. Within the Montreal psychiatric community, his therapeutic allegiances to psychodynamism increasingly marginalized him with the coming of biological psychiatry, while his historical interests were regarded as quaintly but rather irrelevantly antiquarian. At the same time, the steady current of Freudian revisionism running throughout his book caused many psychoanalytic readers in the United States and Canada to qualify their enthusiasm for him. In addition, due to the rise of the so-called new social history within professional historical studies and to the development within Anglo-American psychiatry of debates about the process of decarcerating patients in mental hospitals, the attention of psychiatric historians during the 1970s was riveted on the social and institutional aspects of the field (i.e., on the "rise of the asylum"). In contrast, the sorts of cultural, intellectual, and clinical questions that Ellenberger addressed fell into comparative neglect. Ellenberger was wounded by these circumstances, and for these as well as other reasons he began a process of withdrawal from public view that has continued up to the present. As a consequence, most readers, including many specialists in the field, are unfamiliar with Ellenberger's articles written during the past two decades. Many people, North Americans and Europeans alike, have the impression that he is no longer alive.*

Fortunately, this undeserved obscurity has begun to change. A scholarly conference held recently in Toronto, Canada, and devoted to the history of psychoanalysis was dedicated to Ellenberger.[5] In October 1990, at the first meeting of the European Association of the History of Psychiatry in s'Hertogenbosch, the Netherlands, where nearly 200 psychiatric historians from a dozen countries gathered for the first time, Ellenberger was unanimously elected Honorary Chairman of the organization. And in the United States, a substantial English-language collection of Ellenberger's historical essays, equipped with extensive historiographical and bio-bibliographical apparatus evaluating his work, has just appeared.[6] Most significant have been events in France. From a lifetime of research in European libraries and archives, Ellenberger amassed a formidable collection of historical materials, including roughly 2,000 books and over thirty crates of printed and archival documents. In 1986, Ellenberger, with the guidance of his son Michel Ellenberger, offered the bulk of his personal library and archives to the *Société internationale d'histoire de la psychiatrie et de la psychiatrie* in Paris. The French, who had received *The Discovery of the Unconscious* less ambiguously than the North American medical community, accepted the offer with notable enthusiasm. In March 1992, a special *Centre de recherche et de documentation*, designated officially as the *Institut Henri Ellenberger*, opened in the main library building of the Sainte Anne Hospital in the French capital. This center will house the contents of Ellenberger's collection in combination with other historical materials in what is likely to become a major resource for historians in the future.[7]

These recent developments establish Ellenberger's position as one of the most important commentators on modern psychiatric history. In retrospect, we can see that Ellenberger forms part of a group of brilliant *indépendants*—other figures in the group including Richard Hunter, Ida Macalpine, George Rosen, and Jean Starobinski—who emerged during the 1940s and 1950s at the highpoint of the intellectual and professional prestige of psychiatry in the West. These individuals were trained medically, but they were distanced—in some cases, alienated—from the dominant doctrinal theories and

---

*Editors' Note: On May 1, 1993, while this book was in production, Henri Ellenberger died, at the age of 88.

practices of the psychiatric communities of their day. Furthermore, they tended to be exceptionally creative and cross-disciplinary in their interests. As a result, they were able to formulate their own highly distinctive interpretive perspectives on the historical meaning and evolution of the field. Moreover, Ellenberger in particular anticipates in a striking number of ways many of the most significant developments in present-day psychiatric history writing. In other regards, his writings point forward to fresh areas of inquiry still awaiting exploration. Perhaps more than any other figure canvassed in this volume, Ellenberger merits characterization as the founding figure of European psychiatric historiography. Finally, as I have proposed elsewhere, Ellenberger has managed to achieve a uniquely broad *sociocultural* perspective on the history of the mental sciences and as such may be read as a cultural critic of our psychological century as a whole.[8]

Henri Frédéric Ellenberger was born on November 6, 1905, in southern Africa. Ellenberger issued from a large, French-speaking, Swiss family from the town of Yverdon near Lake Neuchâtel, which since the middle of the nineteenth century had worked as European Protestant missionaries at various locations in the south of Africa. Ellenberger's parents and grandparents on both his paternal and maternal sides had distinguished themselves outside of their religious work through numerous books about the languages and ethnography of native African populations. After passing his childhood in what was then Northern Rhodesia, Ellenberger received his secondary schooling at various locations in France and his undergraduate education at the University of Strasbourg from which he received his baccalaureate degree in *Lettres-philosophie* in 1924. During the late 1920s and early 1930s, he attended medical school at the University of Paris, where he decided almost immediately upon a specialty in psychiatry. He received his medical degree in 1934, writing his dissertation on the affective states of catatonic psychoses.[9]

Fond of France but disadvantaged by the hierarchical Parisian medical system, Ellenberger upon graduation moved to Poitiers in the department of Vienne in west-central France where he spent the remainder of the 1930s. Here he operated a small private practice as a *spécialiste des maladies nerveuses*. During the years in Poitiers, Ellenberger developed a strong interest in transcultural psychiatry—or "ethnopsychiatry" as he has always preferred to call it—a field he helped to pioneer.[10]

In the spring of 1941, due to the military and political situation in France, Ellenberger, with his wife and their four young children, left Poitiers and traveled to Switzerland. For two years during the early 1940s, he worked as senior psychiatrist at the Waldau Mental Hospital near Bern. Then, from 1943 to 1952, he served as associate director, or *Oberarzt*, at the Breitenau Mental Hospital in the beautiful, historic town of Schaffhausen. The Breitenau Hospital was the public psychiatric facility for the town and the canton of Schaffhausen, and Ellenberger worked there with a range of patients including the acutely and chronically psychotic. During the Schaffhausen years, he also became well acquainted with a large number of psychiatry's oldtimers who had been members of the first generation of Swiss psychiatry and psychoanalysis, including Manfred Bleuler, Carl Gustav Jung, Ludwig Binswanger, Alphonse Maeder, Leopold Szondi, and Oskar Pfister. With Pfister, the lay pastor and psychoanalyst who had been on intimate terms for many years with the Freud family, Ellenberger underwent an informal training analysis in Zurich during the early 1950s.

Ultimately, however, the career of provincial asylum doctor and administrator frustrated Ellenberger. Late in 1952, in a major shift in his career, Ellenberger accepted an offer to join the staff of the Menninger Clinic in Topeka, Kansas, in the United States as a professor of clinical psychiatry and special assistant to Karl Menninger. He remained in America for six years. During the 1940s and 1950s, the Menninger Clinic had evolved into the most important facility for the education of mental health professionals in North America while Karl Menninger was at the peak of his prestige in the American psychiatric world. With a close association to the Topeka Psychoanalytic Institute and a large number of European emigré psychoanalysts on its staff, the overwhelming theoretical and therapeutic orientation of the institution during Ellenberger's stay was Freudian.[11]

In Topeka, Ellenberger found almost immediately that he was valued for his multilingualism and his extensive knowledge of developments in twentieth-century European psychiatry. Curriculum records at the Menninger Clinic indicate that in the academic year 1955–1956, he organized for the first time a lecture course entitled ''The History of Dynamic Psychiatry.'' The course, which consisted of forty one-hour lectures, reviewed the origins of modern-day psychiatry from primitive medicine to the Enlightenment, then proceeded to the main theoretical models of dynamic psychiatry in the late nineteenth and twentieth centuries, and concluded with reflections on the contemporary state of theory and therapeutics. The new class was a success, and for the next four years Ellenberger offered the course regularly, polishing his lectures on the subject. These lectures, which are preserved today in handwritten notebooks housed at the *Institut Henri Ellenberger*, represent Ellenberger's first attempt to formulate a comprehensive account of the history of psychiatry; they would later contribute directly to the writing of *The Discovery of the Unconscious*.[12]

Beyond doubt, Ellenberger's years at the Menninger were a highly significant period in his career. However, in the long run, he chose not to remain in the United States. With a diverse and cosmopolitan Continental background, he tired over time of the provincial midwestern American setting. Also, it is likely that he came to feel uncomfortable with the thoroughgoing psychoanalytic environment at the Menninger Clinic, which did not accord well with his own cultivated theoretical and therapeutic eclecticism, and in particular with his enthusiasm for Jungian, existential, and phenomenological psychotherapeutics.[13]

At the same time, there were many things that Ellenberger admired about life in America. Therefore, in 1959, in an effort to combine features of the Old and New Worlds, Ellenberger accepted a position in Montreal, Canada. His French-speaking family, which had remained in Switzerland during the Menninger years, now joined him. From 1959 to 1962, Ellenberger worked at the Allan Memorial Institute, a facility for general psychiatry associated with McGill University. Then, in the early 1960s, he moved to the newly created Department of Criminology at the University of Montreal, where for the next fifteen years he taught courses on the psychology and biology of criminal behavior to students in medicine and the social sciences. (Academic criminology had not previously been a major area of concern for Ellenberger, but in Poitiers and Schaffhausen, he had often provided medico-legal testimony and filed forensic reports. Also, he had developed a strong interest in the emerging subdiscipline of victimology.) During this period, he served as well as a staff psychiatrist at the Hôtel-Dieu in Montreal. Throughout the 1960s, he regularly managed during the summer months to return to Europe to continue his historical researches. It was also during these years, at home in the evenings after full days of medical teaching and practice at the university, that Ellenberger produced the long text of *The Discovery of the Unconscious*, which appeared in print early in 1970. In the spring of 1977, at age 72, Ellenberger retired. Since that time, he has retained his residence in Montreal, and it is here, on the outskirts of the city, that he and his wife, Emilie, live today.[14]

Henri Ellenberger's contribution to psychiatric historiography consists of *The Discovery of the Unconscious* and roughly three dozen historical essays. Reflecting on Ellenberger's *oeuvre* in its entirety, what is perhaps most striking are the many ways Ellenberger sought to broaden how we think and write about psychiatry's past. These enlargements pertain to the subjects, figures, and movements studied, the methodologies employed, and the historical materials consulted by the historian.

To be sure, a small but not insignificant literature about the history of the psychological sciences existed when Ellenberger began his work in the 1950s. Ellenberger was closely familiar with this writing and admired features of it. At the same time, he found much of the extant scholarship deficient. Many of these volumes tended to be factual in nature and hagiographical in conception as well, at times, as nationalistic in tone and intent.[15] Several works represented compilations of essays, while others were useful but very short in length, under 200 pages.[16] Almost all the existing literature offered narrow intellectual-historical accounts of psychiatry based on readings of the most familiar printed texts. Equally important for Ellenberger, the most influential of these studies were cast in one of two historiographical modes, which we might call the rationalist/humanitarian mode or the Freudian teleological mode. These two approaches were clearly exemplified in the two most widely read works in the field during the 1950s and 1960s, Gregory Zilboorg's *A History of Medical Psychology* and Franz Alexander and Sheldon Selesnick's *A History of Psychiatry*.[17]

In retrospect, we can discern several ways—five, to be precise—that Ellenberger sought to expand the inherited textual traditions of psychiatric history. First, he obliterated the common "Whiggish" distinction between the scientific and non-, pre-, or pseudoscientific stages in the history of psychological medicine. Ellenberger had read deeply in the history of the mental sciences, and he came away believing that this essentially positivist division was entirely untenable. More than any scholar before him, he demonstrated the intricate historical interconnections between these different realms.

The opening chapter of *The Discovery of the Unconscious*, for instance, entitled "The Ancestry of Dynamic Psychiatry," presents a discussion of primitive medicine in prehistoric Western societies and present-day preliterate populations. Zilboorg had presented primitive medicine as a background of superstition and irrationality against which to define the coming of the medical Enlightenment. However, for Ellenberger, the shamans and medicine men of primitive peoples were the first true practitioners of psychotherapy. Drawing widely on historical and anthropological evidence from African, Australian, Siberian, Japanese, and Native American societies, he isolated ten varieties of primitive mental healing. He proposed that primitive medicine men operated in essence as intuitive psychosomaticians and as such were often highly successful. Their curative techniques were wholly rational within the belief systems of their time, and they usually involved structured ritualized activities engaged in by specially designated charismatic healers who performed their cures in public, communal settings.[18]

Following his analysis of primitive medicine, Ellenberger considered a series of related past therapeutic practices from diverse cultural settings, including ceremonial temple healing and "philosophical psychotherapy" in the ancient world; the Catholic experiences of confession, demonic possession, and exorcism; and the Protestant practice of the "Cure of Souls."[19] The explanatory worldviews behind these practices, he observed, were very different one from the other; but the psychological factors and forces at play in these methods were often notably similar to those of latter-day scientific psychotherapies. Far from representing an undifferentiated background of ignorance and superstition, many of these teachings offered "a surprisingly high degree of insight into what are usually considered the most recent discoveries in the realm of the human mind."[20] In other words, where many earlier psychiatric historians had envisioned a radical value-laden dichotomy between primitive, religious, and philosophical beliefs on the one hand and modern science on the other, Ellenberger perceived profound continuities across twenty-five centuries of theory and practice.[21]

Another example of Ellenberger's insistent emphasis on the nonscientific origins of modern depth psychological systems can be found in his close attention to the history of mesmerism. An interesting feature of historical accounts of psychiatry is the chronological point at which they choose to begin. Whom do historians interpret as the founding figures of the discipline and where do they locate the key, transformative episodes in the discipline's past? Interestingly, Ellenberger began his history of modern psychiatry not with Sigmund Freud, Wilhelm Griesinger, Philippe Pinel, or Johann Weyer, but with the Viennese physician Franz Anton Mesmer whom he judged a figure of premier importance in the exploration of unconscious mental processes. For Ellenberger, the royal road to the discovery of the unconscious lay through the study of hypnosis, and this hypnotic exploration of the human mind was initiated by Mesmer in the 1770s. Mesmer's work with the hypnotic trance during the late eighteenth century, he showed, was then elaborated upon in Europe and North America during the following hundred years by a diversity of types, including animal magnetists, hypnotists, spiritists, and lay healers as well as independently minded alienists, neurologists, surgeons, and general practitioners. During the 1890s, this rich mesmeric heritage was picked up, systematized, and scientized by the first major dynamic psychiatric theorists. The second and third chapters of *The Discovery of the Unconscious*, then, detail this century-long sequence of research, which incorporated the work of Franz Anton Mesmer, A. M. J. Puységur, Abbé Faria, J. P. F. Deleuze, Alexandre Bertrand, Antoine Despine, John Elliotson, James Braid, James Esdaile, Charles Richet, Ambroise Liébeault, Hippolyte Bernheim, Jean-Martin Charcot, Pierre Janet, Josef Breuer, and Sigmund Freud.[22]

On first glance, it might seem that the work of Mesmer, Puységur, and their followers represented little more than a chapter in the history of charlatanry, but Ellenberger argued otherwise. He demonstrated that the cumulative knowledge produced by several generations of mesmerists represented a full-fledged system of psychology and psychiatry. Their writings document a dual model of the mind, the existence of conscious and unconscious ego activities, and a belief in the psychogenesis of many emotional and physical conditions. They also reveal the utilization of the unconscious for specific psychotherapeutic purposes. Ellenberger went so far as to label their work "the first dynamic psychiatry."[23]

We find this same interpretive gesture in Ellenberger's treatment of so-called Romantic psychiatry. Most Whig historiographies of science and medicine had rejected German *Naturphilosophie* as mystical, metaphysical mush. Ellenberger, however, following the work of the German historian Werner Leibbrand, employed the concept of

"Romantic medicine," which included, he maintained, a distinct Romantic phase of psychiatric history.[24] In the middle section of the fourth chapter of *The Discovery of the Unconscious*, Ellenberger presented in sympathetic detail the medico-philosophical systems of J. C. Reil, J. C. A. Heinroth, K. W. Ideler, and H. W. Neumann as well as Arthur Schopenhauer and E. Hartmann, which again contained, he argued, many "modern" psychological insights.[25] Ellenberger valued the work of the German *Psychikern* highly and proposed that many of the basic psychological concepts associated with Freud and Jung were present in German philosophies of nature and Romantic psychiatry. For many English-language readers, Ellenberger's presentation in 1970 provided an introduction to these important figures.

In short, Ellenberger established that the history of psychiatry has been anything but a clear, continuous, and cumulative evolution from nonscience to science. Rather, primitive medicine, ancient mythology, theology, metaphysics, law, anthropology, literature, academic medicine, popular lay healing, and many other fields had all contributed at different times. Only during the late nineteenth and early twentieth centuries did these diverse strands come together to form what we recognize today as dynamic psychiatry. The constitution of the unconscious in particular had been the collective accomplishment of a diversity of people, including shamans, exorcists, priests, philosophers, novelists, poets, doctors, magnetizers, hypnotists, spiritists, mediums, psychologists, psychiatrists, and psychoanalysts. More than anyone before this time, Ellenberger established the remote and complex multidisciplinary origins of modern psychological medicine.

A second basic way in which Ellenberger sought to expand psychiatric historiography was by bringing to attention individual figures who had been excluded from, or undervalued in, previous historical narratives. Ellenberger, for instance, demonstrated a special awareness of the many minor, contributory figures in the history of the field, which he highlighted in discussions of people such as Ignaz Troxler, Justinus Kerner, James Braid, Ernest Lasègue, Enrico Morselli, Moritz Benedikt, Ludwig Klages, and Arthur Kielholz. Another category, he believed, included figures that had typically been cited but only for a limited portion of their real historical value or for unfounded or uniformed reasons. Pinel and Rorschach, he contended, were examples of these phenomena.[26]

Without a doubt, Ellenberger's most significant effort in this regard concerned his lifelong campaign on behalf of the French psychologist Pierre Janet. Ellenberger was struck by the phenomenon of selective historiographical valorization. Certain figures in psychiatric history, he observed, had been granted the status of major theoreticians and lavished with scholarly attention, while others—he believed, of equal intellectual substance and historical import—languished in mysterious obscurity. Janet was the most prominent example. Throughout his career, Ellenberger polemicized for Janet's recognition as a figure of absolutely first rank in modern dynamic psychiatry who had been unjustly eclipsed by the rise of Watsonian behavioral psychology and Freudian psychoanalysis. To Ellenberger's continual astonishment, Janet was often excluded almost entirely from the existing historical accounts of the field.[27]

Working alone among historians, Ellenberger sought to remedy this situation in a number of ways. In 1950, he wrote a short, informative piece about Janet's little-known psychotherapeutic ideas and practices.[28] More substantially, the second half of *The Discovery of the Unconscious* offers a set of interlocking microbiographies, nearly monographic in length, of the four figures Ellenberger judged to be the main theorists of psychological dynamism in the twentieth century. Tellingly, the first of these chapters dealt with Janet. In 1970, Ellenberger's chapter represented the first detailed account of Janet's life to be given in any language, and it remains to this day the most comprehensive exposition of Janet's ideas in English.[29] In a later publication, Ellenberger highlighted Janet's intimate intellectual associations with the American, especially the Boston, medical community of the early twentieth century.[30] And in 1973, he published a meticulous, comprehensive bibliography of Janet's lifework, which he hoped would precede a future revival of interest in Janetian psychology and which remains an indispensable work of reference for Janet scholars today.[31] In the last half-decade, with the explosion of interest in dissociative disorders, psychological automatisms, and post-traumatic psychopathologies, the renaissance of interest in Janet's work that Ellenberger called for has become a reality. Virtually all of the new medical literature on Janet today acknowledges Ellenberger as the pioneering scholar in this area.[32]

Third, there have been Ellenberger's contributions to the historiography of psychoanalysis. Ellenberger came of age intellectually along with the psychoanalytic movement, and he was very well informed about Freud's writings and the subsequent literature of psychoanalysis. However, most of the voluminous writing on this subject until the 1970s, he observed, consisted of explicative commentary about psychoanalytic theory. What Ellenberger strongly believed was most needed was additional historical data about Freud—the worlds from which he had emerged, in which he had worked, and in which his ideas had been received. In particular, Ellenberger developed a strong interest in reconstructing the complex intellectual universe surrounding the young Freud.

The lengthiest chapter in *The Discovery of the Unconscious*, running to 150 pages with over 540 notes of documentation, dealt with Freud.[33] In this section, Ellenberger offered a large quantity of new information about the scientific, intellectual, and cultural origins of psychoanalysis. He reviewed the Freud family genealogy, explored the life of the professional Jewish intelligentsia in nineteenth-century Vienna, examined Freud's undergraduate and medical school curricula of studies, traced out the course of his academic career, examined his early researches in neuroanatomy and neurophysiology, and studied his personal and intellectual relationships with teachers, colleagues, and family acquaintances. Indeed, on one level *The Discovery of the Unconscious* as a whole may be read as a massive contextualization of Freud's work. In his historical essays, Ellenberger continued this line of research by investigating the role that certain hitherto ignored figures from the nineteenth-century German-language sciences—most notably, Gustav Theodor Fechner and Moritz Benedikt—played in the formation of Freud's thinking.[34] It is a major paradox that Ellenberger, who was not a historian by professional training, went farther than anyone of his generation in recovering what is today termed "the historical Freud."[35]

At the same time, Ellenberger's relationship to Freud was, in a word, ambiguous; and in other areas of his historical writing, he served as an early and influential revisionist critic of psychoanalytic historiography. It was characteristic of Ellenberger to refrain from direct polemics with other historians. However, in an interview in the French magazine *Psychologie* in April 1972, he revealed pointedly that his thinking and writing about Freud had been strongly influenced by the publication of Ernest Jones's three-volume biography during the 1950s.[36] Ellenberger knew Jones slightly, found him personally agreeable, and acknowledged that his biography united invaluably a collection of primary materials about Freud. At the same, many of Jones's interpretations simply did not square with Ellenberger's understanding of psychoanalytic history as he had learned about it in personal conversations during his early adulthood in Switzerland with people such as Oskar Pfister and Alphonse Maeder. Moreover, during the 1960s, a series of publications appeared that uncritically repeated the Jonesian version of events, as if it represented the final, canonical historical account.[37]

Collectively, this "traditional" psychoanalytic historiography (as it has since been labeled, rather derisively) determined the popular and professional view of the history of psychoanalysis during the 1950s and 1960s. Without exception, the scholarship in this category was structured around a psychoanalytic historical teleology in which past psychiatric theory and practice were divided into pre- and post-Freudian periods, early figures were either ignored or memorialized according to the degree to which they anticipated psychoanalytic concepts, and twentieth-century authors were evaluated by the quality of their discipleship with Freud. Also, this literature tended to present Freud heroically, as a lone scientist of the truth who struggled in the first part of his career against ignorance, opposition, and incomprehension and in the second half against a succession of malicious professional enemies. What is more, it routinely offered a radically decontextualized account of Freud's thinking in which the greatest part of the scientific and cultural setting out of which psychoanalysis emerged was blotted out.[38] At its worst, the psychoanalytic history writing of the midcentury era generated the idea that Freud had singlehandedly discovered the unconscious.

In contrast, Ellenberger's work from the 1960s onward is marked by a persistent questioning of the "official" rendition of psychoanalytic history, including an unmasking of what he regarded as the major historical "myths" of psychoanalysis.[39] In retrospect, we can perceive that Ellenberger worked to revise the Freudian historiography of his day in a number of ways: by establishing in detail the rich and independent traditions of theorizing about the unconscious mind preceding Freud; by granting equal space and interpretive weight in the history of psychiatry to alternative, contemporaneous theories of dynamic psychology (i.e., to the theories of Janet, Adler, and Jung); and by critically verifying specific episodes in Freud's intellectual biography.

The most controversial aspect of Ellenberger's work on Freud involved this final approach. In *The Discovery of the Unconscious*, for example, Ellenberger discussed with skepticism the traditional account of such well-known biographical episodes in Freud's life as his slow advancement through the academic hierarchy in Vienna, the negative professional reception of texts like *The Interpretation of Dreams*, and the role of Freud in the Wagner-Jauregg Process over the medical mistreatment of soldiers during the First World War. Ellenberger pursued this line of analysis in greater detail in a study that appeared in the French journal *L'Information psychiatrique* in 1968. Here he offered a revisionist reading of the reception of Freud's well-known lecture on male hysteria to the Vienna *Gesellschaft der Ärzte* in the mid-1880s. Based on the analysis of previously unknown stenographical accounts of the lecture, Ellenberger attempted to establish that the professional reception accorded Freud's presentation was complex, varied, and considerably less censorious than described by Freud and enshrined in the standard historical accounts.[40]

Ellenberger's best-known study in this category concerns his historical reconstruction of the famous case of "Anna O." According to Breuer and Freud in their *Studies on Hysteria* (1895), the case of "Anna O." (Bertha Pappenheim) from the early 1880s led to the development of the so-called talking cure in which the neurotic symptoms of a patient are removed individually by being traced to earlier pathogenic experiences that have remained repressed in the unconscious. In the *Studies on Hysteria* as well as Freud's *History of the Psychoanalytic Movement* (1914) and *Autobiography* (1925), Pappenheim enjoyed a full recovery after her treatment and went on to lead a healthy and productive life. Accordingly, in a half-century of psychoanalytic history writing, "Anna O." 's case was cited as the prototypical instance of a cathartic cure and the foundational case of psychoanalytic theory. However, since the early 1950s, Ellenberger had noted factual inconsistencies in the accounts of Pappenheim's case available in Breuer, Freud, and Jones. Then, beginning in the late 1960s, he researched the case systematically. After a long and detectivelike investigation, Ellenberger located at the Bellevue Sanatorium in Kreuzlingen, Switzerland, a detailed and previously unknown medical file for Bertha Pappenheim, written in Breuer's own hand and dating from 1882. Given the historical importance of the case, this was a major find.

In an article published in 1972 in the *Journal of the History of the Behavioral Sciences*, Ellenberger offered a close, comparative reading of Pappenheim's case as it appeared in *Studies on Hysteria* and in the 1882 report of Breuer that Ellenberger unearthed in Kreuzlingen.[41] In many respects, Ellenberger found, the information in the two documents was similar. On other points, however, the unpublished report diverged dramatically from the printed account of Breuer and Freud. Biographically, the report provided a better sense of Pappenheim's intimate and dependent emotional relationship with her father and of her rivalry with her brother. More importantly, the new document established medically that Pappenheim, far from recovering fully in June 1882, had been hospitalized from July to October of that year at a private clinic for nervous and mental disorders. This institutionalization had occurred at Breuer's recommendation. The patient's neurological symptomatology, the document revealed further, had been more elaborate than previously realized and had included muscular jerks and an acute facial neuralgia. It also indicated that Pappenheim's psychological symptoms had been severe and psychoticlike, often following a cyclical pattern and including at times suicidal behavior. Later, during her months at Bellevue, Pappenheim had been heavily sedated with chloral and morphine to which she developed addictions. Most damagingly, Breuer's unpublished report of 1882 established that the official rendition of this crucial event in the history of psychoanalysis was highly inaccurate, and perhaps deceptively so. As Ellenberger wrote in his sharpest statement in the article, "the famed 'prototype of a cathartic cure' was neither a cure nor a catharsis."[42] Ellenberger did not pursue the matter further, allowing readers to draw their own conclusions; but the implications were seriously subversive.[43]

It is important to note at this point that Ellenberger did not doubt the greatness of Freud's intellectual achievement or the profound cultural impact of his work. Likewise, at no point in his writings, medical or historical, did he criticize psychoanalytic theory proper. Rather, the object of Ellenberger's critical observations in articles such as the one on "Anna O." was what he saw as the historiographical mythologization of Freud that existed during the 1950s and 1960s and that was strongly on display in the United States during Ellenberger's residence at the Menninger Clinic. For some members of the psychoanalytic establishment, Ellenberger's investigations in this direction were profoundly unwelcome.[44] (Dr. Ellenberger informed me in fact that *The Discovery of the Unconscious* was initially rejected by three American publishing houses before finding harbor at Basic Books. He suspected that this was because of the Freudian revisionism in the work.) However, in the long run, Ellenberger believed that people who adhere inflexibly to an uncritical, hagiographical view of a historical figure do little honor to their subject. To demystify a subject is neither to diminish nor to denigrate it. Ellenberger conceived of his scholarship in this area as a clarification of the true nature of Freud's accomplishment.[45]

Next, Ellenberger's historical work is noteworthy for its elaboration of the concept of the paradigmatic patient, the fourth way in which he broadened the scope of professional psychiatric historiography. One of the most significant innovations in *The Discovery of the Unconscious* is its extensive citation of case-historical materials. In the works of Gregory Zilboorg, Erwin Ackerknecht, Franz Alexander and Sheldon Selesnick, and others, the experience of the individual patient was overlooked. These works offered accounts of formal psychiatric ideas in which patients figured at most as the raw and inert "clinical material" from which medical scientists drew their observations and practiced their therapies. In contrast, Ellenberger believed that the case history was a crucially important, but curiously underused, primary source and that the role of the patient was a major, if greatly neglected, factor in the history of psychiatry.

Ellenberger attempted to integrate in various ways the experience of the patient into the story of psychiatric history. Intercalated throughout *The Discovery of the Unconscious* are over five dozen case histories, which Ellenberger translated from European languages and narrated, often at length. The intrinsic interest of these cases is high, and their inclusion imparts a novelistic quality to the book. Additionally, they allow the reader to see the ways in which particular past medical theories have emerged out of specific clinical situations.

Further, Ellenberger over time came to feel that the role of the patient in the history of psychiatry had often been creative in nature. In other branches of medical history, patients played a passive part, as the empirical subjects of analysis studied by physicians. However, in key ways, Ellenberger knew, the structure of doctor-patient relations in psychiatry was fundamentally different.[46] In "Psychiatry and Its Unknown History" (1961), Ellenberger explored the role of the individual patient in the production of past psychological theory.[47] Ellenberger excelled at detecting themes running throughout psychiatric history that other scholars had perceived only passingly in the work of a single figure or text. Among the recurrent patterns that he located in "Psychiatry and Its Unknown History" was "that of the psychiatrist who has for an object of study a certain patient, most often a female patient, generally a hysteric, with whom he establishes unconsciously a rather long, complicated, and ambiguous relationship, of which the final issue will turn out to be highly fruitful for science."[48] The hysterical women in these cases, Ellenberger continued, were usually ill for only a stage of their lives, most often during a vulnerable youthful period. They tended to enter the practices of their physicians at important intellectually formative periods of the doctors' careers, and they often served as the clinical model—the founding case—of their theoretical work. These encounters between doctor and patient were typically based on an emotional and psychological manipulation that was mutual, undeclared, and often unrecognized. Moreover, after these early neurotic illnesses, the hysterical patients in question frequently went on to lead independent and self-expressive lives. Ellenberger illustrated this phenomenon with a series of cases of female patients drawn from the practices of Mesmer, Kerner, Charcot, Janet, Breuer, Flournoy, and Jung.[49] In each of these instances, the "creative" psychiatric personalities of the patient led to intellectual creativity on the part of the physician.

In other essays, Ellenberger took as his subject individual case histories.[50] We already considered his study of "Anna O." As Ellenberger pointed out, it was Pappenheim herself who arrived at a method of removing symptoms through the exploration of past emotional experiences and who presented her "findings" to the doctor. In a separate article, Ellenberger emphasized that "Frau Emmy von N.," another patient in the *Studies on Hysteria*, encouraged Freud to abandon the practice of hypnosis and pointed the way toward the technique of free association.[51] Similarly with Jung's patient Helene Preiswerk: Ellenberger's final historical essay, completed in 1991, returned to the case that Jung grappled with in his medical dissertation of 1902 and that had fascinated Ellenberger since the beginning of his career.[52] Here he proposed that it was Jung's observations of this patient in the 1890s, as she struggled for emotional independence from her family, that provided the germ of Jung's later concept of individuation. Ellenberger hypothesized further that Jung's personal emotional involvement with Preiswerk was revived many years later, when Jung projected his feelings about her onto Sabina Spielrein, his analysand and mistress, and emerged with the idea of the anima.[53] Ellenberger believed strongly that many discoveries in psychiatric history, in both the theoretical and therapeutic realms, owed as much to the patient as the physician. He showed the way toward a historical account of psychiatry that integrates the achievements of the pioneering doctors and the prototypical patients.[54]

Fifth, Ellenberger expanded our conceptualization of psychiatry and its history by exploring the cultural history of psychiatry and the history of psychiatric ideas. These are subjects that Ellenberger believed were exceptionally interesting but almost entirely unexplored. During his undergraduate years at Strasbourg, it will be recalled, he had studied philosophy and literature, and he maintained as well strong interests in religion, mythology, and the visual arts. In his reading, he ranged widely and comfortably across the humanities and, at the height of his abilities, in six languages.

These interests found frequent expression in Ellenberger's historical writings. In *The Discovery of the Unconscious*, Ellenberger interwove a large amount of cultural information with the main historical narrative. In presenting this material, he insisted that it provided much more than simply "background" information. It was a matter rather of psychiatry *in* culture, with psychiatric theories and practices often deriving from, and in turn contributing to, larger cultural developments. More specifically, Ellenberger isolated several modes of interaction between psychiatry and its ambient cultural environments. There was, for instance, direct popularization. In *The Discovery of the Unconscious*, he sketched the popular-cultural history of mesmerism in Germany during the 1820s and 1830s, and he reviewed the spate of novels and plays dealing with hypnotism, hysteria, and somnambulism that appeared in France during the age of Charcot and Bernheim. In other places, he demonstrated that certain poets, novelists, and playwrights, such as Schnitzler and Breton, received their professional training in psychological medicine and then imported this knowledge into artistic productions.[55] In still other cases, he described important cultural representations of psychiatric figures, institutions, and theories.[56]

The most complex forms of interaction between psyche and culture documented in Ellenberger's writings involve the literary construction of psychiatric syndromes and the incorporation of medical models of personality or consciousness into the style of narration or characterization developed in a work of art. In the Romantic and Modernist periods in particular, Ellenberger located complex and culturally productive interactions between psychiatry, psychology, and imaginative literature. We learned earlier that he applied the term *Romantic* equally to poets, painters, and psychiatrists of the first half of the nineteenth century. And in *The Discovery of the Unconscious*, he explored the influence of medical writing about multiple personality on characterization in the stories and novels of E. T. A. Hoffmann, Edgar Allan Poe, Feodor Dostoevsky, Oscar Wilde, and Robert Louis Stevenson.[57] Likewise, in Charcot's work, Ellenberger identified ''the starting point of a whole tradition of psychiatrically oriented writers, such as Daudet, Zola, Maupassant, Huysmans, Bourget, Claretie, Pirandello, Proust.''[58] Furthermore, in an unpublished lecture delivered in 1957 entitled ''Psychiatric Problems as Reflected in German Literature,'' Ellenberger reviewed a sequence of texts (by Goethe, Kant, Lessing, Hoffmann, Kleist, Jensen, Musil, Zweig, Hesse, and Rilke) that analyzed insanity, depicted life in mental institutions, or presented extreme psychological states of the author. In Franz Kafka's *The Trial*, he found an illustration, more powerful than that in any medical text, of the subjective, innermost experience of a patient afflicted with delusions of persecution.[59] In one place, Ellenberger described the complete writings of Daudet, Schnitzler, and Breton as ''potential systems of dynamic psychiatry.''[60]

Elsewhere, Ellenberger traced the history of a single psychological perception as expressed over many centuries in a diversity of cultural discourses. A beautiful example of his work in the cultural history of psychiatric ideas is the essay ''The Pathogenic Secret and Its Therapeutics.''[61] Basically, the article studies the pre-Freudian history of the catharsis concept. The perception that an emotionally laden thought or experience may, if kept secret over a long period of time, exert a deleterious psychiatric effect upon its bearer had found expression in many times and texts, Ellenberger demonstrated in this essay. He discussed the idea in primitive psychotherapeutic activities, Catholic confessional literature, the Protestant theory of the Cure of Souls, the novels and plays of Jeremias Gotthelf, Nathaniel Hawthorne, Henrik Ibsen, and Marcel Prévost, medical writings on magnetism and hypnotism, French and Austrian criminological writing of the late nineteenth century, and the theories of Benedikt, Janet, Freud, and Jung. For each body of writing, he examined the particular emotions suppressed, the clinical effects of the repression, differences in the explanation of the pathogenic mechanism involved, and changes in the prescribed treatments. Illustrating his analysis with short case histories, he reflected in closing on differences in the structure of psychological relations between confessor and confessant, criminal and lawyer, analyst and analysand, and so forth.[62] To Ellenberger, these subjects formed part of the cultural history of the unconscious.

By underscoring the prescientific antecedents of dynamic psychiatry, bringing to light the contributions of new or ignored historical figures, introducing a more critical and factually informed psychoanalytic historiography, insisting on the active and creative role of the individual patient, and studying cultural representations of psychiatry, Henri F. Ellenberger greatly enriched our historical, scientific, and cultural understanding of the psychological sciences. To be sure, Ellenberger cannot be all things to all readers. Among historians of the human mind, Albert Deutsch was more reformist in his motivations, and Walther Riese was a superior medical scientist. Erwin Ackerknecht cut a more venerable academic figure and had many more students, while Richard Hunter and Ida Macalpine integrated more successfully their medical and historical interests. Michel Foucault has had a vastly greater influence upon academic intellectuals, and Jean Starobinski writes and thinks with greater elegance. Nevertheless, Ellenberger's position in the field today remains singular and secure. By any standard, his historical erudition was prodigious. For a full generation, Ellenberger was one of the very few psychiatric historians to immerse himself in quantities of unexplored primary sources. And his very broad, multidisciplinary perspective on psychiatric history has not been captured by any other historian. The chronological sweep of Ellenberger's work, and the trans-European scope of his reading, remain unsurpassed. His linguistic gifts were very considerable. It is also unlikely that we will again be privileged to read a historical commentator who had such an extensive firsthand acquaintance with so many figures from twentieth-century European psychiatry. Above all, Ellenberger, as this review of the five research areas begins to suggest, remains unmatched as a fertile source of ideas for future historical investigation.[63]

In the context of this volume, it is also interesting to speculate on the factors behind Ellenberger's unique achievements. In addition to the fortuitous elements of personal ability and cultural background, it is likely that Ellenberger's historical work reflected to a substantial degree his professional circumstances and ideological temperament. Ellenberger, we have seen, was trained medically, and he earned his livelihood as a psychiatrist working in clinical and institutional settings. These circumstances provided him with extensive firsthand exposure to the psychological theories and psychotherapeutic practices of his time. However, at the same time, Ellenberger was quite mobile professionally and resisted strongly the growing, narrow specialism of the medical world around him. Perhaps most important, he always refused to align himself with any single theory or doctrine but instead throughout his career comfortably combined Janetian, Freudian, Adlerian, and Jungian ideas and practices as well as those of existential and phenomenological psychologies. During an era of psychiatric sectarianism, Ellenberger remained resolutely eclectic. These facts are not irrelevant to an analysis of his historiography. As he learned painfully during the 1970s and 1980s, when he fell into partial eclipse, there exist liabilities to following a solitary path. But, at the same time, this background gave to Ellenberger the simultaneous status of insider and outsider in the modern psychiatric world, a status that provided him at once with the requisite experience and knowledge but also critical distance to do his scholarly work. It is highly improbable that Ellenberger would have written the type of psychiatric history that he did, during the years that he did, without a good measure of professional, intellectual, and ideological independence.

Nor is this quite all. If we are to understand in the broad view the distinctive Ellenbergerian vision of psychiatry, we also need to reflect in closing on those subjects that Ellenberger excluded from historical study. Given the extensiveness of Ellenberger's *oeuvre*, it seems churlish to criticize him for something he neglected to discuss. But one of the most revealing features of his historical work as a whole, I believe, concerns what is missing, that is, the expansion of the historiography of psychiatry that he chose *not* to make.

In *The Discovery of the Unconscious* and throughout his three dozen historical essays, Ellenberger said almost nothing about organic psychiatry, descriptive clinical psychiatry, or behavioral psychology—in other words, about contemporary *nondynamic* psychologies and psychiatries and their histories. There are many conspicuous examples of this: In *The Discovery of the Unconscious*, he discussed the coming of the German organicist tradition in the 1840s and 1850s under the chapter subheading ''the mid-century crisis.'' Wilhelm Griesinger, arguably the most influential mental scientist of the century, received one paragraph of analysis within this section, and that paragraph examined the ignored psychodynamic element in his work. In the same vein, Ellenberger acknowledged the pathbreaking work of Griesinger's followers in the field of cerebral localization (Carl Westphal, Carl Wernicke, and Theodor Meynert) in only a single sentence. In the last chapter of *The Discovery of the Unconscious*, which purported to be a comprehensive chronological review of European psychiatry from the early 1880s to 1945, Ellenberger failed to mention at all Emil Kraepelin's formulation in the 1890s of the two major endogenous psychotic categories of manic-depression and dementia praecox while he cited Pavlov's Nobel Prize–winning research on psychological reflexology only in passing.[64] Similarly, medical events such as the isolation in the 1820s of general paresis as a distinct pathology with cerebral lesions or the discovery of the syphilitic origins of general paresis of the insane in 1906 do not appear in the book. The pattern is unmistakable: However important historically, those physicians who related mental disturbance to cerebral pathology and those therapies that applied chemical or physiological methods to the treatment of mental disease simply were not incorporated into Ellenberger's picture of the disciplinary past.[65]

In pointing out these omissions, it is by no means my intention to belittle Ellenberger's work. After all, the psychological sciences themselves have not managed to achieve a unified theory of mind, so it is scarcely fair to demand that their histories do so. Rather, I make the point to bring into focus the overall identity of Ellenberger's reading of his subject. In a way that he was most likely unaware of himself, Ellenberger was the product of a time, and of a complex of cultures, in which it was possible effectively to equate the history of psychiatry as a whole with the development of the dynamic paradigm. Ellenberger was trained medically in France during the 1930s, when the first wave of Freudian ideas was infiltrating that country. He worked in German-speaking Switzerland during the 1940s and at the Menninger Clinic in the 1950s, two foci of professional interest in psychological dynamism. His writings from the early 1950s onward reveal that he read widely, almost comprehensively, in the contemporary literatures of depth psychology and psychiatry. In reaction to its earlier German somaticist background, the twentieth-century Swiss psychological tradition was overwhelmingly psychodynamic. And Ellenberger personally knew many leading dynamic psychotherapists in Switzerland, France, Austria, Germany, Canada, and the United States. His one personal experience with psychotherapy involved a prominent lay psychoanalyst.

From this perspective, it is ironic that psychoanalytic readers a generation ago received Ellenberger's work as a threat. Since the 1950s, and particularly in the past fifteen years, the theoretical pendulum movement that has characterized the history of psychiatric thought for two centuries has swung in the direction away from psychological dynamism. In the West today, biological psychiatry has found a much greater confidence than earlier in the century and has decisively taken the lead within the mental sciences. Over time, this change in orientation will undoubtedly prompt a rewriting of the history of psychiatry in which, we can well imagine, the story of ''the discovery of the unconscious'' will figure in a relatively minor way, if at all. In the early 1990s, the status of the unconscious as a scientific concept is uncertain, and it appears unlikely that the duality of conscious and unconscious holds the key to the science of the mind of the next generation.[66] However, in Ellenberger's work, if the history of depth psychology is always larger than Freud, the history of psychology and psychiatry is no larger than the dynamic psychiatry of which Janet, Freud, Adler, and Jung were the leading modern medical exponents. To be sure, the unconsciouses created by these theorists differed greatly; but all of the figures studied in Ellenberger's writings, from Franz Anton Mesmer in the 1780s to Eugène Minkowski in the 1940s, believed in the existence of nonconscious ideational processes and in the important, at times decisive, influence of these processes on human thought, feeling, and behavior. Many went a step further and projected a unitary and functionally autonomous entity called *The Unconscious.*

Like the figures and theories about which he wrote so lovingly, Ellenberger, as both historian and psychiatrist, seems to have taken for granted the reality of unconscious mental states. For him, the unconscious mind was not invented, or formulated; it was ''discovered.'' Moreover, it was self-evident to him that the antithesis conscious/unconscious was central to what psychiatry was about and that the exploration of the mysteries of unconscious mentation represented the central intellectual drama in the history of the discipline. Ellenberger's approach to the study of the psyche was a thoroughly humanistic one in which the most important ancillary disciplines were philosophy, anthropology, religion, and the arts—not neurophysiology, endocrinology, pharmacology, and psychiatric genetics. Furthermore, the tone and the scope of his writings, and even the grandeur of his project, suggests that in doing his historical work he saw himself as relating much more than simply the internal evolution of a single medical subdiscipline. For Ellenberger, the progressive discovery of the unconscious mind across the preceding two and a half centuries was part and parcel of the history of modern thought as a whole. It was a chapter in the history of the Western discovery of Self, in the collective growth of self-awareness and the quest for self-knowledge. To probe the unconscious was, in Ellenberger's mind, to explore the human spirit itself.

Whether the turn from Freud and the ascent of genetic, biological, and neuropsychopharmacological psychiatry in recent years represent the end of depth psychology as it was known to Ellenberger's generation, or only a temporary eclipse of it, or the beginnings of a new synthesis in the clinical human sciences, are weighty questions that remain to be settled. They are far beyond the purview of this essay. However, we can begin now to see that the writings of Henri Ellenberger, from the third quarter of the twentieth century, represent the first major historization of that era in which the formulation of models of unconscious cerebration was perceived to represent the major theoretical challenge to psychological theory.[67] In this broad cultural sense, Ellenberger is the most intelligent and comprehensive chronicler to date of the age of the pure dynamic psychiatries. At the end of the twentieth century, as we move away from this stage in the intellectual history of the psychological sciences, we are in an excellent position to appreciate the work of this remarkable man.

Notes

1. Henri F. Ellenberger, *The Discovery of the Unconscious: The History and Evolution of Dynamic Psychiatry* (New York: Basic, 1970), 932 pp.

2. Ellenberger, *La psychiatrie suisse* (Paris: Poirier-Bottreau, [1954]).

3. For a complete historical bibliography, see the addendum at the end of this essay.

4. Stanley Jackson, review of *The Discovery of the Unconscious, Journal of the History of Medicine and the Allied Sciences,* xxvi (1971), 216.

5. The proceedings of the conference have been published as Toby Gelfand and John Kerr (eds.), *Freud and the History of Psychoanalysis* (Hillsdale, New Jersey: Analytic Press, 1992).

6. *Beyond the Unconscious: Selected Essays of Henri F. Ellenberger in the History of Psychiatry,* edited and introduced by Mark S. Micale, translated from the French by Françoise Dubor and Mark S. Micale (Princeton: Princeton University Press, 1993).

7. Also, the French edition of Ellenberger's *A la découverte de l'inconscient: Histoire de la psychiatrie dynamique* (Villeurbanne: Simep-Éditions, 1974) is in the process of being reissued.

8. *Beyond the Unconscious* (1993), introduction, 84–86.

9. Ellenberger, *Essai sur le syndrome psychologique de la catatonie* (Poitiers: Société française d'imprimerie de la librairie, 1933), 131 pp.

10. Ellenberger, "Die Putzwut," *Der Psychologe,* ii (1950), 91–94; 138–147; idem, "Der Tod aus psychischen Ursachen bei Naturvölkern," *Psyche,* v (1951–1952), 333–334; idem, "Der Selbstmord im Lichte der Ethno-Psychiatrie," *Monatsschrift für Psychiatrie und Neurologie,* cxxv (1953), 347–361; idem, "Cultural Aspects of Mental Illness," *American Journal of Psychotherapy,* xiv (1960), 158–173; idem (with E. D. Wittkower, H. B. M. Murphy, and J. Fried), "Crosscultural Inquiry into the Symptomatology of Schizophrenia," *Annals of the New York Academy of Sciences,* lxxxiv (1960), 854–863; idem, "Ethno-psychiatrie" in *Encyclopédie Médico-Chirurgicale* (Paris, 1965), 1: *Psychiatrie,* 37725 A 10, pp. 1–14 and 37725 B 10, pp. 1–22; idem, "Aspects ethno-psychiatriques de l'hystérie," *Confrontations psychiatriques,* i (1968), 131–145; idem, "L'alcoolisme à la lumière de la psychiatrie comparée," *L'Union médicale du Canada,* ciii (1974), 1914–1920; and idem, "Psychiatrie transculturelle" in R. Duguay, H. F. Ellenberger et al. (eds.), *Précis pratique de psychiatrie* (Montreal: Chenelière and Stanké, 1981), 625–642.

11. See Lawrence J. Friedman, *Menninger: The Family and the Clinic* (New York: Knopf, 1990), especially chp. 5.

12. Two of Ellenberger's course lectures were published at the time: "The Ancestry of Dynamic Psychotherapy," *Bulletin of the Menninger Clinic,* xx (1956), 288–299 and "The Unconscious Before Freud," *Bulletin of the Menninger Clinic,* xxi (1957), 3–15, which later appeared with revisions, respectively, as the first and second chapters of *The Discovery of the Unconscious.*

13. For a clear expression of Ellenberger's interest in these last two approaches, see Ellenberger, "A Clinical Introduction to Psychiatric Phenomenology and Existential Analysis" in Rollo May, Ernest Angel, and Henri F. Ellenberger (eds.), *Existence: A New Dimension in Psychiatry and Psychology* (New York: Basic, 1958), 92–124. This volume was highly instrumental in introducing these two movements to North American psychiatrists.

14. For a fuller biographical presentation of Ellenberger, see *Beyond the Unconscious* (1993), introduction, 3–16.

15. Theodor Kirchhoff (ed.), *Deutsche Irrenärzte. Einzelbilder ihres Lebens und Wirkens,* 2 vols. (Berlin: Verlag Von Julius Springer, 1921; 1924); René Semelaigne, *Les pionniers de la psychiatrie française avant et après Pinel,* 2 vols. (Paris: J.-B. Baillière, 1930; 1932); Lowell S. Selling, *Men against Madness* (New York: Greenberg, 1940); Nolan D. C. Lewis, *A Short History of Psychiatric Achievement* (New York: Norton, 1941); Johannes Heinrich Schultz, *Psychotherapie. Leben und Werke grosser Aerzte* (Stuttgart: Hippokrates Verlag, 1952); Walter Bromberg, *Man Above Humanity: A History of Psychotherapy* (Philadelphia: Lippincott, 1954); idem, *The Mind of Man: The History of Psychotherapy and Psychoanalysis* (New York: Harper and Brothers, 1959); Kurt Kolle (ed.), *Grosse Nervenärzte,* 3 vols. (Stuttgart: Georg Thieme Verlag,

1956; 1959; 1963); Jan Ehrenwald, *From Medicine Man to Freud: A History of Psychotherapy* (New York: Dell, 1957); Denis Leigh, *The Historical Development of British Psychiatry* (Oxford: Pergamon, 1961).

16. Erwin H. Ackerknecht, *Kurze Geschichte der Psychiatrie* (Stuttgart: Ferdinand and Enke, 1957; Eng. tr., 1959); Mark Altschule, *Roots of Modern Psychiatry* (New York: Grune & Stratton, 1957); Jerome M. Schneck, *A History of Psychiatry* (Springfield, Illinois: Charles C Thomas, 1960); Nigel Walker, *A Short History of Psychotherapy in Theory and Practice* (London: Routledge & Kegan Paul, 1957); Ernest Harms, *Origins of Modern Psychiatry* (Springfield, Illinois: Charles C Thomas, 1967); Henri Baruk, *La psychiatrie française de Pinel à nos jours* (Paris: Presses Universitaires de France, 1967).

17. Gregory Zilboorg, in collaboration with George W. Henry, *A History of Medical Psychology* (New York: Norton, 1941); Franz G. Alexander and Sheldon T. Selesnick, *The History of Psychiatry: An Evaluation of Psychiatric Thought and Practice from Prehistoric Times to the Present* (New York: Harper & Row, 1966). David S. Werman has shown that the two most commonly assigned texts of psychiatric history in medical schools during this period were Zilboorg and Alexander and Selesnick (see Werman, "The Teaching of the History of Psychiatry," *Archives of General Psychiatry*, xxvi [1972], 287–289).

18. Ellenberger, *Discovery of the Unconscious*, 4–12.

19. Ibid., 13–22, 40–43, 43–46.

20. Ibid., 3.

21. In *Discovery of the Unconscious*, see in particular Table 1–3, p. 47, which explicitly compares these past and present therapeutic modes.

22. Ellenberger, *Discovery of the Unconscious*, 53–181. This line of research had previously been described by other historians, such as Zilboorg in *History of Medical Psychology*, ch. 9 and Bromberg in *The Mind of Man*, ch. 8. It was Ellenberger's accomplishment to reconstruct the story in much greater detail than had been done before and to highlight many new figures, texts, and episodes. For an expression of the influence of Ellenberger on subsequent Mesmer studies, see the excellent collection of essays edited by Heinz Schott and entitled *Franz Anton Mesmer und die Geschichte des Mesmerismus* (Stuttgart: Franz Steiner, 1985). Schott's volume is dedicated to Ellenberger.

23. Ellenberger, *Discovery of the Unconscious*, 100.

24. Werner Leibbrand, *Romantische Medizin* (Hamburg/Leipzig: H. Goverts Verlag, 1937).

25. Ellenberger, *Discovery of the Unconscious*, 199–223.

26. Ellenberger, "Methodology in Writing the History of Dynamic Psychiatry" in George Mora and Jeanne L. Brand (eds.), *Psychiatry and Its History: Methodological Problems in Research* (Springfield, Illinois: Charles C Thomas, 1970), [26–40], 27–28, 33–34; idem, review of Walter Helmut Lechler, *Neue Ergebnisse in der Forschung über Philippe Pinel* in *Journal of the History of Medicine*, xix (1964), 434–435; idem, "The Life and Work of Hermann Rorschach (1884–1922)," *Bulletin of the Menninger Clinic*, xviii (1954), 173–219.

27. For example, in Zilboorg's *History of Medical Psychology*, Janet's work was discussed in two pages (pp. 375–377). In *History of Psychiatry* by Alexander and Selesnick, it received two paragraphs (p. 173). In Dieter Wyss's *Depth Psychology: A Critical History* (New York: Norton, 1966), Janet was dealt with in four sentences (pp. 52, 54, 329, 339), and in Werner Leibbrand and Annemarie Wettley's 670-page *Der Wahnsinn. Geschichte der abendländischen Psychopathologie* (Freiburg: Karl Alber, 1961), he got one sentence (p. 173). Somewhat more satisfactory coverage was provided in Ackerknecht, *Short History of Psychiatry* (1959), 78–80 and Ernest Harms, *Origins of Modern Psychiatry* (1967), ch. 23.

28. Ellenberger, "La psychothérapie de Janet," *L'Évolution psychiatrique*, iii (1950), 465–484.

29. Ellenberger, *Discovery of the Unconscious*, 331–417.

30. Ellenberger, "Pierre Janet and His American Friends" in George E. Gifford, Jr. (ed.),

Psychoanalysis, Psychotherapy and the New England Medical Scene (New York: Science History Publication, 1978), 63–72.

31. Ellenberger, "Pierre Janet, Philosophe," *Dialogue—Canadian Philosophical Review/ Revue philosophique canadienne*, xii (1973), 254–287.

32. On the Janet revival and Ellenberger's place in it, see Paul Brown, "Pierre Janet: Alienist Reintegrated," *Current Opinion in Psychiatry*, iv (1991), 389–395.

33. Ellenberger, *Discovery of the Unconscious*, 418–570.

34. Ellenberger, "Fechner and Freud," *Bulletin of the Menninger Clinic*, xx (1956), 201–214; idem, "Moritz Benedikt (1835–1920)," *Confrontations psychiatriques*, xi (1973), 183–200.

35. Ellenberger was not, however, alone in his research in this direction. See also Maria Dorer, *Historische Grundlagen der Psychoanalyse* (Leipzig: Felix Meiner, 1932); Siegfried Bernfeld, "Freud's Earliest Theories and the School of Helmholtz," *Psychoanalytic Quarterly*, xiii (1944), 341–362; idem, "Freud's Scientific Beginnings," *American Imago*, vi (1949), 163–196; Paul Cranefield, "The Organic Physics of 1847 and the Biophysics of Today," *Journal of the History of Medicine and Allied Sciences*, xii (1957), 407–423; idem, "Freud and the 'School of Helmholtz,'" *Gesnerus*, xxiii (1966), 35–39; Walter Riese, "The Pre-Freudian Origins of Psychoanalysis" in Jules Masserman (ed.), *Science and Psychoanalysis*, i (1958), 29–72; Ola Andersson, *Studies in the Prehistory of Psychoanalysis* (Stockholm: Norstedts, 1962); and Ilse Bry and Alfred H. Rifkin, "Freud and the History of Ideas: Primary Sources, 1886–1910" in Jules Masserman (ed.), *Science and Psychoanalysis*, v: *Psychoanalytic Education* (New York: Grune & Stratton, 1962), 6–36.

36. Ellenberger, "Freud en perspective. Interview par Jacques Mousseau," *Psychologie*, xxvii (1972), 35–43, translated and reprinted as "Freud in Perspective: A Conversation with Henri F. Ellenberger," *Psychology Today*, vi (March, 1973), 50–60. This is a choice document in reconstructing Ellenberger's intellectual biography.

37. Dieter Wyss, *Die tiefenpsychologischen Schulen von den Anfängen bis zur Gegenwart* (Göttingen: Vandenhoeck and Ruprecht, 1961); idem, *Depth Psychology: A Critical History*, translated from the German by Gerald Onn (1966); Marthe Robert, *La Révolution psychanalytique* (Paris: Payot, 1964); idem, *The Psychoanalytic Revolution: Sigmund Freud's Life and Achievement*, translated from the French by Kenneth Morgan (London: George Allen & Unwin, 1966); Alexander and Selesnick, *The History of Psychiatry* (1966); Zilboorg, *A History of Medical Psychology*, 2nd ed. (New York: Norton, 1967); and Jones, *The Life and Work of Sigmund Freud*, edited and abridged by Lionel Trilling and Steven Marcus with an introduction by Lionel Trilling (New York: Basic, 1961). To the best of my knowledge, the only explicit general challenge to the Jonesian historiography of psychoanalysis by a historian of psychiatry during the period preceding Ellenberger's book was Ernest Harms, *Origins of Modern Psychiatry* (1967), ch. 24.

38. Wyss's study, for instance, literally paints a picture of modern psychiatry without a past. Presenting itself as a general historical account of depth psychology, the book absorbs the preceding two and a half millennia of mental medicine into the story of Freud and his followers and rivals. In contrast to Ellenberger, Wyss believed that the development of dynamic psychiatry began in 1892, with the publication of Freud's article on a case of successful treatment by hypnosis. The first sentence of *Depth Psychology: A Critical History* reads "Sigmund Freud was born on May 6, 1856, in Freiburg, a small town in Moravia, where his father was a business man."

39. For a good example of the present generation's indebtedness to Ellenberger, compare him on this point with Frank J. Sulloway, *Freud, Biologist of the Mind: Beyond the Psychoanalytic Legend* (New York: Basic, 1979), Part Three, especially "Catalogue of Freud Myths," 489–495.

40. Ellenberger, "La conférence de Freud sur l'hystérie masculine (15 octobre 1886): étude critique," *L'Information psychiatrique*, xliv (1968), 921–934.

41. Ellenberger, "The Story of 'Anna O.': A Critical Review with New Data," *Journal of the History of the Behavioral Sciences*, vii (1972), 267–279, especially 274–278.

42. Ibid., 279.

43. Subsequent research into the case has revealed that Pappenheim was hospitalized three additional times during 1883–1888 for periods ranging from three weeks to five and a half months. See Albrecht Hirschmüller, *The Life and Work of Josef Breuer. Physiology and Psychoanalysis* (New York: New York University Press, 1989), 115.

44. See above all Kurt Eissler's frantic forty-page defense of traditional psychoanalytic historiography in the light of Ellenberger's work in K. R. Eissler, *Talent and Genius: The Fictitious Case of Tausk Contra Freud* (New York: Quadrangle Books, 1971), Appendix D, "Another Critical View of Freud," 342–380.

45. Interesting, if somewhat unexpected, in view of his psychoanalytic revisionism is Ellenberger's strongly negative reaction to the European and American anti-psychiatric movements of the sixties and seventies. For his thoughts on this subject, refer to Ellenberger, "Psychiatrie ou antipsychiatrie? Enquête sur les courantes de la psychiatrie institutionnelle actuelle en Europe," *L'Union médicale du Canada*, 2 parts, c (1971), 1526–1538; 1737–1749; and idem, "Les courants de la pensée antipsychiatrique," *L'Union médicale du Canada*, cii (1973), 2315–2319.

46. We find here a point on which Ellenberger's personal experience as a clinician informed his historical sensibility.

47. Ellenberger, "La psychiatrie et son histoire inconnue," *L'Union médicale du Canada*, xc (1961), 281–289.

48. Ibid., 281.

49. Ibid., 283–288. Elsewhere in his writings, Ellenberger discusses the creative role of a number of male patients. See *Discovery of the Unconscious*, 18–22, 73, 892, 893 and Ellenberger, review of William G. Niederland, *The Schreber Case: Psychoanalytic Profile of a Paranoid Personality*, *Bulletin of the Menninger Clinic*, xxxix (1975), 598.

50. In *Beyond the Unconscious*, see Section Four, "The Great Patients," Pt. Three, which reproduces all of Ellenberger's essays of this type.

51. Ellenberger, "L'Histoire d''Emmy von N.': Étude critique avec documents nouveaux," *L'Évolution psychiatrique*, xlii (1977), 519–541.

52. Ellenberger, "The Story of C. G. Jung and Helene Preiswerk: A Critical Study with New Documents," *History of Psychiatry*, ii (1991), 41–52.

53. Ibid., 51–52.

54. A programmatic call for a less iatrocentric and more "patient-centered" medical history has since been sounded. See Roy Porter, "The Patient's View: Doing Medical History from Below," *Theory and Society*, xiv (1985), 175–198 and Porter (ed.), *Patients and Practitioners: Lay Perceptions of Medicine in Pre-Industrial Society* (Cambridge: Cambridge University Press, 1985), introduction.

55. See *Discovery of the Unconscious*, passim, but especially ch. 10.

56. Ellenberger, "Charcot and the Salpêtrière School," *American Journal of Psychotherapy*, xix (1965), 253–267.

57. Ellenberger, *Discovery of the Unconscious*, 162–163.

58. Ibid., 99–100.

59. Ellenberger, "Psychiatric Problems as Reflected in German Literature," unpublished lecture presented to the Kansas Modern Language Association, Manhattan, Kansas, 13 April 1957.

60. Ellenberger, *Discovery of the Unconscious*, 898, n. 60.

61. Ellenberger, "The Pathogenic Secret and Its Therapeutics," *Journal of the History of the Behavioral Sciences*, i (1966), 29–42.

62. Ibid., 40–41.

63. Specialists will be aware from my review of the many ways in which a subsequent generation of scholars has developed, and is developing, Ellenberger's ideas. For a detailed accounting of Ellenberger's influence on current-day psychiatric historiography, including references to specific authors and texts, see *Beyond the Unconscious*, introduction and bibliographical essay.

64. Ellenberger, *Discovery of the Unconscious*, 223–228, 241–242.

65. Interestingly, however, Ellenberger's approach to criminology was heavily biological. See Ellenberger, "Introduction biologique à l'étude de la prison," *Quatrième Colloque de recherche sur la délinquance et la criminalité* (Montreal: Société de Criminologie du Québec, 1965), 421–438; idem, "Biocriminogenèse. Aspects biologiques et psychiatriques de la criminalité," *Criminologie en action* (Montreal: Presses de l'Université de Montréal, 1968), 45–48; idem, "Les origines biologiques de la victimologie," *Revue internationale de criminologie et de police technique*, iii (1985), 371–373.

66. For two early questionings of the concept, which appeared as *The Discovery of the Unconscious* was in press, see R. Rabkin, "Is the Unconscious Necessary?" *International Journal of Psychiatry*, viii (1969), 570–578 and R. W. Sperry, "A Modified Concept of Consciousness," *Psychological Review*, lxxvi (1969), 532–536.

67. Pertinent in the light of Ellenberger's work are recent *nondynamic* models of unconscious functioning. See in particular Kenneth S. Bowers and Donald Meichenbaum (eds.), *The Unconscious Reconsidered* (New York: Wiley, 1984), which includes chapters on behavioral, cognitive, and psychobiological paradigms.

Addendum—Henri F. Ellenberger: Complete Writings in the History of Psychiatry

The bibliography below is limited to the writings of Henri Ellenberger of a historical nature. In addition to these, Ellenberger authored over 120 publications on medical topics as well as approximately 190 book reviews, many of which deal with historical subjects. Where possible, I have cited editions of articles in English, although many of these essays also appeared in other languages. Entries that are marked with an asterisk are reproduced in English in *Beyond the Unconscious: Selected Essays of Henri F. Ellenberger in the History of Psychiatry* (1993).

Books

La psychiatrie suisse (series of articles published between 1951 and 1953 in *L'Évolution psychiatrique*) (Paris: Imprimerie Poirier-Bottreau, [1954]).
Criminologie du passé et du présent (Montreal: Les Presses de l'Université de Montréal, 1969).
The Discovery of the Unconscious: The History and Evolution of Dynamic Psychiatry (New York: Basic, 1970). Editions and translations: *The Discovery of the Unconscious: The History and Evolution of Dynamic Psychiatry* (London: Allen Lane, Penguin Press, 1970); *La scoperta dell'inconscio. Storia della psichiatria dinamica*, 2 vols. (Turin: Boringhieri, 1972); *Die Entdeckung des Unbewussten*, 2 vols. (Bern: Hans Huber, 1973), with a reprint in Zurich by Diogenes Verlag in 1985; *El descubrimiento del inconsciente (Historia y evolución de la psiquiatria dinamica)* (Madrid: Editorial Gredos, 1974); *A la découverte de l'inconscient: Histoire de la psychiatrie dynamique* (Villeurbanne: Simep-Éditions, 1974); *Muishiki no Hakken* (Rikido-Seishin-Igaku-Hattatsu Shi, Anri Erenberuga-Cho, Kimura Bin, Nakai Hisao Kenyaku, Kobundo, 1980).

Les mouvements de libération mythique et autres essais sur l'histoire de la psychiatrie, preface by Jacques Dufresne (Montreal: Éditions Quinze, 1978); trans. *I movimenti di liberazione mitica* (Turin: Liguori, 1986).

Articles

"La psychothérapie de Janet," *L'Évolution psychiatrique*, special issue in commemoration of Pierre Janet, xv, no. 3 (July–September 1950), 465–484.

"A propos du *'Malleus Maleficarum,'* " *Schweizerische Zeitschrift für Psychologie*, x, no. 2 (1951), 136–148.

*"The Life and Work of Hermann Rorschach (1884–1922)," *Bulletin of the Menninger Clinic*, xviii, no. 5 (September 1954), 172–219.

"A Psychiatrist's Informal Tour of Europe," *Menninger Quarterly*, viii–ix (1954–1955), 10–23.

*"Fechner and Freud," *Bulletin of the Menninger Clinic*, xx, no. 4 (July 1956), 201–214.

"The Ancestry of Dynamic Therapy," *Bulletin of the Menninger Clinic*, xx, no. 6 (November 1956), 288–299.

"The Unconscious Before Freud," *Bulletin of the Menninger Clinic*, xxi, no. 1 (January 1957), 44–64.

"Psychiatric Problems as Reflected in the History of German Literature," unpublished lecture presented to the Kansas Modern Language Association, Manhattan, Kansas, 13 April 1957.

*"The Scope of Swiss Psychology" in Henry P. David and Helmut von Bracken (eds.), *Perspectives in Personality Theory* (New York: Basic, 1957), 44–64.

"A Psychiatrist's Vacation in Europe," *T. P. R. (Temperature, Pulse, Respiration)*, xviii, no. 7 (November 1957), 5–13.

"A Clinical Introduction to Psychiatric Phenomenology and Existential Analysis" in Rollo May, Ernest Angel, and Henri F. Ellenberger (eds.), *Existence: A New Dimension in Psychiatry and Psychology* (New York: Basic, 1958), 92–124.

*"La psychiatrie et son histoire inconnue," *L'Union médicale du Canada*, xc, no. 3 (March 1961), 281–289.

"L'Existentialisme et son intérêt pour la psychiatrie," *L'Union médicale du Canada*, xc, no. 9 (September 1961), 936–947.

"Histoire de la psychopathologie en Occident," *Critique*, xviii, no. 182 (July 1962), 641–655.

*"Les illusions de la classification psychiatrique," *L'Évolution psychiatrique*, xxviii, no. 2 (April–June 1963), 221–242.

"Les mouvements de libération mythique," *Critique*, xix, no. 190 (March 1963), 248–267.

"L'Autobiographie de C. G. Jung," *Critique*, xx, nos. 207–208 (August–September 1964), 754–779.

*"Charcot and the Salpêtrière School," *American Journal of Psychotherapy*, xix, no. 2 (April 1965), 253–267.

"Mesmer and Puységur: From Magnetism to Hypnotism," *The Psychoanalytic Review*, lii, no. 2 (Summer 1965), 137–153.

*"The Pathogenic Secret and Its Therapeutics," *Journal of the History of the Behavioral Sciences*, ii, no. 1 (January 1966), 29–42.

"The Evolution of Depth Psychology" in Iago Galdston (ed.), *Historic Derivations of Modern Psychiatry* (New York: McGraw-Hill, 1967), 159–184.

*"La conférence de Freud sur l'hystérie masculine (15 octobre 1886): Étude critique," *L'Information psychiatrique*, xliv, no. 10 (1968), 921–929.

*"The Concept of Creative Illness" [1964], *The Psychoanalytic Review*, lv, no. 3 (1968), 442–456.

"La vie et l'oeuvre de Pierre Janet" in *Hôpital Pierre Janet a Hull: Ouverture officielle et journée scientifique* (Hull, 1969).

"Methodology in Writing the History of Dynamic Psychiatry" in George Mora and Jeanne L. Brand (eds.), *Psychiatry and Its History: Methodological Problems in Research* (Springfield, Illinois: Charles C Thomas, 1970), 26–40.

"Histoire de l'anxiété. Contribution de la psychiatrie dynamique" in *Proceedings of the Fifth World Congress of Psychiatry* (Mexico City, 1971), 678–682.

"Discours prononcé par le docteur Henri F. Ellenberger à l'occasion de l'inauguration du nouvel Institut Philippe Pinel de Montréal," *Annales internationales de criminologie*, x, no. 2 (1971), 387–392.

*"The Story of 'Anna O.': A Critical Review with New Data," *Journal of the History of the Behavioral Sciences*, viii, no. 3 (July 1972), 267–279.

*"Moritz Benedikt (1835–1920)," *Confrontations psychiatriques*, xi (1973), 183–200.

"La notion de *Kairos* en psychothérapie," *Annales de psychothérapie*, iv, no. 7 (1973), 4–14.

*"Pierre Janet, Philosophe," *Dialogue: Canadian Philosophical Review/Revue philosophique canadienne*, xii, no. 2 (June 1973), 254–287.

"Psychiatry from Ancient to Modern Times" in Silvano Arieti (ed.), *American Handbook of Psychiatry*, 2nd ed., 2 vols. (New York: Basic, 1974), 1: 3–27.

"Développement historique de la notion de processus psychothérapeutique," *L'Union médicale du Canada*, cv, no. 12 (December 1976), 1820–1830.

*"L'Histoire d''Emmy von N.': Étude critique avec documents nouveaux," *L'Évolution psychiatrique*, xlii, no. 3 (July-September 1977), 519–541.

"Carl Gustav Jung: His Historical Setting" in Hertha Riese (ed.), *Historical Explorations in Medicine and Psychiatry* (New York: Springer Publishing Company, 1978), 142–149.

"Pierre Janet and His American Friends" [1973] in George E. Gifford, Jr. (ed.), *Psychoanalysis, Psychotherapy and the New England Medical Scene, 1894–1944* (New York: Science History Publication, 1978), 63–72.

"From Justinus Kerner to Hermann Rorschach: The History of the Inkblots," unpublished manuscript, available in printed form in Japanese in *Rorschach Japonica*, xxiii (September 1981), 1–8.

"Histoire de la psychiatrie" in R. Duguay, H. F. Ellenberger, et al. (eds.), *Précis pratique de psychiatrie* (Montreal: Chenelière and Stanké, 1981), 1–12.

"Evolution of Ideas about the Nature of the Psychotherapeutic Process in the Western World" [1979] in *History of Psychiatry. Proceedings of the Fourth International Symposium on the Comparative History of Medicine—East and West* (Tokyo: Saikon Publishing Co., 1982), 1–28.

*"The Story of Helene Preiswerk: A Critical Study with New Documents," *History of Psychiatry*, ii, no. 5 (March 1991), 41–52.

7

Jean Starobinski: The History of Psychiatry as the Cultural History of Consciousness

FERNANDO VIDAL

The name of the Genevan critic Jean Starobinski will most likely evoke masterful readings of Rousseau and Montaigne or insightful reconstructions of the world of the Enlightenment. With the possible exception of the history of melancholy, much more rarely will it be associated with the history of psychiatry, or more generally with that of the human sciences. A small number of the critic's contributions to these fields have appeared in some of his books. Most of them, however, remain scattered, and nothing suggests that they are known as widely as they deserve. Yet Starobinski's historical work is exemplary in its perspective on the problematic relations between psychological concepts and experiences, and between medical thought and the larger culture. He is one of those rare scholars who successfully straddle the "two cultures," combining literary elegance with medical training, and a truly cosmopolitan erudition with an uncommon openness to the various humanistic disciplines.[1]

Starobinski's *oeuvre* has won him a wide reputation and several prestigious awards. Whole issues of such different reviews as the Centre Pompidou's refined *Cahiers pour un temps* and the more popular *Magazine littéraire* have been devoted to his work.[2] These honors acknowledge his insights into the fabric of European culture from the Enlightenment to the present, as well as his outstanding literary qualities. Nevertheless, although Starobinski is a major figure of the European intellectual landscape, the reason that the writings to be presented here remain less known and influential than those of other authors included in this volume is perfectly simple.

Starobinski is *not* primarily a historian of psychiatry; his approach and style are not typical of the profession, do not correspond to its major specialized interests, and do not follow prevailing academic currents. Nor are they likely to inaugurate methodologies, lead to crucial empirical findings, or dispense definite interpretive frameworks. The history of science, including that of psychiatry, is inherently porous; its boundaries are, and must, remain open; it is riddled with questions of definition and delimitation; most of its subject matter calls for transdisciplinary research and for extended connections with social and cultural history. The best historical work inventively confronts these challenging features of the discipline, and so does Starobinski's. But his case is more complex.

Starobinski's contributions to the history of psychiatry are not chiefly those of a historian dealing with strictly historical problems but those of a *critic* fascinated, as he says, by the "visible *surface*" where life and creation meet, by the "thin skin of appearance, the exact border at which life and art both deliver their greatest testimony and conceal their secret."[3] Their originality lies in their grasp of the interplay of personal experience, literature and its creation, and the history of concepts and theories; focus on this interplay gives them an unusual psychological depth. As will be shown later, this focus reflects Starobinski's particular viewpoint as a literary critic.

Though essentially a critic, Starobinski does not limit himself to textual analysis. On the contrary, he has "always dreamt of a frontierless history of ideas";[4] hardly ever does he concentrate exclusively on a topic narrowly identifiable as "history of psychiatry," and even his most specialized studies extend beyond the confines of the discipline. He sees the history of ideas as undertaking "to eliminate artificial boundaries and absurd divisions."[5] Starting with a particular theme, the historian explores a whole era, and from the global intuition of a culture, he returns to the details and the examples. Starobinski's books on the Enlightenment and on the "emblems of reason" are brilliant illustrations of this paradigm.[6] His work on the history of psychiatry offers less systematic yet equally insightful and thought-provoking examples. The breadth his work has gained through the pursuit of a frontierless intellectual history is almost as rare as its psychological sensibility, and both are epitomized in his choice of the *essay* rather than the monograph as literary form.

Starobinski's preference for the essay highlights his singularity within the historiography of psychiatry. This choice, which would perhaps suffice to differentiate him from mainstream historians, is consubstantial with his entire manner. Starobinski is a modern master of the essay, which he considers as "the *freest* literary genre."[7] What sets the essay apart from much of academic scholarship is indeed the degree of imaginative freedom, the absence of subservience to any one methodology or specifically disciplinary constraint, and the visible presence of a subjective consciousness. Starobinski reconciles an unassuming exercise of such freedom with an exacting adherence to the standards of historical and linguistic research. He thereby follows his own ideal of the essay as a genre capable of combining "science and poetry," of understanding another language and at the same time inventing its own, of grasping past meanings and yet creating new relations that make sense in the present. The essay, he comments, "requires the simultaneous practice of a hermeneutics and an adventurous audacity."[8] Both are apparent in his writings on the history of the human sciences.

Medicine, Mask, and Melancholy

Jean Starobinski was born in Geneva in 1920. His father, a Polish physician, had arrived there in 1913 to study medicine and stayed after the outbreak of World War I. Starobinski became Swiss only in 1948, yet seemed, from his youth, destined to realize the potential of his native country to function as a crossroads of European cultures. His literary studies between 1939 and 1942 were followed by medical school until 1948; in 1946, he became assistant to his teacher Marcel Raymond, author of the renowned *De Baudelaire au surréalisme* (first published in 1933). From 1949 to 1953, he was an intern in general medicine. His doctoral dissertation on Rousseau came out in 1957, while he was spending a year as intern at a psychiatric clinic.[9] He never became an independent practicing physician. In 1960, he published his medical dissertation on the history of the treatment of melancholy.[10] From 1958 until his retirement in 1985, he occupied a personal chair in the history of ideas at the University of Geneva, where he also taught French literature and the history of medicine. His teaching in medical history included, among other topics, the history of psychiatry in the eighteenth and nineteenth centuries, the humoral doctrine, religious and medical interpretations of madness, the body and the unconscious, mania and melancholy, passion and imagination, nostalgia, dreams, deliria, and bodily illusions.[11]

Much of Starobinski's outlook as a historian may be traced to his discovery of Georges Canguilhem's *La formation du concept de reflèxe* and *Le normal et le pathologique*, and to the years (1953–56) he spent at Johns Hopkins University, where he had been called by the prominent Belgian critic George Poulet. Though a faculty member in the Department of Romance Languages, Starobinski associated with such distinguished historians of medicine and science as Ludwig Edelstein, Owsei Temkin, Richard Shryock, and Bentley Glass, as well as with Leo Spitzer and other participants in the famous "history of ideas" club founded by Arthur Lovejoy. He recalls that the "atmosphere was extremely positive. I had been very edified by Temkin's presence at the Saturday morning ward rounds: a historian of medicine attended the presentation of patients. I endeavored to do the same thing."[12] Since then, he has reached the art of balancing the subjectivity he himself recognizes in criticism with the objectivity that is the ideal of scientific knowledge, and has oriented most of his thinking toward the subtle interrelations and moving boundaries between the subjective and the objective, the inner and the outer, the self and the other, the mind and the body.

This is apparent in all of Starobinski's writings as a critic and a historian, particularly in those (begun in the 1960s) that concern the literary figures of melancholy. But it can be seen emerging in his first pieces on the history of medicine: substantial essay-reviews published in the early 1950s while he was still a practicing physician.[13] Their attention to the anthropological and humanistic relations of medicine, to the interaction of practice and theory, and to the confrontation of natural phenomena and historically contingent knowledge betray the influence of existentialism (Jean-Paul Sartre), phenomenology (Maurice Merleau-Ponty), and the epistemology formulated by Gaston Bachelard in *La formation de l'esprit scientifique* (first published in 1938). They also reveal Starobinski's concern for the relationship between the doctor and the patient, and for medicine as a humane science. These concerns have never disappeared from the critic's horizon.

At the opening of his 1963 *History of Medicine* (a handsomely illustrated work of popularization), Starobinski asserts that medicine—"knowledge turned power"— should not be limited to its technical aspects or to the sick body, but must remain attentive to the "therapeutic relation" and become "an art of dialogue."[14] Almost thirty years later, the question that concludes an essay on Van Gogh's portrait of his physician as melancholy highlights the issue: "This doctor tormented by anxiety witnesses the painter's anxiety: what to do, if the one from whom we expect help is himself in need of help?"[15]

Though in minor ways, Starobinski has never ceased to ponder the emergence of medical power, its relation to other forms of knowledge and healing, and the doubts and objections it has aroused.[16] His critique of psychologism in literary analysis (about which more will be said later) joins his awareness that it is easy to abuse the medical power of diagnosis. And his interest in psychosomatic phenomena is consistent with his belief that most illnesses are "overdetermined," that all end up involving at least "a psychological response to the biological threat," and that medicine should be "multidimensional"; as he remarks, although no disease can be considered merely as a behavior, every disease, up to the extremes of coma and death, is experienced by an individual consciousness.[17]

Starobinski's choice of melancholy as the pivotal theme of his research is related not only to his conception of medicine but also to the nature of his earliest intellectual ventures. Speaking of World War II, of his sympathies for the French Resistance, its philosophers and poets, Starobinski recalls:

> My earliest project, which was to write a phenomenology of masked behavior, was inspired by the lies and masks of the surrounding totalitarianisms. At the beginning, this was not a purely scholarly project, but an attempt at understanding masked behaviors; history was truly involved, in its evil and irrational aspects.
>
> I had initially formed the project, which dissolved, of writing a book on the enemies of masks. . . . At its inception, what became the book on Rousseau alone [*La transparence et l'obstacle*] was conceived as spanning five centuries: from Montaigne to Valéry, through La Rochefoucauld, Rousseau, Stendhal. My first project was to do the history of the exposure of lies.[18]

Many of his numerous studies derived from the unaccomplished project concern the melancholy disposition that, whether genuine or simulated, characterizes the denunciation of illusions. Starobinski's inquiry into melancholy has depicted states of disillusionment and utopian desires of universal reform, the melancholic disappointment with oneself, others, and the world, and the effects of melancholizing on self-consciousness and the making of a literary persona.

Starobinski is most interested in *expression*, in the fact that human beings can give themselves a disguise, a mask, a form. As a young psychiatrist, he discovered "a particular type of man who . . . sees masks everywhere: the melancholic." As he explains,

> Starting with my interest in the mask, I began to investigate the melancholic's experience of the world as it derives from his own internal affect, from the suffering of not being able to adhere to external reality.[19]

The melancholy detachment from reality may go hand in hand with the exposure of worldly lies and illusions; such condemnation, however, must not jeopardize the accuser's disengagement from the world: Thus, the mask-snatcher tends to watch from behind a mask.[20] In short, there is an organic link between the study of melancholy and a "phenomenology of masked behavior."

The combination of Starobinski's youthful project and psychiatric training with intellectual history was stimulated by Panofsky and Saxl's iconological interpretation of Dürer's woodcut "Melencolia I." Their research, exemplary of the approach of the Warburg Institute, eventually grew into *Saturn and Melancholy*, a classic monument of frontierless history.[21] Starobinski wished the study of a nosographical concept to lead from the history of medicine to the history of art, literature, and society. He hoped that such *entretissage*, or intertwining, would bring about a better understanding of phenomena previously known in isolation, that is to say, for him, "partially unrecognized."[22] His contributions to the study of melancholy are characterized by a distinctive blend of historical semantics, medical history, and literary criticism; they have been singled out and praised by Raymond Klibansky, the surviving author of *Saturn and Melancholy* at the time of its publication in French.[23]

Starobinski's first study of melancholy is also the one that can be most easily placed within the limits of the history of medicine and psychiatry. It is a 100-page monograph on the history of the treatment of melancholy from Homer to turn-of-the-century psychiatry, and was initially presented as a doctoral thesis in medicine. The author begins by emphasizing that, from the angle of both the physician and the patient, disease is always a "cultural fact." For the historian of psychiatry, the dependence of illness and medicine on cultural conditions implies a "double variable." On the one hand, in the absence of the concrete patient, retrospective diagnoses have virtually no chances of being valid; on the other hand, today's nosological categories can hardly ever be recognized in those of the past. In the case of melancholy, the centuries-long persistence of the disorder's name veils great variation in the underlying facts: "the medicines prescribed in the course of the centuries apply neither to the same disease, nor to the same causes"; an inadequately explained illness that in addition lacks specific remedies "provokes the successive application of all [potentially or allegedly therapeutic] discoveries as they are made."[24]

Realizing that medical knowledge is historically contingent does not prevent Starobinski from believing in its progress. In his description, the modern notion of depression is narrower and more precise than the older concept of melancholy; the rigorous nosography that gradually replaced "pre-scientific" etiology is accompanied by a courageous acknowledgment that the true causes of the illness remain unknown; a "pseudo-specific and pseudo-causal medication has been superseded by a more modest treatment that admits its being limited to symptoms." This modesty, Starobinski concludes, actually opens the way for the advancement of research.[25]

Starobinski's history of the treatment of melancholy possesses many of his customary qualities: elegance, erudition, breadth, and an intertwining of the histories of science and literature. It also announces the orientation of the critic's later work on the topic. After quoting George Dumas's 1895 remarks that "melancholy does not exist as a mental entity" and that "it is never anything else than the consciousness of the state of the body," Starobinski comments that medicine may indeed act on the body.

> At that date, however, it did not yet have any power over the specific somatic structures that govern the ways in which individuals experience their "inner time," the affective coloring of their horizon, the quality of comfort or malaise accompanying their acts and thoughts. For some more decades, the melancholic would remain the very type of the inaccessible being, prisoner of a gaol the key to which had yet to be found.[26]

Although Starobinski's ending his narrative in 1900 was purely circumstantial,[27] his later work on melancholy did concern the psychological phenomena that remained outside the reach of somatic medicine and found expression in literature and art.

Starobinski has written on the metaphoric transformation of melancholy into black ink in medieval poetry;[28] on how irony enabled Gozzi, Hoffmann, and Kierkegaard to transcend melancholy alienation;[29] on Robert Burton's melancholy utopia;[30] on how Burton's melancholic "depersonalization" became the style of his celebrated *Anatomy of Melancholy*, and on how this style might be comparable to Montaigne's "interminable task of self-description."[31] Montaigne is the subject of a major work where Staro-binski follows through the *Essays* the *"mouvement"* initiated by the question "What happens after melancholy thought has rejected the illusion of appearances?"[32] Rousseau, to whom the critic has devoted many studies, appears at times as a fundamentally melancholy being.[33] Baudelaire's poetics of melancholy was the subject of Starobinski's lessons at the Collège de France.[34] Melancholy dawns at the heart of both Mme. de Staël's conception of literature and the romantic heroization of the buffoon.[35]

Thematic unity around melancholy is accompanied by methodological openness and a "frontierless" perspective. The former is apparent in Starobinski's whole *oeuvre*. It is most explicitly asserted in the domain of literary criticism (see following section), but its defense surfaces elsewhere. For example, in an admiring review of Michel Foucault's *The Birth of the Clinic*, Starobinski perceptively depicts the book's novelty, but is unhappy about its author's "autistic and self-sufficient manner" and points out the value of more "'traditional'" histories that contain "all that Foucault deliberately leaves out."[36]

The "frontierless perspective" manifests itself not only in the variety but also in the treatment of melancholy-related themes. Thus, in one of his articles on nostalgia, Starobinski focuses on the history of the concept, while in another he emphasizes that a proper understanding of nostalgia would involve the history of feelings and *mentalités*, a history of the social structures that make up the concrete background of the history of feelings, the history of science and philosophy, and, finally, considerations on the moral and metaphysical meaning of the nostalgic experience.[37] A glance at how such histories might be brought together is given in a brief paper focused on the spiritualist, anti-Cabanis doctrine about the therapeutic role of language elaborated by Laurent Cerise in his 1842 *Des fonctions et des maladies nerveuses*. As Starobinski explains, the value of language exceeded healing because, in the framework of certain physiological, religious and social doctrines, it appeared as an immanent link between the individual and society.[38] His essay on Van Gogh's portrait of Dr. Gachet emphasizes the painter's identification with his doctor and weaves elements from their lives and personalities with the history of medicine, art, and aesthetics.[39]

Starobinski's study of the problem of "melancholy immortality" focuses on the French physician Jules Cotard's description of the *délire des négations*, a state in which patients believe that they are either incapable of dying, or already dead and fated to eternal survival. In his commentary of the case history that prompted Cotard to elaborate a new clinical category, Starobinski moves from late nineteenth-century psychiatry to the preoccupation with immortality and the "death of God" that permeated philosophy, science, and literature after about 1850 and manifested itself more recently in some of Kafka's writings.[40]

Body and Consciousness between History and Criticism

Starobinski's *oeuvre* is no exception to the fact that the idea of a "frontierless history" tends to remain at the level of a regulative principle of research. Some of his writings are straightforward scholarly commentaries.[41] Others are rather strictly limited to the history of psychological medicine. Thus, his study of chlorosis is motivated by the place of the condition in the work of Balzac, Baudelaire, Zola, the Symbolists, yet it is focused on the history of the term from its creation in the early seventeenth century and its classical background, to the midnineteenth century. The link to literature, however, remains: Starobinski does not fail to observe that, by severing the link between chlorosis and unfulfilled love, melancholy and hysteria, the more accurate modern diagnosis (anemia induced by an iron deficiency) deprived the condition of its literary charms.[42]

Nor does literature play a larger role in Starobinski's history of the word *reaction* from physics to psychiatry. This is an elaborate illustration of how historical semantics may contribute to the history of psychiatry. *Reaction* first acquired wide currency in the action-reaction model amply borrowed from Newtonian mechanics; it entered the political vocabulary after the French Revolution; it became prominent in late eighteenth-century theories of the relations between the *physique* and the *moral*, and was finally assimilated into different varieties of nineteenth-century medicine. The popularity of *reaction* is explained by its convenience: In a Bachelardian vein, Starobinski comments that its use "exempts [its users] from proposing specific and nuanced pathogenic mechanisms or therapeutic operations." After the days of the gentle theory of "moral reaction," according to which the physician heals the patient by imparting confidence and energy, Hippolyte Bernheim (not yet the specialist of suggestion) advocated treating hysteria more vigorously, by eliciting in the patient strong emotional reactions.[43]

Starobinski's overview of Renaissance psychology tacitly involves his interest in the cultural ramifications of psychological notions, while his presentation of medical texts on the passions from Galen to Johannes Müller excludes literature altogether.[44] In an important essay on La Rochefoucauld, however, Starobinski demonstrates how the structure of the moralist's *Maxims* "transcribes" his views about the discontinuous organization of human faculties and passions.[45] Further pieces of "frontierless history" are Starobinski's essays on "the empire of imagination,"[46] on "fury" in literature, religion, and art,[47] and on psychoanalysis and literature,[48] several prefaces to significant works in the cultural history of psychiatry,[49] and minor miscellaneous writings.[50]

Starobinski's research on the consciousness of the body again illustrates his characteristic intertwining of medical and literary history and his effective use of historical semantics. In an original history of the concept of *coenaesthesis*, a term coined in the late eighteenth century, Starobinski traces the idea under different names, follows its vicissitudes into the late 1930s, and concludes that the notion rose with the psychological applications of the reflex arc model and declined with the increasing success of the idea of an interaction between the subject and the environment.[51] Elsewhere, he extends this historical study toward psychoanalysis, existentialism, and literature.

Starobinski's "Brief history of the consciousness of the body" opens with a quotation from the notebooks of Paul Valéry where the poet suggests that the cult of the "machine for living" is the "heresy of the end of time," follows the subject from Descartes through eighteenth- and nineteenth-century medicine and psychology (thus placing in historical perspective Freud's ideas about coenaesthesis and bodily sensation), and concludes by raising the question of the place of Valéry's "heresy" in modern sensibility.[52] One aspect of this sensibility is examined in an article on Valéry's *Monsieur Teste*. Monsieur Teste has generally been seen as the absolute intellectual hero. Yet, like his antithesis Des Esseintes, he ends up having to face his only possible rival: physical suffering. Starobinski quotes again from Valéry's notebooks: "L'homme n'a que lui-même à craindre—son pouvoir de douleur.'' Pain undermines the modern body cult, but also makes possible the total consciousness of the body that was, for Valéry, the ultimate limit of knowledge.[53]

In a detailed textual analysis of *Madame Bovary*, Starobinski studies Flaubert's use of the language of coenaesthesis, in particular of thermic sensations, and demonstrates the reciprocity of the writer's and his character's experiences. In Flaubert's novel, coenaesthesis appears as ''an experience of limits; the moment after,'' he writes, ''the world's contingency will again have the upper hand.'' The awareness of sensation reaches its climax in Madame Bovary's agony, which the critic beautifully describes as ''le sombre bouquet final de la cénésthésie.''[54]

Starobinski's concluding question in his essay on Flaubert is one he has implicitly asked many times. We might think, he says, that the language of the body is the only human expression not contaminated by commonplace. Yet, he asks, ''which *form* will be able to capture it and communicate it to others?''[55]

Melancholy, nostalgia, chlorosis, reaction, coenaesthesis—all these topics manifest Starobinski's fascination with the reciprocal relationship between the mind and the body, and with the confluence of a subjective consciousness (an author's or a character's), an inner state, and external conditions. They all show his concern with the *form* that might capture the feeling and make it communicable.

This question came together with the history of art, literature, and society, as well as with the themes of melancholy, nostalgia, and irony, in Starobinski's elegant and suggestive small book *Portrait of the Artist as Clown*. This essay can be taken as representative of how his criticism meets the dream of a frontierless history of ideas in determining the special flavor of his writings in medical history.

The aim of *Portrait of the Artist* is to define the ''particular quality of the interest that incited writers and painters of the XIXth century to multiply . . . the image of the clown, the acrobat, and the entertainment fair.'' This preoccupation, Starobinski notes, could be explained by the contrast between the circus and the life of an industrializing society. But there must also be a psychological factor: The modern artist identifies with the clown and feels a certain ''nostalgic complicity'' with the world of parade and extravaganza. The theme of the clown is for the artist a parodical way of talking about his condition and of criticizing himself and bourgeois respectability simultaneously.[56]

The ''Criticism of Consciousness''

Portrait of the Artist is not only the historical study of a theme but also an effort to understand what went on in the artist's consciousness, and how this consciousness constructed itself in the process of creation. Such a goal is typical of the so-called Geneva school and of what has been termed ''criticism of consciousness.''[57] No rigorous definition may be given of this school. Each one of its practitioners has emphasized his methodological, stylistic, thematic, and ideological independence.[58] Starobinski himself insists on the ''daring use of various methods'' and has never departed from his own rejection of ''methodolatry.''[59] One of his most elaborate methodological texts, ''The Interpreter's Progress,'' explicitly takes as its starting point a lengthy exercise in critical interpretation.[60] Starobinski's viewpoint thus corresponds exactly to Max Weber's remark that "methodology can only bring us reflective understanding of the means which have *demonstrated* their value in practice by raising them to the level of explicit consciousness."[61] As has been noticed,[62] one can apply to Starobinski what he observes about Leo Spitzer: "His methodology is the description of an intellectual itinerary: it is not a recipe."[63]

The "criticism of consciousness" has been described as being "subjective," as seeking "identification" and "intimacy" with the authors it investigates. "Sympathy," "participation," "coincidence of two consciousnesses," "intersubjective complicity"—such are the words often used to apprehend the approach of the Geneva school. Roland Barthes opposed the "biographic transcendence" of older critical styles to the "immanence" of this newer criticism, which, as he said, aimed less at explaining a text than at making it explicit.[64]

This is not to say that a critic such as Starobinski neglects the world surrounding an author. The point is rather that, for the Geneva school, the "author" is above all "the implied being who gradually assumes form as the work is created"; literature is "a form of consciousness," the "embodiment of a state of mind."[65] Its structures reveal a mental universe. This mental universe, however, does not precede and determine the work: "It is neither before nor after," writes Starobinski's Genevan colleague Jean Rousset, "it is through creation that [the artist] becomes who he is."[66]

Starobinski's criticism attests to his desire to grasp the consciousness of the writers he analyzes, to discover the textual structures that may appear consubstantial with their sensibility and through which they interpret themselves and the world. Thus, the essays collected in *The Living Eye* concern "literary works that manifest the pursuit of a hidden reality" and aim at "following the moving destiny of the *libido sentiendi* in its relation to the world and to other human consciousnesses."[67] Starobinski takes greatest pleasure in discovering the author in the text; and the pleasure is stronger when colored by irony. Not the least of the charms of Foucault's *The Birth of the Clinic* is that it allows the reader to glimpse "the personal and distinctive face of a philosopher-historian whose declared aim is nevertheless to get rid of the subject and subjectivity."[68]

Starobinski's keen "psychological" curiosity accounts for his attention to autobiographical writings, as illustrated in his books on Montesquieu, Montaigne, and Rousseau, and in other lengthy studies.[69] As he acknowledges, his approach is best adapted to texts "whose dominant aim is the revelation of the self."[70] For him, however, psychology does not explicate the text itself; it only brings to light the necessary yet insufficient conditions of creation. As Starobinski comments in relation to the well-documented neurosis of the French writer Raymond Roussel, no matter how revealing, and even though irrefutable as such, psychological interpretations are moved by an "obsessional desire of control" that dooms them to leave out something essential for an understanding of the work of art.[71] The same viewpoint dictates his critical comments on the sociology of literature and his belief that one must try to understand the "inventive marginality" whereby an *oeuvre* stretches beyond given social and psychological structures.[72]

For Starobinski, the work of art is *décentrement;* it may possess a "coefficient of negativity" and exist in opposition to its author's empirical existence.[73] The poetical richness of Baudelaire's *Spleen*, for example, witnesses to a surmounting of melancholy (which generally leads to mutism) through a recreation of the materials of personal experience.[74] The critic thus refuses to state a diagnosis. "I would prefer," he writes, "to say that, with the help of what he called his 'hysteria,' [Baudelaire] admirably mimics the attitudes and inmost mechanisms of melancholy."[75] Starobinski declares not to look for "the man 'behind' the work."[76] To be "free of all biographical anxiety," criticism must "recognize the hypothetical character and the alleged emotional history" of its subjects and "forego constructing an *ego* which is distinctive from the text."[77] To the reproach that his reading of Rousseau is "psychological," Starobinski replies that he wished neither to uncover unavowed motivations nor to reduce complex views to the vicissitudes of unconscious wishes. He compares his approach to Ernst Cassirer's.[78] Cassirer argued for the unity of Rousseau's theoretical writings; Starobinski, for whom the philosopher's early works were "anticipated confessions, reflections of the self,"[79] expanded the argument to the realm of his reveries and self-presentation. Accordingly, rather than participate in the controversy on Rousseau's illness, he reconstructs "what disease was for Rousseau's own consciousness."[80]

Starobinski's writings betray his attraction toward psychoanalysis. He has long been in contact with psychoanalysts but has been neither analyst nor analysand. Psychoanalysis seems to him untestable, and its argumentative structure, suspicious. Nevertheless, he is interested in it as a system of thought and has, as a historian, written on its relationship to literature.[81]

As a critic, Starobinski finds in Freud a lesson in the technique of exegesis and liberally adopts the psychoanalytic language for his own interpretive purposes. Yet he does not proclaim its timeless validity. As he emphasizes in a penetrating study on psychological inhibition and social prohibition in the work of Madame de Charrière, psychoanalytic language limits itself to bringing past mentalities and sensibilities closer to us.[82] For him, the distinguishing trait of criticism is precisely that it reaches beyond psychological and historical determinants, toward the individual's self-construction. Literature is for Starobinski a way of surpassing one's anonymously determined destiny as natural and social being,[83] and that is why he opposes treating it as a symptom, or "as a mask behind which lay[s] a psychological truth open to self-empowered interpretation."[84] He systematically asserts the difference between the present and the past, himself and the authors he analyzes. "Distance" is for him a crucial notion.[85]

Starobinski's fundamental problem has been defined as, How to relate to that which proves to be radically other?[86] In the quest for an answer, he gives up the claim to pure identification with his analysands. He frequently describes himself as listening to others and letting them speak their own tongues: hence the key role of quotation in his writing. This attitude is part of what Starobinski calls the "critical relation"—the ceaseless movement between intuitive identification with an individual consciousness and the panoramic view of the context and the cultural patterns in which a work is embedded.[87] Criticism thus belongs to a specific level, irreducible to either history or psychology; historical information by itself is as insufficient for interpretation as psychological data alone. Thus, it would be as absurd to reduce Albert Camus's *The Plague* to its medical sources as it would be ignore that, well beyond any "clinical verdict," Mme. de Staël's attitude toward suicide manifests a whole conception of art and literature that relates, in complex ways, to the writer's own life.[88] As in the case of the "artist as clown," what counts is the relation between being and creating, poetics and existence.

Language as Transparency and Obstruction

Starobinski's apparently distant attitude stems from his insight into the mediated nature of the affective and intellectual experience of past humanity. He owes to medicine his realization of the integral place of the body in the makeup of individual self-awareness: "Our consciousness is from the beginning engaged in a body and in an experienced situation."[89] A sharp attention to the inescapable presence of the body has become the common denominator of his approach to psychosomatic medicine, coenaesthesis, and melancholy and other psychological states, and it also accounts for some of his inquiries into literary texts. But all we can know of bodily and mental states is what has been stylized or symbolized.

Starobinski's "distance," therefore, proceeds from an understanding that the other, the great writer or an anonymous individual of the past, can be apprehended only through an intermediary that gives him an objective form. This intermediary is always a language: verbal, pictorial, architectural, musical. The critic and the historian, in their advance toward a particular mind, are intercepted by forms and traditions. As Starobinski puts it, for them,

> sentiments do not exist before they attain linguistic status. Nothing is perceptible of a feeling ahead of the point where it is named, designated and expressed. It is therefore not the affective experience itself that is offered to us: only the part of it that has passed into a style can appeal to the historian.[90]

Starobinski remarks that after the feeling has been named, its verbalization becomes a constitutive part of the affective experience.[91] As a historian, he knows he cannot go beyond words, and that is why so much of his work may be legitimately placed in the great French tradition of a "stylistics of existence."[92] As a critic, however, even in his historical writings, he steadily reaches toward the "'truth'" of what shows through the surface of expression.[93]

Awareness of the barrier of language—language as a means to reach awareness: These are the two poles of history and criticism that Jean Starobinski tries to reconcile. The *oeuvre* that has resulted, concentrated with fascination on the "thin skin of appearance" where text and life meet, points in a direction that converges with the vanguard of psychiatric history.

The history of psychiatry is no longer confined to narrating the discipline's progress, from the primitive and the Oriental, through the "great decline" of early Christianity and the "restless surrender to demonology," to the humanizing of the asylum, and the elaboration of scientific nosographies, nosologies, and therapies.[94] Studying the emergence of psychiatry as a profession, doing the sociology of mental illness and psychiatric institutions, questioning biographical and historical legends, following (with or without Foucault) the dynamics of reason and unreason, and tracking what he characterized as society's "consciousness of madness," are all among the enterprises of contemporary historiography. Most of the time, however, the focus has remained on the diverse agents of medical and administrative authority: Theories and therapies are theirs; they design hospitals and dictate regimens; they write the notebooks, memoranda, reports, and books that make up the bulk of the historian's research material. Typically, what the patients have had to say is known through case histories designed to illustrate the workings of etiology, diagnosis, treatment, and, often, the well-founded character of their authors' medical choices. Yet enough may be known to incorporate otherwise the patient's own "voice" into the history of psychiatry.

Henri Ellenberger, a pioneer in this domain, demonstrated the patient's active role in psychiatric discovery.[95] Roy Porter has advocated recapturing the patient's point of view and listening to the "stories of the insane."[96] Recovering the human substrate of the history of psychiatry has inherent limitations. The "mad" who left written testimonies must have been literate and articulate; the actual corpus of such writings includes no women and hardly anyone from the lower orders.[97] Yet the "stories of the insane," beyond what they tell about the conditions of treatment, the relations between patient and doctor, or the manufacturing of madness, should offer a glimpse into an individual's psychological and social experience.

Jean Starobinski has not only contributed to place psychiatric and psychological thought in cultural context but has also approached the intellectual frontier where the history of psychiatry tends to become the history of experience. For him, the very act of writing an autobiographical testimony is part of the construction of the self, and this applies to discoursing on one's own malady. The "consciousness" to which he pays so much attention in his criticism is for him fashioned in the process of creation and becomes central to what can be known about the writer. Whether it be Rousseau's *Confessions* or Daniel Paul Schreber's *Memoirs of My Nervous Illness*, the text, with its rhetoric, rhythm, and themes, may function as a translucent window of language through which to apprehend experience. Nevertheless, precisely because it witnesses to the surpassing of the past and to the active making of the present, the text is an obstacle to apprehending raw personal experience. Through the "critical relation" he chooses to establish with his authors, Jean Starobinski demonstrates that only that part of psychological life that has "passed into a style" is accessible to the historian. But he also proves that the careful analysis of this "style" is crucial for going as far as possible toward the experiencing consciousness and for placing it within the social horizons it both reflects and transcends.

Notes

A shorter, somewhat different version of this chapter appeared as "Jean Starobinski and the History of the Human Sciences," *History of the Human Sciences*, v (1992), 73–85. I have referred to translations only when relevant to the presentation. See the Addendum for fuller references.

1. "In straddling C. P. Snow's two cultures, Starobinski has made a virtually unique contribution to contemporary thought." Michael Shepherd, "Jean Starobinski," *Lancet*, 4 April 1987, 798. A bibliography of Starobinski's writings is included in *Cahiers pour un temps / Jean Starobinski* (Paris: Centre Georges Pompidou, 1985), 283–301. Vincent Barras, "L'histoire de la médecine chez Jean Starobinski," *Courrier du Groupe d'études du XVIIIe siècle* (Geneva), no. 9, May 1992, 23–26, is an updated list of his publications in the history of medicine (excluding the more literary studies). Most directly relevant to our topic are: François Azouvi, "Histoire des sciences ou histoire des mots?" in *Cahiers pour un temps*; Vincent Barras, "Entretien avec Jean Starobinski," *Médecine et Hygiène*, xlviii (1990), 3294–3297, 3400–3402; Claudio Pogliano, "Il bilinguismo imperfetto di Jean Starobinski," *Intersezioni*, x (1990), 171–183. The best general overview is Claudio Pogliano, "Jean Starobinski," *Belfagor*, xlv (2) (1990), 157–180. Staro-

binski effectively discusses the bilingualism of modern culture in "Langage scientifique et langage poétique," *Diogène*, no. 100 (1977), 139–157. For his view of the relation between literary criticism and the methods of history, sociology, psychology, and formal analysis, see his "Considerations on the present state of literary criticism," *Diogenes*, lxxiv (1971): 57–88.

2. *Cahiers pour un temps*, and *Magazine littéraire* (Paris), no. 280, September 1990.

3. Starobinski, "Réponse de J. Starobinski" in *Prix Rambert 1965. Feuille centrale de Zofingue* (1965), 28.

4. Jacques Bonnet, [Interview with J. Starobinski] in *Cahiers pour un temps*, 21.

5. Starobinski, "Histoire des idées et critique littéraire," *Bastions de Genève*, no. 10 (1962–63), 6–19, 7–8.

6. *L'invention de la liberté* (Geneva: Skira, 1964); *1789. Les emblèmes de la raison* (Paris: Flammarion, 1973). See discussion by Hans Robert Jauss, "Jean Starobinski et l'archéologie de la modernité" in *Cahiers pour un temps*.

7. Starobinski, "Les enjeux de l'essai," *Revue de Belles-Lettres* (Geneva), 106e année (1983), no. 2–3, 93–105, 102.

8. Ibid., 105.

9. *Jean-Jacques Rousseau: la transparence et l'obstacle* [1957], followed by *Sept essais sur Rousseau* (Paris: Gallimard, 1971).

10. *Histoire du traitement de la mélancolie des origines à 1900* (Basle: Documenta Geigy / Acta Psychosomatica, no. 4, 1960).

11. *Programme des cours de l'Université de Genève* (1963–1965). Apart from *Histoire du traitement* and other works cited below, Starobinski's writings in medical history include "Descartes et la médecine," *Synthèses* (Brussels), vii (1953), 333–338; "Molière et les médecins," *Symposium Ciba*, xiv (1966), 143–148; "D'Agrippa de Nettesheim à Montaigne: l'embarras des médecins devant l'origine de la semence," *Gesnerus*, xl (1983), 175–183; (edited with Marc Cramer and Marco-Antonio Barblan), *La Faculté de Médecine de Genève, 1876–1976* (Geneva: Médecine et Hygiène, 1978).

12. Barras, "Entretien," 3294–3295. Although it does not mention Spitzer, Starobinski's research on the history of concepts (melancholy, nostalgia, civilization, action, and reaction) observes Spitzer's faith in the central relevance of historical semantics for the understanding of culture; cf. Leo Spitzer, *Essays in Historical Semantics* (New York: S. F. Vanni, 1948). For Starobinski's appreciation of other aspects of Spitzer's work, see "Leo Spitzer et la lecture sylistique" in *La relation critique* (Paris: Gallimard, 1970).

13. Starobinski, "Une théorie soviétique de l'origine nerveuse des maladies" [on A. D. Speransky, *Grundlagen der Theorie der Medizin*], *Critique*, no. 47 (1951), 348–362; "La 'sagesse' du corps et la malade comme égarement: le 'stress' " [on Hans Selye, *The Physiology and Pathology of Exposure to Stress*], ibid., no. 59 (1952), 347–360; "Le passé de la médecine" [on Henry E. Sigerist, *A History of Medicine*, vol. 1], ibid., no. 70 (1953), 256–270; "La connaissance de la vie" [on Georges Canguilhem, *Essai sur quelques problèmes concernant le normal et le pathologique* and *La connaissance de la vie*], ibid., no. 75–76 (1953), 777–791; "La médecine psycho-somatique" [on Franz Alexander, *La médecine psychosomatique*, and Thérèse Benedek, *Les fonctions de l'appareil sexuel et leurs troubles*], ibid., no. 81, 165–181; "Des taches et des masques" [on Hermann Rorschach, *Psychodiagnostik*, Ewald Bohm, *Lehrbuch der Rorschach-Psychodiagnostik*, Françoise Minkowska, *Le Rorschach*, and Roland Kuhn, *Ueber Maskendeutungen im Rorschachen Versuch*], ibid., no. 135–136, 792–804. Revised versions of the last two articles are included in *La relation critique* under the titles, respectively, "La maladie comme infortune de l'imagination. (La médecine psychosomatique)" and "L'imagination projective. (Le test de Rorschach)."

14. Starobinski, *Histoire de la médecine*, with iconography prepared by Nicolas Bouvier (Lausanne: Éditions Rencontre, 1963), 6. This work appeared in English translation as *A History of Medicine* (New York: Hawthorn Books, 1964).

15. Starobinski, "Une mélancolie moderne: le portrait du docteur Gachet par Van Gogh," *Médecine et Hygiène*, 49e année (1991), 13–16.

16. Starobinski, "Médecine et anti-médecine," *Cahiers de la Faculté de médecine* (University of Geneva), xiii (1986), 11–22; "Le médecin, le patient et le bon Dieu," *Campus* (University of Geneva), no. 7 (November–December 1990), 20–21.

17. Starobinski, "La leçon de la nostalgie," *Médecine de France*, no. 129 (1962), 6–11, 10–11.

18. Michel Contat, "Jean Starobinski sur la ligne Paris-Genève-Milan" [an interview], *Le Monde*, 28 April 1989, 24.

19. *Jean Starobinski. La maschera e l'uomo*, text of an interview carried out by Guido Ferrari for the Swiss-Italian Television in 1986 (Bellinzona: Edizioni Casagrande, 1990), 17, 18.

20. Cf. Starobinski's remarks on Burton's "pseudonymous mask" in "Démocrite parle. L'utopie mélancholique de Robert Burton," *Le Débat*, no. 29, March 1984, 49–72. See also Starobinski, "Stendhal pseudonyme" in *L'Oeil vivant* (Paris: Gallimard, 1961).

21. Erwin Panofsky and Fritz Saxl, *Dürers "Melencolia I." Eine quellen- und typengeschichtliche Untersuchung* (Leipzig: B. G. Teubner, 1923); Raymond Klibansky, E. Panofsky, and F. Saxl, *Saturn and Melancholy. Studies in Natural Philosophy, Religion and Art* (London: Thomas Nelson & Sons, 1964).

22. Bonnet, [Interview with J. Starobinski], 21–22.

23. Klibansky, "Avant propos" in *Saturne et la Mélancolie. Études historiques et philosophiques: Nature, religion, médecine et art*, trans. F. Durand-Bogaert and L. Evrard (Paris: Gallimard, 1989). This edition superseded the original English one, since Klibansky supplied corrections, additions, new illustrations, and a thoroughly revised version of the Aristotelian "Problem XXX.I," source of the traditional link between genius and melancholy.

24. Starobinski, *Histoire du traitement*, 9, 86.

25. Ibid., 10. See also the brief "Mania and depression" in Michael Shepherd and Olivier L. Zangwill (eds.), *Handbook of Psychiatry*, vol. 1, *General Psychopathology* (Cambridge: Cambridge University Press, 1983).

26. Starobinski, *Histoire du traitement*, 91.

27. It was agreed that another author would write for Geigy's "Acta Psychosomatica" the twentieth-century sequel (he never did).

28. Starobinski, "L'encre de la mélancolie," *Nouvelle Revue Française*, xi (1) (1963), 410–423.

29. Starobinski, "Ironie et mélancolie: Gozzi, Hoffmann, Kierkegaard," *Sensibilità e razionalità nel Settecento* (Florence, Sanzoni), August 1967, 423–462. Almost identical text in *Critique*, nos. 227 and 228 (1966), 291–308, 438–457. On Kierkegaard, see also Starobinski, "Les masques du pécheur et les pseudonymes du chrétien," *Revue de théologie et de philosophie*, 3e série, xiii (1963), 334–346.

30. Starobinski, "Démocrite parle."

31. Starobinski, "La mélancolie de l'anatomiste," *Tel Quel*, no. 10 (1962), 1–29. Starobinski has also written a short presentation of Robert Burton, *L'utopie, ou la république poétique* (Paris: Obsidiane / L'Age d'homme, coll. Acedia, 1992), portions of Burton's preface to *The Anatomy of Melancholy*, translated and annotated by Louis Evrard.

32. Starobinski, *Montaigne en mouvement* (Paris: Gallimard, 1982), 7. The English version misses the point entirely. Starobinski writes that Montaigne's initial question is: "une fois que la *pensée mélancolique* a récusé l'illusion des apparences, qu'advient-il ensuite?" The English mistranslates: "Once *pessimistic philosophy* has repudiated illusory appearances, what then?" *Montaigne in Motion*, trans. A. Goldhammer (Chicago: University of Chicago Press, 1985), ix. (Emphasis mine.)

33. Starobinski, *La transparence et l'obstacle*.

34. Starobinski, *La mélancolie au miroir. Trois lectures de Baudelaire* (Paris: Julliard, 1989).

35. Starobinski, "Suicide et mélancolie chez Mme de Staël," *Preuves*, cxc (December 1966), 41–48; "Note sur le bouffon romantique," *Cahiers du sud*, lxi (1966), 270–275; *Portrait de l'artiste en saltimbanque* (Geneva: Skira / Paris: Flammarion, 1970).

36. Starobinski, "Gazing at Death" [review of M. Foucault, *The Birth of the Clinic*], *New York Review of Books*, 22 January 1976, 18–22, 21. The "'traditional' " history mentioned is Erwin H. Ackerknecht's *Medicine at the Paris Hospital*.

37. Starobinski, "La nostalgie: théories medicales et expression littéraire," *Studies on Voltaire and the Eighteenth Century*, xxvii (1963), 1505–1518; "Le concept de nostalgie," *Diogène*, no. 54 (1966), 92–115 [developed version of "La nostalgie," with a new introduction]. These studies are currently being expanded into a book (to appear in Paris, Éditions du Seuil) that will give more room to the literary dimension of nostalgia.

38. Starobinski, "Sur la fonction de la parole dans la théorie médicale de l'époque romantique," *Médecine de France*, no. 205 (1969), 9–12. The therapeutic role of language and the relation of therapist to patient are also dealt with in Starobinski, "Descartes et la thérapie épistolaire," *Documenta Geigy* (1969), issue "Le verbe en médecine," 2–3.

39. Starobinski, "Une mélancolie moderne."

40. Starobinski, "L'immortalité mélancolique," *Le temps de la réflexion*, iii (1982), 231–251. Pages 232–236 reproduce Cotard's 1880 report "Du délire hypocondriaque dans une forme grave de la mélancolie anxieuse." Starobinski establishes a connection between Cotard's syndrome and Baudelaire's "Spleen" in "Les proportions de l'immortalité" in Vittore Branca, Carlo Ossola, and Salomon Resnik (eds.), *I linguaggi del sogno* (Florence: Sansoni, 1984), 240–241, 245. Of related interest: Starobinski, "Rêve et immortalité chez Baudelaire,"*Corps écrit*, no. 7 (1983), 45–56. The anthropological dimension of Kafka's writings has long interested Starobinski; see, for example, Franz Kafka, *La colonie pénitentiaire. Nouvelles suivies d'un Journal intime*, preface and translation by J. Starobinski (Fribourg: Egloff, 1945).

41. See, for example, Starobinski, "L'*Essai de Psychologie* de Charles Bonnet: Une version corrigée inédite," *Gesnerus*, xxxii (1975), 1–15, and "Le 'médecin croyant' et le théologien genevois. Une lettre écrite en 1802 par M. F. R. Buisson à Pierre Picot," ibid., xlix (1991), 333–341. These annotated editions witness to Starobinski's perennial interests: The authors studied were all deeply concerned with the relations body-soul and life-afterlife. In his letter to the Genevan Protestant theologian Picot, the French Catholic physician Buisson advocated the alliance of theologians and doctors against the ideas that dominated the Paris School of Medicine (*idéologie*, Pinel's anticlericalism, Cabanis's monistic materialism).

42. Starobinski, "Sur la chlorose," *Romantisme*, no. 31 (1981), 113–130.

43. Starobinski, "Le mot réaction de la physique à la psychiatrie," *Diogène*, no. 93 (1976), 3–30. The history of the "action-reaction" couple is the subject of a book to be published after the one on the concept of nostalgia, also in Paris by Éditions du Seuil. For the stylistic and rhetorical ways in which the concepts of action and reaction became embedded in literary and scientific discourse, see Starobinski, " 'Action et réaction' chez Diderot" in Catherine Lafarge (ed.), *Dilemmes du roman. Essays in Honor of Georges May*, Stanford French and Italian Studies, vol. 65 (Saratoga: Anma Libri, 1989).

44. Starobinski, "Panorama succinct des sciences psychologiques entre 1575 et 1625," *Gesnerus*, xxxvii (1980), 3–16; "Le passé de la passion. Textes médicaux et commentaires," *Nouvelle revue de psychanalyse*, xxi (1980), 51–76.

45. Starobinski, "La Rochefoucauld et les morales substitutives," *Nouvelle Revue Française*, xiv (3) (1966), 16–34, 211–229. See also the introduction in La Rochefoucauld, *Maximes et Mémoires* (Paris: Union Générale d'Éditions, coll. 10/18, 1964).

46. "L'empire de l'imaginaire," part II of *La relation critique*, includes two previously published historical essays, "Jalons pour une histoire du concept d'imagination" and "Sur l'histoire des fluides imaginaires. (Des esprits animaux à la libido),"and the modified versions

of two essay-reviews of the 1950s, "La maladie comme infortune de l'imagination" and "L'imagination projective" (see note 13).

47. Starobinski, *Trois fureurs* (Paris: Gallimard, 1974) includes "L'épée d'Ajax" (on Sophocles' tragedy), "Le combat avec Légion" (on Marc V, 1–20), and "La vision de la dormeuse" (on Fuseli's "The Nightmare"); see also Starobinski, "La littérature et l'irrationnel," *Cahiers roumains d'études littéraires*, ii (1974), 4–15.

48. Starobinski, "Psychanalyse et littérature," part III of *La relation critique*, includes "Psychanalyse et connaissance littéraire," "Hamlet et Oedipe," and "Freud, Breton, Myers." See also "Le corps animé," *Nouvelle revue de psychanalyse*, no. 12 (1975), 137–143, introduction to an excerpt of one of Johann Eduard Erdmann's 1852 *Psychologische Briefe*, partially quoted by Freud in the *Interpretation of Dreams*. Starobinski also translated into French a 1907 letter of Josef Breuer to Auguste Forel concerning Anna O. and the origins of psychoanalysis: Erwin H. Ackerknecht, "Lettre à Auguste Forel," *Mercure de France*, xxxlii (1964), 309–312.

49. Starobinski, "Segalen aux confins de la médecine" in Victor Segalen, *Les cliniciens ès lettres* [1902] (Montpellier: Fata Morgana, 1980); Préface in Hans Prinzhorn, *Expressions de la folie. Dessins, peintures, sculptures d'asile [Bildnerei der Geisteskranken* (1922)], trans. A. Brousse and M. Weber (Paris: Gallimard, 1984); "Préface: Le salut à la statue" in Joseph Popper-Lynkeus, *Fantaisies d'un réaliste [Phantasien eines Realisten* (1899)], trans. C. Heim (Paris: Gallimard, 1987). The preface to Segalen is actually a solid thirty-six-page study.

50. See the brief, light, and very free essays (most of them related to Starobinski's favorite "psychological" topics) contributed between 1989 and 1992 to the Italian magazine *Sfera*, and now gathered in a fifty-five-page, not-for-sale volume, *Jean Starobinski* (Rome: Sfera / Editrice Sigma Tau, 1992). The essays are "Le philosophe couché" (on the consciousness of the body); "Les antidotes de la peur" (mainly on Rousseau); "La dissimulation tragique" (which discerns, *in fine*, the turn-of-the-century theme of hysteria in Hofmannsthal's character of Electra); "Vide et création" (which touches on melancholy); "L'attraction en tant que retour à l'unité" (focused on Poe's "Eureka"); "Force et faiblesse psychologiques" (through La Rochefoucauld, Pierre Janet, and Roger Caillois); "La Machine de Descartes" (on Descartes's physiology).

51. Starobinski, "Le concept de cénésthésie et les idées neuropsychologiques de Moritz Schiff," *Gesnerus*, xxxiv (1977), 2–19.

52. Starobinski, "Brève histoire de la conscience du corps" in Robert Ellrodt (ed.), *Genèse de la conscience moderne* (Paris: Presses Universitaires de France, 1983), 215.

53. Starobinski, "Monsieur Teste face à la douleur" in *Valéry, pour quoi?* (Paris: Les impressions nouvelles, 1987), 99.

54. Starobinski, "L'échelle des températures. Lecture du corps dans *Madame Bovary*" in Raymonde Debray-Genette et al., *Travail de Flaubert* (Paris: Seuil, 1983), 61, 63.

55. Starobinski, "L'échelle des températures," 77.

56. Starobinski, *Portrait de l'artiste en saltimbanque*, 6–8; see also "Note sur le bouffon romantique."

57. See J. Hillis Miller, "The Geneva School: The Criticism of Marcel Raymond, Albert Béguin, Georges Poulet, Jean Rousset, Jean-Pierre Richard, and Jean Starobinski" in John K. Simon (ed.), *Modern French Criticism. From Proust and Valéry to Structuralism* (Chicago: University of Chicago Press, 1972); Sarah N. Lawall, *Critics of Consciousness. The Existential Structures of Literature* (Cambridge: Harvard University Press, 1968); Georges Poulet, *La conscience critique* (Paris: José Corti, 1971). On Poulet, who coined the expression "Geneva School," see Starobinski, "Le rêve de Georges Poulet," *Le Monde*, 21 August 1992, 10.

58. See Franco Giacone "L''école de Genève:' Mythe ou realité?" [Part I] *Micromégas*, ii (1) 1975, 81–101 [interviews with M. Raymond, J. Rousset, and J. Starobinski]; [Part II] ibid., ii (2), 67–91 [interviews with G. Poulet and J.-P. Richard].

59. Starobinski, "The Meaning of Literary History," *New Literary History*, vii (1) (1975), 83–88, 87, 86.

60. Starobinski, "Le progrès de l'interprète" in *La relation critique*.

61. Max Weber, "Critical Studies in the Logic of the Cultural Sciences" [1905] in E. A. Shils and H. A. Finch (eds.), *Max Weber on the Methodology of the Social Sciences* (Illinois: Free Press, 1949), 115.

62. Philip Stewart, "The Critical Tautology" [reviews of Starobinski, *La relation critique* and *La transparence et l'obstacle*], *Diacritics*, Spring 1975, 2–6.

63. Starobinski, "Leo Spitzer et la lecture sylistique," 66.

64. Roland Barthes, "Les deux critiques" in *Essais critiques* (Paris: Seuil, 1964).

65. Lawall, *Critics of Consciousness*, 267; Hillis Miller, "The Geneva School," 279.

66. Jean Rousset, *Forme et signification. Essai sur les structures littéraires de Corneille à Claudel* (Paris: José Corti, 1962), ix.

67. Starobinski, *L'Oeil vivant*, 16, 18.

68. Starobinski, "Gazing at Death," 22.

69. Starobinski, *Montesquieu par lui-même* (Paris: Seuil, 1953), *Montaigne en mouvement, La transparence et l'obstacle*. The main studies are "Jean-Jacques Rousseau et le péril de la réflexion" and "Stendhal pseudonyme," both in *L'Oeil vivant*; "Le dîner de Turin," exemplary detailed analysis of an episode from Rousseau's *Confessions*, part (b) of "Le progrès de l'interprète" in *La relation critique*; and "La lance d'Achille," part I of "Le remède dans le mal: la pensée de Rousseau" in *Le remède dans le mal. Critique et légitimation de l'artifice à l'âge des lumières* (Paris: Gallimard, 1989).

70. Claude Reichler, "Entretien [avec] Jean Starobinski," *Repères (Revue romande)*, no. 12 (1985), 96–115, 101.

71. Starobinski, "Raymond Roussel et le mythe de la défaillance fatale," *Les lettres nouvelles*, xxxix, October 1963, 207–209, 209.

72. Starobinski, "Sur les conditions de travail de la sociologie littéraire," *Études littéraires*, iii (2), August 1970, 167–172.

73. Starobinski, *La relation critique*, 63.

74. Starobinski, "Les proportions de l'immortalité," 240–241.

75. Starobinski, "Les rimes du vide. Une lecture de Baudelaire," *Nouvelle revue de psychanalyse*, xi (1975), 133–143, 143, n. 1.

76. Giacone, "L'École de Genève,' " Part I, 90–91.

77. Starobinski, "Considerations on the present state of literary criticism," 74–75.

78. Starobinski, Preface to Ernst Cassirer, *Le problème Jean-Jacques Rousseau*, trans. M. B. de Launay (Paris: Hachette, 1987), xvii–xviii. Cf. Peter Gay's discussion in his Postscript to Cassirer, *The Question of Jean-Jacques Rousseau*, trans. P. Gay, second edition (New Haven: Yale University Press, 1989), 132–133.

79. Starobinski, "Lire Rousseau" in Jean-Jacques Rousseau, *Les Confessions et autres écrits autobiographiques* (Lausanne: La Guilde du Livre, 1962), xii.

80. Starobinski, "Sur la maladie de Rousseau" in *La transparence et l'obstacle*, 438.

81. "Psychanalyse et littérature," part III of *La relation critique*, includes "Psychanalyse et connaissance littéraire," "Hamlet et Oedipe," and "Freud, Breton, Myers."

82. Starobinski, "Les *Lettres écrites de Lausanne* de Madame de Charrière: Inhibition psychique et interdit social" in *Roman et lumières au XVIIIe siècle* (Paris: Éditions Sociales, 1970).

83. Starobinski, "Psychanalyse et connaissance littéraire," 284.

84. Starobinski, preface in *The Living Eye*, trans. A. Goldhammer (Cambridge: Harvard University Press, 1989), viii.

85. Georges Poulet, "Jean Starobinski et le thème de la distance" in *Cahiers pour un temps*.

86. Poulet, *La conscience critique*, 237.

87. See in particular Starobinski, "Le voile de Popée" in *L'Oeil vivant*.

88. Starobinski, "Albert Camus et la peste," *Symposium Ciba*, x (2) (1962), 62–70; "Suicide et mélancolie chez Mme de Staël."

89. Starobinski, "Merleau-Ponty: 'Je ne peux pas sortir de l'être,' " *Gazette de Lausanne*, 27–28 May 1961, 13 and 19, 13.

90. Starobinski, "Le concept de nostalgie," 92.

91. Ibid., 93.

92. Michel Foucault on Philippe Ariès: ". . . il a fondé le principe d'une sylistique de l'existence—je veux dire d'une étude des formes par lesquelles l'homme se manifeste, s'invente, s'oublie ou se nie dans sa fatalité d'être vivant et mortel." Quoted in Didier Eribon, *Michel Foucault* (Paris: Flammarion, 1991), 132.

93. Starobinski, "La nostalgie," 1506.

94. Some of these expressions come from Gregory Zilboorg, *A History of Medical Psychology* (New York: Norton, 1941).

95. Mark S. Micale, "Henri F. Ellenberger: The History of Psychiatry as the History of the Unconscious," this volume.

96. Roy S. Porter, *A Social History of Madness. Stories of the Insane* (London: Weidenfeld and Nicolson, 1989).

97. Porter, *Mind-Forg'd Manacles. A History of Madness in England from the Restoration to the Regency* (Cambridge, MA: Harvard University Press, 1987), 269 (from ch. 5, "The Voice of the Mad").

Addendum—Jean Starobinski: Writings in the History of Psychiatry

At the risk of betraying the unity of Jean Starobinski's *oeuvre*, this bibliography has been limited to those writings that seem best to fit the professional boundaries of the history of psychiatry. Two other bibliographies may be consulted: the comprehensive one published in *Cahiers pour un temps / Jean Starobinski* (Paris: Centre Georges Pompidou, 1985), 283–301, including the rubrics "Mask and Melancholy" and "History of Medicine and Psychological Thought," and Vincent Barras's "L'histoire de la médecine chez Jean Starobinski," *Courrier du Groupe d'études du XVIIIe siècle* (Geneva), no. 9, May 1992, 23–26.

.*Histoire du traitement de la mélancolie des origines à 1900* (Basle: Documenta Geigy / Acta Psychosomatica, no. 4, 1960), 100 pages [Simultaneously issued in German]; trans. *Storia del trattamento della malinconia delle origini al 1900*, trans. F. Paracchini (Milano: Guerini e associati, 1990).

"La nostalgie: théories médicales et expression littéraire," *Studies on Voltaire and the Eighteenth Century*, xxvii (1963), 1505–1518.

[Translation of a 1907 letter of Josef Breuer to Auguste Forel concerning "Anna O." and the origins of psychoanalysis] Erwin H. Ackerknecht, "Lettre à Auguste Forel," *Mercure de France*, xxxii (1964), 309–312.

"Le concept de nostalgie," *Diogène*, no. 54 (1966), 92–115 [Development of "La nostalgie"]; trans. "The Idea of Nostalgia," *Diogenes*, 54 (1966), 81–103.

"Suicide et mélancolie chez Mme de Staël," *Preuves*, cxc (December 1966), 41–48. Also in *Madame de Staël et l'Europe* (Paris: Klincksieck, 1970), vol. 1.

"Sur la fonction de la parole dans la théorie médicale de l'époque romantique," *Médecine de France*, no. 205 (1969), 9–12; trans. "The role of language in psychiatric treatment in the French Romantic age. A note on Dr. Laurent Cerise," *Psychological Medicine*, iv (1974), 360–363.

"Descartes et la thérapie épistolaire," *Documenta Geigy* (1969), issue "Le verbe en médecine," 2–3.

The following essays are collected in *La relation critique* (Paris: Gallimard, 1970): Part II, "L'empire de l'imaginaire"; "Jalons pour une histoire du concept d'imagination"; "Sur l'histoire des fluides imaginaires"; "La maladie comme infortune de l'imagination. (La médecine psychosomatique)"; "L'imagination projective. (Le test de Rorschach)." Part III, "Psychanalyse et littérature"; "Psychanalyse et connaissance littéraire"; "Hamlet et Oedipe"; and "Freud, Breton, Myers," trans. "Psychoanalysis and Literary Understanding" and "Hamlet and Oedipus" in *The Living Eye* [selected chapters from *L'Oeil vivant* and *La relation critique*], trans. A. Goldhammer (Cambridge: Harvard University Press, 1989).

"Le corps animé," *Nouvelle revue de psychanalyse*, no. 12 (1975), 137–143.

"Le mot réaction de la physique à la psychiatrie," *Diogène*, no. 93 (1976), 3–30; trans. "The Word Reaction: From Physics to Psychiatry," *Diogenes*, 93 (1976), 1–27.

"Gazing at Death," *New York Review of Books*, no. 21–22, 22 January 1976, 18–22. [Review of M. Foucault, *The Birth of the Clinic*.]

"Le concept de cénésthésie et les idées neuropsychologiques de Moritz Schiff," *Gesnerus*, xxxiv (1977), 2–19.

"Panorama succinct des sciences psychologiques entre 1575 et 1625," *Gesnerus*, xxxvii (1980), 3–16.

"Le passé de la passion. Textes médicaux et commentaires," *Nouvelle revue de psychanalyse*, xxi (1980), 51–76.

"Sur la chlorose," *Romantisme*, no. 31 (1981), 113–130.

"L'immortalité mélancolique," *Le temps de la réflexion*, iii (1982), 231–251; trans. (slightly modified): Pages 231–238: "Der 'Verneinungswahn,' " § 1 of "Melancholie und Unsterblichkeitswahn bei Baudelaire" in *Kleine Geschichte* (see below).

"Mania and depression" in Michael Shepherd and Olivier L. Zangwill (eds.), *Handbook of Psychiatry*, vol. 1, *General Psychopathology* (Cambridge: Cambridge University Press, 1983), 42–44.

"Brève histoire de la conscience du corps" in Robert Ellrodt (ed.), *Genèse de la conscience moderne* (Paris: Presses Universitaires de France, 1983), 215–229; trans. "A Short History of Bodily Sensation" in Michel Feher (ed.) *Fragments for a History of the Human Body*, Part II (New York: Zone, 1989); "Kleine Geschichte des Körpergefühls" in *Kleine Geschichte* (see below).

"L'échelle des températures. Lecture du corps dans *Madame Bovary*" in Raymonde Debray-Genette et al., *Travail de Flaubert* (Paris: Seuil, 1983). Also in *Le temps de la réflexion*, i (1980), 145–183; trans. "Die Skala der Temperaturen—'Körperlesung' in *Madame Bovary*" in *Kleine Geschichte* (see below); *La scala delle temperature*, translation and postscript by Carlo Gazzelli (Genoa: Il Melangolo, 1984).

"Démocrite parle: l'utopie mélancolique de Robert Burton," *Le Débat*, no. 29 (1984), 49–72; trans. (expanded): "Democrito parla: l'utopia malinconica di Robert Burton" in Robert Burton, *Anatomia della malinconia. Introduzione*, trans. F. Fonte Basso and G. Franci (Venice: Marsilio editore, 1983).

Préface in Hans Prinzhorn, *Expressions de la folie. Dessins, peintures, sculptures d'asile* [*Bildnerei der Geisteskranken* (1922)], trans. A. Brousse and M. Weber (Paris: Gallimard, 1984).

"Monsieur Teste face à la douleur" in *Valéry, pour quoi?* (Paris: Les impressions nouvelles, 1987), 93–119; trans. "Monsieur Teste Confronting Pain" in Michel Feher (ed.) *Fragments for a History of the Human Body*, Part II (New York: Zone, 1989); "Herr Teste und der Schmerz," expanded in *Kleine Geschichte* (see below).

Kleine Geschichte des Körpergefühls, trans. I. Pohlmann (Konstanz, Universitätsverlag Konstanz, 1987; reissued, Frankfurt am Main: Fischer Taschenbuch Verlag, 1991). Includes the four essays cited above. "Baudelaire: Schwindelgefühl und literarisches Schaffen," § 2 of "Melancholie und Unsterblichkeitswahn bei Baudelaire" (see above "L'immortalité

mélancolique'') translates, with some alterations, ''Rêve et immortalité chez Baudelaire,''
    Corps écrit, no. 7 (1983), 45–56.

''Force et faiblesse psychologiques,'' *Sfera*, no. 21, July–August 1991; reprinted in *Jean Staro-
    binski* (Rome: Sfera/Editrice Sigma Tau, 1992 [not for sale]), 39–45; trans. ''Der Mensch
    und seine Kräfte. Von La Rochefoucauld bis Roger Caillois,'' *Neue Zürcher Zeitung*, 17–
    18 August 1991, 58.

''Une mélancolie moderne: le portrait du docteur Gachet par Van Gogh,'' *Médecine et Hygiène*,
    xlix (1991), 13–16.

III

THE PSYCHOANALYTIC STRAIN

8

A History of Freud Biographies

ELISABETH YOUNG-BRUEHL

Psychoanalysis is unique among the sciences for many reasons, but certainly the most important is its completely exceptional mode of transmission from one generation of practitioners and researchers to the next. It is the one science, even the one type of psychology, that is practiced upon its future practitioners as the key ingredient of their training. Not simply a course of study nor even an apprenticeship is required of the future practitioners, but insight in the science's own terms, and self-alteration. Psychoanalysis is not learned, it is incorporated and an identification is formed with it.

In their training all analysts must, in effect, or perhaps one should say in affect, recapitulate both the founding father's analysis, which he, uniquely, conducted upon himself, and their own analysts' analyses. They all know that a self-analysis cannot, considered in light of Freud's own theory as well as his practice, be complete, so they are all automatically supercessors, better trained than their masters' master, but they are all also, nonetheless, lesser, for he is the unsurpassed genius.

This last observation brings me to a second reason why psychoanalysis is unique among the sciences (including other types of psychology). That is, the founder has never been made historical by a successor, never been equaled or even approximated as a contributor to psychoanalysis. There is no Einstein for this Newton. On the contrary, in their contributions to psychoanalytic method, theory, and metatheory, psychoanalysts for some six generations have had, before they can truly begin, to go back and confront the master's vast opus, and, as they became available, his almost equally vast correspondences and, eventually, even large libraries of commentaries on his person and his work. It is not surprising, therefore, that psychoanalysis is a science that not only cannot hold up the banner of Progress with any confidence but is full of rebellions—frustrated rages, in fact—against the very patriarchal achievements without which it would not exist. During Freud's lifetime, schisms and reassertions of the true—if not fixed or far followed—path alternated, and since Freud's death the patterns of these possibilities have been replayed again and again. But in these past decades there has, of course, been no Freud but only claimants to his legacy to indicate the true path, and, further, the process of identification has become progressively less and less with *Freud's* science (in a personal sense) and more and more with a literature about Freud.

For a related reason, psychoanalysis is—thirdly—unique among the sciences as the one without major contributions to its own history as a science, and also without major contributions to the history of its own history, or, that is, without any historiography.[1] What I mean is not just that psychoanalysis after Freud's death in 1939 has no history—although this is certainly true; but the more striking fact is that the history of psychoanalysis that has so far been written is not really history, it is biography, a subspecies of history, and, further, much of it is the type of biography for which Freud himself was the originator, that is, psychobiography.[2]

Let me indicate briefly what this state of affairs implies by noting that the first history of psychoanalysis was written in 1914, entitled, without ceremony, *On The History of The Psychoanalytic Movement*, and penned by Freud himself. With this book the history of psychoanalysis began as a type of autobiography, and so it continued until Freud's death, as the title of his next history, *An Autobiographical Study* (1925), shows. Later, when history writing fell to the first generation of heirs, it became a type of biography—of Freud. Ernest Jones's *The Life and Work of Sigmund Freud*, the most fully documented and the most official of the first generation's histories, became, in turn, the precipitant for a third type of history: critiques of Jones's biography, or what might be called second-order biographies. In these subsequent biographies, written with increasing frequency by nonanalyst historians, Jones's idealization of Freud has been rejected, and, particularly in the medium of psychobiography, a much more contextualized and conflicted and complicated founder has emerged.

Biographies of Freud, both of the Jones vintage and of the later, more critical sort, have had a greater role in the development of psychoanalysis since the Second World War than biographies of seminal figures have ever had in the developments of other sciences. Freud's life and the life of psychoanalysis were and still are intertwined in a unique way. This is so for the reasons I have been noting: Freud made his discoveries partly on himself; his autobiographical writings, which conveyed his self-created image of himself, were then key texts in the intellectual and organizational history of his science; and, finally, he established psychobiography and the psychoanalytic theory of creativity. However, among these factors, the first remains key. The most written-about and debated moment in the history of psychoanalysis remains the moment declared to be the origin of psychoanalysis, that is, the period of Freud's self-analysis, of *The Interpretation of Dreams*, and of his letters to Wilhelm Fliess. The whole of psychoanalysis, in Freud's lifetime and after, seems to rise up out of the legendary beginning, the moment of founding. And it is no exaggeration to say that each and every Freud biographer has based his or her assessment of psychoanalysis *tout court* on an assessment of the originary period.

The story of this phenomenon in the cultural history of science began after the Second World War, when psychoanalysts in Europe and America began to turn their attention to how their science, without its founding father, should be prepared for its second half century and transmitted to new generations, particularly after the great damage done to its followers and its aspirations during the *Nazizeit*. Analysts who had known Freud personally in Vienna or Berlin wrote textbooks for the extrafamilial analysts who were founding training institutes in London, New York, Boston, Washington, Buenos Aires, Delhi—all around the world. Otto Fenichel produced *The Psychoanalytic Theory of the Neuroses* (1945), Frieda Fromm-Reichmann reached out to nonanalytic practitioners with *Principles of Intensive Psychotherapy* (1953), Hermann Nunberg revised and expanded his 1932 *Principles of Psychoanalysis* (1955), and Robert Waelder slowly assembled the materials for his *Basic Theory of Psychoanalysis* (finally published in 1960), which includes a revealing "List of the Most Common Misunderstandings of Psychoanalytic Concepts." Between 1945 and 1960, the production of textbooks was meant both to teach and to prevent misunderstandings. The biographical studies of Sigmund Freud written by analysts during the same period—to which I will return in a moment—had the same two purposes.

But it is important to realize that the first postwar analytic textbooks and biographies were launched into an atmosphere created by a spate of nonanalytic popular biographies. Helen Walker Puner, an associate editor at *Parent's Magazine*, wrote *Freud: His Life and His Mind* (1947) for her magazine's audience, and Emil Ludwig, a prolific journalist, wrote his *Sigmund Freud* (1947) for a similarly uninformed general audience. Only the first of these two books had a significant afterlife, but both were works suited to that period of American arrogance in intellectual and technological matters. Puner assumed that most of Freud's work was already outmoded and that more recent psychoanalysis was more scientific, both less like a religion and less reflective of the personal faults of the founder, a man as "fallible and frail as other men," a man possessed by secret father-hatred and repudiation of his Judaism. The combination in Puner's work of celebration and debunking condescension became quite typical of the nonanalytic biographical literature, as did her tendency to psychoanalyze Freud with amateur versions of his own techniques.[3]

Works like Puner's and Ludwig's struck fear into the communities of Viennese emigrés in England and America, particularly those associated with Anna Freud, who had assumed the role of chief protector of her father's memory. After Freud's death in 1939 and through the period of these first postwar popular biographies, Anna Freud had stood strenuously opposed to any kind of biographical inquiry into his life. But 1946 had also brought a challenge to her convictions. Marie Bonaparte came to London bearing a packet full of Freud's letters to his friend and fellow explorer of biological-psychological territories, Wilhelm Fliess, letters written during Freud's "self-analysis" in the originary decade of psychoanalysis. Despite her fear that the letters would be misunderstood and misused, Anna Freud decided, in consultation with her siblings, that the letters should be published. Ernst Kris, one of the Viennese trainees, was designated the editor and assigned the task of a thorough biographical introduction.

Working with Kris richly informed Anna Freud about the complexities of biographical writing. Kris had to work on himself, in a self-analysis and in analysis with Anna Freud, as he wrote, and others involved in the project were similarly unsettled by the difficulties of being objective about their hero. Max Schur, Freud's physician during 1938–39, vacillated frequently between the idea that Freud's physical symptoms at the turn of the century were psychosomatic and the idea that they were not. Siegfried Bernfeld, another Viennese colleague, contributed important material from his series of historical essays on Freud's prepsychoanalytic neurological work, but he grew restive when confronted with Anna Freud's anxieties and discretions.[4] Wilhelm Fliess's son Robert sometimes expressed to Kris the opinion that his father was a paranoiac and sometimes backtracked to protect him. The only one of Freud's associates who wrote biographically in relative isolation from the Anna Freudians and the Fliess project in these years was Hanns Sachs, a member of Freud's original circle, whose two studies,

Freud: Master and Friend (1944) and *Masks of Life and Love* (1948), are among the most interesting—obviously partisan, but understated and unpretentious—works of the period.

While the letters to Fliess were being prepared for publication, the Puner and Ludwig biographies appeared—without so much as a mention between them of Freud's crucial friendship with Fliess. The Freudians could see clearly how keeping letters out of the public domain would increase the distortion and reliance on anecdote in biographies, but they could also see how an irresponsible biographer might use the letters sensationalistically. Finally, without enthusiasm, Anna Freud came to the conclusion that an authoritative full-scale biography might forestall future falsifications. An additional advantage would be that one person, a sifter and a winnower, would act as recipient for all who wanted to tell their anecdotes about Freud, thus preventing betrayals or civil wars among the Freudians. Discussions about such a biography and possible biographers began in the Freud family circle even before Ernest Jones, one of Freud's earliest associates and the preeminent member of the British psychoanalytical group, was approached for the task by an American publisher.

Despite the Freud family's misgivings about Jones's past hostilities toward Freud, Jones became the biographer designate and began work in 1951, just as James Strachey was launching upon the monumental editing and translating project later called *The Complete Psychological Works of Sigmund Freud* (in twenty-three volumes, 1953–1966). Both the biographer and the translator, who exchanged information as they worked, had to develop the basic ingredient of scholarly biography: a detailed, reliable chronological frame. Their joint work, together with Kris's on the Fliess letters, set the standard for future biographies, and also established a key feature of them: All the researchers considered the founding decade of psychoanalysis, 1895–1905 (and especially 1896–1897), to be the crux of biographical inquiry, and it appeared in their standard-setting works as both the great creative period and the great "psychoneurotic period" (in Jones's phrase), the psychoanalytic *mysterium tremendum*.

As he worked, Jones took enormous (and rather self-deceiving) pride in his accuracy, and he keenly pointed out in his voluminous correspondence with Anna Freud how inaccurate other biographers—including Ernst Kris—had been. Gradually cured of her skepticism, Anna Freud complained to Jones about Siegfried Bernfeld's loose interpretations in a paper on Freud's cocaine use, and about a hated piece on Freud's "Irma dream" by her Vienna trainee and fellow child analyst Erik Erikson: "It should be your role to silence all the other biographers who have to invent half their facts" (to Jones, 19 September 1952).[5] She became more and more deeply absorbed in Jones's work, feeling as he sent chapter after chapter, that she was discovering her father: "I thought that I knew my father better than anybody, but I do not think it any more," she told Jones (to Jones, 14 February 1954). Jones relished her praise and enjoyed spending paragraphs demolishing inferior works like Puner's. Together the coworkers even summoned a little humor about the stream of other biographical work, which continued unchecked by Jones's efforts. "I wonder if a book entitled Lies about Freud would sell? It would be easy to concoct" (to Anna Freud, 3 December 1957).

The Jones biography, which eventually ran to three volumes, was a collaborative venture from the start. Martha Freud supplied memories and some of her husband's courtship letters; the Freud children read the manuscript as it evolved (the oldest, Martin, was even inspired to his own work, *Sigmund Freud, Man and Father*, 1958); and all participated in delicate discretionary decisions, including one that resulted in a version of Freud's death that completely protected Max Schur from any possible charge of euthanasia for administering a lethal dose of morphine when Freud was *in extremis*. But it was Anna Freud who most clearly assumed the role of biographer *manqué* and also *grise*. She had many times refused importuning publishers who had wanted her to write about her father, insisting that this was the last thing in the world she either could or would think of doing, but in the role of conscience to Jones, to whom she had (in her own technical term) "altruistically surrendered" this self-forbidden work, she was so comfortable that she agreed to translate his first volume into German.

Jones's pages are vivid with details only his direct sources could have supplied about Freud's domestic and work routines, his friendships and working relationships, his organizational tribulations, and his travels. Protecting the family's privacy produced some strange disbalances—there is almost as much about Freud's dogs as there is about his children and grandchildren; the reader gets no real sense of the complexity of the Freud family and household and the many crises and strains weathered while the children were growing up; Martha Freud becomes more and more enigmatic as the story unfolds. Jones's own feelings about others of Freud's colleagues produced some distortions (for example, no inquiry into the nature of Sándor Ferenczi's mental condition in his last year, which Max Schur had told Jones was probably an "organic psychosis" linked to pernicious anemia); and the institutional history of psychoanalysis is very lightly filled in, while the episodic schisms are covered in the kind of strategic (as opposed to theoretical) detail Jones, a great combatant himself, enjoyed. There is a compelling history of Freud's unfolding discoveries, but not much sense of how his mind worked, the character of his thought, or the intensity of his often lonely battle for his cause. In the first volume, which ends as psychoanalysis has been created, his life and work dimensions are carefully interwoven, but this achievement is lacking in the later volumes, as Jones elected to alternate between life sections and work (or thematic) sections. Unrealistically, Jones tended to see Freud's struggle and growth as completed by the end of the originary decade, and after that he often idealized his subject as a serene, always composed patriarch.

It is, nonetheless, one of the great virtues of Jones's massive work that it is a psychobiography, but a very restrained one and one that does not lose sight of the current historical contexts (as do so many works by analysts who are recapitulating psychoanalysis in the manner I noted before). Jones had such an abundance of material that he did not suffer the temptation to invent or to speculate at each step of the way, but he also had so much that he knew clearly how much he lacked, how much was missing, lost, or unavailable. He wrote as a historian, without the idea, so common among later psychoanalyst-biographers, that biography writing and doing analysis are similar kinds of activities. He did not, for example, interpret blanks in his documentation as secrets or resistances; he knew that many of the most important things in people's lives are never recorded and also that many records vanish for reasons that have nothing to do with the biographical subject's unconscious life. Occasionally, he felt that he was in the presence of a secret, as he noted of Freud's adolescence (vol. II, pp. 409, 455), but he was content to say so without trying to paint a keyhole on the closed door.

As soon as Jones's biography was completely available (1957) and both it and Freud's centenary (1956) had been celebrated in an outpouring of small biographical speculations, some by others of Freud's early associates, a new phase of biographical study began. From about 1960, the publication date of a selection of Freud's letters, edited by his son Ernst Freud, until the mid-1970s, every biography both set out from and contended with Jones's biography.[6] This was a reactive period and not one of new discoveries or interpretative innovation, for the materials available to others were less than those known to Jones. In New York, a Sigmund Freud Archives was set up under the direction of a Viennese analyst named K. R. Eissler, and most materials not available to Jones went into the closed archives, out of the reach of biographers not sanctioned by the Freud family or Eissler. The field was, thus, divided into insiders and outsiders, a situation bound to foster resentment.

Although it was not published until 1972, Max Schur's *Freud Living and Dying* is the ultimate insider's biography of the late 1960s, the period when Schur began work. Schur had prepared a lengthy medical memorandum about Freud for Ernest Jones, and he had been drawn into the biographical arena while he negotiated by mail about Jones's use of the memorandum. What fascinated Schur was Freud's attitude toward death, which Schur tracked from the period of the Fliess letters into the 1920s theory of the "death instinct" and up to the year of Freud's dying. The biography is very uneven—Schur himself did not live to finish it—but it contains some of the most insightful reflections to be found on the influence of Freud's personality on his theories. And it also contains a sampling of Freud's letters, cited only in German, as an appendix—another sign that the Freud circle gave special documentary access to its own.

During the fifteen years or so after the Jones biography, while Schur was the only biographer with further access to documents, the main biographical mode was "assessment of influence." In this mode, the outlines of Freud's life were taken as a settled matter, and interpretation of his personal and intellectual significance seemed the job in need of doing. And assessing Freud's influence became one of the key modes—the other was assessing Marxism's (not Marx's) influence—for portraying the course and meaning of the twentieth century in the third quarter, its period of prolonged "Cold War" and of booming consumer culture in America and Western Europe.

Lionel Trilling's "Freud and the Crisis of our Culture" (1955) was a brilliant, distinguished harbinger of this phase, but the Frankfurt School Marxist Eric Fromm's title, *Sigmund Freud's Mission: An Analysis of his Personality and Influence* (1959), was much more typical in its polemical purposes and tone. (For his main historical argument, that Freud's psychoanalysis became a religious movement for a secularized and disoriented and consumption-driven urban middle-class elite, Fromm acknowledges his debt to . . . Helen Walker Puner.) Of this vast assessment literature, however, the one book that has lived on and is kept in print is Philip Rieff's *Freud: The Mind of the Moralist* (1959).

Rieff's work has not had its staying power, I think, because of its portrait of "the mind of Freud," which is a portrait too admiring to be acceptable in any American reading atmosphere since the early 1960s, even though Rieff explicitly distinguished it from Jones's idealization (for which "the writer was too near his subject," "he compelled the reader to venerate the man as well as respect the ideas"). Rather, what has remained challenging about Rieff's work is the ardor and intensity with which he sought "psychological man," an ideal type whom Rieff hoped would show himself courageously able to live a truly liberated life, a life free from all constraints of authoritarian community life (whether religious or political) and from external moral imperatives, a life of unsentimental autonomy. Even while he insisted that Freud was not a moral messenger, Rieff nonetheless felt compelled to set Freud up as the very model of this modern man and to "draw the implications" (his own recurrent phrase) of Freud's personal and scientific example for a new morality, nondoctrinaire and stemming from analytic introspection. Rieff's image of Freud demanded—in contrast to Fromm's—that Freud be considered apart from the psychoanalytic movement he founded and apart from the popular expropriations of Freudianism that had, actually, prepared the way for "psychological man" to emerge as a possibility. For Rieff, everyman had the potential to be his own cultural hero. And it seems to me that there is such a deep affinity between this idea and the individualism (of the rugged sort or the more refined Emersonian sort) of American mainstream culture, that Rieff's vision of "psychological man" could reverberate, even among those who had far less admiration for Freud, right into the quite different sort of extreme individualism and nonmoralistic moralism that now goes under the name "postmodernism."

The general "assessment of influence" cultural-historical approach to Freud became more intense as the 1960s unfolded in all their upheaval and torment, and Freud's cultural speculations, particularly *Civilization and Its Discontents*, gathered to themselves much more nonanalytical interest than his clinical and more technically metapsychological contributions. For many of the rebellious "baby boom" postwar generation, Herbert Marcuse's *Eros and Civilization* (1955, but only in mass market paperback after 1961), with its invocation of "polymorphous" sexual liberation, was more compelling than any assessment of Freud's influence, any text of Freud's own, or any image, like Rieff's, of Freud the man. For these rebels, biography in general was too "role model" oriented. But during this period of ferment, two important tributaries of biographically focused critique did arise and branch off from the growing Freud assessment literature. One concerned Freud's Jewishness and the influence of his religious heritage and national character on his work; and one focused on his psychology of women. The latter was fed by one of the most widely read books of the mid-1960s, Betty Friedan's pioneering *The Feminine Mystique* (1963), but it did not really grow into a rushing torrent until the end of the decade.

The Jewish stream, however, was woven into an intense Jewish identity quest that concentrated during the Eichmann trial in 1961 and gathered momentum through the 1967 Middle East War.[7] The progenitor of this stream is David Bakan's 1958 work *Sigmund Freud and the Jewish Mystical Tradition*, which was reissued as a paperback in 1965; many works followed until a dip in trajectory was signaled by the re-emergence, in the mid-1970s, of images of Freud as a Jewish self-hater, exactly the character who had starred in Puner's popular post–war volume. But this whole stream of inquiry then had a revival in the 1980s, and typical of this new era is D. B. Klein's *The Jewish Origins of the Psychoanalytic Movement* (1981). The literature is very repetitive in its claims about the importance of Freud's Jewishness for psychoanalysis, but recent emphasis has shifted to the biographical question of whether Freud's upbringing had actually been as Reform or unreligious as he liked to present it. The historian and future biographer Peter Gay in *A Godless Jew* (1987) supports this position, whereas two publications focusing on Freud's late work *Moses and Monotheism*, Emanuel Rice's *Freud and Moses* (1991) and Yosef Yerushalmi's *Freud's Moses* (1991), took new information about Freud's parents into account and presented him as more shaped by Orthodoxy than the Gentile Jones or the Freud children—or Freud himself—had admitted.

The second wave of Jewish-influence biographers has tended to focus on Freud's later years, the years of Hitler's prewar power and promulgation of anti-Semitism. But this was precisely the period in Freud's life that a small but vociferously critical group began, in the later 1960s, to see as the period of Freud's deradicalization. Critics who admired the early Freud, the id-theorist, the pioneering discoverer of the unconscious whose complex genius was so clear in the massive volume by Didier Anzieu called simply *L'Autoanalyse* (1959; 1975 edition in English) found his later work, with its growing emphasis on ego-psychology, too conservative. These critics, mostly Kleinians (in Britain and America) and Lacanians (in France) among analysts, mostly radical Marxists among nonanalysts, set up "ego psychology" and the progressive bureaucratization of psychoanalytic societies as the twin signs of an anti-liberationist turn in psychoanalysis, and they held Freud's own allegedly retreating last years responsible for the turn.

As this critical spirit was gathering force, Henri Ellenberger published a huge tome called *The Discovery of the Unconscious* (1970). Many of the biographical claims in Ellenberger's work have now, after two decades, become staples in Freud portraits. Chiefly, thanks to Ellenberger, the milieu into which Freud first launched his psychoanalytical studies on hysteria is now generally thought to have been both more ready for psychoanalysis—that is, there were more precursors of Freud's ideas abroad than Jones had acknowledged—and less monolithically disparaging or critical. Ellenberger gave tremendous impetus to a mode of Freud biography that flourished ten years later, one that stressed contextualizing Freud, putting him in his intellectual milieu, showing his influences and debts, questioning Freud's own and Jones's versions of the history of psychoanalysis and even of particular cases. Ellenberger was a very respectful critical historian, but not hindered by the Jonesian conviction that the psychoanalysis that appeared in the miraculous discovery decade of the 1890s was completely *sui generis*.

In the mid-1970s, the revisionary period forecast by the late 1960s critiques of Freud and of psychoanalysis began in earnest. There were two ruling assumptions in this period. The first was that Freud was an authoritarian who suppressed dissent in his movement and induced in his followers a spirit of orthodoxy. The second assumption, really a corollary of the first, was that the Freudian biographers of Freud were also authoritarians who had been keeping secrets about the master or idealizing him, suppressing his weaknesses as a person and as a psychologist. This second assumption was reinforced as publications of Freud's correspondences appeared in German and then in English (with Oskar Pfister in 1963, Karl Abraham in 1966, Arnold Zweig in 1968, Lou Andreas-Salomé in 1972, and Carl Jung in 1974) and also when two other key correspondences, with Sándor Ferenczi and Ernest Jones, did not appear. The published collections were both biographically stimulating and frustrating for their glaring omissions of letters and deletions within letters. The Sigmund Freud Archives in New York came to be widely perceived as the institutional equivalent of the protective, idealizing Freud family: Both were reactionary and dedicated to embalming both Freud's story and the story of psychoanalysis, particularly of the heretics and dissidents within psychoanalysis who, had they not been crushed by the orthodoxers, would have made psychoanalysis a progressive force.

A particular battle exemplified the scene: Paul Roazen, a young Harvard-trained historian, published *Brother Animal* in 1969, a book dedicated to showing that Viktor Tausk, one of Freud's early disciples, had been a genius whose unorthodox views Freud had repudiated and whose very sanity he had helped destroy. This book was a more focused version of an argument that Roazen then made more diffusely in *Freud and His Followers* (1975), a book that both beneficially headed the business of biography writing toward the second generation of Freudians (where it eventually flourished in the 1980s) and established a tone of aggrieved outsiderdom combined with slipshod scholarship that had a baleful influence on future nonanalytic and non-Freud-circle biographers. K. R. Eissler responded to the Tausk study with a book twice as long, called *Talent and Genius* (1971), in which Tausk was shown to be merely talented, Freud got the designation genius, and Paul Roazen was made out to be a charlatan. (Eissler made many rich contributions to the Freud biography literature, all of them, strangely enough, in the form of replies to alleged and sometimes actual charlatan biographers and other ignorant writers, but his work is, unfortunately, skewed by its defensive stance.[8])

Debunking had, of course, always played a role in the Freud biographical literature, particularly in the popular, amateur ranges where Helen Puner had set the postwar tone. The debunking of this period was done, however, not by journalists but by academics, many of them trained in history and the social sciences, and it was connected to the larger cultural phenomenon of a ''baby boom'' generation, graduate-schooled in the late 1960s, deconstructing and reevaluating the historical work of the elders who had dominated intellectual life in the 1950s and 1960s. The most significant biography of this sort was Frank Sulloway's *Freud: Biologist of the Mind* (1979), which contains an elaborately constructed argument that Freud, far from being an isolated and lonely heroic genius, was a man in step with the biological and evolutionary thought of his time, a man whose theories, in all their deep contradictoriness and inconsistency, bear within them all the fallacies of nineteenth-century natural science. Sulloway's work is both enormously informative about the history of science and quite tone-deaf to psychoanalysis—it willfully reduces Freud's work to its biological dimensions and then calls the impoverished result ''psychoanalysis.''

Much more publicly important—and, eventually, important for the internal reform of psychoanalysis—was the debunking done in the the late 1960s and early 1970s by feminists. Kate Millett's attack on Freud throughout the pages of *Sexual Politics* (1971), for example, set a standard for rejection of psychoanalysis among radical feminists. Freud's views on female psychology, read as a function of Freud's supposed misogyny, became targets for many polemics, and older works like Simone de Beauvoir's *The Second Sex* (1949) and Viola Klein's *The Feminine Character* (1946) were rediscovered and reissued to increase the volume and to hammer home the basic claim that Freud had conflated ''sex'' (the biological or anatomical) and ''gender'' (the social) in female development. From many different angles, the ''phallocentrism'' (a word originally coined by Ernest Jones) of Freud's views was noted, and, generally, the period of infant development prior to the differentiations Freud described, the pre-Oedipal, came to be the only period feminists judged uncorrupted by Freudian misunderstandings. Not coincidentally, the pre-Oedipal period became the focus, then, of feminist efforts to find a time of innocence, and thus of fresh possibility, prior to what came to be called "the social construction of gender." Eventually, however, this important but sometimes wild critical assault was tempered, and by the late 1970s Freud was being read with much greater appreciation—and in a way that actually moved psychoanalytic practitioners to a major reconsideration of Freud's views on female psychology and that also exploited rising psychoanalytic interest in the pre-Oedipal period.[9]

But it is interesting to note that, although the vast preponderance of biographical work on Freud is by men, feminists have not used the genre for their critique. There were, however, three biographical speculations by women in this period: two were French, Marthe Robert's *From Oedipus to Moses* (1974; English, 1976), and Marie Balmary's *Psychoanalyzing Psychoanalysis* (1979; English, 1982), and one German, Marianne Krüll's *Freud and His Father* (1979; English, 1986). These works shared with Helen Puner's postwar volume the assumption that Freud hated his father and also hated being a Jew, the son of a Jewish father. But they came out differently. For example, Robert felt that Freud, trying to free himself of a paternal "mediocrity who did nothing to overcome the confinement of his existence within the intolerable limits of inferior birth," wanted to be a self-created man, "the son not of any man or country but like the murdered prophet [Moses] only of his work." And she felt that his failure was reflected in his clinical doctrine of the Oedipus complex. But Marianne Krüll felt that Freud had succeeded, that in his last book he had settled accounts with his father and with his secret wish not to have been born a Jew. This late triumph left the Oedipus complex doctrine unrevised, however, and Krüll viewed it as an impediment to a truer psychoanalysis, one that would be more attentive to the importance of "the social environment in the socialization of man" and less fixated on intrapsychic conflict.

Krüll noted in the preface to the 1986 translation of her book that she had not been a feminist in 1979, when the German edition was published. But she had since been converted—by her good friend Sigmund Freud's granddaughter, Sophie Freud—and had realized in retrospect that "I unconsciously took a woman's stand against the extremely patriarchal Oedipus theory. I also believe that my picture of Freud as a frightened and bewildered, yet courageous and curious, little boy is a view not easily reached by most men, and also not by those women who accept their subordinate role in our male society." This supposedly feminist view of Freud embroiled in his father rivalry and denigrating women as a consequence has its counterpart in the trend that appeared in this period among male biographers. While the female expositors were focusing on Freud's father-relationship, the men argued that Freud's relationship with his mother had been misconstrued by Jones, Schur, and all other orthodox Freudians. As Peter Homans, a Chicago-based sociological commentator, has said in summary: "Jones's exclusively Oedipal interpretations of Freud's relationships and conflicts have made it difficult to introduce the idea of earlier developmental lines into the study of Freud's life, such as the persistence of maternal motifs in his intimate dealings with other men."[10] (I think one can see—in retrospect—a foreshadowing within this contra dance of biographical concerns much of the 1980s general cultural ferment over who is to blame for *la condition masculine*—indulgent mothers or unsatisfactory, uninvolved fathers. As this debate was also common in the early 1950s under the popular title "Momism," it is not surprising that there is an underground channel, so to speak, connecting the two eras in the specific little exemplary domain of Freud biography.)

Devotees of the Chicago analyst Heinz Kohut's "self psychology," including

Kohut himself, have developed the idea that Freud's creativity was a matter of his narcissistic transferences and displacements—a carrying over into his entire creation of his bond to his adoring mother.[11] On the other hand, the pre-Oedipal motif has been worked out by Kleinian expositors such as Richard Wollheim in his *Sigmund Freud* (1971), and from thence it has filtered into the work of Peter Gay, whose *Freud* (1988) will be considered later. Among French biographers influenced by Lacan, Sigmund Freud's first two years of life with his mother are floridly imagined, but there is also a very clear and interesting Lacanian work of the period, O. Mannoni's *Freud* (1968; English 1971). Mannoni's book is quite unusual for its freedom from chronology; it does offer a narrative of Freud's life, but its order is really thematic, and it makes a truly rare and admirable effort to show how Freud thought his way from one facet of his evolving system to another, how and why he revised his ideas so frequently.

In general, it can be said of this third period in the history of postwar Freud biographies that every school of psychoanalysis—and this was a period of proliferating schools—had its Freud biography and that each sectarian Freud biography showed how Freud could best be understood in the terms of the school. Just as the proliferation of schools and the consequent battles among and splittings within psychoanalytic institutes stimulated abundant polemics, it also stimulated reworkings of almost every important item in the history of Freud biography. Dreams from *The Interpretations of Dreams*, many times written about, were written about again; Freud's case studies were raked over and reanalyzed from new perspectives; all the schisms in the history of psychoanalysis were rediagnosed by the latter-day schismatics and schism-haters. Similarly, the trend established by Paul Roazen in the late 1960s of writing about Freud's followers grew in this period, and many early analysts were treated biographically, with their adherent or schismatic relations to Freud figuring largely in their stories.

The political and polemical agendas behind psychobiographies became quite widely recognized by the late 1970s, when deconstructionism, embraced as a dispeller of illusions about objectivity, took over as the critical method of choice in universities. Also helping to raise consciousness about the battle for Freud were various types of hermeneutical views of psychoanalysis itself, that is, visions of it as a symbol system and as a method for culture-decoding rather than as a type of natural science. The key methodological problem of psychobiography was also widely recognized—although such recognition has not yet informed a major historiographical work on psychoanalytic biography and history writing. That problem is that all types of psychobiography, no matter what their brand of theory, are rooted in the research that relates to childhood, and childhoods, particularly ones lived in eras when childhood was not subject to the sort of study Freud and his followers developed, are notoriously wrapped in obscurity. For Freud's own childhood, the source is Freud himself in the medium of his self-analysis. Birth records may show the number and ages of his parents' children, but only the analyst of himself could say, "I welcomed my one-year-younger brother (who died within a few months) with ill wishes and real infantile jealousy, and . . . his death left the germ of guilt in me."[12]

In the 1970s, revisionists trained their detective work on the next best thing to new material about Freud's childhood experiences: They sought out archives in Moravia and Vienna for facts about the Freud family during Freud's childhood. On the basis of such facts as the existence of a third woman (perhaps a third wife) in Freud's father, Jacob's, life, many speculations were built. When letters from Freud revealing his infatuation at age fifteen with a girl named Gisela Fluss (and with her mother) surfaced, his adolescence became a new focus of interest—and biographers, according to their theories, saw in Freud's letters to two adolescent friends, Emil Fluss and Eduard Silberstein, replays of Freud's pre-Oedipal or of his Oedipal psychodynamics.[13]

The one good product of the search for new facts, particularly when it has combined with a growing recognition of how difficult it is to reconstruct a nineteenth-century childhood, has been a growing tendency to place Freud in his historical contexts more carefully. Writers with this kind of methodological sophistication are often indebted to the work of Henri Ellenberger or to the methodological critique in the French philosopher Paul Ricoeur's *Freud and Philosophy*; but the most important progenitor of this tendency among historians was Carl Schorske in his influential essay collection called *Fin-de-Siècle Vienna* (1980). Recently, Schorske's follower William McGrath, who published *Freud's Discovery of Psychoanalysis* in 1986, has provided important information and interpretation about Freud's relation to liberal political currents in his day and about his search for a political place to stand in the rising anti-Semitic tide of the 1890s. McGrath's notion that Freud tended to reduce political perplexities into psychological dilemmas and fashion theory out of his retreat from the political perplexities strikes me as unsupported by his careful exegesis, but his work is nonetheless important for this salutary contextualizing trend.

Ronald W. Clark's *Freud: The Man and His Cause* (1980), the first full-scale biography to incorporate the new Freud family data and Freud's adolescent letters, is eight years older than Peter Gay's *Freud: A Life for our Time* (1988), which benefited from the new research and documentation but also suffered from the atmosphere created during the intervening years by the escalating debunking trend. Clark's book, thus, lacks the magisterial set-everything-right tone of Gay's encyclopedic book, but it did not, on the other hand, conduct an unspoken argument with the *dramatis personae* in a media event, Janet Malcolm's *In the Freud Archives* (1984). This volume, by a New York journalist, tells the story of how K. R. Eissler at the Sigmund Freud Archives took under his patronage a young psychoanalytic candidate, Jeffrey Masson, to make of him the future Archives director, and then was astonished as Masson turned into a Freud detractor and eventually the author of *The Assault on Truth* (1984), an argument that Freud intentionally suppressed his early "seduction theory" (the idea that Oedipal love stories represent stories of real, not fantasized, incestuous relations) because of a "personal failure of courage."

Also in the cast of this melodrama, which was magnified in the manner of the 1980s media, so preoccupied with scandal and celebrity making, is Peter Swales, a young Welshman with no formal connection to psychoanalysis and no university training, an autodidact, who has developed a renown both for his remarkable archival detective work and for his debunking biographical speculations. Swales, who is on a mission to prove that Freud and the Freudians were and are, simply, crazy, wrote a series of papers, most of them privately published, which now turn up in all biographical studies, where they are either dismissed as wild, as they are in Gay's book, or treated with a kind of reverence, as they are in J. N. Isbister's *Freud* (1985), a dreadfully bad volume in which hostile speculations about Freud that had been mounting up since Helen Puner's time are simply asserted, without evidence, but with the authority of Swales. The two key interpretive ideas of Puner's work—that Freud hated his Jewish father and that he made of psychoanalysis a new religion, a religion of sexuality—appear in Isbister as facts.[14] The book is full of ponderous absurdities like this: "Psychoanalysis was for Freud a means whereby he could vicariously enjoy sexual gratification with women."

Peter Gay's *Freud: A Life for Our Time* begins with a list of biographical problem areas and solves each one as judiciously as possible. As far as evidence can show, no, Freud did not (*pace* Swales) have an affair with his wife's sister Minna; no, the libido theory is not indebted (*pace* Swales, again) to Freud's cocaine use, etc. Like the Jones biography, but after the end of Anna Freud's reign as biographical conscience, the Gay biography is dedicated to accuracy and to overcoming the Helen Puners of its day. Also like Jones, Gay is an insider biographer, with more access to the Archives than those whose hashes he set out to settle, which makes him—depending on the assessor's point of view—more reliable, more beholden, or more resented.

Building on his treasure of sources and using his own previous studies of Freud and of psychoanalysis, Gay presented a Freud who is fallible but basically a son of the Enlightenment, a rigorous scientist, a rationalist with uncanny insight into the irrational. He is a son also of his mother, and (in the manner of all biographies by men after the late 1970s) he was chiefly limited by being "unconsciously eager to leave some of his ambivalence about his mother unanalyzed" (p. 89) while he concentrated on his father and his Oedipus complex. This is Jones's Freud brought up to date in terms of the evolving biography literature, the evolving psychoanalytic concern with the pre-Oedipal period, and the evolving debunking tendency—but this last in a very curious way. Gay's *Freud* is not focused on the originary decade of the founding of psychoanalysis. Indeed, it took Jones a third of his pages to arrive at *The Interpretation of Dreams*, but Gay gets there in less than a sixth of his. And this is not because Gay has made an argument to the effect that concentrating on the discovery of psychoanalysis is, in some way, distorting the whole story or falling into the genetic fallacy. Rather, it seems to me, his rapid acceleration acknowledges that the 1890–1900 terrain has become too polemic-strewn and contested for leisurely narrative passage. Gay traveled by train, photographing through the windows, outlining, and then conducted his quarrel with his biographer predecessors indirectly, in the long bibliographic essay situated at the end of his trip. But this tactic entailed that he did not get to the level of querying why the founding decade of psychoanalysis has become so critically embattled, or, even more specifically, to querying why we are now, for example, hearing accusations that Freud, by abandoning "the seduction theory," and psychoanalysts by following him, neglect seduction and child abuse; why we are now hearing charges that a frustrated or mother-fixated Freud overplayed or made a religion of sexuality, which is certainly not as important as he said it was, and so forth.

The result of Gay's attitude is that he does not rise to the level of interpreting the possible meanings of his own subtitle, "A Life for Our Time." And the unexamined shadow of the Freud debunking in the early 1980s that falls so heavily over the key first chapter and the rapid first part of Gay's book also marks it off decisively from Ronald Clark's opener, written a decade earlier. But, in general, the two biographies show clearly what different biographical methods and priorities can reveal of the same subject. Clark, who is not analytically trained, lingers over the details of the recent archival research into the Freud family in Moravia and Vienna, concentrating two pages on the newly discovered (perhaps) wife of Jacob Freud; Gay, who is analytically trained but lacks the restraint shown by Jones, simply states that Jacob had three wives and moves right along past family matters to get to the kinds of analytic themes he relishes—

Freud's deep ambivalence toward Vienna, Freud's many "mistakes in remembering his childhood" (alleged on p. 11 without documentation). Clark devotes four pages to Freud's infatuation with Gisela Fluss and his inexperience with women, citing many letters; Gay disposes of the Gisela episode in two brisk paragraphs, asserting flatly and blandly that it was a "belated Oedipal infatuation." Clark is very knowledgeable about the history of science, so when he introduced Freud's cocaine experiments in the early 1880s he gave background about the drug and cited Freud's letters about how it affected him; Gay concentrates thematically on how Freud displaced his annoyance at failing to discover cocaine's anesthetizing properties onto his fiancée, who drew him out of his laboratory at the key wrong moment. Clark quotes an ebullient letter of Freud's about his joy on receiving a stipend to study in Paris with Charcot and his anticipation of a six-week stay en route with his fiancée; Gay remarks the visit to Martha Bernays in passing and gets Freud to Paris as quickly as possible.

In short, while Clark enjoyed Freud's family and love relations, as well as his scientific development, and looked always for the affective side of his subject, Gay was quick and perfunctory on both love and science while he built up his psychodynamic picture. Clark quoted Freud when he wanted to show Freud's feelings, while Gay went straight past feelings to alleged unconscious complexes, offering one-sentence quotes as evidence. But the balance in these books begins to shift as Freud's life unfolds: Gay is better informed about psychoanalysis after the originary decade, and he gives a richer clinical and theoretical picture of its unfolding than Clark is able to provide or than had been provided by any biography adopting Jones's method of treating life and work separately.

These two full-scale biographies of the last decade show, I think, that the limitation upon Freud biographies is no longer chiefly a matter of materials—of unavailable or unrecovered documents and letters—or a matter of sectarian theories circumscribing portraits. Good Freud biography requires, like any good biography, accuracy without defensiveness (which means both using strict evidentiary rules and analyzing as a cultural historian, not just reacting to, ongoing polemics). But, in this case it also requires relinquishing the idea that theories—much less a whole science like psychoanalysis—can be explained by or reduced to motivations, as though a theory and a symptom were the same thing. The great weakness in the whole of the Freud biographical literature, in my estimation, is that it is all skewed in the same two ways. First, it is focused on the originary decade of Freud's science to the neglect of his later work and to the neglect of a sense for the evolving whole of his work; and second, the originary decade is itself constantly read simplistically as a record of or a product of Freud's childhood, which has meant that Freud has not emerged as a character, a man with an adult character, a man who could be *portrayed* not just analyzed with more or less sophisticated versions of his own theories. Both of these limitations are reflected in the persistent idea that Freud's "self-analysis" was confined to the period of the Fliess correspondence and *The Interpretation of Dreams*, whereas it seems obvious that self-analysis was Freud's constant mode and that his later work was as deeply indebted to his *changing* conception of himself as it was to his continued clinical experience. But important self-analytical results from Freud's later years, particularly those concerning his narcissism, have consistently been overlooked by his biographers.

For the history of psychoanalysis, the fixation to Freud himself and, even more particularly, to the originary decade of Freud's discoveries, has meant that later developments, during Freud's lifetime and especially since, are virtually without history. One can hope that Gay's biography, so encyclopedic and yet so superficially responsive to the moment with which its subtitle—*A Life for Our Time*—seeks to link it, will simply signal that in our time we do not need more biographies of Freud. What we need is a much higher degree of self-consciousness among cultural critics about why and in what changing terms Freud has been so fought over, and fought over with such clamor that it is nearly deafening to turn an ear—analytic or otherwise—on the battleground.[15]

It is not surprising, of course, that the man who gave theoretical formulation to the phenomenon of "transference"—to the capacity all people have for playing out upon a later stage their earlier, and often quite unknown, dramas of love and hate and love-and-hate—should be a "transference object" for a particular class of analyst and non-analyst biographer-historians and also more generally across our polysemic culture. We need a history of this transference object. The history might be called *F---d*, to acknowledge that this figure is so familiar that any literate person can fill him in acrostically, with a flourish of feeling—positive, negative, in-between, or studiously indifferent; but also to acknowledge that this figure is unknown, a space onto which innumerable stories of individual and cultural desire have been projected, a palimpsest so run-together that each layer of stories carries an imprint of all the others. Such a history would be very valuable as a deep sounding of how twentieth-century people have wanted to understand themselves and to be understood. But more narrowly, and more to the purpose of the volume you are now reading about discovering the history of psychiatry, *F---d* might help psychoanalysis's history dissolve its Oedipus complex and develop beyond biography.

Notes

1. Perhaps a sign of historiography to come is given by John E. Toews's review essay "Historicizing Psychoanalysis: Freud in His Time and for Our Time," *Journal of Modern History*, xliii (September 1991), 504–545.

2. There is an extensive, helpful, and very opinionated review of the literature, including much but not all of the biographical literature, on Freud in Peter Gay's *Freud: A Life for Our Time* (New York: Norton, 1988).

3. Other examples of amateur psychoanalyzing are numerous; see, for one, Maurice Natenberg's *The Case History of Sigmund Freud* (1955), in which Freud appears as a severe neurotic with a fantastic delusional system.

4. Bernfeld's essays are listed in Gay's bibliography (see note 2); a biography of him by Philip Utley is in preparation.

5. These letters and a more extensive discussion of the history of the Jones biography can be found in my *Anna Freud: A Biography* (New York: Summit Books, 1988).

6. See *The Letters of Sigmund Freud*, selected and edited by Ernst Freud (London: Hogarth, 1960), and also Ernst Freud's collaborative work with his wife, Lucie Freud, and Ilse Grubrich-Simitis on *Sigmund Freud: His Life in Pictures and Words* (London: Andre Deutsch, 1978), a superb edition.

7. For a superficial review see Justin Miller, "Interpretations of Freud's Jewishness, 1924–1974," *Journal of the History of the Behavioral Sciences*, xvii (1981), 357–374.

8. Eissler also produced *Viktor Tausk's Suicide* in 1983. There is much valuable biographical information in his *Sigmund Freud und die Wiener Universität* (1966), but I find his most interesting contribution to be a reflection on Freud's adolescence in *The Psychoanalytic Study of the Child*, xxxiii (1978).

9. For a brief history of relations between psychoanalysis and feminism, see Elisabeth Young-Bruehl and Laura Wexler, "On 'Psychoanalysis and Feminism,' " *Social Research*, lix (Summer 1992), 453–483.

10. Peter Homans, *The Ability to Mourn: Disillusionment and the Social Origins of Psychoanalysis* (Chicago: University of Chicago Press, 1989), 17.

11. Heinz Kohut, "Creativeness, Charisma and Group Psychology: Reflections on Freud's Self-Analysis" in J. Gedo and G. Pollock (eds.), *Freud: Fusion of Science and Humanism* (New York: International Universities Press, 1976), 379–425.

12. Freud's letter of 3 October 1897 in *The Complete Letters of Sigmund Freud to Wilhelm Fliess, 1887–1904* (Cambridge: Harvard University Press, 1985), 168.

13. See *The Letters of Sigmund Freud to Eduard Silberstein, 1871–1881* (Cambridge: Harvard University Press, 1990).

14. The nadir of the history of Freud biographies was reached—one can hope—when Helen Puner's book was republished, with an introduction by Paul Roazen: *Sigmund Freud: His Life and Mind* (New Brunswick, NJ: Transaction Publishers, 1992).

15. There are gestures in this direction in Homans's book (see note 10) and in a not very good, but suggestive British work: Barry Richards, *Images of Freud: Cultural Responses to Psychoanalysis* (New York: St. Martins Press, 1989).

Bibliography

Anzieu, Didier. *L'auto-analyse: Son rôle dans la découverte de la psychanalyse par Freud.* Paris: Presses Universitaires de France, 1959.

Bakan, David. *Sigmund Freud and the Jewish Mystical Tradition.* Princeton: Van Nostrand, 1958.

Balmary, Marie. *Psychoanalyzing Psychoanalysis.* Baltimore: Johns Hopkins University Press, 1982 (originally 1979).

Beauvoir, Simone de. *The Second Sex.* New York: Knopf, 1952 (originally 1949).

Clark, Ronald. *Freud: The Man and His Cause.* New York: Random House, 1980.

Eissler, Kurt R. *Talent and Genius.* New York: Quadrangle Books, 1971.

Ellenberger, Henri. *The Discovery of the Unconscious.* New York: Basic Books, 1970.

Fenichel, Otto. *The Psychoanalytic Theory of the Neuroses.* New York: Norton, 1945.

Freud, Ernst, ed. *Letters of Sigmund Freud.* New York: Basic Books, 1961.

Freud, Ernst, ed. *Sigmund Freud: His Life in Pictures and Words.* London: Andre Deutsch, 1978.

Freud, Martin. *Sigmund Freud: Man and Father.* New York: Vanguard, 1958.

Freud, Sigmund. "On the History of the Psychoanalytic Movement," *The Standard Edition of the Complete Psychological Works of Sigmund Freud.* xiv. London: Hogarth, 1957.

Freud, Sigmund. "An Autobiographical Study," *Standard Edition.* xx. London: Hogarth, 1959.

Friedan, Betty. *The Feminine Mystique.* New York: Norton, 1963.

Fromm, Erich. *Sigmund Freud's Mission.* New York: Harper & Brothers, 1959.

Fromm-Reichmann, Frieda. *Principles of Intensive Psychotherapy.* London: Allen & Unwin, 1953.

Gay, Peter. *A Godless Jew—Freud, Atheism and the Making of Psychoanalysis.* New Haven: Yale University Press, 1987.

Gay, Peter. *Freud: A Life for Our Time.* New York, Norton, 1988.

Homans, Peter. *The Ability to Mourn: Disillusionment and the Social Origins of Psychoanalysis.* Chicago: University of Chicago Press, 1989.

Isbister, J. N. *Freud.* Cambridge: Blackwell's, Polity, 1985.

Jones, Ernest. *The Life and Work of Sigmund Freud.* New York: Basic Books, 1953–57 (3 vols).

Klein, D. B. *Jewish Origins of the Psychoanalytic Movement.* Chicago: University of Chicago Press, 1985.

Klein, Viola. *The Feminine Character.* London: Routledge & Kegan Paul, 1946.

Kris, Ernst et al., eds. *The Origin of Psychoanalysis: Letters to Wilhelm Fliess, Drafts and Notes, 1887–1902, by Sigmund Freud.* New York: Basic Books, 1954.

Krüll, Marianne. *Freud and His Father.* New York: Norton, 1986 (originally 1979).

Ludwig, Emil. *Doctor Freud.* New York: Hellman, Williams, 1947.

Malcolm, Janet. *In the Freud Archives.* New York: Vintage, 1985 (originally 1983).

Mannoni, Octave. *Freud.* New York: Random House, 1971.

Marcuse, Herbert. *Eros and Civilization.* Boston: Beacon Press, 1955.

Masson, J. M. *The Assault on Truth: Freud's Suppression of the Seduction Theory.* New York: Viking Penguin, 1985, with new preface (originally 1984).

McGrath, William. *Freud's Discovery of Psychoanalysis.* Ithaca: Cornell University Press, 1986.

Millett, Kate. *Sexual Politics.* New York: Doubleday, 1970.

Nunberg, Herman. *Principles of Psychoanalysis.* New York: International Universities Press, 1955.

Puner, Helen Walker. *Freud: His Life and Mind.* New York: Howell, Soskin, 1947.

Rice, Emanuel. *Freud and Moses: The Long Journey Home.* Albany: State University of New York Press, 1990.

Richards, Barry. *Images of Freud.* New York: St. Martin's Press, 1989.

Ricoeur, Paul. *Freud and Philosophy.* New Haven: Yale University Press, 1971.

Rieff, Philip. *Freud: The Mind of the Moralist.* New York: Viking Press, 1959.

Roazen, Paul. *Brother Animal: The Story of Freud and Tausk.* New York: Knopf, 1969.

Roazen, Paul. *Freud and His Followers.* New York: Knopf, 1975.

Robert, Marthe. *From Oedipus to Moses.* Garden City, NY: Anchor Books, 1976 (originally 1974).

Sachs, Hanns. *Freud: Master and Friend.* Cambridge: Harvard University Press, 1944.

Sachs, Hanns. *Masks of Life and Love.* Cambridge: Sci-Art Publishers, 1948.

Schorske, Carl. *Fin-de-Siècle Vienna.* New York: Vintage Books, 1981.

Schur, Max. *Freud: Living and Dying.* New York: International Universities Press, 1972.

Sulloway, Frank. *Freud: Biologist of the Mind.* New York: Basic Books, 1979.

Swales, Peter. "Freud, Minna Bernays, and the Conquest of Rome: New Light on the Origins of Psychoanalysis," *The New American Review,* Spring/Summer, 1982.

Trilling, Lionel. *Freud and the Crisis of our Culture.* Boston: Beacon, 1955.

Waelder, Robert. *Basic Theory of Psychoanalysis.* New York: International Universities Press, 1960.

Wollheim, Richard. *Sigmund Freud.* New York: Viking Press, 1971.

Yerushalmi, Yosef. *Freud's Moses.* New Haven: Yale University Press, 1991.

9

"A Whole Climate of Opinion": Rewriting the History of Psychoanalysis

JOHN FORRESTER

> to us he is no more a person
> now but a whole climate of opinion
>
> under whom we conduct our different lives:
> Like weather he can only hinder or help
>
> W. H. AUDEN, "In Memoriam Sigmund Freud"

If Auden's diagnosis is accurate, writing the history of psychoanalysis is rather like writing the history of twentieth-century cultural weather: Its presence is so constant and pervasive that escaping its influence is out of the question. And precisely because of its inescapable character, it cannot be isolated from the myriad striking events that can more straightforwardly be singled out as part of the histories of science, of medicalization, of great ideas, of cultural movements, of modernization, of all the other movements to which it might apparently belong. Freud, it seems, is like electric light—the twentieth century is unthinkable without it, but not many histories of the twentieth century pause to evoke the customary and natural darkness of all previous generations dispelled forever by light bulbs, car headlights, flashing neon tubes, and the nighttime flicker of movie and TV screens. There is, of course, a history of electricity in which names such as Maxwell and Edison figure prominently; but theirs is not the only history of electricity, nor is it the most important history. Likewise, there are histories of psychoanalysis where it belongs alongside radiotherapy and hypnosis, alongside energetics and the advent of causal medicine, alongside brain anatomy and the history of linguistics, alongside Durkheimian sociology and intelligence testing; but these assembled together do not make up the most important history.

Whether or not one assents to Auden's portrait of Freud as the weathervane of the twentieth century, the tone of his tribute unmistakably captures a striking feature of the historiography of psychoanalysis: its personal tone. Auden's poem depicts Freud's death as first and foremost his own personal loss:

> so many long-forgotten objects
> revealed by his undiscouraged shining
>
> are returned to us and made precious again;
> games we had thought we must drop as we grew up,
>   little noises we dared not laugh at,
> faces we made when no one was looking.

Of all the histories of psychoanalysis, the first was, in one sense of the term, undoubtedly the most unabashedly and explicitly personal: Sigmund Freud's "On the History of the Psycho-Analytic Movement." This work contained some of Freud's most astringent criticism and intolerant ostracism. It is a personal vendetta conducted in the Olympian impersonal voice that only autobiography, that completely unanswerable genre, can adopt. The history of psychoanalysis, Freud implies, is inextricably the history of refusals, resistances, and the necessary regroupings of the orthodox. What is more, the scathing attacks on the renegades and heretics were not only an attempt to preempt the judgment of history; they were also intimately entwined with a reordering of psychoanalytic concepts. Out of Freud's diatribe against Jung would develop the concepts of narcissism and the necessity to revise his first dualist theory of drives; out of his diatribe against Adler would develop the musings on the essential nature of femininity that came to fruition in some of his best-known and most notorious papers, those written under the sign of penis envy.[1] Controversies were perennially not only occasions for rewriting the history of psychoanalysis, as the expelled—Rank, Ferenczi (almost)—retrospectively had their earlier work removed or downgraded, but also, and *necessarily* so, occasions for major conceptual clarification. It is not for nothing that the history of psychoanalysis appears to be synonymous with the history of its splits, schisms, and dissidents.

However, Freud did not have to wait until he had dissenting followers for the process of rewriting the history of psychoanalysis to take place. From the outset, the interpretations upon which psychoanalysis was founded were reinterpretations of the treatments of patients, of the significance of nonsensical past events, and of the validity of childhood memories. Inasmuch as psychoanalytic writing embodies a specific theory about the relation of the present to the past, Freud's scientific style preempts the rational reconstruction of the historical development of his concepts. To understand the concept of repression, one follows his account of its genesis out of the experience of the resistance of patients. And to give an account of the "resistance" of patients, one must follow Freud in recounting the history of doctor-patient relationships at the end of the nineteenth century, including therein the ideal of the transparency and absolute authority of the relationship between hypnotist and subject in hypnosis.[2] The rational reconstruction of concepts and the personal narrative of Freud's experience as a therapist, indeed as a sexed being, are entwined. Freud "discovered" that he could not analyze himself without knowledge of his patients, nor could he analyze his patients without knowledge of himself; the historian is placed in the position of both having to treat psychoanalytic concepts as strictly personal documents and as governed by the architectonic of a theoretical system.

Three classic studies of the history of psychoanalysis illustrate the intertwining of personal, contextual, and conceptual, despite their idiosyncratically fastidious conceptions of the historian's task: Jones's biography of Freud;[3] Ellenberger's study of the development of dynamic psychiatry, in particular the systems of Freud, Pierre Janet, Carl Jung, and Alfred Adler, in the nineteenth and early twentieth centuries;[4] and Jean Laplanche and J.-B. Pontalis's conceptual dictionary of psychoanalytic concepts.[5]

Jones attempted to write a traditional neo-Victorian life-and-work of his subject, and went as far as to divide volumes II and III into separate sections dealing with the "Life" and the "Work". However, even Jones found it impracticable to separate the Life and the Work in Volume I, which deals with "the young Freud" from his birth to the publication of *The Interpretation of Dreams* at the age of 43. He established what has since become the psychoanalytically orthodox version of this early history: the intimate connection of Freud's inner personal life and the outer work of theory building, medical practice, and publishing. The self-analysis—as Jones described it—of the late 1890s became the historical linchpin for biographers and historians of science alike. "Once done it is done for ever": this was Jones's view of the self-analysis that revealed a New World as definitively and epoch-transformingly as the voyage of Christopher Columbus. This view is that of the first generation disciple of his Master. And psychoanalysts themselves—most eminently and illuminatingly Wladimir Granoff[6]—have questioned first whether an account that is such a naked transference, such a naked apology for both disciple and master, can stand as history, let alone as psychoanalytically sophisticated history, and second whether any other account is feasible.

Those who have since followed the biographical path have enthusiastically pursued the goal of rendering a life of Freud that is also the key to the conceptual development of psychoanalysis, not only because of a psychoanalytical *parti pris* in favor of seeking the causes of the outer trappings of life in the inner vicissitudes of personal history but also because of a nervous eschewal, often going as far as an energetic repudiation, of psychoanalytic visions of a life in favor of more traditional biographical approaches. Even those, such as Ola Andersson and Henri Ellenberger, whose works in the 1960s had provided firm foundations for the early intellectual history of Freud's work in the 1890s, found in previously unpublished documents concerning early patients of Breuer's and Freud's—Bertha Pappenheim and Fanny Moser—material for a revisionist account of this early history.[7] Biographical history could now compete with case history, as well as with Freud's accounts of psychological mechanisms. Since these works of the 1960s, Gerhard Fichtner, Albrecht Hirschmüller, and others have worked along similar lines, making available a new level of detail and mastery of previously inaccessible sources.[8]

The edge of iconoclasm in these new and detailed historical studies was to be expected: History from below, as the contemporaneous social history proclaimed itself, was self-consciously an attempt to revise and unsettle the stories told by those with an interest in a stable version of the past. The iconoclasm is explicit in the work of Swales.[9] In particular, Swales has demonstrated that controversial and always interesting results are to be had from combining techniques of close reading that both mimic and repudiate those of Freud with high-class sleuthing: delving in the archives and hotel registers of fin-de-siècle Austro-Hungary, interviewing and coaxing the memories of the descendants of forgotten or previously unknown historical participants in Freud's early work.

It is Swales more than anyone else who has struck a chord in Freud studies to which there is an immediate response on the part of the general reader who is intensely aware that psychoanalysis reveals hidden truths and that, if they are hidden, these truths of psychoanalysis must surely be worth hearing: Did Freud have an affair with his sister-in-law, arrange for her to have a secret abortion, and then use these skeletons in his closet as the foundations upon which to build a theory about skeletons in the closet?[10] Did Freud owe so much to his one-time friend Fliess that, rather than admit his debt, he planned to murder him?[11] Once we know exactly where and when Freud masturbated in an Alpine meadow, Swales implies, we will be less tempted to take seriously his theories of the importance of masturbation fantasies and their relation to childhood.

These iconoclastic studies, invaluable for the evidence they have produced and the dramatically new picture they paint of the milieus in which psychoanalysis arose, are as psychoanalytically *parti pris* as Ernest Jones, Max Schur, Kurt Eissler, and other psychoanalytically orthodox historians. Like the analysts at work on the self-deluding memories of their patients, the iconoclasts often aim to deprive psychoanalysis of firm foundations by demonstrating the tendentiousness of its own history. In a very different vein, the contextualists, of whom Ellenberger is the doyen, also are at odds with the history the psychoanalysts tell.

Once one establishes, as Ellenberger and others attempt to, that psychoanalysis is only one among many similar projects, both in space—the synchronic Europe-wide invention of dynamic psychiatry, of psychotherapies, of discourses on sexuality—and in time—the reinvention of the secret therapeutic mysteries and sects of the Pythagoreans, the mesmerists and popular hypnotists and healers—then its claim to its unique position can no longer be upheld. Not only that: Other contextualist arguments—such as Carl Schorske's and William McGrath's[12]—paint psychoanalysis as only comprehensible within the wider context of the pressure-cooker of fin-de-siècle Vienna. Psychoanalysis, like so much else in the declining years of the Hapsburg empire, was a nonpolitical means for achieving the frustrated political and class aims of the first generation of the new bourgeoisie. In more recent years, a new twist has been given to the politically sensitive question that ran like a red thread through the early dealings of Freud with his disciples and on into the Nazi era that transformed the demographics of psychoanalysis: Is psychoanalysis a Jewish science? Whereas Schorske emphasized the frustrations of the Viennese liberal bourgeoisie, more recent cultural historians emphasize the fact that this liberal bourgeoisie was overwhelmingly Jewish: The Jews became the numerically preponderant group in the cultural renaissance of Vienna, despite making up only ten percent of the overall population. Over half of the doctors and lawyers in Vienna in 1890 were Jewish. And:

> [Freud] was born a merchant's son in the Bohemian crownlands; 85 per cent of the Viennese *Gymnasiasten* with this background were Jewish. At his school . . . 97 per cent of merchants' sons were Jewish, and of those pupils born in the Bohemian crownlands, 73 per cent were Jewish. . . . He chose to do medicine at university; 78 per cent of the "liberal bourgeois" sector—into which Freud had, of course, been born—among *Maturanten* who opted to study medicine were Jewish. A staggering 93 per cent—76 Jews as opposed to only 5 non-Jews—of the merchants' sons in the *Gymnasien* sample who chose medicine were Jewish. He went on to become a practising physician. . . . Jews comprised 65 per cent of all former *Gymnasiasten*

from a liberal bourgeois background who went on to be doctors and lawyers. . . .
Freud, at least, could hardly have been anything else but Jewish, in the Viennese
context.[13]

Such studies of the delicate position of these Jews in the liberal professions have also
found in the autobiographical odyssey of *The Interpretation of Dreams* the model for
a search for a new identity for those Jews in flight from their truncated Jewish identities;
it "could provide a rallying point for both Jews and non-Jews who rebelled against the
prevailing tendency to assign social identities on the basis of religious affiliation."[14]

But if the specificity of psychoanalysis, if not its originality, is to be sought here in
Vienna, such arguments increase the urgency of the question: Can the enduring fascination of psychoanalysis—of Freud's grandiose autobiography—in interwar America,
in postwar France, in late twentieth-century South America also be found in the obligation imposed on the newly educated urban professional classes to undertake the Great
Modernist Trek in search of a secular identity?

Hence there is a historiographic tension between the need to find an explanation for
the emergence of psychoanalysis in Vienna (rather than somewhere else) and the need
for a historical characterization of psychoanalysis that will also explain its rapid dissemination and acceptance in Western culture in the early years of this century. Curiously enough, this problem of the universality of the appeal of a theory and a movement
whose specific and unique historical origins are pinpointed more and more accurately
is the structural duplicate of an even deeper historiographic problem: the question of
Freud's originality. Looking forward from Freud's Vienna, we see psychoanalysis dis-
seminating out to other cultures and institutions; looking backward from Vienna's
Freud, we see myriad diverse progenitors and precursors.

As I have already implied, iconoclasm makes itself felt, in the history of psychoanalysis as in so many other areas in the history of science, in the attempt to demonstrate
the commonplace character, even ubiquity, of a scientist's most distinctive claims. The
unconscious, it is argued, is a product of Romantic thought, if not earlier;[15] infantile
sexuality had been recognized as common, even by doctors, for decades, if not centuries
before Freud.[16] But, it is riposted, Freud's originality did not stem from his discovery
of these "facts", just as Newton's did not stem from his "discovery" of gravity, but
in his systematizing of them, in the manner in which he transformed and undercut earlier
conceptions of sexuality and the mind.[17] The history of Freud's precursors has been
and will inevitably be a burgeoning and sizable part of the historiography of psychoanalysis. However, the significance of each precursor diminishes the more names are
added to the list: Each precursor transforms Freud's significance from being that of a
discoverer (who is then shown not to be one by the precursor-hunting historian) to that
of being the conduit for the heterogeneous cultural resources of his—and our?—times.

If the French tradition of epistemology was to produce the *Vocabulaire* of Laplanche
and Pontalis, which I shall discuss shortly, the most representative, and revealing, product of the equivalent Anglo-American tradition of history of science was Frank Sulloway's *Freud. Biologist of the Mind*. If the French tradition errs by ignoring context in
favor of conceptual analysis, Sulloway attempted to reduce conceptual development to
intellectual context: in his case, to exactly that intellectual context to which a historian
of science whose training had been in the familiar territories of the physical and biological sciences would appeal. Sulloway discovered that psychoanalysis was an offshoot

of the biological sciences of the nineteenth century that had never freed itself from the parent plant. Ignoring the fact that, just to count crude heads for a moment, there are seventy-five instances of Freud quoting Goethe in the *Standard Edition*, seventy-four quotes from Shakespeare, and only twenty-one mentions of Darwin, Sulloway proposed that psychoanalysis was a crypto-biology, a sort of sociobiology *avant la lettre*; and, most triumphantly, he used the gaps in the evidence for this view as proof of a cover-up, proof of the sustained effort (to what end?) of Freud and his disciples to promote the myth that psychoanalysis is not an art of interpretation and a science of mental life, but a self-deluding conceptual system intended to answer biological problems. Rereading Sulloway's rewriting of history, one cannot but feel that the iconoclasm of the biographical detectives had become intertwined in an unfortunate manner with the somewhat self-contradictory conviction that no psychology is worthy of the name unless it is really a biology (as with the sociobiology of the era). Certainly, the closure of historical development produced by his argument that Freud was mired in the neo-Lamarckian biology of fin-de-siècle Vienna does not help explain how psychoanalysis as an endemic practice and as a cultural system ever came into being.

At the opposite pole to the contextualist histories we find the third of my classic studies in the history of psychoanalysis, which at first blush does not appear to be history: Laplanche and Pontalis's *Vocabulaire de la Psychanalyse*, first published in French in 1967. Organized as a lexicon, or manual of conceptual terms, it is focused primarily on the conceptual development of Freud's terminology, although certain terms from later analysts, notably Lacan and Klein, are found. In the process of teasing out the subtleties of the changes in these concepts, the authors give a most thought-provoking and textually accurate internal history of the science of psychoanalysis, so that every student of Freud's writing is indebted to them and will be for many years. However, to call their work "history" raises interesting questions, not only about the relation between the "internal" and the "external" histories of science—as historians of science have, in something of a mood of resignation, become used to calling one of the oldest and most important debates in their field—but about the nature of psychoanalytic knowledge itself and its relation to the discipline's history.

While in no sense taking away from Laplanche's and Pontalis's independence and originality, the very possibility of their project of a conceptual dictionary of Freudian terms is to be found in the conditions of psychoanalysis in postwar France. The very idea of a conceptual dictionary of such subtlety and sophistication could only be attempted and brought to fruition in a psychoanalytic environment that was open to alliances less with medicine than with the "human sciences": the dictionary could thus be constructed employing the techniques of the historian of philosophy and the French tradition of the epistemology of the sciences (a very different tradition from the philosophy of the sciences in postwar Anglo-American intellectual life, where history of science was a burgeoning discipline in its own right, always more contextualist and eager to distance itself from the overly formal account of the sciences associated with Viennese logical positivism and the falsificationism of Karl Popper). This atmosphere of philosophical sophistication and textual enthusiasm for close and accurate commentary on the Freudian *textes* (as the French, and later the English-speaking commentators, would call them) was provided by the "return to Freud" of Jacques Lacan, with its mistrust of the medicalization of psychoanalysis in favor of alliances with the proto-structuralism of the "conjectural sciences": ethnology, linguistics, and cybernetics.

If Jones's official biography of Freud was in part written by the disciple wishing to cast his own life—as early follower and bearer of the psychoanalytic Good News to England, as mainstay of the International Psychoanalytic Association for some forty years—together with that of the Master in the heroic mode, and in part to establish an abundantly researched official history to pit against the tendentious popularizations; if Ellenberger's history was that of an eclectic psychiatrist wishing to rescue his discipline from narrow-minded commitment to any one system of dynamic psychiatry; then Laplanche and Pontalis were attempting to establish the historical baseline for a discipline that has a very curious and distinctive relation to its own history. The works of Jones and Ellenberger illustrate how the "history" of psychoanalysis is inextricably bound up with a conception of what psychoanalysis is *and should be*; the work of Laplanche and Pontalis demonstrates how a specific conception of what psychoanalysis is and should be is built upon a definitive and historically defensible reading of Freud.

It was almost certainly the example of Lacan's return to Freud and the sophisticated exegetical enterprises associated with the energetic dissemination of psychoanalysis in France in the 1950s and 1960s of which Laplanche and Pontalis's work was among the most distinguished, together with the burgeoning quasi-analytic textual procedures of Jacques Derrida, that led Michel Foucault in 1968 to write his essay, "What is an author?" Almost in the style of an analytic philosopher, Foucault clarified the various usages of the term *author*, which range from the tautological—well captured by Aldous Huxley's bon mot: "*The Odyssey* was written by Homer or by some one with the same name"—via the material sense ("The author asserts her moral right") to the more interestingly transdiscursive senses. Names such as Dickens or Darwin are transdiscursive not only because they have *oeuvres* associated with them, so that *The Descent of Man* is evoked by the name Darwin as much as *The Origin of Species*, but also because they are associated with texts and social movements that go beyond "mere" or tautological authorship, or even possession of a "corpus": there is a Darwinian revolution, there is Dickensian London. Authors of founding religious texts—such as Mohammed or Joseph Smith—have an equally transdiscursive function, in part because of their ambiguous relationship to their "coauthors," in part because their texts become "canonical"—unquestionably imbued with a truth whose extraction requires exegesis and commentary. In addition to such transdiscursive authors, Foucault concentrates on the new breed of nineteenth-century writers who gave rise to "discursive practices"; these authors "produced not only their own work, but the possibility and the rules of the formation of other texts."[18] The work of Freud and Marx are the best examples: Their work is not just the first in a series, but is distinctly separated off as unique and foundational in relation to all other texts that followed. In this respect, so Foucault argues, Freud's work is different from the works of other authors in the history of science.

While doubting whether the history of science displays no other founding authors of the ilk of Marx and Freud—one could point to the relation of British mathematical natural philosophy in the eighteenth century to Newton, or to certain fundamentalist Darwinians of the last two decades—the distinctiveness of psychoanalytic communities with respect to Freud is unquestionable. The preservation and teaching of the theories of Sigmund Freud are often enough enshrined as formal aims in the statutes of psychoanalytic societies and institutes; every student of psychoanalysis spends some years mastering Introductory, Intermediate, and Advanced Freud. Here, mastering means what it might mean in a practical art such as painting, or building a computer: being able to put oneself in the position of Freud to enact the interpretations or the conceptual developments oneself, as if the student were doing them for him- or herself.

At the very same time, the student must undertake a training analysis and must perform, and have performed upon him or her, what Freud performed upon himself: the act of analysis. The training analysis is closely linked to a more specific feature of Freud's psychoanalytic writing: its autobiographical character. This personal tone, the fact that every reader, certainly every early follower, is obliged to establish a personal relationship with the theory, means that histories of psychoanalysis often read as if they are accounts of Freud's autobiography—as if they are biographies of Freud and his extended analytic family.[19] And hence the history of psychoanalysis for the period following Freud's death appears to lose its guiding thread or its *raison d'être*: The history of psychoanalysis is the story of Freud's autobiography. Or, by extension, the history of psychoanalysis is a family saga, the history of the family he created. Genealogical researches—that mode of historical knowledge dear to aristocrats and those in search of their personal "roots", but a mode that is anathema to professional historians—and accounting of debts and inheritance—more usually the domain of the historians of royalty and of industrial empires—can become the framework for the history of the dissemination of psychoanalysis: informal gossip about analytic filiation—who frequented which couch, who is the analytic mother and father of whom; informal gossip about who is the true legatee of the symbolic legacy of theory and of the true method of psychoanalysis.

This singular and unique importance of Freud for the history of psychoanalysis prompted Derrida to ask a searching question about the distinctive relation of psychoanalysis to its founder: "How can an autobiographical writing, in the abyss of an unterminated self-analysis, give birth to a world-wide institution?"[20] Derrida's numerous writings on psychoanalysis—on the interconnection of autobiography with theory, of telepathy and the analyst's use of the first person pronoun, of family dynamics and institutional affiliation[21]—raise the question of the distinctiveness of the institutional character of psychoanalysis: Is it a revival of an ancient model of an esoteric therapeutic philosophical sect, à la Ellenberger? Is its insistently reflexive character the harbinger of the deconstructionist or postmodern world of the end of the twentieth century?

In an obvious sense, the institutional history of psychoanalysis begins with Freud's relationships with his followers, and there have been useful and major studies of the family networks and subnetworks, from Roazen's studies of the external forms of discipleship, via Roustang's more psychoanalytically oriented, but no less critical, studies of the structure of relationship, the structure of mastery and slavery, necessary to the formation of psychoanalytic institutions, to more contextually embedded accounts of specific psychoanalytic cultures.[22] And it is when one places these contextualized histories of national cultures of psychoanalysis alongside the studies that focus on Freud that one senses that in the historiography of psychoanalysis there are two distinct genres: on the one hand, *Freud studies*, which is more biography than history, more the struggle over the legacy than a social history of a new profession; and on the other hand, the histories (always plural) of psychoanalysis in its local habitats and microcultures.

However, one should not presume too quickly that it is only the figure of Freud that leads to history ending up as a cross between myth and family romance; the most accomplished of psychoanalytic histories to date, Elisabeth Roudinesco's monumental

La Bataille de Cent Ans. L'Histoire de la Psychanalyse en France, 1885–1985, quickly dispels such an illusion. Each of the two volumes of Roudinesco's generously conceived and culturally catholic history has a hero: The first volume, covering the period from Charcot to the early years of the Société Psychanalytique de Paris, appears to have Freud as its hero. Her study of the early years of French psychoanalysis, from 1885 to 1939, is a study in cultural misappropriation, of the image of the cosmopolitan universalist Freudian theory refracted in a chauvinistic, anti-Semitic, and sexually repressive French society. Hence the Freud who appears in this history is present only as a negative contrast to the false Freuds, those invoked in France in this period as the inventor of an unconscious that Roudinesco argues is only an *"inconscient à la française"*. Implicit in the second volume is the possibility of the emergence of a Freud who is now faithfully reflected by his disciples—this is the Freud of Laplanche and Pontalis, of an exegetical attention to detail that has produced a document such as B. This and P. Theves's lengthy study of the translation of Freud's "Die Verneinung", a four-page paper he published in 1925. This and Theves scrutinize and compare, line by line, word by word, particle by particle, the seventeen different translations of these four pages that French psychoanalytic culture has produced.[23]

However, the living hero of Roudinesco's second volume is not this textually embalmed and sacred Freud, but Jacques Lacan, magician and charlatan, grand theorist and transgressor of all psychoanalytic etiquette. It is tempting, though not perhaps safe, to draw the historical conclusion: It is only when there is a figure as dominating as Lacan in any given psychoanalytic culture that the spell cast by Freud can be conjured away. Perhaps one method of internal transformation open to psychoanalysis is neither the repudiation nor the forgetting of Freud; perhaps Freud is as flexible as Jesus or Newton, allowing a plethora of faithful versions to flourish in his many mansions. Another lesson is equally clear: It is possible for the story of a psychoanalytic culture to be told that is not a version of Freud's family romance. Someone else's will do just as well.

Roudinesco's history is by quite a margin the most comprehensive and subtle general history of a psychoanalytic culture to date. Only the summation of research done on the early American enthusiasm for and co-option of Freud's work bears any comparison. Together the American and French histories raise the question: Will the history of psychoanalysis always be best done within the framework of national cultures?

Schorske and McGrath had provided an account of the place of psychoanalysis within Viennese culture that can only hold for a very specific time and place; at the same time, they supported an older, *Marxisant* or *sociologisant,* view of psychoanalysis as the apolitical discourse that tempts the bourgeoisie away from the privileged arena of political struggle and conflict. It is as if Vienna exported one brand of International to subvert the effects of the other. Left-leaning bourgeois groups have, throughout the twentieth century, viewed with suspicion those who would place their inner personal hygiene alongside of the plight of the masses. The attractions of the theories and movements associated with both Marx and Freud have been one of the cultural constants in Western intellectual circles of the twentieth century, as have, inevitably, been the attempts at Freudo-Marxist synthesis, from Wilhelm Reich to Jürgen Habermas, from Herbert Marcuse to Louis Althusser.

Similarly, it is transnational media that may be extensively implicated in the creation of the image of charismatic scientists, from the late nineteenth century on. Certainly, in the late 1910s and 1920s Freud joined Einstein and a few other contemporary scientists in the novel role of a charismatic figure for the daily press and weekly reviews; an analysis of the function of such charismatic figures, from Darwin to Hawking, will aid in the understanding of the popular dissemination of psychoanalysis. Roudinesco's history of psychoanalysis in France gives ample details of this popularization for one culture,[24] and there is an illuminating study by D. Rapp of England in the 1920s.[25] There is also a fine study of American psychiatry—that is, psychoanalysis—as portrayed in the Hollywood cinema from the 1930s to the 1980s, which both shows how rich a resource for twentieth-century cultural history the cinema is, and how central a part of popular culture psychoanalysis had become from the early 1930s on,[26] one dream industry feeding off the other. Yet the connections between these national cultures are, in this respect, essential to explore, a fact that the transcultural media of film should alert us to, together with a sense of the international character of so much of the history of medicine in the period.

If the history of the rise of French psychoanalysis to cultural prominence can be written as the history of a cultural movement, relatively independent of preestablished professional organizations, the American example provides a clear contrast. From the 1920s until 1989, when a civil suit required the American Psychoanalytic Association to change its regulations, the American psychoanalytic profession required all psychoanalysts to be medically qualified. Thus, in the United States, the history of psychoanalysis was intimately part of the history of medicine, in particular of the history of psychiatry. For a period, from the late 1930s (at the latest) to the 1960s, psychoanalysis was an indispensable part of the American psychiatrist's training and authoritative knowledge, and certainly a crucial component of his or her social status. With the introduction of psychotropic drugs in the 1950s and 1960s, with the shift, on the part of those concerned less with symptom alleviation and cure and more with the welfare of patients in institutions (a shift well marked in the historiography of psychiatry with the work of Michel Foucault, Klaus Doerner, and Andrew Scull)—in other words with the rise of drug psychiatry and social psychiatry as two sides of one coin—the mid-century psychoanalytic hegemony, which had been so successful in part because it appeared to fuse attention to the symptom with concern for the patient, was undermined, set to one side, and, finally, with the rise of a victorious and philistine organic psychiatry of the 1980s, virtually eliminated. The decline and fall of American psychiatric psychoanalysis has yet to be written.

Even before it has been written, its main outlines pose questions for the historiography of psychoanalysis: Given that the relations of psychiatry and psychoanalysis were halfhearted on both sides in the beginning of the century, should we reconsider the question of the history of psychoanalysis in its relations to medicine in general? One immediate way to do so would be to consider the relations of psychoanalysis with other branches of medicine, in particular with general practice. However, the background to this exploration would be an analysis of the varieties of medicine that emerged in the late nineteenth century. First, there is the clinical art of medicine, transformed, no doubt, from the beginnings of the nineteenth century on, by the supremacy of the clinical examination, pathological anatomy, and the post mortem, but still dominated by the individual contact between the doctor and the patient, no matter how subordinated to general principles and laws governing the behavior of organs; second, the rise of public health medicine, of epidemiology and state-centered sciences of hygiene: sanatory and miasmic medicines, vaccination, the statistical ordering of the population, and the imperative to render the health of the nation visible and public; third and imperialistically, the rise of scientific laboratory-based medicine, from the laboratories of Bernard, Koch, and Pasteur[27] to the test and drug-based medicine of the twentieth century, in which the doctor can only act on the patient's behalf once the patient's body has become fully integrated within and tamed by the barrage of tests and safeguards of the laboratory—situated either in a hospital, or in an industrial plant for the manufacture of magic bullets.

However, one of the consequences of the rise of scientific medicine was a crisis in the very idea of the doctor-patient relationship. Doctors refused to be stampeded by the enthusiastic Pasteurians into exchanging the white coats of a scientific priesthood for the more traditional sacerdotal accessories; organizations of doctors opposed to scientific medicine were started, articulating for the first time an ideal of the unique relationship the doctor has with the patient: unique and confidential, to be protected from the universalizing, statistical requirements of populational medicine and hygiene and from the requirements of public testing and standardization of the laboratory. From whence was created one reactive modern ideal of the doctor-patient relation, an intimate relation of trust, confidence, and secrecy. This is the doctor we find inhabiting the family dramas of Freud's near contemporaries, Ibsen, Chekhov, and Schnitzler (the last two of whom were practicing physicians). It would be a mistake to conceive of the doctors who are so prominent in these plays—these pillars of bourgeois society, often psychotherapists *avant la lettre*—as traditional doctors; these are the *new* general practitioners of a medical world that is divided and at odds with itself, now scientific, now priestly.

Viewed within this admittedly tentative sketch of the cartography of medicine in the modern era, psychoanalysis would not appear as a wing of the newly professionalizing medical subspecialities such as psychiatry or neurology so much as a reaction to the more widespread problems general practitioners faced when confronted with a shift toward public and scientific legitimations for their ancient art. Hypnosis and suggestion, quite clearly the historical antecedents of much psychoanalytic practice,[28] can be viewed as revivals of folk medical practices, as the rough and ready rural technique of the founder of the Nancy School of suggestion, Ambroise Liébeault, shows. The history of psychoanalytic practice—as is suggested by Carlo Ginzburg's speculative study of the new sciences of the end of the nineteenth century concerned with clues and signs derived from medical diagnostics—may owe much to the resurfacing of "popular" practices and rules of thumb, becoming acceptable because of the pressure that the rise of scientific medicine placed on more traditional conceptions of the physician-client relationship.[29]

The work of Michael Balint at the Tavistock Institute in London in the early 1950s is salutary in this respect. Employing a psychoanalysis divested of all technical terms for their scrutiny of the day-to-day work of general practitioners within the British National Health Service, Balint and his nonanalytically trained GP colleagues put together a conception of the long-term function of the doctor as being primarily engaged in establishing working relationships, the joint capital of a medical mutual investment company, with patients that allowed the business of medicine, such as organizing the illness into an agreed-upon diagnosis and finding the correct dosage of the "drug doctor" (the principal element in the GP's pharmacopoeia), to proceed smoothly.[30] Freud's view—often instantiated in later present-centered histories, that psychotherapy was as old as illness and that "we doctors could not give it up if we wanted to, because the other party to our methods of healing—namely the patient—has not the slightest intention of doing without it"[31]—was thus expanded: The demand addressed to each and every doctor has always been initially psychotherapeutic in character, whatever the manifest "presenting symptom." It is one of the principal functions of psychoanalysis to retain and to bring to the center of every doctor's attention the psychotherapeutic function that every visit to the doctor entails and awakens. In this way, instead of the "collusion of anonymity" and ensuing irresponsibility that the modern institutions of hospital, clinic, specialist, and laboratory have created, the GP—whose speciality is "the total personality," or who in the United States practices medicine first and foremost on the family—will serve as a conduit both for modern medical science and for the ancient and perennial medical function that has been crystallized by psychoanalysis: the transference relationship.

Such a historiography—yet to be written in any detail—would pay attention to the vexed question of the relationship between psychoanalysis and deep cultural movements, yet would retain some sense of the relationship between psychoanalysis and the changing character of the medical profession. Psychoanalysis began with the medical interpretation of Aristotle's concept of catharsis that Josef Breuer and Bertha Pappenheim accepted and applied to their relationship. However, many interpretations of the cultural significance of psychoanalysis in the twentieth century prefer to align it with ethical transformations and the advance of secularization, rather than with medicine, as if they recognized psychoanalysis to have an ethical rather than medical lineage. It is to these interpretations that I will now turn.

Ernest Gellner accepts the significance of psychoanalysis[32]—he accepts Auden's view that we live in a Freudian climate; but he locates its significance in the domain of secular anxiety consequent upon the processes of modernization, the luxury of Western societies, and the increasing ineptitude of religious institutions and consolations. Psychoanalysis emerged as a secular procedure with the authority of science that offered hope to those in trouble with their fellow humans. Gellner pinpoints psychoanalysis as the leader, perhaps even the loss leader, of those twentieth-century movements that we can gather together under the name of "therapy service industries." These industries service what Philip Rieff, in one of the most acute of all commentaries on Freud and his institutional creations, called "psychological man." Characterizing psychoanalysis as "a popular science of morals that also teaches a moral system,"[33] Rieff pinpointed its "ethic of honesty" as an alternative to the inefficient and toxic moral commitments of modern society: beyond political man, the public man of action and virtue; beyond religious man, who, in Western society, is always against this world; beyond *homo economicus*, the avaricious self-interested calculator invented by the Enlightenment, is psychological man, whose only ideal is one of experimental insight leading to self-mastery.

Rieff's fruitful essays on Freud and the "triumph of the therapeutic" in the mid and late twentieth centuries are extended and placed in a different context by Alasdair MacIntyre's *After Virtue*,[34] in which he proposes that historical cultures are in part defined by their stock of *characters*, which, as the masks worn by moral philosophies, partially define the possibility of public and private action. These masks constitute the moral and social ideals of the epoch; a character "morally legitimates a mode of social existence. . . . So the culture of Victorian England was partially defined by the *char-*

acters of the Public School Headmaster, the Explorer and the Engineer; and that of Wilhelmine Germany was similarly defined by such *characters* as those of the Prussian Officer, the Professor and the Social Democrat.'' For the twentieth century, MacIntyre isolates three characters: the rich aesthete-hedonist, the manager, and the therapist.

> The manager represents in his *character* the obliteration of the distinction between manipulative and nonmanipulative social relations; the therapist represents the same obliteration in the sphere of personal life. . . . Neither manager nor therapist, in their roles as manager and therapist, do or are able to engage in moral debate.[35]

In parallel with MacIntyre, Rieff noted how the analyst is able to escape from the moral debates of the religious and the nonprofessional precisely because ''his is not a therapy of belief but one which instructs how to live without belief.''[36]

MacIntyre pinpoints the same ideal as Rieff perceived in Freud's vision of the ''secular spiritual guide,'' the analyst functioning as physician and priest to each and every family;[37] even Lacan could wax eloquent on the ideal represented by psychoanalysis:

> Of all the undertakings that have been proposed in this century, that of the psychoanalyst is perhaps the loftiest, because the undertaking of the psychoanalyst acts in our time as a mediator between the man of care and the subject of absolute knowledge.[38]

It is instructive, if somewhat surprising, that the final works of Michel Foucault led him to a similar relocation of the historical significance of psychoanalysis as to be found in an ethical domain. Foucault's odyssey recapitulates, in miniature, some of the main themes in the historiography of psychoanalysis.

In *Madness and Civilization*, he located Freud as the perfected end point of the alienation of the madman—thus as the riposte and culmination of nineteenth-century psychiatry; in *The Order of Things*, psychoanalysis, through its founding concept of the unconscious and its recognition of the Other, represents ''a perpetual principle of dissatisfaction, of calling into question''[39] of the human sciences in general, rather than the medical domain. As Foucault turned away from the archaeology of concepts to the genealogy of practices, so psychoanalysis became less a subversive principle than a propitiously typical, because purged and purified, element in the apparatus of knowledge-power that emerged in the nineteenth century to become dominant in the welfare states of the twentieth. Psychoanalysis is quite clearly the most sophisticated and effective—because so liberal—incitement to talk about sexuality, to codify it and to recognize it as the core of the subject's being. Foucault's projected six-volume history of sexuality was thus conceived of as an archaeology of psychoanalysis, asking how it had become possible for us, we Freudians, to say *this*, to act in *this* way.

However, in seeking the genealogy of psychoanalytic practice in the development of confessional techniques, Foucault was drawn further back in time, expanding his notion of the confessional to include larger features of Christianity and its long alliance and conflict with the state. He came to be more concerned with the extended matrix of individualization of intimate knowledge, produced by pastoral techniques, and the methods of subjectivation—a method of producing a subject of moral truth and action. Foucault evoked a long tradition of the hermeneutics of the self which, starting with the early Christians and passing through Freud, required an extended purification of any trace of desire, no matter how distorted, and which in the process specified the singularity of that individual. Simply through the juxtaposition of this hermeneutics of the self with the ''aesthetics of the existence'' of the Ancient World, a way of life that depended solely ''on certain formal principles in the use of pleasures,''[40] Foucault was in search of an ethic for the conduct of life that was outside that tradition whose modern and ubiquitously influential representative, he implied, was psychoanalysis and the practices it required of the subject. To show both the significance and the historical limitations, perhaps even cultural perversity, of psychoanalysis, Foucault proposed the category of the pastoral as best suited to focus attention on the distinctiveness of the ethos of the post-Ancient moral universe.[41] This distinctive ''oriental'' (i.e., Judeo-Christian) pastoral power—self-sacrificing, salvation-oriented devotion to the individual[42]—eventually separated itself from political power in the nineteenth century via ''an individualizing 'tactic' which characterized a series of powers: those of the family, medicine, psychiatry, education, and employers.''[43] Hence to psychoanalysis as the most distinctively modern ''technology of the self.''[44]

These analyses of Gellner, MacIntyre, and Foucault, half historical, half moral reflections on the sensibility of the age, are, insofar as they are historical, oriented toward being a characterization of the psychoanalytic clientele: patient-centered history. But the ''patient'' has been transmuted into a representative, perhaps the quintessential, character of our time: a subject in therapy, in search of authenticity and satisfactions primarily in its private life and its pleasures.[45] This history is, then, part of a panoramic history of sensibilities.[46] The attention of literary and film theorists, of essayists and novelists throughout this century, also points to the fact that the innovative recounting and writing of the individual life made possible by psychoanalysis—in the form of case history, of memoir, of fictionalized analysis, of stream of consciousness modernist prose à la Woolf and Joyce, or of the Hollywood movie à la Hitchcock or Brian de Palma, and confessional sexual fantasy à la Nancy Friday[47]—constitutes the mythical genre of our time.[48]

Looking to the other side of the psychoanalytic mirror, to the history of the analyst, it is not clear yet whether, beyond its place in the history of science, of ideas, of sexuality, psychoanalysis belongs to histories of the medical-industrial complex, to those of the service and leisure industries, or is a part of the media. Shamanic doctor, secular priest, unadorned and simple therapist, even scientist, as the early analysts so unproblematically assumed: These are the figures of the history that has been and is in the process of being rewritten. Auden's certainty about Freud's ineluctable presence, as the climate of opinion, in our culture may meet with our assent; the historians of psychoanalysis have not as yet proved less shamanlike than our meteorologists, both ancient and modern. Whether they will is an interesting question.

Notes

1. See Lisa Appignanesi and John Forrester, *Freud's Women* (London: Weidenfeld & Nicolson; New York: Basic, 1992), 397–429.

2. See Carroll Smith-Rosenberg, ''The Hysterical Woman: Sex Roles and Role Conflict in Nineteenth-century America'' (1972) in Smith-Rosenberg, *Disorderly Conduct: Visions of Gender in Victorian America* (New York: Knopf, 1985; New York: Oxford University Press, 1985),

197–216; A. de Swaan, "On the Sociogenesis of the Psychoanalytic Situation," *Psychoanalysis & Contemporary Thought*, iii (1980), 381–413.

3. Ernest Jones, *Sigmund Freud. Life and Work*, 3 vols. (London: Hogarth Press, 1953–57).

4. Henri F. Ellenberger, *The Discovery of the Unconscious. The History and Evolution of Dynamic Psychiatry* (London: Allen Lane, 1970).

5. Jean Laplanche and J.-B. Pontalis, *The Language of Psychoanalysis* (1967), trans. Donald Nicholson-Smith (London: Hogarth Press and the Institute of Psycho-analysis, 1973).

6. Wladimir Granoff, *Filiations* (Paris: Editions de Minuit, 1975).

7. Ola Andersson, *Studies in the Prehistory of Psychoanalysis* (Stockholm: Scandinavian University Books, Svenska Bokförlaget/Norstedts-Bonniers, 1962); idem, "A Supplement to Freud's Case History of 'Frau Emmy v. N.' " in *Studies on Hysteria 1895*," *Scandinavian Psychoanalytic Review*, ii (1979), 5–15; Henri F. Ellenberger, "The Story of 'Anna O.': A Critical Review with New Data," *Journal of the History of the Behavioral Sciences*, viii (1972), 267–279.

8. Gerhard Fichtner, *Freuds Patienten* (Tübingen: Institut für Geschichte der Medizin, Dec. 1979), mimeo; G. Fichtner. and A. Hirschmüller, "Freuds 'Katherina'—Hintergrund, Entstehungsgeschichte und Bedeutung einer frühen psychoanalytischen Krankengeschichte," *Psyche*, xxxix (1985), 220–240; Albrecht Hirschmüller, *Freuds Begegnung mit der Psychiatrie. Von der Hirnmythologie zur Neurosenlehre* (Tübingen: Edition Diskord, 1991); Hirschmüller, "Freuds 'Mathilde': Ein weiterer Tagesrest zum Irma Traum," *Jahrbuch der Psychoanalyse*, xxiv (1989), 128–159; Hirschmüller, *Physiologie und Psychoanalyse in Leben und Werk Josef Breuers*, [*Jahrbuch der Psychoanalyse*, Suppl. 4], (Bern: Hans Huber, 1978), trans. *The Life and Work of Josef Breuer. Physiology and Psychoanalysis* (New York: New York University Press, 1989).

9. Peter Swales, "A Fascination with Witches," *The Sciences*, xxii (*no. 8* November 1982), 21–25; idem, "Freud, Breuer and the Blessed Virgin" (privately printed, 1986); idem, "Freud, His Teacher, and the Birth of Psychoanalysis" in Paul E. Stepansky (ed.), *Freud. Appraisals and Reappraisals. Contributions to Freud Studies*. vol. i (Hillsdale, New Jersey: Analytic Press, 1986), 3–82; idem, "Freud, Katharina, and the First 'Wild Analysis,' " in Paul Stepansky (ed.), *Freud. Appraisals and Reappraisals. Contributions to Freud Studies*. vol. iii (Hillsdale, New Jersey: Analytic Press, 1988), 79–164; and a series of Swales's papers, previously privately printed, now published in Laurence Spurling (ed.), *Sigmund Freud. Critical Assessments. vol. i. Freud and the Origins of Psychoanalysis* (London: Routledge & Kegan Paul, 1989).

10. Peter Swales, "Freud, Minna Bernays and the Conquest of Rome: New Light on the Origins of Psychoanalysis," *The New American Review*, i (1982), 1–23; idem, "Freud, Martha Bernays and the Language of Flowers, Masturbation, Cocaine, and the Inflation of Fantasy" (privately printed, 1983).

11. Swales, "Freud, Fliess and Fratricide; The Role of Fliess in Freud's Conception of Paranoia" (1982) in Laurence Spurling (ed.), *Sigmund Freud. Critical Assessments. vol. i. Freud and the Origins of Psychoanalysis* (London: Routledge & Kegan Paul, 1989), 302–329.

12. Carl E. Schorske, *"Fin-de-Siècle" Vienna: Politics and Culture* (New York: Knopf, 1980). William J. McGrath, *Freud's Discovery of Psychoanalysis. The Politics of Hysteria* (Ithaca: Cornell University Press, 1986).

13. Steven Beller, "Class, Culture and the Jews of Vienna, 1900" in Ivar Oxaal, Michael Pollak, and Gerhard Botz (eds.), *Jews, Antisemitism and Culture in Vienna* (London: Routledge & Kegan Paul, 1987), 39–58, this passage from pp. 57–58; see also Michael Pollak, "Cultural Innovation and Social Identity in *Fin-de-Siècle* Vienna" in Oxaal, Pollak, and Botz (eds.), *Jews, Antisemitism and Culture in Vienna*, 59–74.

14. Pollak, "Cultural Innovation and Social Identity," 69–70.

15. L. Whyte, *The Unconscious before Freud* (London: Methuen, 1962).

16. K. Codell Carter, "Infantile Hysteria and Infantile Sexuality in Late Nineteenth-century German-language Medical Literature," *Medical History*, xxvii (1983), 186–196; Stephen Kern,

"The Discovery of Child Sexuality: Freud and the Emergence of Child Psychology, 1880–1910" (Ph.D. diss., Columbia University, 1972), Diss Abs X1970 p. 205; Stephen Kern, "Freud and the Discovery of Child Sexuality," *History of Childhood Quarterly: The Journal of Psychohistory*, i (1973), 117–141; see also Frank Sulloway, *Freud. Biologist of the Mind* (London: Burnett Books, 1979).

17. See, for instance, the thoughtful Arnold I. Davidson, "How to Do the History of Psychoanalysis: A Reading of Freud's *Three essays on the theory of sexuality*" in Françoise Meltzer (ed.), *The Trial(s) of Psychoanalysis* (Chicago: University of Chicago Press, 1988), 39–64; on the distinctive character of the unconscious, see John Forrester, *Language and the Origins of Psychoanalysis* (London: Macmillan; New York: Columbia University Press, 1980), 4–6, 57ff., 179–180.

18. "What is an author?" in Michel Foucault, *Language, Counter-memory, Practice*, ed. D. Bouchard, trans. S. Simon (Ithaca: Cornell University Press, 1977), 131.

19. See Elisabeth Young-Bruehl, "A History of Freud Biographies," this volume.

20. Jacques Derrida, "Spéculer—sur Freud" in Jacques Derrida, *La Carte Postale* (Paris: Flammarion, 1980) 277–437, this passage from p. 325; *The Post Card. From Socrates to Freud and Beyond*, trans. Alan Bass (Chicago: Chicago University Press, 1987), 257–409, this passage from p. 305, trans. modified.

21. Jacques Derrida, "Freud and the Scene of Writing" (1965) *Yale French Studies*, xxxxviii (1972), 74–117; "Le Facteur de la Vérité" in Jacques Derrida, *La Carte Postale* (Paris: Aubier-Flammarion, 1980), 441–524; *The Post Card. From Socrates to Freud and Beyond*, trans. Alan Bass (Chicago: Chicago University Press, 1987), 411–496; "Télépathie," *Cahiers Confrontation*, x (Automne 1983) 201–230; reprinted in Derrida, *Psyché. Inventions de l'Autre* (Paris: Editions Galilée, 1987) 237–270; Derrida, "My Chances/*Mes Chances*: A Rendezvous with Some Epicurean Stereophonies" in Joseph H. Smith and William Kerrigan (eds.), *Taking Chances: Derrida, Psychoanalysis and Literature* (Baltimore: Johns Hopkins University Press, 1984), 1–32; *Psyché. Inventions de l'autre* (Paris: Galilée, 1987).

22. For the United States, see J. C. Burnham, *Psychoanalysis and American Medicine, 1894–1918: Medicine, Science and Culture* (New York: International Universities Press, 1967); G. E. Gifford (ed.), *Psychoanalysis, Psychotherapy and the New England Medical Scene, 1894–1944* (New York: Science History Publications, 1978); Nathan G. Hale, *Freud and the Americans* (New York: Oxford University Press, 1971); John Seeley, *The Americanization of the Unconscious* (New York: International Universities Press, 1967).

23. Bernard This and P. Theves, *Die Verneinung. S. Freud (1925–1975). Nouvelle traduction, étude comparée de quelques traductions et commentaires sur la traduction en générale*, *Le Coq-Heron*, lii, Bulletin du group d'étude du Centre Etienne Marcel, Paris, 1975.

24. Elisabeth Roudinesco, *La Bataille de Cent Ans. L'Histoire de la Psychanalyse en France*, Vol. I. *1886–1925* (Paris: Editions Ramsey, 1983, reprinted by Seuil, 1986; Eng. trans. 1990).

25. D. Rapp, "The Reception of Freud by the British Press: General Interest and Literary Magazines, 1920–1925," *Journal of the History of the Behavioral Sciences*, xxiv (1988), 191–201.

26. Krin Gabbard and Glen O. Gabbard, *Psychiatry and the Cinema*, foreword by Irving Schneider (Chicago: University of Chicago Press, 1987).

27. See Bruno Latour, *The Pasteurization of France* (Cambridge: Harvard University Press, 1988).

28. See Ellenberger, *The Discovery of the Unconscious*; Allan Gauld, *The History of Hypnotism* (Cambridge: Cambridge University Press, 1993); Mark Micale, "Hysteria and Its Historiography: A Review of Past and Present Writings, I & II," *History of Science*, xxvii (1989), 223–261, 319–351; Micale, "Hysteria and Its Historiography: The Future Perspective," *History of Psychiatry*, i (1990), 33–124.

29. Carlo Ginzburg, "Clues: Morelli, Freud and Sherlock Holmes: Clues and Scientific

Method'' in Umberto Eco and Thomas A. Sebeok (eds.), *The Sign of Three. Dupin, Holmes, Pierce* (Bloomington: Indiana University Press, 1983), 81–118.

30. Michael Balint, *The Doctor, His Patient and the Illness* (London: Pitman Medical, 1957); see Thomas Osborne, ''Mobilizing Psychoanalysis: Michael Balint and the General Practitioners,'' *Social Studies of Science*, xxiii (1993), 175–200.

31. Freud, ''Interview with Adelbert Albrecht,'' *Boston Transcript*, 11 September 1909, reprinted in Hendrik M. Ruitenbeek (ed.), *Freud as We Knew Him* (Detroit, Michigan: Wayne State University Press, 1973), 22–27, this passage from p. 23.

32. Ernest Gellner, *The Psychoanalytic Movement, or the Cunning of Unreason* (London: Paladin, 1985).

33. Philip Rieff, *Freud: The Mind of the Moralist* (New York: Viking Press, 1959), 300.

34. Alasdair MacIntyre, *After Virtue* (London: Duckworth, 1985), 27 ff.

35. Ibid., 30.

36. Rieff, *Freud: The Mind of the Moralist*, 305.

37. Ibid., 302.

38. Jacques Lacan, ''The Function and Field of Speech and Language'' (1953) in Lacan, *Ecrits* (Paris: Seuil, 1966), 321; *Ecrits: A Selection*, trans. Alan Sheridan (London: Tavistock, 1977), 105.

39. Michel Foucault, *The Order of Things* (1966), (London: Tavistock, 1970), 373.

40. Ibid., 89.

41. John Forrester, ''Michel Foucault and the History of Psychoanalysis'' in Forrester, *The Seductions of Psychoanalysis. Freud, Lacan and Derrida* (Cambridge: Cambridge University Press, 1990), 286–316.

42. Michel Foucault, ''The Subject and Power'' (1983) in Hubert L. Dreyfus and Paul Rabinow, *Michel Foucault. Beyond Structuralism and Hermeneutics*, 2nd ed., with an afterword and an interview with Michel Foucault (Chicago: University of Chicago Press, 1983), 214.

43. Ibid., 215.

44. See Michel Foucault, ''Technologies of the Self'' in Luther H. Martin, Huck Gutman, Patrick H. Hutton (eds.), *Technologies of the Self. A Seminar with Michel Foucault* (London: Tavistock, 1988), 16–49.

45. Richard Rorty, ''Freud and Moral Reflection'' in Rorty, *Essays on Heidegger and Others. Philosophical Papers*, vol. 2, (Cambridge: Cambridge University Press, 1991), 154.

46. Cf. Peter Gay, *The Bourgeois Experience: Victoria to Freud*, 2 vols. (New York: Oxford University Press, 1985–7).

47. Nancy Friday, *Women on Top. How Real Life has Changed Women's Fantasies* (London: Hutchinson, 1991).

48. The recent literary study of psychoanalysis and the literary deployment of psychoanalysis is too extensive to survey here; two important contributions are Shoshana Felman, (ed.), *Yale French Studies Nos. 55/56; Literature and Psychoanalysis. The Question of Reading: Otherwise* (New Haven: Yale University Press, 1977) and Daniel Gunn, *Psychoanalysis and Fiction* (Cambridge, Cambridge University Press, 1990).

10

Philip Rieff: The Critic of Psychoanalysis as Cultural Theorist

KENNETH S. PIVER

To be a prophet is to assert that there is no way out of tradition.

PHILIP RIEFF, *Freud: The Mind of the Moralist, 1959*

The moment a man questions the meaning and value of life he is sick, since objectively neither has any existence.

SIGMUND FREUD, *Letter to Marie Bonaparte*

If they are ill, they can be cured. But if they are not ill, I know not what to do.

Reb. SIMEON B. LAKISH, *Midrash Rabbah: Exodus XLV.3*

Beyond all the particularities of therapeutic techniques and psychological complexes, there lies at the center of the Freudian text, according to Philip Rieff, an answer to a question of such tremendous significance that it has been resisted by some of the greatest minds of this century; not least, Freud himself. As one of the foremost scholars of the cultural significance of Freud and his theory, Rieff in recent years has come to assert the provocative, yet highly problematic, idea that Freud has reduced the "parent" question of humanity, i.e., "Am I Thy master or art Thou mine?" to merely "a question of parents" and thus resisted his own greatest insight.[1] For over thirty years, Philip Rieff has been minding the mind of Sigmund Freud in an attempt to find his way closer to a response to this question at the core of all received notions of culture, character, and conduct. To this end, since the publication of the now classic exegesis *Freud: The Mind of the Moralist* in 1959, Rieff has been probing the tension between instinctual candor and the renunciations essential for civilized culture. From that work hence, it is my theory that Rieff has slowly, and more or less wittingly, evolved from a primarily analytical interpreter of the cultural significance of psychoanalysis into a classically conservative prophet of cultural demise.

Freud's primary concern both as theorist and clinician centered on the tension between "repression" and the expression of human instinctuality, and it is here that Rieff has found clues to both Freud's and his own moral vision.[2] If one reads the Rieffian *oeuvre* with this dialectic in mind and monitors the oscillations in his relationship to Freud, as well as his own ideal type, *psychological man*, insight into the direction and significance of Rieff's entire theory of culture can be gleaned. While Rieff's conversion can be detected most clearly in his relationship with Freud's "analytic attitude," it is also simultaneously reflected through changes in his style and verse. As analytic scholarship becomes "committed," Rieff's style grows increasingly cryptic, aphoristic, and vitriolic. Moreover, his published work, while growing meager in output, gradually becomes more polemical in tone and intent with enigmatically religious overtones. Thus, I intend to illustrate how these stylistic and methodological changes are consistent with the theoretical ones. It appears that the modality for Rieff's conversion was his attempt to articulate a theory of culture.

Philip Rieff's formal academic training began as an undergraduate at the University of Chicago, which he now refers to in his ever increasingly ironic and ever decreasing irenic tone as "that Baptist institution where Jews teach Catholicism to communists."[3] Having left the university before finishing his bachelor's degree to volunteer for the Lincoln Battalion during the Spanish Civil War, upon his return Rieff was placed directly on the faculty of Chicago due to the outstanding nature of his brief work as an undergraduate. From this auspicious beginning, Rieff has gone on to lead a no less impressive academic career. Following interludes at Berkeley, Brandeis, and Harvard, Rieff has been a professor at the University of Pennsylvania for over thirty years where he holds both the title Benjamin Franklin Professor of Sociology and a rare University Professorship. He was a Fulbright professor at Munich from 1959 to 1960, a Guggenheim Fellow in 1970, Visiting Fellow at All Souls College, Oxford, from 1970 to 1979, and a Rockefeller Fellow at Bellagio in 1992. Additionally, Rieff has delivered many distinguished lectures, including the Gauss at Princeton, the Terry at Yale, and the Presidential at Toronto.[4]

It is indisputable that Rieff's first major work, *The Mind of the Moralist*, played a critical role in Freud's acceptance into the American academic canon and has since become required reading for all serious students of Freud.[5] As one of the original theorists to recognize that Freud's vision *in toto* constituted a theory of culture, and therefore had moral and ethical implications, Rieff was also one of the first to attempt the type of exegetical interpretation of Freud that now has become commonplace.[6] Throughout the sixties, which included the appearance of his second book, *The Triumph of the Therapeutic*, Rieff was recognized as a leading authority on Freud often grouped with Herbert Marcuse, Erik Erikson, and Erich Fromm. Subsequently, several important studies of Freud have appeared that posit that their entire project is framed in Rieffian terms.[7] Moreover, such recognized contemporary critics as Christopher Lasch, through his theory of a "narcissistic" culture, and Alasdair MacIntyre, in his celebrated *After Virtue*, cite the importance of Rieff's influence on central issues in their work.[8] In particular, *The Mind of the Moralist* continues to be referenced primarily in terms reserved for works of the highest order, such as "after Rieff's work, there is very little more to be said on this subject."[9] The range of Rieff's influence is further discernible through the fluid manner in which his terms and ideal types, such as the "analytic attitude," "psychological man," or various references to the language and "triumph" of the therapeutic are used in discourse, often without reference to their progenitor. At its most extreme, Rieff engenders a veneration almost unsettling in this disillusioned day and age.

Despite these tangible academic accomplishments and a notable range of influence, Rieff's current renown is incommensurate with his intellectual achievement.[10] While other academics from this era have maintained a level of public exposure equal to or perhaps greater than their contributions, Rieff has fallen into relative anonymity. Indeed, in a recent interview, he describes himself as "an obscure academic."[11] In the fifties and sixties, however, as a well-recognized expert on Freud, Rieff participated openly in the public discourse and wrote for such mainstream intellectual fare as *Commentary, Encounter,* and *Partisan Review,* and the original editions of his books were published by houses regularly involved in commercial trade.[12] Rieff, himself, was an editorial consultant for Schocken, Beacon, and Harper & Row during this time, as well as the founding editor of *Daedalus.* His prose style was signified in the first two decades of his career by a lucid syntax, terms that could be readily understood, and a mood basically indicative of the analytic and critical attitude of our psychological century, a posture he considered "the only attitude available to intellectuals living in a world 'spent of sacred forces.' "[13]

Rieff, like Herbert Marcuse, Erik Erikson, and Norman O. Brown, achieved marked publishing success on the American scene in the sixties, which one reviewer attributed to "his style, the content of his writing, and his sensitivity to the conditions of his readers."[14] Those familiar with Rieff's more recent published work would find such commentary remarkable. Beginning with his third book, *Fellow Teachers,* Rieff enters what I would like to propose is his "prophetic" phase, whereupon his readership paid him the compliment of what Karl Menninger teaches is the fate of all cautionary admonishers and dire predictors in our age: "They hang prophets. Or ignore them which is worse."[15] Rieff has clearly paid a price in popularity for the changes in his work, but there have been theoretical reasons, from his perspective, for risking that fate. Rieff's personal maturation provides a microcosmic view of the struggle and transformation that the entirety of his published work addresses. Never has a more thoroughly self-conscious cultural theorist attempted to expose the perils of the pervasiveness of self-consciousness. With the recent issuing of his collected papers, *The Feeling Intellect,*[16] and the projected release of the summation of his sociology of culture, *Sacred Order/ Social Order* as our background, I will retrace Rieff's scholarly conversion in an endeavor to spark a broad reengagement of this vital, yet problematic, figure.

An Early Encounter with Freud

Around 1959, three seminal books on the cultural and social significance of Freud were published marking a watershed in the academic and public response to Freud and psychoanalysis.[17] Rieff's was among them, bearing the enigmatic title *Freud: The Mind of the Moralist,* along with Herbert Marcuse's *Eros and Civilization* and Norman O. Brown's *Life Against Death.*[18] An infatuation with things Freudian from all sides of the academic spectrum had built to a crescendo by the end of the fifties. On the one hand, many intellectuals were disillusioned with Marxism in the wake of publications by Lionel Trilling and Hannah Arendt, as well as the open disclosure of the enormities of Stalinism.[19] Brown and Marcuse clearly encountered each other on the road from political to cultural radicalism, i.e., from Marx to Freud.[20] Simultaneously, as the shock of the horrors of nazism sank in, numerous intellectuals began defining their understanding of contemporary Western culture in terms of the "crisis" of normative authority in modernity, a potentially irreconcilable break from the past. In the latter group, Rieff at the beginning of his career seems to have encountered *himself* on the road from Nietzsche to Freud.

Early in the text of *The Mind of the Moralist*, the eventual focal point of Rieff's lifelong interest in Freud is foreshadowed: "Without gauging the critical function of repression in the Freudian scheme, we cannot perceive either the hidden weight of Freud's moralizing or his appeal to modern minds, suspicious of all moralizings."[21] From Rieff's perspective, memory for Freud is not a passive response but rather embodies moral choices characterizable as a series of acceptances and rejections; thus, repression becomes an "infallible index of ethical import." Harold Bloom agrees, positing in *Ruin the Sacred Truths* that the concept of repression is the true center of Freud's vast speculative project and, moreover, is profoundly Jewish in its normative implications.[22] With the perspective of repression as a moral indicator, Rieff asserts that the most ambitious theme in the entire Freudian text hinges on the theory that the rise of the neuroses was due to the exhaustion of Judeo-Christian culture.[23] Rieff implies that as a theorist "who knew that his science was as much medicine as philosophy," Freud deals explicitly with the study of human conflict and therefore, despite the proposed neutrality of his theory, could not avoid drawing morals from his diagnoses and influencing attitudes through his interpretations. Freud himself Rieff calls "a statesman of the inner life, aiming at shrewd compromises with the human condition, not at its basic transformation . . . a moralist without even a moralizing message."[24]

Rieff insists that Freud considered instinctual renunciation indispensable to culture. However, Freud thought the failure of traditional religious proscriptions to remain compelling was the primary etiology of the neurotic symptoms his patients and his peers presented. Failing as a system of repressions, traditional religious culture continued to exist only as a problem.[25] Rieff views Freud, being a man of culture and more psychologically Jewish than his doctrine allowed, as capable of admiring the repressions.[26] Yet, Freud sought to lower what he considered to be the now hypocritically high demands of the superego, believing nothing could possibly be gained by a victory purchased through the sacrifice of mental health.[27]

In response to the dynamic before him, Freud proposed through the "analytic attitude" and technique of psychoanalysis a system through which rational inspection aimed at making a peculiar peace between the instincts and their repressions. According to Rieff, Freud teaches us to avoid putting too much faith in either our instinctual desires or man's highest moral ideals opposing them, and thus, is the quintessential realist, envisioning no salvation and waiting for no ultimate cure.[28] The dictum, that all one can hope for from psychoanalysis is the transformation of "hysterical misery" into "common unhappiness," expresses Freud's ultimately prudent goal.[29] Freud's way of mitigating the problem before him was through a rational, technical knowledge of the inner workings of the mind. Self-criticism was to be replaced by analytical self-examinations of motives, contradictions, and defenses. Through limited commitments, partial syntheses, and a detached relationship to communal purposes, the "analytic attitude" aims only to increase man's sense of well-being with the ultimate goal of leaving the inner life undisturbed.[30] There are no ultimate winners, but for Freud this is better than serial losers. He, therefore, in a resigned master-stroke against all traditional visions from the Socratic to the Christian, created an entirely new definition of health.

Rieff wrote his famous final chapter "The Emergence of Psychological Man" as a coda to the main text of *The Mind of the Moralist* to announce an ideal type, which he saw emerging with the advancement of Freudian theory. Rieff presents his ideal type as the fourth in a paradigmatic series that has dominated Western culture.[31] These include political man out of classical, pagan antiquity; pre-Enlightenment, religious man formed from Judaism and received primarily through Christianity; the short-lived economic man of the Enlightenment; and finally psychological man. Under Freud's tutelage, the latest prototype lives by none of the ideals of his predecessors, having abandoned the traditional dichotomizing of human action into categories of "higher" and "lower."[32] Psychological man, through his "analytic attitude," lives by an insight aimed at a technological mastery of the self and a tolerance of ambiguities, "a stable life in an unstable world."[33] Rieff's original contribution to cultural theory was to articulate a now commonplace idea: the extent and significance of Freud's influence upon Western sensibility. Among countless subsequent commentators ranging from George Steiner to Jacques Derrida, there is now a general acceptance that the modalities of individual thought and public discourse in the latter half of the twentieth century could characterize it as the "Age of Freud." This implies at least that the modern self-understanding has become more privatized and individual; hence, when people ponder the meaning of life and, moreover, how they should act, it is likely done from a psychological perspective rather than a religious, political, or communitarian one.[34] By positing psychological man as having learned to "withdraw from the painful tension of assent and dissent," Rieff hints at a metastasizing moral cancer that has left us all terminally ill,[35] making the hospital the archetypal institution of modern Western culture.

At this early stage of his career, Rieff appears ambivalent toward Freud and psychological man. He clearly is a great admirer of Freud and defends him throughout the book against his critics. Rieff repeatedly reminds the reader that Freud thought some degree of instinctual censorship, particularly involving the sexual drives, was necessary for culture. Moreover, it was exactly through a series of renunciations that Freud thought culture was created, and unlike the neo-Freudians, Rieff reads Freud, the moralist, as being cautious with respect to tinkering with the mechanism of repression.[36] Rieff's admiration for these insights does not blind him either to the shortcomings of Freud's theory or its very radical implications. With respect to its particularities, Rieff is critical of what he perceives as the sexist indictment of women as intellectually inferior in Freud's work, appears skeptical of the reality of infantile sexuality and the role of the Oedipus complex, and suggests that Freud's symbolism, for example in dream interpretation, is too generalized to be convincing.[37] More important, Rieff is critical of Freud's consistent expectation of the sinister and dark motivation behind all human action, suggesting that for Freud to uncover an acceptance behind every rejection is to be incredulous of human goodness.

Rieff is most critical of Freud's inability to grasp the ultimately *unrepressiveness* of modern culture. The serial inversions Freudian theory creates startle Rieff: Moral ideas are named as the problem of life, and thus the object of the psychiatrist's examinations, rather than the basis of the solution to the problem.[38] He waxes philosophic: "If every limit can be seen as a limitation of personality, the question with which we may confront every opportunity is: after all, why not?"[39] In Rieff's view, psychoanalysis finds no more reason to be obedient than to rebel, and it is in this sense that

Freudianism carries nihilistic implications. While Rieff understands that Freud did not create psychological man *sui generis*, he appears convinced of the primacy of ideas and presents psychological man as fundamentally a product of the Freudian articulation. He asks: "Imagine an entire society dominated by psycho-therapeutic ideals?"[40]

Rieff's response to his own rhetorical postulate remains, at this stage in his career, primarily analytical, while the tenor of the work in general reflects a certain resigned acceptance of the state of things. He neither defies nor heralds the emergence of psychological man. Rather, *Freud: The Mind of the Moralist* is an announcement, done with great insight and eloquence, but also with a distinct absence of polemic and alarm. In an early review of the book, John Dollard wrote, "the great value of this work is that it represents an appraisal of Freud as a social scientist by a social scientist."[41] Rieff's social scientific approach, at a time when the fledgling social sciences were attempting to gain respectability by approximating the natural sciences, is reflected in his ambivalence toward his ideal type, his admiration of Freud's analytical insight, and his reluctance to offer "therapies."

At this juncture, Rieff appears openly to count himself among the deconverted and admits "having had the American experience of detachment from all communities."[42] In a rare moment of revealing candor in this early work, Rieff divulges that it is "exhilarating and yet terrifying to read Freud as a moralist." He further implicates himself in the modern experience by following with: "To be less vulnerable to the arrows of sickness that fortune inevitably shoots at us, and that we, by virtue of our particular constitution, invite—this is as much good health as any one of us educated by Freud can wish for."[43] The sole hint of a reactionary tendency in Rieff is buried in the chapter "Religion of the Fathers" when he cautiously submits that "religion, with its symbols of remembrance, may be that very submission to the past that will preserve in us some capacity for a radical criticism of the present."[44] However, Rieff, like Freud, foresees at this point no real reconciliation between his character type and society and no ultimate cure for man's dis-ease. While Rieff remains reticent, others in response to the announcement of his ideal type suggested that if the dominant character type is really what Rieff calls psychological man, then "the consequences for western society are quite incalculable."[45]

Toward a Theory of Culture

Openly billing the book as a "calculus of the incalculable," Rieff's next foray into the cultural significance of the analytic attitude, *The Triumph of the Therapeutic: Uses of Faith After Freud*, appeared in 1966.[46] Rieff confesses he felt obliged to amplify his concept of psychological man in response to the aforementioned appraisal, and herein his slow, and as yet subtle, change can be first detected. Beginning the work with the now familiar lines from Yeats and Weber regarding the center's inability to hold and the "sensualists without heart," Rieff acknowledges that, like all moderns, he has become a participant-observer in the transition out of one culture and into another. At this point in his career, Rieff describes his task as the *analysis* of "doctrinal as well as organizational profiles of the rage to be free of the inherited morality, the better to see how these differ from what is being raged against."[47] Moreover, he suggests that sociology, "like psychiatry when it is not lost in a particular patient," is ultimately concerned with ''whether our culture can be so reconstructed that faith—some compelling symbolic of self integrating communal purpose—need no longer superintend the organization of personality.''[48]

In the *Triumph of the Therapeutic*, we catch the first glimpses of what would become the core of Rieff's later theory of culture. In these early observations, Rieff notes ''a culture survives principally by the power of its institutions to bind and loose men . . . with reasons which sink so deep into the self that they become commonly and implicitly understood.''[49] Curiously, he refers to this condition as an order of *therapy*.[50] But Rieff admits there are two meanings of ''therapy'' as he uses it, and the contrast of meanings is the perspective needed to understand the main moral implications of Freud's achievement.[51] In his peculiar and ironic usage, there exist both ''therapies of commitment,'' epitomized by the *Therapeutae* described by Philo,[52] and ''analytic therapies,'' exemplified by the posture of his re-christened psychological man—the *therapeutic*. Cultures based on therapies of commitment are defined through their public symbolics: a system of prohibitions and permissions, in return for some assurance of salvation. The great Western symbolics, particularly the Jewish/Christian and Greek, were constituted by militant and repressive ideas, with limited releases, opposing the infinite range of enactable human behaviors.[53] These proscriptions (e.g., ''thou shalt nots''), enunciated by the sacral elites, are intended to be *therapeutic* by enabling the satisfactory functioning of the community and deterring the psychological decompensation of its members.[54] In sum, previous character types in Rieff's vision are described as being personified by a moral artistry of trained deprivations from the multitude of desires Freud called instincts.

Therapies of commitment, in Rieff's thinking, are what all cultures before modernity were based on, being both authoritarian and symbolic, while analytic therapies are inherently anti-authoritarian and suffer from symbolic impoverishment.[55] Freud believed that traditional therapies of commitment—call them faiths—were no longer compelling and therefore could not enter deeply enough into individual psyches to be effective. According to Rieff, Freud's is the greatest theory of deconversion, and psychoanalysis became the symbolic mode for a particular type of ''negative community.'' In the age of analytic psychologizing, self-awareness supersedes devotion to any commanded ideal model of right and wrong. With the perspective of the analytic attitude, the main character type of the negative community, the therapeutic, in opposition to earlier ascetic paragons, must keep all options open because the criterion for judgment has shifted merely to the degree of psychological effectiveness. Jeffrey Abramson summarizes the concept well: ''Such a virtuoso is at once radically knowledgeable about the origin of his or her own desires, unburdened of moral constraints that cannot survive negotiations with reason, and situated in a world no longer by reference to gods or traditions, but solely in terms of what science can reveal about who one is.''[56]

Based primarily on Freudian postulates, analytic therapies redefine the nature of individual character and therefore public culture. Whereas older committed modes of therapy are generative, each person born not once but twice, analytic therapies are simply informative. In fact, Rieff implies that the latter may be so profoundly informative they preclude all forms of commitment.[57] As successors to the clerics and founding members of the emerging negative communities, psychiatrists and intellectuals know that membership requires few dues.[58] As Allan Megill accurately expresses in his study *Prophets of Extremity*, ''a therapeutic thinker, by definition, seeks to attack received ideas, to demolish previous platitudes.''[59] Rieff opines: ''Despite a massive effort by professional psychoanalysts to remain clinical therapists rather than culture critics, there is nothing in psychoanalysis that makes them any less so.''[60] Thus, modern therapeutic culture appears to be based merely on the exigencies of individual desires recreated into needs, and it is in this sense that Freud's psychology begins, according to Rieff, to matter culturally.

While an ironic tone punctuates the treatise, Rieff's approach in the *The Triumph of the Therapeutic* remains primarily analytic and ''scientific,'' as we can see in his comment that ''however one may judge the validity of the multiple truths at which science and history arrive, my interest is in their social viability.''[61] Though he suggests that ''viewed traditionally the continuing shift from a controlling to a releasing symbolic may appear as the dissolution of culture,'' his opinion on this point remains provisional. Furthermore, Rieff's own complicity is suggested in the following passage:

> I, too, aspire to see clearly, like a rifleman, with one eye shut; I, too, aspire, to think without assent. This is the ultimate violence to which the modern intellectual is committed. Since things have become as they are, I, too, share in the modern desire not to be deceived.[62]

Rieff's ambivalence is further exemplified in his ironic assertion that ''to call corrupt a culture purchased at a lower cost to our nerves, and at larger magnitudes of self-fulfillment, would show a lamentable lack of imagination''[63] and in his admission that *The Triumph of the Therapeutic* was not meant as a defense of the culture that was dying. Moreover, Rieff responds to the allegation that his cultural diagnoses could appear quasi-apocalyptic by questioning: ''But what apocalypse has ever been so kindly? What culture ever attempted to see to it that no ego is hurt?''[64]

One commentator on the *The Triumph of the Therapeutic* observes that ''just who the therapeutic is and how he came to be is more than difficult to understand. That we are left with confusion is in part a function of Rieff's heavy use of irony and his insistence on using words in such an idiosyncratic manner.''[65] Thus, numerous critics by the early 1970s had made the grave misprision that Rieff was unequivocally a proponent of psychological man and his therapeutic ethic.[66] However—and this will prove enigmatic as we chart Rieff's evolution—Rieff does put stock in the analytic attitude's ability to protect us from corporate fanaticism. In fact, he fears the converse: ''To raise up faith from its stony sleep encourages the possibility of living again through the nightmare history of the last half century.''[67] Rieff's ability at times to be cautiously optimistic about the analytic attitude may reflect the unprecedented abundance that characterized America from the end of World War II through the midsixties. Although he is able to see where Freud's disciples have erred, when Rieff does appear sanguine about psychological man it is from a distinctly Freudian perspective.[68] He maintains emphatically that those who call for the release of the repressions do not understand that the Freudian doctrine was never to be put into systematic service either to control or release, under pain of ceasing to be analytic.

Despite Rieff's open disavowal of this position, *The Triumph of the Therapeutic* has also been read as a defense of traditional culture, a type of antidote to Norman O. Brown's sensualist *Life Against Death*.[69] This may be closer to the truth, but Rieff's main fault in this work is that he does not make clear exactly how the therapeutic differs from psychological man. The darkening of his irony portends a growing fear of the decomposition of his ideal type into a corrupt hedonist and the analytic attitude into the "ecstatic attitude." This may be what he implies by the "triumph of the therapeutic."[70] Rieff's potentially negative assessment of the self-forgiving ethos of modernity appears to lie in the way that idioms of analytic therapy have made their way into such inappropriate spheres as education and religion.[71] It becomes clear that Rieff is growing increasingly dissatisfied with the potential merits of his ideal type and the prospect of a society resembling more and more the type of hospital-culture that Goethe was the first to fear.[72] In *Humboldt's Gift*, Saul Bellow's protagonist, Charlie Citrine, gives an impromptu reading of *The Triumph of the Therapeutic* that addresses this theme:

> It says that psychotherapists may become the new spiritual leaders of mankind. A disaster. . . . According to this author, when culture fails to deal with the feelings of emptiness and the panic to which man is disposed (and he does say disposed) other agents come forward to put us together with therapy, with glue, or slogans, or spit, . . . poor wretches are recycled on the couch.[73]

Despite enough available evidence to make a case for either argument, it is my opinion that at this stage in his career Rieff has tried to adopt an unsentimental attitude toward both the old and the new: an analytic, social-scientific approach. While lamentations are apparent in the tone of the work, Rieff still appears to be proposing no counterreformation. In the years since the publication of *The Mind of the Moralist*, his style has grown increasingly poetic, and at times aphoristic, but on the whole I agree with Frank Kermode's characterization of *The Triumph of the Therapeutic* as "perfectly lucid."[74] One reader, commenting on his initial exposure to Rieff through *The Triumph of the Therapeutic*, wryly remarked that it was "a fascinating work which merited translation into English."[75] Although this comment is overdetermined for that particular text, the quip is particularly well suited for all of Rieff's subsequent writing.

A Grand Inquisitor

Public response to *The Triumph of the Therapeutic* included numerous suggestions that the work was "prophetic," while an article in *The American Scholar* further claimed that Western culture was in a "state of unconditional surrender" to Rieff's ideal type.[76] In Rieff's next significant publication, *Fellow Teachers*, his partiality toward the old, despair regarding the new, and dire predictions for the future become patently obvious. The original version of this extended essay appeared in the 1972 summer-fall edition of *Salmagundi* entitled "Psychological Man: Approaches to an Emergent Social Type."[77] Herein, Rieff parodies an actual interview with Boyers and Orill, the journal's editors:

> It is possible that my invitation to come to Skidmore on 26th March, 1971, to be publicly interviewed, was based on a happy misunderstanding? Did you imagine that I am a herald of the therapeutic? I am neither for nor against my ideal type. Nor am I Freudian or anti-Freudian, Marxist or anti-Marxist, Weberian or anti-Weberian, I am a scholar teacher of sociological theory; as such, I try to help myself and my students to see not only what the theorist has seen, but through him to see what is at stake in his vision.[78]

Upon reading the text of any edition of *Fellow Teachers*, which was expanded to book form in 1973 and reissued with the subtitle "Of Culture and Its Second Death" in 1985, it becomes clear that Rieff's claim of analytic neutrality is disingenuous. Both a marked increase in acerbity and abstruseness signify the work. Boyers and Orill believe Rieff's misgivings about their interpretation of his writings are without foundation; however, they express something quite extraordinary: "it is our conviction that Rieff's writing, presently studied in detail by only a few, eventually will find acceptance as the single most penetrating effort of cultural analysis produced by an American in recent times."[79]

Fellow Teachers, ostensibly a commentary on the state of crisis in American universities, is a pretext for Rieff's indictment of modern culture and his elegy for the culture that is passing.[80] Rieff's decrial of modernity, now referred to as an "anticulture," is detailed through his juxtaposition of the dominant motifs of the dying culture and the emergent, and his anger is focused on the intellectual elite who he feels have abandoned their duties. In this sense, Rieff's *Fellow Teachers* is reminiscent of two earlier interwar cultural treatises: Julien Benda's reactionary text *La Trahison des Clercs* (*The Great Betrayal*) and Johan Huizinga's *In the Shadow of Tomorrow*.[81] Also, *Fellow Teachers* has been compared frequently to Alan Bloom's best-selling rehash of Chicago Great Books theory, *The Closing of the American Mind*.[82] However, *Fellow Teachers*, despite having made many of the same points but with greater poignancy and deeper implication fifteen years earlier, has received scant recognition.[83] Yet, the obscurity of the book has plausible explanations involving its vociferous tenor and impenetrable style.

In *Fellow Teacher*, Rieff introduces his definition of what constitutes a *true* culture using these terms: *interdicts, transgressions*, and *remissions*. Rieff by now believes that the greatest indication of the truth of a concept is in its limiting potential. He argues that there can be no culture without an authority that prescribes right and proper demands (interdicts) and refers to these as those eternally given "Nots." In credal organizations, earlier referred to as therapies of commitment and now openly defended by Rieff, interdicts carried the weight of the possibility of transgression, more commonly remembered as "sin." To allow the paradigm to remain both viable and humane, there is also the inner modality of "remission," when what is not to be done is done, yet forgiven, due to justifiable circumstances. Because therapy has become the "greatest conceptual term . . . for the justification of all immediacies,"[84] remission has grown so pervasive in modernity that it has come to connote, for Rieff, a condition that is permissive and anarchic.[85] In the age of the therapeutic no god of commandments can survive, and thus, in their "moral modesty," therapeutics will know that everything is possible because they are inhibited by no compelling reason. Put most crisply by Rieff: "The moral life begins with renunciation; the therapeutic life begins with the renunciation of renunciation."[86]

Although Rieff suggests psychiatrists and psychotherapists would be heralders of the movement toward release, it is more the general transformation that concerns him. He sees both the therapeutic attitude and the hypercritical, scientific style, most notably in the academy, as pushing culture toward the first true instance of barbarism:

> The line that divides culture from barbarism in this century . . . is between the teaching of our inherited interdicts, so deep that men are not free to become neurotic,

and the preaching of endless remissions so that men are free to become what they are not. That freedom is deadly.[87]

Freud's continuing influence on Rieff is apparent through the emphasis Rieff puts on the depth of the interdicts, evoking the dictum that "if we are aware of our repressions, we are no longer repressed."[88] By the time he wrote *Fellow Teachers*, Rieff seems to have become entirely incredulous of human goodness, something the younger Rieff found to be a fault in Freud. Rieff submits that a first step toward preventing the barbarians from storming the gates would be for his fellow teachers to recognize that "our barbaric enlightenments have deinhibited the agency of inhibition: the super-ego."[89] Yet he continues to insist that Freud indulged no mystique of change. Freud is characterized as "our last grand theorist, gifted with a capacity to defend high culture in its failures, against infinite openings of possibility,"[90] and Rieff submits further that, except perhaps in the case of Dora, Freud believed that what was moral was self-evident. Conversely, and thus confusingly, he also posits that Freud is the ultimate murderer of Moses,[91] the greatest human theorist of the interdictory.

Whereas in *The Triumph of the Therapeutic*, Rieff explores the dynamic between therapies that control and those that release, it is evident in *Fellow Teachers* that he has taken sides with the culture that seeks to preserve controlling symbolics: "To teach is to conserve the related benefits and penalties of our inherited existence. . . . How dare we dismiss the authority of the past as if we understood it? From the past we gain our regulating weight, to hold against the lightness of our acts."[92] Although the text of *Fellow Teachers* provides a convincing case for Rieff's evolving despair, he also illustrates one of the "penalties of our inherited existence" in the following passage:

> For the safety of our own souls, to prevent the mental disease of praxis, we teachers of various theories have to imagine truths still to be stable old men, never fickle young women ever itchy to bed down with the latest winners in the perpetual intellectual-political style show.[93]

Rieff's patently sexist comment, an unequivocal response to Nietzsche's opening words of *Beyond Good and Evil*, "supposing truth is a woman—what then?," reminds the reader that the "authority of the past" also carries some very distasteful motifs belying his otherwise compelling arguments. This and other similar passages in *Fellow Teachers* provide stark contrast to the author of *The Mind of the Moralist* who was critical of Freud's sexism and illustrates the problematic nature of the conversion under discussion. However, later in the work, Rieff states that "I have not the slightest affection for the dead church civilization of the West. I am a Jew. No Jew in his right mind can long for some variant of that civilization,"[94] implying that he is interested in a peculiar form of meta-history. As Berel Lang explains, it is "a premise of conservative episte-mology that we do not have to know all the facts in order to know some of them."[95] Moreover, he posits that Rieff has become "too stern a witness even as elegist to speak only good of the dead."[96]

Rieff's stylistic changes in *Fellow Teachers* appear to be deliberately exacerbated:

> We teachers are called to represent the god-terms, in all their marvellous indirec-tions, inhibiting what otherwise might be too easily done. Even Christ as he revealed, precisely in order to reveal, concealed. . . . Concealment is the most nec-

essary pedagogic art, without which there are no revelations. If I have written anything worth rereading, then it is necessary and right that you should misunderstand
me.[97]

As both the style and the title of *Fellow Teachers* imply, Rieff has decided to address
a highly particularized, academic audience. The cryptic mode, as well as the fact that
the work was mainly completed in a self-imposed exile at All Souls College, Oxford,
is symbolic of his retreat from the public discourse. Moreover, Rieff opts to bury his
most revealing remarks in the recesses of the many detailed footnotes in *Fellow Teachers*, aware that they will be overlooked by all but the most careful readers. These facts,
along with his choice of Christ as his analogy, signal a movement away from an analytic
to a more committed mode of scholarship. The opaque quality of the treatise also
conveys Rieff's desire for his work to have enduring influence in an increasingly dis-
posable knowledge industry. Frank Kermode may also be right in claiming that Rieff's
style has "a smack of Carlyle, an extravagance to match the extremity of the opinions
it conveys" and attributes Rieff's grandiloquence to the obvious anger of "a prophet
who knows his fellow teachers will not listen to him."[98]

Many commentators have proposed that *Fellow Teachers* was written in reaction
to the cultural turmoil of the late 1960s.[99] Indeed, Rieff makes clear in a theoretical
point about the increasing remissive/permissive quality of our culture that "behind the
hippies are the thugs."[100] Within the university, the late sixties and early seventies were
a determining period. It was not the students alone, but the teachers, including numerous
scholars of Freud, who successfully attacked the canonical wisdom that had informed
the character of Western universities since their inception in medieval Europe. By being
taught criticism and critical methods before any loyalty to that which is criticized,
students, Rieff believes, are being "transgressively" educated.[101] In a book not known
for its brevity, Rieff puts succinctly the consequences: "Authority untaught is the condition in which a culture commits suicide."[102] The profusion of visible, voluble anti-
authoritarian behavior in the late sixties obviously affected Rieff deeply, although any
attempt to historicize him is dangerous owing to his Olympian viewpoint. Rather, I
believe a profoundly interior conversion has been at work and that *Fellow Teachers* is
a snapshot of the transition. While his new attitude is unmistakable, Rieff clings neu-
rotically to modernity by his assertions that he is taking no side, and through comments
like this:

> . . . I prefer a more humane, less dynamic world, deeply graven interdicts etched in
> superior and trustworthy characters. Do not count on me; I am not one of those
> characters . . . I am at one, with all you heterodoxologists. For me, too, orthodoxies
> of all sorts smell of the narrowness that they permit in their characters.[103]

I am not sure we should take Rieff at his word here. I am inclined to believe Norman
O. Brown may be right to accuse the Rieff of *Fellow Teachers* of being akin to Dostoevsky's Grand Inquisitor. Brown, described by Rieff as a "rhapsody of transgressions," agrees that *Fellow Teachers* marks the beginning of a transsubstantiation, in
the Augustinian/Jamesian sense: "I have a feeling that second birth is precisely what
is happening to Philip Rieff. . . . This piece of writing feels as if it were an explosive
birth of a nova, a new star which sheds light all over the place. What will come of
it?"[104]

A Period of Transition

It has been twenty years since Rieff published his last major work, *Fellow Teachers*. During this long period, the unobtrusive reissuing of his three books by the University of Chicago Press has provided Rieff a forum for some of his most significant statements—particularly a difficult, yet revealing, epilogue added to *Freud: The Mind of the Moralist* in 1979, entitled "One Step Further," and new prefaces to *The Triumph of the Therapeutic* and *Fellow Teachers*. However, these inconspicuous arenas have left these statements in large measure unread and virtually unreviewed. This relative dearth of publishing may be related to the fact that Rieff considers himself to be a "rewriter." Moreover, Rieff appears to have come to the decision that there are certain benefits to keeping his opinions to himself, and also hints that his retreat is a continuing reaction to the hypertrophy of second-rate publications: "Why publish? With so many authors, who remains behind to read?"[105]

While Rieff denies his defense of the dying culture in *Fellow Teachers*, he takes up the question unequivocally for the first time in "One Step Further." Juxtaposed to the more patient tone of the famous text to which it is appended, it becomes immediately clear, as one critic who agrees with my thesis states, there was once "a younger Philip Rieff more at peace with the ascendency of psychological man."[106] Psychological man is now described as one "whose passion in life is lowering what is high and raising what is low" and whose conceit is "to think that life is no longer a question of making right responses to inescapable answers already given."[107] However, the first appearance of an entirely unconditional attitude on Rieff's part is obfuscated by a deliberately impenetrable style. Moreover, while "One Step Further" comprises a supersessive reading to the entire original work, Rieff claims that his purpose in this epilogue is the same as when he first "stopped rewriting the book in 1958: to see what might be seen through Freud's vision faceted toward the right conduct of our lives."[108] Although he used a similar phrase in the first preface, the content, style, and tenor of "One Step Further" belie his assertion, and Rieff obscures the fact that his criteria for "right conduct" have changed considerably over twenty years. It is possible that Rieff was originally hiding his moralizing purpose, but my guess is that a deep inner conversion is occurring. Rieff's other explicit purpose for adding this epilogue supports this theory: to show that " 'repression' cannot be abolished; and why not."[109]

In "One Step Further" Rieff returns to a theme first intimated in *Fellow Teachers*: the open equation of repression with revelatory *truth*. According to Rieff, repressions cannot occur except in responsive *defense* of the interdicts from which they derive:

> If we are not obedient to the interdicts, then we are not cultured. It is from the interdicts that repressions gather their energy. Only then can repressions subserve interdicts. Interdicts are the primary forms of high culture, not the arts and sciences.[110]

The familiar term *values* represents for Rieff "the modern code for the educated belief that the central repressions . . . cannot hold us close enough to what they really are—the unavoidable refinements of a commanded life."[111] In opposition to the psychological men and women engulfing Rieff, he believes a culture without repressions would be suicidal, closing the "sacred" space between every desire and its object. He reminds us that Freud was far more cautious than his successors, having realized that to grow "healthier" is not necessarily *to be* better. Yet, by translating true guilt into "the pure sense of guilt without any content,"[112] Rieff believes Freud formulated not only the most meaningless concept in the entire Freudian canon but illustrated his resistance to the source behind those "unavoidable refinements of a commanded life." Rieff seeks in this enigmatic epilogue to show a series of details in Freud's theory that illustrate how Freud allowed references to this source, i.e., a god-term, even into his own theory of unbelief.

To this end, Rieff postulates a god-term of his own, *the repressive imperative*: "that authority, external to all negational recognitions of it, which splits good and evil."[113] In a revealing passage from Freud's *The Ego and the Id*[114] Rieff sees recognition of this unalterable authority in Freud's concept of "the third unconscious." Here is Rieff's oblique interpretation of Freud's classic text:

> By such a maneuver and others more mythic—all styles of cognitive avoidances, of negational recognitions of what is called by Freud, above, the "third *Ucs*."— the repressive imperative being minded, becomes visible in the darkest moments of depth psychology. Carried backward and forward upon his momentarily perceived paradox, of the unrepressed repressive, Freud wheeled helplessly, a virtuoso rider more commanded than commanding. Being conscious or not: the ground of Freud's truth split beneath him. In fear, Freud retreated immediately from the third unconscious, his commanding truth. He withdrew into his inveterate talent for repressing the repressive, lest this characteristic of being take over the life of his work.[115]

In the passage under discussion, Freud suggests that a third unconscious is perhaps necessary to postulate because, he believes, there might be a repressive aspect of the unconscious, a part of the ego, that does not coincide with the repressed and does not, like the preconscious, become conscious upon being activated. To explain Freud's idea, Rieff in "One Step Further" lays out an obscure map of the mind: The first unconscious coincides with the id, which is "beyond good and evil," while the second unconscious corresponds to primal repression. Rieff interprets the third unconscious as the moral sensibility engraved in our mind that "does not need an issue of some right disgraced to be activated"[116] and thus is that heretofore unnamed source that makes primal repression operate before any idea can occur unacceptable enough to repress. Rieff's quasi-psychoanalytic interpretation of the great analyst as analysand is that Freud's obscure enunciation of such an obvious god-term is his greatest negation.

Rieff repeatedly asserts that Freud refused to see the truth before him: that repressions were in service to revelation, the interdicts. Along with the third unconscious, Rieff enumerates other examples of Freud's resistance to his own ultimate insight including the unanswered wondering Freud does about why the superego "often displays a severity [for] which no model has been provided by the real parents"[117] and about why it seems perfectly human to feel always in the wrong. Being able to offer only mythic portrayals of the "primal" crime, Rieff suggests that Freud made over into a negational faith, an *idée fixe*, that the revelatory truth asserted by Judeo-Christian culture was finally on its way to being completely abolished. But Rieff argues that this is an "illusory hope" and that Freud's therapy must be interminable "because of the interminability of that which it addresses." He avers, "the repressive imperative cannot be repressed. Mind can only fall asleep to It."[118] With these pious proclamations, Rieff participates in a language of faith, once called a "therapy of commitment," and can no longer be considered a virtuoso interpreter neutrally analyzing both old and new. Rather, by his own rules voiced in the 1959 edition of *The Mind of the Moralist* (the opening epigraph of this essay), Rieff appears to have evolved into an idiosyncratic prophet, because the thesis of "One Step Further" is that no matter how hard psychological man tries "there is no way out of tradition," i.e., repression, as a negational recognition of revelatory truth, cannot be abolished. Although Rieff would still protest the designation of prophet even today, with "One Step Further" he has at least met the criterion previously set by himself.

In his 1987 article "For the Last Time Psychology: Thoughts on the Therapeutic Twenty Years After," Rieff's attitude toward his ideal type has become decidedly hostile.[119] He admits in this screed that to add these afterthoughts directly to *The Triumph of the Therapeutic* would be too easily contrasted with the original text. Moreover, Rieff is more concerned than ever about the therapeutic's role in transforming the social order. By this stage in his career, Rieff believes the therapy of all therapies is ultimately violence, while sacred fear is the only cure for a neurotic and therapeutic health which appears a horror in all of its transgressive possibilities. Rieff wonders when rape will be divorced from its origin in sin and find its way into *DSM-III* under the registration "paraphilic coercive disorder."[120] He is particularly critical of liberation movements, especially for sexual freedoms, and his attitude is quite pitiless:

> In his hospital theaters, some of them made over from churches and synagogues, and in such television dens he calls home, most of all during the last twenty years in political movements of "liberation" from everything sacred, from anything absolutely prohibited, the therapeutic in his infinite role-faiths knows he has become the most pious fraud on earth; a pious fraud who celebrates his fraudulences.[121]

> Faith entails doxologies. Therapy entails opportunities of sensual satisfaction, each are like serial monogamies, which are like adulteries—which are not to be done, no more than murders or abortions or homosexualities.[122]

What we have here is truly unique. These are prophetic ejaculations whose message is no different from those in the Prophets section of the Hebrew Torah, the Epistles of Paul, or the Surahs of the Koran, yet they are delivered in the hybrid language of a modern sociologist with more than healthy doses of both irony and sarcasm. The accusations of hypocrisy, the reiteration of the interdicts, the condemnation of the infidels, are motifs from another world. Thus, Rieff, over the course of his career, appears to have written himself out of one world and into another. Many have rightly and consistently accredited Rieff since the beginning of his career with uncanny prognosticatory ability, but he appears most prophetic in his later work through his conservative defense of the interdictory order he considers sacred. Great prophets such as Isaiah, Jesus, and Mohammed have always been profoundly concerned with the fulfillment of the Law and vehemently opposed to its abrogation, and they warned that the consequences of transgression were severe. Although I am not comparing Rieff in stature, I am suggesting a common purpose.

While Rieff's language of faith and defense of traditional culture have become undeniable during this period of transition, as late as 1987 he still felt the need to maintain that he has not taken sides in the struggle,

I have aimed to take no sides in the permanent culture class wars between insider-winners, who believe in nothing sacred, and outsider-losers who abide in an order that is nothing if it is not sacred. More precisely, I have aimed to take both sides, and ask no vexing questions in the old ladder languages of the faith that was and is the question in these wars.[123]

Despite Rieff's unequivocal attitude expressed in "One Step Further" and "For the Last Time Psychology," his two most significant statements during the eighties, he appears to fear that the intellectual climate cannot tolerate his unequivocal language of faith. Hence, Rieff feels compelled either disingenuously to deny his intentions or to obscure them through an opaque and crypto-Freudian presentation. Rieff must believe that if he were to engage his readers entirely directly, he would be laughed out of court. As Jerry Muller rightly asserts, Rieff's ultimate goal is to convince them they would be "laughing in the dark."[124]

Toward a Rieffian Psychiatry

Rieff's latest publication, "The Newer Noises of War in the Second Culture Camp: Notes on Professor Burt's Legal Fictions," appeared in the Summer 1991 edition of the *Yale Journal of Law and the Humanities*. It may be read as an adumbration of the first part of a forthcoming trilogy constituting the summation of his sociology, *Sacred Order/Social Order*.[125] The leitmotif of this article, and the proposed three-volume series of which it is a fragment, is that Rieff finally admits his position. There is no more equivocation here and no feigned indifference. Rieff has decidedly chosen sides in the "culture-class wars" that he has renamed *Kulturkampf*. He now opts openly to defend a culture with interdictory heights and transgressive depths, with true guilt rather than "the pure sense of guilt without any content" and with a social order that reflects its derivation from a sacred order. In opposition, Rieff sees the therapeutic as attempting to create something unprecedented, a social order entirely divorced from the sacred.

   In *Sacred Order/Social Order*, Rieff will elaborate a Viconian theory of culture based on the assumption that moderns live more or less synchronically in three cultures at once, numbered first, second, and third. Rieff's historical perspective is based on the theory that to understand the synchronic place where we are we must have a chronological sense of where we have been.[126] The first culture refers to those all but dead paganisms, ranging from aboriginal Australia to philosophical Athens, yet always centered around mythic, primordial taboos and inhabited by a pantheon of gods. The second culture is constituted by the faiths out of Jerusalem (e.g., Judaism, Christianity, and Islam) that display the aforementioned interdictory-remissive-transgressive paradigms deriving from the "Authority above all authorities." The third culture, which is predominant in both modernity and moderns, was announced most concisely by Nietzsche's three short words in section 125 of *The Gay Science*: "God is dead."[127]

   Put more simply, the three cultures are pagan, monotheistic, and modern. Rieff also refers to these cultures as first world, second world, and third world (deliberately misleading puns) because he believes the historical task of culture, until the third, has been to translate invisible sacred orders into habitable social orders.[128] He submits that the leitmotifs of the three cultures (first, second, third) are fate, faith, and fiction. The direction that the dominating third culture is taking us in Rieff's view is ever deeper into the abyss of transgressions of which Auschwitz is considered prototypal, and he now views the Holocaust as the seminal moment of the third culture/world. Later abysses on the horizon may appear more pleasant in their subtleties but will be no less horrible in their essence. A younger, less troubled Philip Rieff once considered the analytic attitude of psychological man as a potential safeguard to the "nightmare history" of the first half of the twentieth century. The once-upon-a-time social scientist interested in neutral hermeneutics and *analysis* of changes in the psychohistorical process now sees the analytic attitude as anathema in all shapes and forms from therapy to criticism.

Rieff reveals in the Yale essay that the *Kulturkampf* takes place within each person, as well as without, and refers to this condition as the *psychomachia*. It is of course Rieff's interior war that I have really been charting in these pages. He seems finally to have negotiated a peace within and, moreover, to have decided to risk being unequivocal about this fact:

> That I call the third culture an anti-culture suggests, of course, my adamantine membership in the second culture; or what one of the more creative and liberated members of the third culture may diagnose as a case of faith-fixation that needs therapy. So to dissolve into a playful adieu that enchanting sense of membership in an order at once sacred and social . . . and [which] affirms the truth of human identity as established first in *Genesis* 1:26–27.[129]

This is the most unqualified assertion of Rieff's personal faith I have found in his writings, and its ultimate intention is indisputable. Throughout his most recent works there are numerous references to the oneness of the divinity and the truth of the interdicts. While scriptural prooftexts abound in Rieff's latest writings, it is important to note that these are gleaned from both testaments of the Bible. Hence, he appears to be practicing a uniquely Rieffian brand of syncretism. Born a Jew, Rieff avers "When I read Hopkins, as when I hear a Bach Mass, I am an honorary Christian."[130] He explains that traditional theologies are but one form of address to sacred order and not necessarily the most illuminating, due to problems with bad faith.[131] In a recent interview, he further illustrates the point: "Lincoln was as profoundly faithful to sacred order as any non-churchgoer can go. . . . I run him a close second in that category."[132]

Rieff's present vision can only be understood as a variant reading of the Judeo-Christian tradition, a language of faith in Abraham's God, and thus amounts to no less than a "sacred sociology." According to Rieff, sacred, or second world, sociology began with the authors of the Pentateuch and the author of *The Republic*.[133] Being a minority tradition in that discipline, it would be "no 'New Christianity,' " such as Comte and Saint-Simon put forth and would include an eclectic range of theorists in its canon. Rieff explains further that "All second world traditions have embarrassingly candid loyalists, such as de Maistre, and brilliantly lyric traitors, such as Nietzsche."[134] Most importantly, Rieff admits that his sacred sociology implies a willingness to take up sides to fight for the traditions of the second world: "To read our worlds at war is to participate unavoidably in the fighting . . . There is no neutral ground to be found in this or any other world."[135]

In these latest works, Rieff's style remains profoundly epigrammatical; he has even taken to writing in numbered paragraphs with italicized, aphoristic titles. He also capitalizes such god-terms as Highest Authority, a symbolic trend first detectable in "One Step Further." These stylistic symptoms are directly related to the conversion that Rieff seems finally ready to admit. They also imply the ascendance of Nietzsche's influence upon Rieff's thought and the decreased influence of Freud. Whereas the style of the *The Mind of the Moralist* in part mirrored the lucid, analytic style of Freud, Rieff's work now has come to resemble most conspicuously that of Nietzsche. Although Rieff seems to have caught up with himself since *Fellow Teachers*, his peripatetic rhythm reflects the urgent, yet melancholic style of Nietzsche, a fragmentation that could be characterized as *bricolage*. For pedagogic and opposed purposes, Rieff ironically mirrors the discordant, schizoid nature of modernity.

Two of Rieff's most formidable opponents in the *Kulturkampf* are the poststructuralists Jacques Derrida and Michel Foucault, the latter having had a profound, yet troubling, effect on the historiography of psychiatry. Rieff rarely attacks these theorists directly, preferring to "draw hermeneutic circles" around them through exegeses of texts regarded as central to the modern canon.[136] Throughout his career, Rieff has been as comfortable interpreting Joyce, Stevens, and Duchamp, as the Torah, Augustine, and Paul. In a passage entitled *Derrida as Illustrator* in "The Newer Noises of War in the Second Culture Camp," Rieff describes Derrida as a not particularly "lyrically persuasive" third world leader who flouts the policing character of all second culture elites. He quotes from *The Truth in Painting* wherein Derrida ironically states that "everything comes down to one of those reading exercises with magnifying glass which calmly claim to lay down the law, in police fashion indeed."[137] In response to Derrida's taunt, Rieff reveals the ultimate intentions of his positive hermeneutical style based on close readings: "We professionals of the reading discipline: we are the real police. As teaching agents of sacred order, and inescapably within it, the moral demands we must teach, if we are teachers, are those eternal truths by which all social orders endure."[138]

Rieff is still able to understand the intentions of both sides of the *Kulturkampf*, but he is no longer willing even to pretend to take both sides and ask no vexing questions in the old style. Rieff openly admits that he considers Michel Foucault his "opposite number in these theoretical matters."[139] Megill, in describing his own view, characterizes Rieff's as well:

> For if one adopts, in a cavalier and single-minded fashion, the view that everything is discourse or text or fiction, the *realia* are trivialized. Real people who really died in the gas chambers at Auschwitz or Treblinka become so much discourse. . . . we ought to read Foucault, and the prophets of extremity in general, not literally but ironically. We ought to take them not as our guides but as our opponents.[140]

Conversely, Foucault made his opposition to Rieff clear in a debate by proxy during an interview in 1983. Responding to Rieff's idea that repression is truth, Foucault retorts that "the important question here, it seems to me, is . . . whether the system of constraints in which a society functions leaves individuals the liberty to transform the system" and "as to credal assumptions, I don't think that Rieff and I would agree on their value or on their meaning or on the devices by which they are taught."[141] Rieff must take on the poststructuralists because their "hermeneutics of suspicion" by definition aims to clear away the proscriptions behind all credal assumptions. For Rieff, this would mean the dissolution of culture, not only a viable one now, but the true one. Where Rieff would have interdicts only apparently alterable over time, Foucault would agree to have rules; but only if those rules were never raised above rules to the level of sacred interdicts. "But," Rieff teaches, "restrictions without either interdictory or taboo predicates do not long exist."

In his latest work, Rieff wonders openly: "Who in the third world can imagine a universal, unchangeable rule?"[142] In rhetorical response to his own query, Rieff suggests: "Even Freud thought there were certain permanent rules—the incest taboo, for example—which were universal." Although Rieff would like somehow to reclaim a part of Freud for his side in the *Kulturkampf*, he sadly identifies Freud as the "greatest theorist of our therapeutic transition from second worlds to third." Throughout his career, Rieff has identified the theory of repression as the *crucial problem* of the man he first called moralist. He continues on the theme originally voiced in "One Step Further" by asserting in his latest, and as yet unpublished work, the following daring conclusion:

> I have speculated that had he dare look, Freud would have discovered revelation beneath its transparent disguise, the second unconscious, in the third. Mere speculation of course. Petty Pascal that I am, I would wager on this sure thing: not repression but revelation; not the immense disorder of truths; not this culture consuming itself at the historic end of its theological tether. Had he dared look down far enough, Freud would have discovered that he had the world upside down. But then Freud would have ceased to be an "infidel Jew" and made his way toward the sacred order of Israel.[143]

Rieff believes that within the concept of the repressive repressed we may find the skeleton key that could unlock the meaning of third culture authority, call it modern or therapeutic. Freud's role in our psycho-"therapeutic" century has been crucial, particularly, according to Rieff, through his ingenious and influential repressions of revelation: "The revelational father unacknowledged, except as 'primal repression,' modern sensibility has been achieved at the cost of critical insensibility. . . . Critical intellect rubs near criminal impulse."[144]

Rieff remarks that "public therapy was never imagined, in Freud's wildest dreams of conquering the 'third unconscious,' Freud's name for sacred order."[145] Following a trend that began with *Fellow Teachers*, Rieff has become even more openly critical of "public therapies" in the name of one or another "lifestyle," reserving his sternest comments for homilies on homosexuality and abortion. Illustratively, of the 1991 St. Patrick's Day parade protests in New York by Irish homosexuals, Rieff comments:

> The green gays understand the *kulturkampf*. They want the language of absence to legitimate their transgression. That is never to say that the green gays, even celebrants of that abomination, should be excommunicated. Though they have set the mark upon themselves and gone the way the transgressive world goes, the purpose of the Church is to bring its wayward and their worlds back and forward to The Way. That purpose calls for pastoral priests trained in a truer psychiatry than the profession of psychiatry now has to offer.[146]

Rieff has often referred to sociology and psychiatry as sister disciplines, and in the last sentence above, he hints at what a Rieffian, or sacred, psychiatry might be. This is an "exhilarating, and yet terrifying" concept, and it appears that Rieff may have taken another page from Freud, who also saved his most prophetic remarks for the end of his career, and who ironically asked of himself in *The Future of An Illusion* "what can it matter to him in his old age when he is certain to be beyond the reach of all favor or disfavor?"[147] At a minimum, Rieff seems ready to reopen the now essentially closed debate over whether psychiatry should play a role in "curing" homosexuality.

With these intimations of a "sacred psychiatry," a highly provocative theory of repression, and an evolving lifelong encounter with Freud, the question raised is what role, if any, Philip Rieff will play in the future of psychiatry and the cultural impact of its historiography? In his recent and celebrated volume, *The Spiritual Life of Children*, Robert Coles, the eminent Harvard psychiatrist, speaks to the problem: "Rieff's work has been enormously helpful to those of us who want to balance a great respect for psychoanalytic work with serious reservations about what has emerged, intellectually and culturally, in its name these past decades."[148] Both clinicians and historians of psychiatry have been forced to play a central role in understanding the tangled agon between wishes and their renunciation and, thus, clarifying the tension between cultural responsibility and meaningful individual freedom, "since things have become as they are." Yet, can we tolerate the presence of such a syncretic and deeply faithful figure as Rieff within this discourse or has the category of the sacred been so deconstructed that it is no longer a viable distinction worthy of discussion? Perhaps Rieff's vision is too narrow and "moralistic." His brand of soul-making precludes many currently accepted behaviors, and he dismisses modern theories that excuse "transgressions" as products of social and economic deprivation. On the other hand, can we survive a culture governed by such therapeutic modalities as Rieff describes? Perhaps Rieff can help us work our way out of our present cultural crisis. We are surely in desperate need of balances against the destructive movements whose ranks are legion. In Philip Rieff, we have an individual of overwhelming intellectual range and erudition who stands at the opposite pole of the contemporary social construction/social control debate, within and beyond the history of psychiatry.

Notes

I would like to express my deep gratitude to Philip Rieff, without whom, of course, this project would not have been possible. Professor Rieff personally introduced me to many of the questions discussed herein, tirelessly corrected my theoretical errors in both classroom and tutorial, and it is difficult to express adequately my great appreciation for the support, as well as documentary access, that he has provided. I take full responsibility for any misrepresentations. I would also like to express my great thanks to Tom Mazur, D. Psych., whose editorial assistance was invaluable.

1. Philip Rieff, *Freud: The Mind of the Moralist*, 3rd ed. (Chicago: University of Chicago Press, 1979), 389.

2. Jeffrey Abramson, *Liberation and Its Limits: The Moral and Political Thought of Freud* (Boston: Beacon Press, 1984), 3.

3. Philip Rieff, "Aesthetics of Authority: Sacred Order/Social Order before Tocqueville and After," Copyright. Philip Rieff, 1990: 23. An abridgment of Part II of a projected three-volume series entitled *Sacred Order/Social Order: Image Entries to the Aesthetics of Authority* (Chicago: University of Chicago Press, forthcoming). On file with author. Permission to cite from the manuscript for this work is required and has been received from the author.

4. This information was gleaned primarily from the Curriculum Vitae of Philip Rieff. On

file with author. Herein, Rieff reveals a clue to the conversion under discussion when he lists on his C.V. that in 1986 he was the second annual Presidential Lecturer at the University of Toronto, while the first annual Lecturer was Cardinal Ratzinger and the third was Cardinal Willebrandts.

5. See Jerry Muller, "A Neglected Conservative Thinker," *Commentary*, xci, no. 2 (1991), 50.

6. Ibid., 50.

7. See particularly, Barry Richards, *Images of Freud: Cultural Responses to Psychoanalysis* (New York: St. Martin's Press, 1989), and Judith Van Herick, *Freud: On Feminity and Faith* (Berkeley: University of California Press, 1982).

8. See Christopher Lasch, *The Culture of Narcissism* (New York: Norton, 1979), and Alasdair MacIntyre, *After Virtue*, 2nd ed. (Notre Dame: University of Notre Dame Press, 1984).

9. Don Browning, *Generative Man: Psychoanalytic Perspectives* (Philadelphia: Westminster Press, 1973), 32.

10. Muller, "Neglected Conservative Thinker," 49.

11. Stephen Goode, "America's Most Conservative Professor," *Insight*, viii, no. 12 (1992), 14.

12. Christopher Lasch, "The Saving Remnant," *New Republic*, 19 November 1990, 34.

13. Ibid., 34.

14. Browning, *Generative Man*, 16–17.

15. Karl Menninger, *Whatever Became of Sin?* (New York: Bantam Books, 1978), 1.

16. Philip Rieff, *The Feeling Intellect: Selected Writings*, edited by Johnathan Imber (Chicago: University of Chicago Press, 1990).

17. Norman O. Brown, "Rieff's Fellow Teachers," *Salmagundi*, Fall (1973), 34.

18. See Herbert Marcuse, *Eros and Civilization: A Philosophical Inquiry into Freud* (Boston: Beacon Press, 1962), originally published in 1955. And Norman O. Brown, *Life Against Death: The Psychoanalytic Meaning of History* (Middletown: Wesleyan University Press, 1959).

19. Muller, "Neglected Conservative Thinker," 50.

20. Carl Schorske, "A Life of Learning" in Larry May (ed.), *Recasting America* (Chicago: University of Chicago Press, 1989), 101.

21. Rieff, *Freud: The Mind of the Moralist*, 37.

22. Harold Bloom, *Ruin the Sacred Truths* (Cambridge: Harvard University Press, 1987), 152.

23. Rieff, *Freud: The Mind of the Moralist*, 291. As Rieff points out, we learn from Freud's autobiography that he deliberately abstained from reading Nietzsche in fear of not being original.

24. Ibid., x–xi.

25. Ibid., 291.

26. Ibid., 61.

27. Ibid., 324.

28. Browning, *Generative Man*, 41.

29. Stephen Frosh, *The Politics of Psychoanalysis* (New Haven: Yale University Press, 1987), 67.

30. See generally, Rieff, *Freud: The Mind of the Moralist*, 329–57, and Browning, *Generative Man*, 32–60.

31. Rieff, *Freud: The Mind of the Moralist*, 329–57.

32. Ibid., 356.

33. Cited in Browning, *Generative Man*, 55.

34. Ibid., 13.

35. Michael Beldoch, "The Therapeutic as Narcissist," *Salmagundi,* xx (1972), 135.

36. Ibid., 197.

37. See Rieff, *Freud: The Mind of the Moralist*, in general.

38. Ibid., 253.

39. Ibid., 328.

40. Ibid., 329.

41. John Dollard, "Society, Too, is on the Couch," *New York Times Book Review* 22 March 1959, 7.

42. Rieff, *Freud: The Mind of the Moralist*, xx.

43. Ibid., *xi*.

44. Ibid., 299.

45. Gordon Wright and Arthur Mejia, *An Age of Controversy: Discussion Problems in Twentieth-Century European History* (New York: Dodd, Mead, 1972), 416.

46. Philip Rieff, *The Triumph of the Therapeutic: Uses of Faith After Freud*, 2nd ed. (Chicago: University of Chicago Press, 1987). Originally published in 1966.

47. Ibid., 5.

48. Ibid., 5.

49. Ibid., 2.

50. Ibid., 15.

51. Ibid., 74.

52. To feel the depth of Rieff's irony, see "On the Life of the Therapeutic" in *Three Jewish Philosophers* (New York: Atheneum, 1969), 42–51.

53. Philip Rieff, "Toward a Theory of Culture: With Special Reference to the Psychoanalytic Case," reprinted in *The Feeling Intellect*, 323.

54. Rieff, *Triumph of The Therapeutic*, 36.

55. Ibid., 74–76.

56. Abramson, *Liberation and Its Limits*, 2.

57. Rieff, *Triumph of the Therapeutic*, 77. Also, see generally Browning, *Generative Man*.

58. Rieff, *Triumph of the Therapeutic*, 85.

59. Allan Megill, *Prophets of Extremity: Nietzsche, Heidegger, Foucault, Derrida* (Berkeley: University of California Press, 1985), 346.

60. Rieff, *Triumph of the Therapeutic*, 33.

61. Ibid., 25.

62. Ibid., 13.

63. Ibid., 12.

64. Ibid., 27.

65. "The Therapeutic as Narcissist," *Salmagundi*, 20 (1972), 135.

66. See, among many, Browning, *Generative Man*, 32–59; and Menninger, *Whatever Became of Sin*, 251n.

67. Rieff, *Triumph of the Therapeutic*, 4.

68. Browning, *Generative Man*, 45.

69. Robert Weisburg, "Bloom, the philosopher behind Bennett, . . ." *Stanford Daily*, 21 April 1988, 6.

70. Frosh, *Psychoanalytic Politics*, 221.

71. MacIntyre, *After Virtue*, 26.

72. Rieff is fond of saying, "I have never had an original idea in my life. I owe my every thought to some predecessor." [*Fellow Teachers*, (Chicago: University of Chicago Press, 1985)]. While Rieff obscures his own originality in style and method in this comment, his real intention is to abjure "creativity" in the sense of even conceiving of a proscribed or never before considered act. However, in this case, Rieff properly cites Goethe as the progenitor of the concept of a hospital culture when he quotes from his *Italienische Reise*: "Speaking for myself, I too believe that humanity will win in the long run; I am only afraid that at the same time the world will have turned into one huge hospital where everyone is everybody else's humane nurse." Cited in *Triumph of the Therapeutic*, 24n.

73. Saul Bellow, *Humboldt's Gift* (New York: Penguin Books, 1973), 175.

74. Frank Kermode, "That Uncertain Feeling," *Times Literary Supplement*, 13, June 1975, 639.

75. Muller, "Neglected Conservative Thinker," 49.

76. See Aristides, "Incidental Meditations," *The American Scholar*, Spring 1976, 173–174.

77. See *Salmagundi*, no. 20, Summer–Fall 1972. In this edition, articles by the following authors, among others, respond directly and indirectly to Rieff and his ideal type: Michael Beldoch, Norman Brown, Peter Sedgwick, Jack Jones, and Michel Foucault.

78. Rieff, *Fellow Teachers*, 1.

79. Robert Boyers and Robert Orill, "Introduction," *Salmagundi*, 20 (1972), 3.

80. Berel Lang, "About the Dead Speak——— (only, mainly, some, no) Good," *Salmagundi*, lxxi (1986), 232.

81. Julien Benda, *La Trahison Des Clercs* (Holland: Bernard Grasset, 1927); Johan Huizinga, *In the Shadow of Tomorrow* (London: William Heinemann, 1936).

82. Alan Bloom, *The Closing of the American Mind* (New York: Simon & Schuster, 1987).

83. Weisburg, "Bloom, The philosopher behind Bennett," 6.

84. Rieff, *Fellow Teachers*, 23.

85. Brown, "Rieff's Fellow Teachers," 42.

86. Rieff, *Fellow Teachers*, 208.

87. Ibid., 53.

88. Lang, "About the Dead Speak," 232.

89. Rieff, *Fellow Teachers*, 43.

90. Ibid., 216.

91. Ibid., 99.

92. Ibid., 15. See further, in general, Milan Kundera, *The Unbearable Lightness of Being*, English translation (New York: Harper & Row, 1984).

93. Rieff, *Fellow Teachers*, 16.

94. Ibid., 51.

95. Lang, "About the Dead Speak," 230.

96. Ibid., 231.

97. Rieff, *Fellow Teachers*, 9, 10.

98. Kermode, "That Uncertain Feeling," 639.

99. See Weisburg, "Bloom, the philosopher behind Bennett"; Lang, "About the Dead Speak"; and Kermode, "That Uncertain Feeling."

100. Rieff, *Fellow Teachers* 169–70.

101. Ibid., 215.

102. Ibid., 12.

103. Ibid., 87.

104. Brown, "Rieff's Fellow Teachers," 44. The second birth would be the opposite of Augustine's concept of the second death described in the *City of God*. Rieff's social-psychological description of that second death is "such a repression of the primary sense that we feel ourselves free from membership in the eternal life of sacred order." See Rieff's *Fellow Teachers*, particularly the "Pretext of Prooftexts," vii–xxii.

105. Cited in Lasch, "The Saving Remnant," 32.

106. Mark Edmundson, "Freudian Mythmaking: The Case of Narcissus," *Kenyon Review*, x, no. 2 (1988), 20. See further, Edmundson, *Towards Reading Freud: Self-Creation in Milton, Wordsworth, Emerson and Sigmund Freud* (Princeton: Princeton University Press, 1990).

107. Rieff, *Freud: The Mind of the Moralist*, xxiii–xxv.

108. Ibid., 358.

109. Ibid., *xxv*.

110. Rieff, *Fellow Teachers*, 69.

111. Rieff, *Freud: The Mind of the Moralist*, 361. A perhaps apocryphal story is told of an

occasion when Rieff was giving a talk to a group of young students from a local Yeshiva and had briefly covered his conception of Freudian repression. Continually attempting to move on to other subjects, he was repeatedly brought back to the issue of repression by a particularly curious young Jew who simply could not grasp the concept but seemed desperate to understand it. Having patiently tried to explain it several times, Rieff finally in desperation blurted out the truth behind his own concealment: ''Orthodox Jews don't need repression!''

112. Ibid., 363.

113. Ibid., 367. Rieff's term, I suspect, is a play on Kant's *categorical imperative*.

114. On Freud's theory of the possibility of a *third unconscious*, see Sigmund Freud, *The Ego and the Id* with a biographical introduction by Peter Gay (New York: Norton, 1960), 9–10. When I asked this distinguished editor and Freud scholar, Peter Gay, his thoughts on Freud's ruminations of the possibility of a *third unconscious*, he said that he had never heard of it, and, moreover, wondered what the first and second unconsciousness might be. While these term appear starkly in this volume of *The Ego and Id*, perhaps this great admirer of Freud resisted and thus repressed Freud's god-term as much as or more than Freud, himself.

115. Rieff, *Freud: The Mind of the Moralist*, 368.

116. Ibid., 369.

117. Ibid., 380.

118. Ibid., 395.

119. Philip Rieff, ''For the Last Time Psychology: Thoughts on the Therapeutic Twenty Years After,'' reprinted in *The Feeling Intellect*, 351–365.

120. Ibid., 362.

121. Ibid., 354.

122. Ibid., 353.

123. Rieff, *Triumph of the Therapeutic*, xiii.

124. Muller, ''Neglected Conservative Thinker,'' 51.

125. Philip Rieff, ''The Newer Noises of War in the Second Culture Camp: Notes on Professor Burt's Legal Fictions,'' *Yale Journal of Law and the Humanities*, 3 (1991), 315–388. Copyright Philip Rieff. I have received permission to quote from this work as well as the other published and unpublished parts of the forthcoming *Sacred Order/Social Order* (Chicago: University of Chicago Press, forthcoming).

126. Philip Rieff, ''Worlds at War: Illustrations of an Aesthetics in Authority; Or, numbered notes toward a trilogy of which the general title is *Sacred Order/Social Order*.'' On file with author.

127. Friedrich Nietzsche, *The Gay Science* (New York: Vintage, 1974), 181.

128. Rieff, ''Worlds at War,'' no. 12.

129. Rieff, ''Aesthetics of Authority: Tocqueville and After,'' 23.

130. Rieff, ''Newer Noises of War in the Second Culture Camp,'' 378.

131. Philip Rieff, ''By What Authority? Post-Freudian Reflections on the Repression of the Repressive as Modern Culture,'' reprinted in *The Feeling Intellect*, 334.

132. Goode, ''America's Most Conservative Professor,'' 29.

133. Rieff, ''Newer Noises of War in the Second Culture Camp,'' 326n.

134. Ibid., 326n.

135. Ibid., 326.

136. See Muller, ''A Neglected Conservative Thinker,'' 51–52, and Rieff, *Fellow Teachers*, 14, 19.

137. Cited in Rieff, ''Newer Noises of War in the Second Culture Camp,'' 324.

138. Ibid., 324. George Steiner characterizes Rieff's quasi-rabbinic form of hermeneutics in the following comment: ''Be it in a specifically religious, for us Judeo-Christian sense, or in the more general Platonic-mythological guise, the aesthetic is the making formal of epiphany. There

is a "shining through." *Real Presences* (Chicago: University of Chicago Press, 1989), 226. Steiner is one of the few theorists whose work resembles Rieff's in any way, particularly in its normative implications. For more on the opposing forms of hermeneutics, see, generally, Giles Gunn, *The Culture of Criticism and the Criticism of Culture* (New York: Oxford University Press, 1987), and Megill, *Prophets of Extremity*.

139. Rieff, "Aesthetic of Authority: Tocquevile and After," 46.

140. Megill, *Prophets of Extremity*, 345.

141. Michel Foucault, *Foucault Live* (New York: Semiotexte, 1989), 220–221. For more on the debate between Rieff and Foucault, see *Homosexuality: Sacrilege, Vision, Politics*, ed. George Steiner, *Salmagundi*, Fall 1982–Winter 1983, no. 58–59.

142. Rieff, "Newer Noises of War in the Second Culture Camp," 324.

143. Rieff, "Aesthetics of Authority: Tocqueville and After," 43.

144. Rieff, "Aesthetics of Authority: Tocqueville and After," 41.

145. Ibid., 367.

146. Ibid., 368. Rieff's vociferous condemnation of homosexuality may involve personal reasons of which I am unaware. However, theoretically, I believe it stems from his insight into sexuality as the main mode of personal rebellion, humans at their most symbolic. Freud's influence is crucial here. Rieff suggests that Freud "has made the greatest single contribution to the understanding of civilization—not merely to the understanding of our own" through illustrating that the significance of sexual life, despite his belief in sublimation, is embodied in the fact that civilization is permanently opposed by sexuality. See *Freud: The Mind of the Moralist*, 339–342.

147. Sigmund Freud, *The Future of An Illusion* (New York: Norton, 1960), 45. Rieff's personal biography, also, provides some insight into the conversion under discussion. On the verge of becoming a septuagenarian, Rieff has decided to forego becoming emeritus at the University of Pennsylvania in favor of accepting an appointment in the Department of Psychiatry at the Medical College of Pennsylvania.

148. Robert Coles, *The Spiritual Life of Children* (Boston: Houghton Mifflin, 1990), 340.

IV

HISTORICAL THEMES AND TOPICS

11

"Les mythes d'origine" in the History of Psychiatry

PATRICK VANDERMEERSCH

Not every science finds its own history very interesting. The more exactly it defines itself, the more it experiences itself as being timeless, because the objectivity of the research results it obtains is not dependent upon historical factors. Being dependent on history: Is this not placing oneself in the hands of chance? Naturally it is nice when you can say something about the history of your own science. But "real" scientists usually busy themselves with their discipline's history only after having reached the age of retirement. For the training of younger colleagues they find an understanding of the history of their own profession not so necessary. And when there are books published about their discipline's history, they are usually deluxe editions that can be given as a gift, and in which the illustrations, the binding, and the quality of print are deemed more important than the soundness of the text.

Psychiatry is an unusual contradiction to this rule. In general it has had a great deal of interest in understanding its own history. It is true that there are some exceptions, namely, whenever this discipline takes as its model the exact sciences and tries, for example, to follow the timelessness of physics, holding this timelessness in higher regard than physics itself. The famous *Comprehensive Textbook of Psychiatry* began to stress more and more the biological approach in its fourth edition and decided to move the chapter on the history of psychiatry from the front to the back. In the fifth edition the chapter was rewritten in such a way that it abandoned the attempt to interpret this history and chose instead simply to report historical fact.[1] But this is an exception. Not only is there a short historical sketch in most psychiatric textbooks, but, it could be argued, no other discipline produces so many volumes on the history of its own profession. It suggests that understanding psychiatry's place in history is an essential for success in the field; and perhaps this is indeed the case.

In the historical writings of psychiatry there are many stories that might be called myths. They are first of all myths in the ordinary sense: that is to say, fictions. In this sense, Pinel's liberation of the alienated of Bicêtre from their chains is a myth, as J. Postel has rightly pointed out; the ceremonial scene immortalized by Tony Robert-Fleury in his famous painting of 1878 never actually took place.[2] But the history of psychiatry also includes stories in the sense of *"mythes d'origine."* Their function is the legitimization of the present. Pinel's story also has this second function, but perhaps a clearer example can be found in the accounts of demonology that most historical surveys continually return to and in which honor was brought to the name of Johann Weyer (1515–1588). His fame was secured as one of the "founding fathers" of psychiatry in his battle against the simplistic belief in sorcery and his attempt to rescue witches from the stake by declaring that they were sick and mentally incompetent to stand "trial."[3] Some scholars still refer to Weyer today.[4]

This distinction is important when we want to discuss the truth or falsehood of a particular myth. Two questions must be asked: Did what is described in the myth actually occur? and Why have people attached a mythical function to a certain figure? A story may stand the test of a historical critique, but then there is still the question of why the historically true story was rescued at a particular moment from oblivion in an attempt to validate the present through the past. Whether Johann Weyer actually existed can be a question that an exact and scientifically responsible body of research can undertake. It can attempt to establish his real achievements. Yet, such research says nothing about his mythical function. That has to do with the moment when and the reasons why one returns to Johann Weyer and connects him to the history of psychiatry. Was the link with the past correct? Why did people—in this case, in the middle of the nineteenth century—need to dig up this story about Johann Weyer? Was there perhaps a crisis in the legitimization of psychiatry that had to be more precisely defined, a problem to be solved or concealed with the introduction of the myth?

If we look at myth and the formation of legend in this way in the historical writings of psychiatry, we are confronted with two sorts of historical questions. There is, first of all, the critique of the sometimes all-too-beautiful stories that people tell one another about the history of their own discipline, which find their prototypes in the "life stories" of famous psychiatrists who follow the footprints of René Semelaigne.[5] Here questions arise such as whether Pinel really freed the alienated of Bicêtre from their chains, or if the rotating chair was invented by Horn or by Darwin and whether it was widely used. Beside that question is another concerning whether the use of myths really establishes what they pretend to establish. In this context it is essential to study when the myth came into existence and to examine the situation at the time that needed legitimization.

The Problematic Identity of the Psychiatric Discipline

In the case of psychiatry, one particular example of the phenomenon of *mythes d'origine* springs to mind. Very often the story that is told comes from a historical period in which there was still no real, acknowledged "psychiatry," but a period in which it was understood as being practiced implicitly. In this sense there is a significant difference between the myth of Pinel as a liberator of the alienated and that which made Weyer the father of psychiatry because he fought a battle against the belief in witchcraft. Pinel has indeed played a substantial role in the development of psychiatry as a unique discipline, if we consider the manner in which psychiatry has developed from the end of the eighteenth century until the present. The formation of myth concerning Johann Weyer, however, worked in a completely different way. It suggests that in the time of Weyer, when there was no acknowledged psychiatry, psychiatry should have already existed.

Now one can, it is true, establish that a similar retrospective projection of their own discipline to the far past has been accomplished by a number of the sciences. The positive sciences have themselves done it. It is not difficult, after all, to consider Thales of Milete and Democritus as the forefathers of chemistry and physics. Medical graduates still take the Hippocratic oath. For psychologists and pedagogues it is even more self-evident. When they attempt to sketch a historical survey of the theories of their disciplines, they can do nothing other than discuss the thought of Plato, Locke, and Rousseau, even if the work of these thinkers was more clearly understood as belonging to the philosophical discourse.

And yet there is still a fundamental difference in the case of psychiatry. There is more at stake here than the fact that psychiatry had to wait a long time before it was recognized in its autonomy. The identity itself of the psychiatric discipline appears more problematic. An essential problem involved the attempt to define the psychiatric field. Not only did the field of psychiatry become ever greater—this was not such a problem in so far as expansion generally gave the impression that psychiatry was heading in the right direction—but it was becoming incoherent. Moreover, its directions were continually shifting their focus. Patients who were considered the prototypes of psychiatric patients in the past lost their psychiatric status, such as in the case of epileptics. Others whose behavior was considered in earlier times to have nothing to do with mental illness have become, in recent years, legitimate psychiatric patients, as in the case of addicts and sexual deviants. The question could be asked whether a well-formulated definition of the object of psychiatry could be given. Does the discipline rest on a coherent common principle? Undoubtedly, psychiatrists deal with the most diverse sorts of business and they are very busy. The only question is whether we can consider all the things they do as psychiatry. Or, in other words: Can psychiatry be defined in another way than by formulating it on the basis of what psychiatrists do? Or, again, the question can be put otherwise: Does the appraisal described in the *DSM-III* rest on anything else than the accidental concurrence of circumstances that have placed a heterogeneous group under the heading of a single profession? In the attempt to wrestle with these questions, a number of myths were created, myths that were used to establish the proper terrain of psychiatry.

A second problem arises alongside the first, which also relates to the production of myths. The social acceptance of psychiatry has repeatedly been challenged, and this once again called for a new confirmation for which specific myths were created. And so it was necessary, at a certain moment, to paint a picture of the benevolent, fatherly philanthropist; and this equally in the case of Pinel as of Weyer.

In the background of this uncertainty about the proper identity and social image of psychiatry lies an enormous problem concerning the medical character of psychiatry. In part, it finds itself interwoven with the previous two problems. In another way it functions as a veil to conceal these problems. The medical character of psychiatry is thus also a dominating frame in which the different myths function.

The Mythical Establishment of the Medical Character

For how long has psychiatry existed? The question is important when we attempt to discuss the mythical reconstruction of a prehistory of psychiatry. We must, therefore, mark the boundaries between prehistory and history. It is not without reason that historical surveys usually take as their criteria the existence of a distinct, recognizable, and socially accepted structure for the care of the mentally ill. The fact that the word *psychiatry* was designed and was socially acknowledged; that certain institutions appeared expressly for the treatment of the mentally ill; that particular legislation was erected for their intake, their residence, and dismissal; that there emerged a distinct discipline that recognized the ''mad'' as a single group; that the discipline had its own textbooks, its own journals, and that specialists emerged with their own particular training for the care of the ''alienated'': this is the psychiatry whose members will repeatedly contend that their identity had always had to exist.

Historically, the birth of this psychiatry must be situated in the transition between the eighteenth and nineteenth centuries. As might be anticipated, controversy about the attribution of the discovery quickly arose. There were good reasons to think that the process was first carried out in England with the establishment of the Retreat in York by Samuel Tuke, and to think that Pinel learned the basis of his ''moral treatment'' there. As one might expect, Pinel disputes this version, contending that he was really the author of this treatment,[6] which, in return, provoked sharp criticism in the English press.[7] Regardless of that, Pinel was very quickly received—elsewhere and in England itself—as the greatest philanthropist that had ever concerned himself with the situation of the mentally ill, deserving a central place in the history of psychiatry, even if one maintained that the reformations in England and France ran parallel to one another and that they, for the most part, developed independently of one another.[8]

The discussion surrounding the attempts to attribute the birth of psychiatry to one of these figures should not allow us to forget the ambiguity that was connected with the identity of psychiatry as a distinct discipline from the very beginning. The argument for the declaration of the autonomy of psychiatry was the ''moral treatment.'' People were convinced that the mentally ill could be cured if they were submitted to an extremely intensive program of what, at present, we would call ''psychological influence.'' It was thought, therefore, that the mentally ill must be isolated in separate institutions and be subjected to the imposing authority of a single man who, by his *présence*, could aid the mentally ill in their internal struggle to put aside their sick ideas.

The classical formulation of the ideal of moral treatment was introduced by Pinel with an account that could be considered as the first *mythe d'origine* of psychiatry. Pinel tells of an incident in which one of his friends was driven by severe depression to attempt suicide. The man was found lifeless in a forest, with one of Plato's dialogues in his hands concerning the immortality of the soul.[9] After this account, which Pinel titled ''Histoire d'une manie où le traitement moral auroit été nécessaire'' follows his famous definition of the moral treatment:

> In the treatment of his mania, it was in my power to use a great number of remedies; but I lacked the most powerful of them all, which one can simply find in a well-ordered hospice, the one which consists in the art of subjugating and taming the alienated, to put it in this way, by placing him in a strict dependency upon a man who, by his physical and moral qualities, is apt to exercise on him an irresistible empire and to change the vicious chain of his ideas.[10]

When one considers the account, it is difficult to find a single reason in it to speak of the birth of a medical discipline. Everything in Pinel's book could be said to point to the contrary. Certainly, Pinel knew that it was sometimes thought that physical causes could be attributed to mental illnesses, and more precisely he was well informed about the theories that attributed a dominating role of the nervous system and the brain in this field.[11] With a sense of duty, Pinel measured with great precision the skulls of the mentally disturbed and compared them with the measurements of what, without argument, one has to accept as the ideal form of the human head, the statue of Apollo in the Paris museum.[12] The conclusion of this research is unconvincing: Pinel doesn't want to exclude the legitimacy of such research, but he himself had few results. "Moral affectations" like overambition, religious fanaticism, or an unhappy love affair appeared to him more profound causes of mental illness, and since they usually occurred long after skull-formation is completed, he didn't expect a priori that much from further skull research.[13]

With these remarks Pinel dismisses the biological argument as grounds for a medical conception of psychiatry, but he nevertheless does not say that it is nonmedical. The responsibility for this reticence lies in the broad conception of medicine during the French Revolution, which was not narrowly organic, but had to be understood, since the work of Cabanis, as the intimate unity of body and soul, and as such must be considered the final achievement of human sciences.[14]

What springs to mind from our point of view is that Pinel breaks through the clear division between pathology and normality. The insane are seen as driven by motives that linger in everyone's heart. The difference is only one of degree.

Pinel's point of view would quickly be abandoned. It is understandable that the story of his deceased friend with Plato in hand did not become a founding myth. It was totally at odds with the development of psychiatry in its medical direction in which "medical" would from then on mean "organic" and in which the boundaries between normality and pathology would be firmly established.

It is worthwhile to consider the way in which this development proceeded. Esquirol further developed the idea of psychiatric institutions and stated that it was absolutely necessary that in the institution there would be one, and only one power figure. The following famous words are his:

> The doctor has to be, in some way, the principle of the life of a hospital for the alienated. It is by him that everything has to start its movement. He has to regulate all actions as he is called to be the regulator of all thoughts. It is to him, as to their centre that all things that interest the inhabitants of the establishment have to refer. . . . He has to be invested with an authority that no one can subtract himself from.[15]

Esquirol was, then, also strongly against the thought that the power inside the institution should be divided. This still does not provide a substantial argument to make psychiatry a medical discipline. Why must the doctor be the personage that represents this absolute authority? No explicit answer was given. In many countries there was the opposite reaction against the fact that doctors took it upon themselves to dispense the moral treatment. This was especially so everywhere philosophy and religion were not in discredit, unlike in France. Philosophers, jurists, and even the clergy themselves claimed to be at least as good as medical men in the practice of the moral treatment.[16] Even in

France itself there were voices calling for this. Above all, the return of religion as foundation for authority must have been the source of unlimited irritation for French doctors. For they saw themselves as the heirs of the anticlerical Enlightenment *par excellence.*[17]

Unfortunately for them, the moral treatment failed. In a desperate attempt to make the moral treatment still more effective and efficient, sometimes cruel means were grasped at.[18] Protest arose against the inhumane manner by which patients were administered the therapeutic psychological shock for a cure that never seemed to arrive, especially when the brutality was becoming even more explicitly defended as in the work of F. Leuret.[19]

In this context two myths were created, which from that day forward can be repeatedly found in any historical survey of psychiatry: one about Pinel and the other concerning demonology. Pinel was in the first place a doctor, elevated to the status of a philanthropist. As a reaction against the charges of brutality in the moral treatment, the portrait of its founder as the figure who liberated the mentally ill from their chains was spread.[20] There was added to this that he had done so because he had recognized that they were "sick." The medical image of Pinel was also emphasized.[21]

The stories concerning demonology had an analogous mythical function. From about 1840 a number of psychiatrists themselves began to be interested in the history of Christianity, and in particular in its darker period in which belief in possession by the devil, in sorcery, and in witchcraft had arisen. Parchappe wrote a long commentary on *Malleus maleficarum*, the famous book written in 1486 that provided the Catholic Inquisition with rules for the indictment, trial, judgment, and punishment of witches. Calmeil authored a book that employed an aggressive tone and that was to become very popular: *On Lunacy from the Point of View of Pathology, Philosophy, History and Law, from the Renaissance of the Sciences in Europe until the Nineteenth Century. Description of the Big Epidemics of Simple or Complicated Delirium Overwhelming the People of Earlier Times and Dominating the Monasteries. Exposition of the Judgements Unjustly Passed because of Ignorance of Madness.*[22] His work contained more than a thousand pages on such topics as "The Demonopathy of the Nuns at Cambray," "A Case of Hystero-Demonopathy at the Monastery of St. Brigit," "The Theo-choreomany [the religious mania of dancing] in Some Religious Sects," and so forth. A plethora of articles followed in the wake of Calmeil's book. It is in this context that Johann Weyer was made the father of psychiatry.[23] The message that was sounding through was clear: It was absurd nostalgia to cling to anything that has to do with a religion that in earlier times and in such a terrible manner had something to do with obscurantism, and on the grounds of superstition had brought innocent souls to be burned at the stake. If this is the case, people had better put their trust in doctors.

The medical character: The portrait that was painted by these myths included everything except that of an expert, with a technical competence on the level of the human body. It is a picture of someone who people themselves can rely upon, without individuals being able to say precisely why. The *mythes d'origine* have then also the function in the support of these images. The reference to religion, earlier the very foundation of authority, in combination with the image of genuine humanity, helped the physician to provoke the transference of the patient's deep-rooted feelings of dependency.

The Myths Concerning the Enlargement of the Psychiatric Field

Also originally absent in the early days of psychiatry was the organic position that dominated psychiatry in the second half of the nineteenth century. In France this development was connected with the name of J. Moreau (1804–1884); in Germany with that of W. Griesinger (1817–1868). One might think that from here on the development of psychiatry should follow in a straight line, in keeping with the singular organic perspective. The creation of myth would now disappear, or so one might expect.

Nevertheless, this was not the case. J. B. Friedreich found it necessary to begin his *Historisch-kritische Darstellung der Theorien über das Wesen und den Sitz der psychischen Krankheiten*[24] with a review of the *"psychische Theorie"* (psychical theories), which ends with the perspective that psychiatric disturbances in the literal sense of the word were "spiritual" disturbances. He heavily underlined where such a conception leads: "When individuals now add there a strong dose of occultism, mysticism, and an all too sweet piety, one arrives at the conception that the source of the psychic illness (*psychische Krankheiten*) inherent in the repudiation of rationality and morality, lies in the passions and in the sins.'[25] He also sounds a clear warning: Belief in psychic causality is not only false, it can even be dangerous.

While citing his less somatically one-sided colleague F. Groos (1768–1827), Friedreich reacts militantly against his adversaries. That is, against Catholic belief and its Pope looking down from his high-handed and apostolistic Petrus position upon Galilei. Once such belief sought its salvation in images of Mary and holy water, while the only true religion according to Groos—and Friedreich—is that human beings conform to their own will in the universal will of nature.[26] The voice of Cabanis seems to be heard here.

It is surprising to find this message at a moment when psychiatry began to follow the promising organic way. But one must not forget two things: No matter how enthusiastically the first positive results in brain research were welcomed—research concerning dementia paralytica in particular—it gave no perspective in regard to therapy.[27] The second half of the nineteenth century saw the establishment of psychiatric institutions. People had anticipated only the best from them. Yet the massive building work was accompanied by sad resignation. For after the failure of the moral treatment, for which these institutions were built, there followed a sense of defeatism that was a consequence of the belief in organic causality. In these institutions there were biological laboratories where brain dissections were performed. These laboratories were certainly busy places, but the patients experienced few benefits from them, in fact it was quite the contrary. The belief in biological causality had as a consequence of its main principle the disappearance of the psychological position that was in a certain way present in the moral treatment. The fact that the expectations people had placed in anatomical research were not realized did not change much. The success of the discoveries, such as in dementia paralytica, provided few benefits for the largest group of patients, those we would now call psychotics, but who, at the time, were all placed together under the extremely broad category of paranoia. The organic explanation, therefore, was still trusted by many as a matter of belief.[28] A lot needed to be demonstrated if psychiatry wished to be a science, and in this context there followed a number of mythical accounts that attempted to depict the stupidity of belief in psychological causality.

There is another paradox. No matter how much people in the second half of the nineteenth century put their faith in the organic approach, there was also an expansion of the psychiatric field that took place during that period, encompassing a number of illnesses for which no organic causes could be found, as in the case of monomania and neurosis.

The fact that the psychiatric field was expanded to cover monomania was an object of controversy. That the most normal-looking people could possess a partial form of delusion, that it could break out in well-determined circumstances, and that the existence of the delusion could only be diagnosed by a doctor—no, the ordinary man would not believe that. This would mean in concrete terms that many criminals would be declared ''mentally incompetent to stand trial'' in the courts. Alarm was aroused by the specter of crazed murderers being set free thanks to medical expertise. It is not our intention here to investigate how monomania has survived through the detours of history up to the present day in accepted categories such as pyromania and kleptomania. Let us just mention that Prichard's understanding of ''moral insanity'' lead to our understanding of ''psychopathy,'' that interest in cases of sexual deviancy was awakened, and that sexology was made a psychiatric affair.

What strikes us more here is that we also find at the birth of the concept of mono-mania a mythical story, in which the themes of a philanthropic doctor and the unhealth-iness of religion return. It concerns a certain ''Sergeant Bertrand,'' who disinterred a number of bodies between 1847 and 1848 in order to cut them into pieces, and—according to the story that is usually told—to have sexual intercourse with them.[29] The fact that the man was condemned was, for L. Lunier, an expert who disagreed with his colleagues, the occasion to write an article to argue once again for an understanding of monomania and, in that way, to ''defend the valiantly conquered terrain.''[30] A real doctor, Lunier reasoned, would have manifest more understanding for Bertrand, and equally more for society as a whole. Bertrand should not be sent to prison where he would be released again after a year—he should not be imprisoned at all. Instead, he should spend a much longer period of time in the hands of a well-meaning doctor. The mythical image of the philanthropic doctor does not fail to appear in the story, nor is the extremely critical reference to religion absent. Lunier pointed out that Bertrand was a seminarian, which, according to him, added strength to his melancholic disposition and made him sexually more excitable.[31] He adds that the case of Bertrand did not really surprise him, because in the four or five cases of necrophilia that he was familiar with in the literature, there were three priests or at the very least ex-seminarians involved. He concludes his article with the accounts of several of these stories, and a reference to the legendary figure of Gilles de Rais, the companion of Joan of Arc, who murdered dozens of children for the sake of sexual pleasure.

Alongside monomania the neuroses form the second field of problems annexed by psychiatry. Neurology was clearly distinguished from psychiatry in its infancy, and this was certainly the case in France. In this sense one could not have expected that Charcot's research at the Salpêtrière in Paris would have lead to an expansion of the psychiatric field. In the neurologists' search for an anatomical basis of hysteria, they were forced to draw the opposite conclusion of what they were looking for: they were forced to recognize the autonomy of psychic causality. This result did not take away from the fact that one could still refer to hysteria as an illness. To support their position, these neurologists looked back on the history of the church to demonstrate how frequently this illness had been misrecognized. In the same manner as Calmeil had done before them, J. M. Charcot and P. Richer devoted a large section of their *Études cliniques sur l'hystéro-épilepsie ou grande hystérie* to religious phenomena of the past, which they suggested contained unrecognized cases of hysteria.[32] A book concerning *Les démoniaques dans l'art* followed in the same spirit.[33]

With Freud and the spread of psychoanalysis in psychiatric circles the field of the neuroses was also recognized as within the psychiatric domain. Psychoanalysis was itself for decades after the 1940s the basic principle that would structure the psychiatric field, and this applied equally to its therapeutic methods as well as its systematic diagnostics. The history of psychiatry was rewritten in this new perspective by G. Zilboorg and G. Henry, in which they reiterated and detailed the myths both concerning demonology and those associated with it.[34]

Why did these myths continue to exert such a profound influence? One might think they would now disappear. W. Leibbrand and A. Wettley brought the theme of demonology back to modest proportions in their *Der Wahnsinn* and rightly said that it is singularly impossible to write a history of psychiatry as a discipline. The only possible thing to write is a history of insanity.[35] The same applied for F. Alexander and S. Selesnick, who were convinced that it was only after Freud that one can speak of a "real," valuable psychiatry. They criticized the way in which the battle against demonology, and in particular the figure of Weyer, were usually portrayed.[36] When H. Ellenberger decided to write a history of psychiatry that would retrace the footprints of Freud, he nevertheless returned to the demonological theme. Searching the prehistory of the Freudian concept of the transference, Ellenberger looked for its origins in hypnosis and mesmerism. He returns to the time in which Mesmer was placed on a commission in Bavaria to give an opinion on the famous exorcist Gassner.[37] It is here that Ellenberger makes explicit use of a *mythe d'origine:* "The emergence of dynamic psychiatry can be traced to the year 1775, to a clash between the physician Mesmer and the exorcist Gassner.[38]

Again and again you find in the textbooks that psychiatry arose out of the fact that illuminated minds left the obscurantism and the blind faith of religion behind them. Thereafter the illuminated minds were the real philanthropists, while religion, in spite of all appearances, housed much violence. Admittedly, it is often put less brutally. With regard to religion a "benevolent neutrality" is the polite position to take. However, even today the statement can appear rather brash. Whoever takes the last edition of the *Comprehensive Textbook of Psychiatry* in hand may be surprised at how the preface begins:

> It is a curious truth that the vast majority of scientists who have ever lived are living now. The fact reveals two important facets of science: It is relatively young, and its recent growth has been exponential. Historically, there had long been a tension between scientific inquiry and theological truth. These latter truths were often revealed and not subject to rational inquiry. The church was far more powerful than science, and it held the position that if logical inquiry contradicted revealed truth, then the results of the logical inquiry were false.[39]

Conclusion

It might appear fitting to claim that psychiatry is dependent on medicine in so far as psychiatry evolved from the question of whether psychic disorders can be accounted for physically or not. History teaches us, nevertheless, that psychiatry originated from a completely different conception. Moreover, psychiatry enlarged its field in a period when there was indeed widespread belief in biology, but it occurred by the annexation of two forms of pathology for which there was no precise organic explanation: monomania and neurosis. What was it, then, that brought this diverse set of "problems" together in such a way that we may consider them as psychiatric "illnesses"? How did the apparent unity that we find so neatly classified in the *DSM-III* come into existence?

It is on this point that the *mythes d'origine* shed some light on a part of the question. When one delves into their effect, one discovers in the end that it is a matter of the discovery of the susceptibility to the transference. Psychiatry was born of the moral treatment, out of the experience of how strongly people are inclined to give up their independence for the esteem of an authority figure.

This is not to deny how important biological determinants can be for psychiatry. Nevertheless, history shows us that the success of biology was, in the first place, largely dependent on the measure by which it was an object of belief; and then, again, above all in the measure of the trust that people were willing to place in the figure of a doctor. What supported this trust? It was clearly the myths, as is seen in their extremely harsh treatment of religion and in their cultivation of images of philanthropy in the psychiatric field. In order to know how this worked—and perhaps still works—one should ask two questions, which fall outside the scope of this paper. First of all, further analysis is necessary of the conception of the transference, which emerged with the discovery of psychoanalysis but which is naturally not a question of *creatio ex nihilo*. One should examine the reasons why particular forms of transference are evoked, maintained, and manipulated in a certain society at a particular moment. Second, there is great need to submit the idea of "religion" to further research. It is research that should not take as its starting point a definition of religion stemming from its function today, in the wake of the Enlightenment and secularization, as a remainder of what it formerly was. Whoever begins with the conception of religion as being "other than the secular" can naturally not follow our perspective and ask: What happened when religion was no longer the factor that provided both a certain conception of life and a foundation for authority in the West? It is neither nostalgia nor the zeal for restoration that motivates us to ask this question, but the attempt to come to terms with the situation that secularization has placed us in; a problem that the existence of psychiatry can sometimes be regarded as part of the solution for, and sometimes as the symptom.[40]

Notes

1. Harold I. Kaplan and Benjamin S. Sadock, *Comprehensive Textbook of Psychiatry* (Baltimore: Williams & Wilkins, 4th ed. 1985, 5th ed. 1989).

2. Jacques Postel, *Genèse de la psychiatrie. Les premiers écrits de Philippe Pinel* (Paris: Le Sycomore, 1981), 62.

3. P. Vandermeersch, "The Victory of Psychiatry over Demonology: The Origin of the Nineteenth-Century Myth," *History of Psychiatry*, ii (1991), 351–363.

4. An English translation of his work has recently appeared: G. Mora (ed.), *Witches, Devils and Doctors in the Renaissance. Johann Weyer, "De praestigiis daemonum"* (Binghamton, New York: Medieval and Renaissance Texts & Studies, 1991). The preface by John J. Weber puts it clearly: "An early classic of psychiatry, it is difficult to understand why such a seminal work was not available to English-speaking readers earlier" (p. v). In his introduction G. Mora is nevertheless cautious: "Weyer's role as a pioneer of modern psychiatry is more difficult to assess than his place in the history of witchcraft" (p. lxxvii).

5. R. Semelaigne, *Les grands aliénistes français* (Paris: Steinheil, 1894); *Aliénistes et philanthropes. Les Pinel et les Tukes* (Paris: Steinheil, 1912); *Les pionniers de la psychiatrie française avant et après Pinel*, 2 vols. (Paris: Baillière, 1930–32).

6. P. Pinel, *Traité médico-philosophique sur l'aliénation mentale ou la manie*. (Paris: Richard, Caille et Ravier, An IX), 47–50: "Les médecins anglais ont-ils publié les rèles du traitement moral?"

7. See David Hack Tuke, *Chapters in the History of the Insane in the British Isles*, 1st ed. (London: 1882; reprint, Amsterdam: Bonset, 1968), 142–145.

8. "... as a matter of fact the course of French and English reform in the treatment of the insane was entirely distinct and independent." Ibid., 146.

9. Pinel did not tell us, unfortunately, which dialogue it was. Was it the Phaedon, or was it the Phaedrus?

10. Pinel, *Traité médico-philosophique*, 57–58.

11. Pinel cites for the case the theories of Greding. Ibid., 112.

12. Ibid., 113–118.

13. "Dans le recensement des aliénés que je fis à Bicêtre l'an 3 de la République, je reconnus que les causes déterminantes de cette maladie sont le plus souvent des affections morales très vives, comme une ambition exaltée et trompée dans son attente, le fanatisme religieux, des chagrins profonds, un amour malheureux. ... Ces notions préliminaires indiquent d'avance combien doivent être rares les lésions ou difformités du crâne parmi les aliénés, puisque dans l'âge adulte l'ossification des os de la tête est complète, et que les affections morales ne peuvent l'altérer. Il restait seulement à constater cette vérité par des ouvertures des corps très multipliées, et des recherches exactes." Ibid., 110–111.

14. P. Vandermeersch, "De religie en het ontstaan van de psychiatrie" (Religion and the Birth of Psychiatry) *Tijdschrift voor Theologie*, xix (1979), 329–351.

15. J. E. D. Esquirol, art. "Maison d'aliénés," *Dictionaire des sciences médicales*, vol. xxx (Paris: Panckoucke, 1818), 84.

16. The division of power was self-evident in Germany. See Jacobi, "Bemerkungen über die Bedeutung des Ausdrucks 'Seelenstörung' in der Psychiatrie, und über die Mitwirkung der Geistlichen bei Behandlung von Irren, durch *Nasse's* Schrift: 'Ueber die Behandlung von Gemüthskranken und Irren durch Nichtärzte' veranlasst," *Allgemeine Zeitschrift für Psychiatrie*, i (1844), 353–422. In Belgium there was also the call, for it was all but self-evident that the moral treatment should not be trusted to doctors: P. J. Maes, *Considérations sur les maisons d'aliénés en Belgique* (Bruges: Imprimerie Vandecasteele-Werbrouck, 1845), 96–98. For a French reaction concerning the state of affairs in other countries, see M. Falret, *De l'utilité de la religion dans le traitement des maladies mentales et dans les asiles d'aliénés* (Paris: Imprimerie de Bourgogne et Martinet, 1845).

17. Still in 1853 we find warnings against possible claims of the clergy on moral treatment: D. H. van Leeuwen, *Rapport sur la fondation, la construction et l'organisation des meilleurs asiles d'aliénés en France et ailleurs, présenté au comité des états de l'île de Jersey, chargé de prendre en considération le sort des aliénés de l'île* (Jersey: Le Lievre, 1853).

18. J. Postel, "Naissance et décadence du traitement moral pendant le première moitié du XIXe siècle," *Evolution psychiatrique*, xliv (1979), 585–616.

19. F. Leuret, *Du traitement moral de la folie* (Paris: Baillière, 1840).

20. J. Postel, "Philippe Pinel et le mythe fondateur de la psychiatrie française," *Psychanalyse à l'Université*, iv (1979), 197–244.

21. The process demanded some time. The next citation is typical: "Pinel, although his writings would have made him eminent as a physician had he never rendered his name illustrious in reference to the insane, did not, as the study of his life abundantly proves, liberate the patients from Bicêtre from their chains in direct consequence of his medical knowledge of insanity, but mainly, if not entirely, from the compassion which he felt for their miserable condition. His knowledge, great before, was vastly increased after he had placed the patients in a more favourable state for medical observation; in fact, it is obvious that the opportunities of scientific research, and specially of observing the satisfactory progress of those labouring under the disease, were greatly augmented from the moment he introduces a humane system of treatment." Daniel Hack Tuke, *Chapters in the History of the Insane*, 146.

22. L.-F. Calmeil, *De la folie considérée sous le point de vue pathologique, philosophique, historique et judiciaire, depuis la renaissance des sciences en Europe jusqu'au dix-neuvième siècle; Description des grandes épidémies de délire simple ou compliqué, qui ont atteint les populations d'autrefois et regné dans les monastères. Exposé des condamnations auxquelles la folie méconnue a souvent donné lieu* (Paris: Baillière, 1845). Reprinted with a foreword by M. Collée (Marseille: Lafitte Reprints, 1982).

23. See Vandermeersch, "The Victory of Psychiatry over Demonology."

24. J. B. Friedreich, *Historisch-kritische Darstellung der Theorien über das Wesen und den Sitz der psychischen Krankheiten* (Leipzig: Otto Wigand, 1836).

25. Ibid., 1.

26. Ibid., 3–4.

27. J. Postel, "La paralysie générale" in J. Postel and Cl. Quétel, *Nouvelle histoire de la psychiatrie* (Toulouse: Privat, 1983), 322–333.

28. G. Lantéri-Laura and G. Bauttier, "L'évolution des idées sur le système nerveux central et ses rapports avec les développements de la psychiatrie contemporaine" in *Nouvelle histoire de la psychiatrie*, 413–430.

29. G. Lantéri-Laura, *Lectures des perversions. Histoire de leur appropriation médicale* (Paris: Masson, 1979), 17–18. The formation of myth has gone further: It was said that Bertrand always dug up young women and that his intentions were expressly sexual, which does not at all fit with the story.

30. L. Lunier, "Examen médico-légal d'un cas de monomanie instinctive," *Annales médico-psychologiques* v (1948), 351–379. "N'oublions pas avec quelle difficulté a prévalu la doctrine de la monomanie, et combien encore de nos jours cette folie partielle est niée et méconnue par certains magistrats. Pour conserver le terrain si laborieusement conquis, il ne suffit donc point de dire: Cet homme est aliéné: il faut avant tout le démontrer" (p. 351).

31. "Bertrand a été élevé dans un séminaire, et cette circonstance, assurément, n'était guère propre à éloigner de son esprit les idées mélancholiques qui y avaient pris racine. Ce genre d'éducation a peut-être aussi développé chez lui une excitabilité des organes génitaux, comme cela n'est que trop commun, si l'on s'en rapporte aux écrits des médecins qui font autorité en pareille matière." Ibid., 369.

32. J. M. Charcot and P. Richer, *Études cliniques sur l'hystéro-epilepsie ou grande hystérie* (Paris: Delahaye et Lecrosnier, 1881).

33. J. M. Charcot and P. Richer, *Les démoniaques dans l'art* (Paris: Delahaye et Lecrosnier, 1887). Recently reedited (Paris: Macula, 1984).

34. G. Zilboorg and G. Henry, *A History of Medical Psychology* (New York: Norton, 1941). For a critique of the way in which they refer to demonology, see P. Vandermeersch, "The Victory

of Psychiatry over Demonology,'' 352–353. For a critique of the way they cite Pinel and in particular their confusion between the first and second edition of his *Traité médico-philosophique sur l'aliénation mentale ou la manie,* see J. Postel, M. Postel, and P. H. Privat, ''Les deux introductions au *Traité médico-philosophique* de Pinel,'' *Annales Médico-psychologiques* cxxix (1970), 15–48.

35. W. Leibbrand and A. Wettley, *Der Wahnsinn. Geschichte der abendländischen Psychopathologie* (Freiburg: Karl Alber, 1961).

36. F. Alexander and S. Selesnick, *The History of Psychiatry: An Evaluation of Psychiatric Thought and Practice from Prehistoric Times to the Present* (New York: Harper & Row, 1966). We have used the French translation, as its footnotes correct many inaccuracies: *Histoire de la psychiatrie. Pensée et pratique psychiatrique de la préhistoire à nos jours* (Paris: Collin, 1972). Concerning Weyer, see pp. 105–106.

37. Ellenberger emphasizes the story, as he also does with the figure of Mesmer.

38. H. Ellenberger, *The Discovery of the Unconscious. The History and Evolution of Dynamic Psychiatry* (London: Allen Lane, 1970), 53.

39. Harold I. Kaplan and Benjamin S. Sadock, *Comprehensive Textbook of Psychiatry,* 5th ed. (Baltimore: Williams & Wilkins, 1989).

40. P. Vandermeersch, *Psychiatrie, godsdienst en gezag* (Psychiatry, Religion and Authority), (Louvain: Acco, 1984).

12

"*Le geste de Pinel*": The History of a Psychiatric Myth

DORA B. WEINER

The French do not know the founder of psychiatry in their own country. All that most textbooks tell us about Philippe Pinel (1745–1826) is that he was the first to liberate the insane from their chains, at Bicêtre Hospice in Paris at the height of the French Revolution. Yet recent scholarship and documentary evidence definitively discredit that legend, known in France as "Pinel's gesture." The facts do not support it, yet the legend persists. It has a life of its own because, like all fairytales, it hides a deeper meaning. This chapter explores the reasons why a crudely manufactured myth has overshadowed Pinel's innovative and creative achievement, leading one of the foremost French historians of psychiatry of our own age to announce a new attitude when he writes: "Our generation has stopped adoring [Pinel] and has begun to read him."[1]

More than any other public medical figure 200 years ago, Pinel offered society assurance that mental illness is treatable and sometimes curable. To this end he advocated close and extended observation of, and carefully structured conversations with each patient so as to understand the natural history of the illness and to arrive at individual case histories. He used the precipitating event, the duration of each illness, and his analysis of the affected mental faculty to fashion a diagnosis. He then subdivided his patients into categories and used the accommodations and facilities of the asylum to further therapy. Pinel insisted on the prohibition of physical violence against patients and on a drastic reduction in bloodletting for therapeutic purposes; he was skeptical of drugs, preferring natural remedies. He paid serious attention to the complaints of the poor as well as the rich and stayed at the sickbed to help his indigent patients die. Owing to an unfortunate and thoughtless translation into English, his psychologically sensitive approach to the mentally ill has become known as "moral treatment." The fact is that he attempted to raise the rejected madmen and madwomen housed in the kingdom's public institutions to the dignified status of medical patients in the newly formed French republic.[2] In that sense, and in that sense only, did he liberate the insane men at Bicêtre from their chains.

Pinel has remained controversial: He was a public servant, clinician, author, and professor living in Paris during the Revolution and Empire, and therefore his every word and action were intertwined with the political events of twenty-five turbulent years. Even though he had little interest in politics and never took an active part, he was forced to make choices, express allegiances, and side with or against successive ruling powers. Political regimes have therefore claimed or rejected him, historians have faulted him for loyalties or fickleness, and the informed public has judged his person, his work, and even his contribution to medicine in political terms. Certain of his critics seem determined to disparage the man in every possible way.

In order to understand the long life of the myth, it will be useful to view Pinel in relation to four general themes of great importance to him, to psychiatry, and to French history. These themes are the Catholic religion, the revolution in the medical sciences at the end of the Enlightenment, French educational politics in the Revolutionary and Imperial era, and the impact of anatomo-pathology on psychiatry in the early decades of the nineteenth century. But the reader should first be introduced to the myth.

In *Le sujet de la folie* and some complementary articles, Gladys Swain, the brilliant French psychiatrist, has shown how Dr. Scipion Pinel (1795–1859), the professor's eldest son, and Dr. J. E. D. Esquirol (1772–1840), his favorite pupil and spiritual heir, began the process of constructing a sentimental symbol.[3] In 1823, with Pinel increasingly incapacitated by successive strokes, Scipion published a brief piece on "The removal of the chains," supposedly extracted from his father's papers. "Pinel's gesture" is here described for the first time.[4] Here towers the tall, muscular Chevingé, liberated from chains by Pinel, the lifelong bodyguard and servant who presumably saved the doctor from deranged inmates more than once.[5] The main episode in Scipion's story is Pinel's defense of his patients' right to personal freedom at Bicêtre in 1794.

In an embellished version presented to the Royal Academy of Medicine in 1836, Scipion portrayed Pinel confronting the cruel, paraplegic Georges Couthon, a member of the autocratic Committee of Public Safety, who came to inspect the situation of the chained "wild beasts."[6] In the story, Pinel heroically faces Couthon, demanding that all the unfairly restrained madmen be instantly freed. He risked his life in defying the powerful Jacobin. But nothing in Couthon's biography, Pinel's writings, or contemporary accounts corroborates this visit. In fact, Couthon seems to have been out of town at that time.[7]

Scipion's motivation in publicizing his father's fearless attitude was undoubtedly complex. He was surely keen on diverting attention from the father's emphasis on psychologic factors in illness. That emphasis was embarrassing to a son who was convinced that mental illness is caused by diseased brains. Scipion, fifty years his father's junior, lived in a different scientific, cultural, and political world. But we also know that Scipion had money troubles and that he borrowed heavily, using his father's property and good name to obtain credit; he even appropriated Pinel's library while the father was still alive. The total lack of letters or other personal documentation forces us to leave the two men's feelings toward each other to conjecture.[8]

The same is true of Pinel's relationship to Esquirol. It suited the ambitious younger man to see the image of his teacher reduced to a symbolic gesture. Pinel had been his mentor, sponsor of his private mental institution since 1802, president of his thesis committee in 1805, his chief at the Salpêtrière from 1811 to 1825. They collaborated closely until Esquirol was a mature man in his fifties. Yet Pinel, sounding both proud and patronizing, continued publicly to call Esquirol his "student."

In 1817, under the restored Bourbon monarchy, Esquirol began offering clinical lectures on mental illness at the Salpêtrière, and he took the first step in a lifelong course of action to win political attention for the mentally ill. At the behest of the minister of internal affairs, he undertook a nationwide survey, visiting all the institutions throughout France where mental patients were then confined. Esquirol painted a dramatic picture:

> I have seen them naked, clad in rags, having but straw to shield them from the cold humidity of the pavement where they lie. I have seen them coarsely fed, lacking air to breathe, water to quench their thirst, wanting the basic necessities of life. I have seen them at the mercy of veritable jailers, victims of their brutal supervision. I have seen them in narrow, dirty, infested dungeons without air or light, chained in caverns where one would fear to lock up the wild beasts that luxury-loving governments keep at great expense in their capitals.[9]

Pinel is not mentioned in this text, which implies that his reforms had remained fruitless. The need for a rescuer was evident and urgent.

Esquirol claimed that role for himself. In 1822 he was appointed inspector general of medical faculties, and in 1825 medical director of Charenton Hospice. He became the main architect of the national law of 1838 that instituted departmental asylums for all needy French mental patients and that is still in force today. It is surely significant that the only important formative role by Pinel that Esquirol still acknowledged in the 1830s was that of Pinel's famous book on mental alienation. But in the revised version of the myth that appears in Esquirol's *Treatise on Mental Maladies* of 1838, Pinel, referred to as the "learned doctor," was seen as a tool of anti-governmental rebellion. We read: "The ideas of the time perverted the importance of breaking the chains that degraded and troubled the madmen at Bicêtre. The success of the learned doctor and friend of misfortune turned into a trophy for the agitators."[10] Esquirol the royalist dissociated himself from Pinel the republican.[11]

Had the myth of the chainbreaker been merely the work of two envious "sons," it could not have prevailed for over a century. To understand its deep meaning for other Frenchmen, we need to explore the main themes upon which the myth touches. The first was the Catholic religion: We must analyze its relationship to Pinel and to the nascent psychiatric specialty.

In the region between Toulouse, Albi, and Castres where Pinel spent the first twenty-eight years of his life, the religious past is still a major concern. Even today, conversation turns easily to the cruel suffering of the people during the Albigensian Crusade, during the religious wars of the Reformation, or after the revocation of the Edict of Nantes. Pinel's family was Catholic, but his mother's ancestors came from Protestant Castres: Her parents converted when the Edict was revoked in 1685.[12] Local Protestants did not emigrate in large numbers but continued to inhabit Pinel's native region, shielded by their Catholic neighbors.[13] As a boy, Pinel learned the need for tolerance and for accommodation with powerful political and religious forces. He learned that lesson mainly from the village teacher, Jean Pierre Gorsse (173?–1772), who became a family friend and a role model for the boy. Gorsse had graduated from the Jesuit college at Albi; but by the time Pinel was ready for college, the Jesuits had been expelled from France. Through this teacher's influence Pinel was awarded a scholarship to attend the seminary of the Fathers of the Christian Doctrine at nearby Lavaur. To accept the scholarship, Pinel needed to receive the tonsure and a recently discovered document indeed tells us that he did.[14] Pinel studied as a tonsured clerk, free of charge, until he completed the Master of Arts degree. He then prepared for the doctorate in theology and it is only around the time of his twenty-fifth birthday that he switched to medicine. Critics from the political Right criticize Pinel bitterly for this "treason," for having "thrown the cassock into the flames." Critics from the Left welcome the change. Both identify psychiatry with left-wing politics.

Did Pinel transfer any aspect of his religious upbringing to his medical teaching and practice? In his writings he never adduced the authority of the Old or New Testament, any saint, dogma, or belief. Nor did he ever utter any moral judgment of a patient that might indicate his own position with regard to Catholic dogma. What Pinel did share with the Catholic faith was a lifelong commitment to help the suffering poor. He served for thirty years as physician-in-chief of Salpêtrière Hospice, caring for indigent, old, and sick women patients. He often stayed at their bedside to help them die. In doing so, he brought the finest humane aspect of Catholic charity to clinical medicine. He also developed the individual doctor-patient relationship into a long-term collaborative undertaking. Swain discovered that the German philosopher Georg Wilhelm Friedrich Hegel appreciated the fact that Pinel's concept of "*manie périodique*" offered the therapist the opportunity to gain the patient's confidence and over time to establish a collaborative therapeutic relationship during the patient's lucid intervals.[15] Pinel's use of repeated, probing, personal conversations with his mental patients grew into an important part of "psychologic treatment." His long years of experience with the personal advice and guidance lavished by the Fathers of the Christian Doctrine on their young students leads one to conclude that nascent psychiatry in France owed an important debt to Pinel's clerical past.

Pinel's serious involvement with science, particularly natural history, is another aspect of his work that belies the simpleminded heroism of the myth. Pinel came to Bicêtre after years of work in zoology at the Paris Botanical Gardens, work that resulted in eight important papers published in the *Journal de physique* and led to his election to the Academy of Sciences in the section for anatomy and zoology in 1803. His work is based on comparative anatomy and on the close observation of animal behavior. It also shows a sustained interest in taxonomy and classification.[16] Pinel applied these interests to the mentally ill men at Bicêtre whose health became his main responsibility once he was appointed as "*médecin des infirmeries*." For nineteen months he spent many hours every day observing the behavior of each individual patient and he repeatedly talked to each man so as to understand his personal history. His notes then enabled him to chart the natural history of the disease and arrive at a diagnosis. To depict Pinel as an idealistic and somewhat simpleminded liberator is to ignore historic facts.

The third, and central, part of Pinel's thought and work, trivialized or simply ignored by the advocates of the myth, concerns the teacher and writer. He elaborated his clinical method in three books that complement each other. For his students he wrote a textbook, the *Philosophic Nosography*,[17] presenting a classificatory framework of all diseases. The *Medico-Philosophic Treatise on Mental Alienation* explicated a part of the nosologic picture, namely the nervous illnesses, then called "neuroses."[18] And in *Clinical Medicine* Pinel illustrated how he combined attention to physical and psychologic illness at the sickbed, integrating the perceptions, diagnoses, and therapy of the psychiatrist and physician into a humane public medicine.[19] This exceptional patient-centered approach impressed Pinel's contemporaries, who often stressed his "kindness." The students prized his skill in honing their clinical acumen.

The *Treatise on Insanity* became world-famous. The *Nosography*, though widely used for at least twenty years in six successive editions, did not stand the test of time. We shall see that critics attacked Pinel's classification, particularly his first class of diseases, the "essential fevers." In fact the initial attack, by an adherent of John Brown (1735–1788), the advocate of "excitement" as the clue to illness and health, appeared soon after the *Nosography*'s publication.[20]

But it is the last phase of Pinel's life, when the Royalist government dismissed him from the medical faculty, when the idol of the young, François Broussais (1772–1838), ridiculed the *Nosography*, when the medical thesis of A. L. J. Bayle (1799–1858) seemed to demonstrate the reliability of the anatomo-pathologic method even in psychiatry, that Pinel's credit fell, and the myth of the liberator established itself. We now turn to the political fortunes of the myth.

Politics was an essential element of the myth. It transformed Pinel's medical message into a controversial claim because he raised questions in the public mind about the rights of the mentally ill, their involuntary confinement, their claim of innocence for crimes by reason of insanity—questions involving the Rights of Man. "Man is born free, yet everywhere he is in chains," Jean Jacques Rousseau had written at the beginning of the *Social Contract*. These chains became identified with those shackling the insane—an identification that transformed Pinel into a political revolutionary.

In nineteenth-century France, the politics of the Rights of Man reached far beyond the struggle for freedom of assembly, speech, and religion. Rather, the fight for individual freedom became part of the confrontation between the Catholic religion and Science, including medical science, and extended from Napoleon's Concordat with the Holy See in 1802 to the separation of state and church in 1905. No nineteenth-century French scientist or physician could escape involvement in that duel: whether it was François Vincent Raspail, the microscopist, who languished in jail in the 1830s as president of the Society for the Rights of Man, or Ernest Renan who lost his chair at the Collège de France in 1862 because he published a factual biography of Jesus, or Claude Bernard who was given a state funeral in 1878 so as to preclude a solemn commemoration of Pope Pius IX—great scientific figures were pushed or used for political ends throughout the nineteenth century. Pinel was no exception.

The battle between Left and Right, claiming the brilliant clinician and learned doctor as one of theirs, began while Pinel was still alive. The regime of Charles X was evidently frightened by student agitation, in the early 1820s, in favor of broader suffrage and a constitution guaranteeing freedom of assembly, expression, religion, and the press. The University of Paris, particularly its medical faculty, was a hotbed of political protest in which Pinel's son Charles (1802–1871), a law student, was involved. Under a pretext, the reactionary minister of education, Jacques Joseph Guillaume Pierre Corbière, closed and then purged the medical faculty on 21 November 1822. On 2 February 1823, Pinel was placed on emeritus status, on half-pay, together with ten eminent colleagues also perceived as liberal heralds of revolution.[21] The Bourbons—the Right—thereby rejected Pinel.

Three years later, politics intruded into Pinel's very funeral at the Père Lachaise cemetery. Etienne Geoffroy St. Hilaire spoke, representing the Academy of Sciences,[22] then Etienne Pariset, for the Academy of Medicine,[23] followed by Léon Louis Rostan, for the Salpêtrière staff. "When no one came forward for the medical faculty," wrote the anonymous author of a "Notice" in the *Archives générales de médecine*, "M. Cruveilhier [Jean Cruveilhier, the distinguished anatomist] made his way through the crowd and improvised a speech full of warmth and feeling. It is said that an eyewitness, seeing the Faculty thus remain silent among this justified and universal sadness, remarked that [the Faculty] was attempting to dismiss Pinel a second time."[24] Cruveilhier, a member of the *Congrégation*, the arm of Catholic reaction, had let his personal decency and admiration for Pinel silence his political allegiance. Not so Cruveilhier's teacher, the king's powerful first surgeon, Guillaume Dupuytren, who concluded an obituary "Notice" in the *Journal des Débats*, claiming Pinel for the Right: "He was a Christian," wrote Dupuytren, "and of his free will he died a Christian."[25] Pinel was too important a figure to abandon to the Left. (Whether Pinel in fact received extreme unction has not yet been established.)

As for the abolition of chains and the claim of priority so often made for (not by) Pinel, the documents give a clear picture—more precise than historians have hitherto realized. Since so much ink has flowed on this subject of chains, and they are the theme of the self-perpetuating myth discussed in this chapter, it is worth establishing a definitive record of the facts and their sources. To begin with, we have testimony about the orderly St. Prix ward for mentally ill men at Bicêtre, run by Jean Baptiste Pussin (1745–1811), soon to become Pinel's assistant. This evidence comes from a wholly trustworthy source, the site visitors of the Duke de La Rochefoucauld-Liancourt's Poverty Committee of the National Assembly who inspected Bicêtre in May 1790. They reported that "the number of [violent patients] is small and varies with the seasons: only ten out of 270 were chained the day of our visit."[26]

What is most surprising, given the ubiquitous propaganda for Pinel as the "chain-breaker," is that, when he initially arrived at Bicêtre on 6 August 1793 as "physician of the infirmaries," Pinel accepted the traditional use of chains to restrain the violent insane as a matter of course. In his "Memoir on Madness" of 11 December 1794, he mentioned without further comment that three of his patients had been shackled for fifteen, twenty-five, and forty-five years, respectively.[27] It was his talented assistant Pussin who, evidently on his own initiative, first freed the insane men at Bicêtre from their fetters in Prairial, Year V [May–June 1797].[28] At that time Pinel had been gone from Bicêtre for two years. The doctor praised Pussin's exemplary accomplishment in the second edition of the *Treatise* in 1809, mistakenly giving the date "4 Prairial, Year VI" for Pussin's historic initiative, adding that he followed his assistant's example "three years later."[29]

Both men knew that some mental patients need to be restrained if they become violent and destructive or suicidal, or threaten the lives of others. And all humane persons object to the weight of iron shackles and the unnecessary pain they inflict as well as the degradation they imply. Why Pinel did not take immediate action remains unexplained and reprehensible. When he and Pussin eventually dispensed with chains, they substituted straitjackets when needed, a fact that is attested to repeatedly in the contemporary official literature. Thus the Paris Hospital Council report of 1803 simply stated that the condition of the mentally ill at Bicêtre "has been improved, quite apart from the abolition of chains."[30] The second report, in 1816, reveals a new interest in the mentally ill. A thirteen-page chapter deals with mental hospices, and Pinel's innovative methods of management and therapy are discussed at length. A separate paragraph concerns Pussin and chains. Since this official statement has hitherto passed unnoticed, it is here translated *in extenso*.

> The idea of chaining the mad so as to dominate and confine them more easily had been adopted in all insane asylums in Paris and all other European establishments. A dedicated, intelligent and courageous supervisor who recently died, M. Pussin, brought about a useful and humane change. His efforts were entirely successful. The excitement of maniacs subsides instead of growing when they are not chained. They are now restrained, even during their most violent attacks, in a straitjacket made of strong cloth, with sleeves longer than the arms that can be tied at their ends. The sleeves can be used to fasten the inmates to their beds, without shackling their limbs.[31]

Pinel's and Pussin's contemporaries attributed a specific role to each man and distinguished clearly between Pinel, who reflected on theory and improved management as well as therapy, and Pussin, who initiated the removal of chains or their replacement with straitjackets. Scipion Pinel must not have known this report or he would have hesitated to publish his tall tale.

While the myth was gradually taking hold, Pinel's scientific teachings were being seriously challenged by young medical investigators. Scientists were now searching for the seat of diseases, in the tradition of Giambattista Morgagni. They analyzed tissues, following Xavier Bichat; explored physiologic functions with François Magendie; sought to establish neurologic localization with the phrenologists Gall and Spurzheim; scanned physiognomy with Camper and Lavater. They relied on physical diagnosis with the help of Auenbrugger's percussion and Laënnec's stethoscope. Eager researchers dissected brains to locate the causes of delirium, depression, retardation, and other mental disturbances. Pinel was looking increasingly old-fashioned.

The first skirmish in the battle to dethrone the old master had occurred as early as 1802. That year Gaspard Laurent Bayle (1774–1816) defended his thesis entitled "Considerations on Nosology, Medical Observation and Practice"[32] before a jury that included Pinel. Bayle's argument directly attacked nosology, and thus the author of the popular *Nosography*, and questioned the concept of species if applied to diseases. Bayle argued that species in medicine are based on subjective criteria and not on objective characteristics like those presented by animals, plants, or minerals. A physician observing a sick person selects signs and symptoms that he believes indicate the presence of a specific illness, then he combines a number of similar cases to conceptualize a species of disease. Thus he uses a double abstraction. Bayle then dismissed Pinel's classification of "discrete" and "confluent" smallpox as two different species of the disease, arguing that they belong to the same species because the inoculation of one can produce the other. And the transmission of such characteristics is a basic scientific criterion for identifying a species.[33]

Fortunately for the historian, Bayle's friend R. T. H. Laënnec was present and he took stenographic notes.[34] Bayle's argumentativeness had annoyed Professor Petit-Radel, so Pinel intervened in a conciliatory tone: "I feel great esteem for your personal qualities and your learning," Pinel told the candidate, "let us amicably discuss a few points on which we differ," and he suggested the two species of smallpox for discussion. Bayle explained his position, driving home the argument that Pinel failed to adhere to the rules of natural history, rules by which he himself taught medicine should be guided. Pinel was multiplying species of diseases unnecessarily, argued Bayle. Pinel defended himself, saying that such specificity was helpful in guiding therapy (which was, of course, beside the point), he interrupted Bayle several times and almost lost his temper. Bayle insisted, with some insolence, that he be heard. "You are right," conceded Pinel, "everyone must be allowed to state his argument freely." The battle was won. In the course of the discussion Pinel made one crucial concession: "The aim of classification is to aid memory," he stated. "That is the aim of methods in medicine."

"This discussion remains memorable to many physicians who were Bayle's contemporaries," commented Bayle's nephew, A. L. J. Bayle in 1855. The *Nosography* had found its first critic.

Yet it is significant that G. L. Bayle, like so many of Pinel's students, was more indebted to his teacher than he realized. In Bayle's most important work, the *Researches on Pulmonary Phthisis* of 1809–1810, he defined the lesion in the lung as a constantly developing entity, thus incorporating Pinel's vision of the changing clinical reality in the natural history of diseases. Even the critics among Pinel's students were touched by his teaching, and Pinel's students numbered in the thousands.[35]

This was also true for François Joseph Victor Broussais, the combative Breton military doctor who dedicated his thesis on "hectic fevers" to the professor in 1803. His book on *Phlegmasias* of 1808 is also faithful to Pinel's and Xavier Bichat's teachings.[36] But Broussais belonged to Esquirol's generation, and by the time he reached prominence as professor at the Val-de-Grâce in 1815, the Paris teaching hospital for military doctors, he had elaborated a new doctrine. He now explained most illnesses as varieties of inflammation, mainly of the gastrointestinal tract. The inflammation was caused by irritation and indicated a disturbance of function and usually a disease he called "gastro-enteritis." Broussais called his doctrine "physiologic medicine," and, in order to make it prevail, he launched a frontal attack on Pinel's classificatory category of "essential fevers": Fevers were only symptoms, Broussais rightly maintained. His gift of eloquence and his youthful, aggressive energy (in contrast to the professors at the medical faculty most of whom were aging) attracted the students in droves. Broussais's *Examination of the Widely Adopted Medical Doctrine* of 1816 was a brutal pamphlet. "Within ten years, [he] made Pinel's *Nosography* age by a century," comments Ackerknecht.[37]

The third and most serious scientific challenge to Pinel's preeminence, after those by G. L. Bayle and Broussais, occurred in 1822 when Antoine Laurent Jessé Bayle (1799–1858), Gaspard Laurent's nephew, defended a thesis entitled "Research on Mental Illness."[38] Bayle had observed and autopsied almost 200 mental patients under the eye of his mentor A. A. Royer-Collard (1768–1825), the medical director of Charenton Hospice. In his thesis Bayle presented six patient histories. All of these persons had suffered from increasingly severe paralysis and dementia—these illnesses had fre-

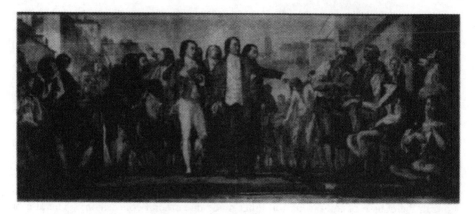

Figure 1. Philippe Pinel (1745–1826). "Pinel Orders the Removal of Iron Shackles from the Insane Men at Bicêtre Hospice." Painting by Charles Müller, 1849. Lobby, National Academy of Medicine, Paris.

quently been observed to be concurrent. Bayle now revealed that, on autopsy, the arachnoid membrane in the patients' brains showed increasingly severe inflammation, and he concluded that "chronic arachnoiditis exists and is the cause of a symptomatic mental alienation."[39] (Actually he could not prove a cause, but only a correlation.) He enlarged upon his observations in *Nouvelle doctrine des maladies mentales* in 1825 and *Traité des maladies du cerveau et de ses membranes* in 1826. Bayle's discovery "strengthened somaticist tendencies," comments Ackerknecht, it "was the end of ancient psychiatry."[40]

While the young generation was thus challenging Pinel's leadership, Scipion's story of the myth had been quietly working its way into powerful circles. Immediately after his father's death, in 1826, Scipion provided Georges Cuvier, the permanent secretary of the Academy of Sciences, with the notes for the official eulogy.[41] From there the myth and "Pinel's gesture" found their way into Etienne Pariset's tribute in the Academy of Medicine.[42] In 1836 Scipion read his expanded version of the myth to this academy, as we have already mentioned. As luck would have it, the Academy of Medicine soon thereafter planned to move into permanent quarters, rue des Saints Pères, where it wished to decorate its meeting hall with paintings of heroic medical deeds. Larrey performing surgery on the battlefield was an obvious theme, but how did "Pinel Orders the Removal of Iron Shackles from the Insane Men of Bicêtre" become the second choice?

The documents are somewhat inconclusive. But it is a fact that the secretary of the Academy of Medicine, Dubois d'Amiens, had heard Scipion's paper, and correspondence between him and the ministry of internal affairs indicates that the artist to execute the paintings for the academy, Charles Müller (1815–1892), was easily chosen.[43] How Müller was commissioned to immortalize the Pinel myth we do not know. The Academy—and the paintings—moved to 16, rue Bonaparte in 1902, and now a huge canvas of eighteen feet by eight feet, depicting an event that never happened, greets the visitor in the lobby of the Paris Academy of Medicine. On this canvas a youthful Pinel strides through some classical buildings, followed by an awed crowd and accompanied by a young associate who can only be Esquirol. Pinel, extending his arm in a commanding gesture, directs an employee (Pussin?) to unlock the irons on the wrists of an emaciated old man.

But history played a strange trick, and the image of Pinel as the herald of liberty, commissioned under the July Monarchy, was not unveiled in the meeting hall of the rue des Saints Pères until after the "February Revolution" of 1848, under the Second Republic. An anonymous newspaper article proclaimed "Pinel's triumph," editorializing: "One day Providence sent Pinel: his great genius brought about this transformation." The republic had gained an official medical hero.[44]

Müller's painting was followed in 1856 by a portrait showing Pinel in his professorial robes, "offered to the Imperial Academy of Medicine by his family, his friends and his students." Responsible for this initiative was Dr. Casimir Pinel, the son of Philippe's brother Louis, who signed himself "Pinel nephew."[45] In 1856, the academy also acquired a bust of Pinel by P. Robinet, now standing in the lobby under Müller's canvas. These two works of art resulted from acts of familial piety and do not carry a political connotation.

Not so the canvas by Tony Robert-Fleury (1837–1912) that adorns the entrance to the Charcot Library at the Salpêtrière, where it was inaugurated in 1878. Here the Third Republic paid tribute to its hero with a painting entitled "Pinel Delivering the Insane."

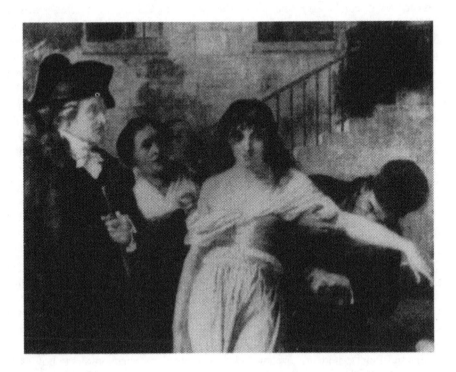

Figure 2. Philippe Pinel (1745–1826). "Pinel Delivering the Insane." Detail from a painting by Tony Robert-Fleury, 1878. Charcot Library, Salpêtrière Hospital, Paris.

Even though the word "*aliénés*" is in the masculine, the canvas shows a distraught young woman, behind her a female attendant, with a man unlocking a broad girdle that restrains the patient at the waist. In contrast to its counterpart at Bicêtre, this painting has historic veracity, for Pinel did order the chains removed at this hospital. Furthermore, the woman standing behind the girl unquestionably portrays Marguerite Pussin, since 1802 the supervisor of the mentally ill woman;[46] her husband, Jean Baptiste, had the keys to the shackles. Madame Pussin's head is centrally placed in this scene, close to the doctor's and higher than her husband's, which is virtually invisible behind the girl's arm. Madame Pussin's face expresses concern for the young woman and she appears personally involved in the liberation that Pinel has ordered. The artist judged— rightly, in my opinion—that this woman was an important actress in these proceedings.

It is remarkable how often and warmly Pinel praised Madame Pussin. In his "Memoir on Madness" of 1794 he wrote a whole paragraph on the improvement of the food at Bicêtre under her stewardship, praising "the succulent and tasty soup" . . . it had saved his life that year when he was recovering from typhus. Ten years later, in the twenty-four-page foreword to the second edition of *Clinical Medicine*, he stressed four areas of recent improvements at the Salpêtrière, three of them concerning food, laundry, and cleanliness.[47] Pinel repeatedly recorded his appreciation for her skill in managing recalcitrant patients. (There is an obvious parallel between Mme. Pussin and her contemporaries, Mrs. Dunston, the matron at St. Luke's Hospital in London, and Katharine Jepson at the York Retreat as portrayed by Samuel Tuke.)

As for Monsieur Pussin, Pinel's repeated praise made him overbearing—witness the following, hitherto unknown story. We find Pussin, together with Pinel and at least eighty French physicians, surgeons, and pharmacists among the corresponding members of the Société de médecine de Bruxelles in 1808. The exact date of their election cannot be ascertained from the surviving documents.[48] The picturesque popular diarist known as "Père Richard," a longtime employee at Bicêtre, mistook Pussin's membership certificate for a medical degree. He recounts that he himself "handed Pussin his diploma of doctor of the faculty of medicine of Brussels."[49] And, indeed, Pussin appears in the account books of the Salpêtrière as "physician of the madwomen" with a salary of 1,200 francs, half of that of Pinel and 200 francs more than Pinel's medical assistant A. J. Landré-Beauvais.[50] It is surprising that the administration—and Pinel—condoned this arrangement.

In addition to paintings, Republican Paris had other ways of honoring the famous liberator: A *rue Pinel* was inaugurated in the 13th arrondissement on 9 April 1851 (in connection with his birthday on the 20th), a *place Pinel*, also near the Salpêtrière, on 26 February 1867, and finally a postage stamp for 8 francs was issued on 25 January 1958.[51] And the Société médico-psychologique periodically honored the founder of the psychiatric profession in France, on the 100th and 150th anniversaries of his death.[52] Great specialists and others gathered on these occasions to offer paeans of praise in which the myth of the liberator provided a predominant theme. One exception was an excellent paper on the Wild Boy of Aveyron presented in 1976 by T. Gineste and R. Mises where the empathy and creative involvement of Dr. J. M. G. Itard, "Victor's" teacher (and Pinel's student), overshadows the professor's rejection of the boy as an incurable idiot.[53] A bicentennial celebration of the meeting between Pinel and Pussin is being planned at Bicêtre Hospital in June 1993.

The crowning effort of the Société médico-psychologique to honor the founder of psychiatry in France resulted in a statue of Pinel by Ludovic Durand erected near the entrance portal to the Salpêtrière. Paid for by public subscription, it portrays a youthful, elegant man holding links of a broken chain. At his feet cower two young girls, overcome with emotion, who look up at him in surprised gratitude. Statues of *Science* and *Bienfaisance* flank the liberator. And to underscore the political meaning of the event, the Society unveiled the statue on *13* July 1885, thus linking the breaking of chains with the storming of the Bastille.[54]

Thus the memory of Philippe Pinel has been kept alive in a historiographic controversy that would have perplexed him. Pinel himself is partly responsible, because his writings do not provide precise answers regarding either his politics or his religious convictions. He accepted hospital appointments, professorships, a seat in the Academy of Sciences, the Legion of Honor, and the Cross of St. Michael from the successive Jacobin, Thermidorian, Napoleonic, and Bourbon regimes. He served as consulting physician to Napoleon from 1808 on. He personally brought his twelve-year-old son to be baptized in 1807, yet four years later he buried his wife under a tombstone without a cross. He became indifferent to religion after leaving the study of theology in April 1770, and disgusted with politics after witnessing the death of Louis XVI under the guillotine on 21 January 1793.

It should by now be clear that the controversy over the Pinel myth conceals a much more important debate over this innovator's historic importance and influence. Indeed, in the medical field, two different approaches to mental illness have confronted each other ever since the defense of A. L. J. Bayle's thesis in 1822. Edward Brown called them "psychiatry's research programs."[55] Neuroanatomists who seek to understand the pathology of the human mind by studying the dead brain have been vying with the adherents to Pinel's approach, the advocates of psychologic investigation and treatment. In the 1820s, the young generation was swayed by the rise of a positivist and solidist fashion in medical theory and practice. Meanwhile, the myth of the chainbreaker flourished. Pinel, the innovative clinician, was forgotten and Esquirol became known as the real founder of psychiatry in France. The psychologic approach to mental illness did not again become popular in France until the era of Charcot.

Paradoxically, the strongest recent criticism of Pinel and of the mental hospital comes from sociologists, many of them Marxists, spearheading "anti-psychiatry." These thinkers, brilliantly led by Michel Foucault and Klaus Doerner, see physicians (and psychiatrists in particular) as members of the bourgeois establishment who have, since the early nineteenth century, used huge numbers of indigent patients for research and experiment. According to this argument, these doctors have exploited these patients for their own careers or for profit while claiming the advancement of knowledge as their avowed goal. The doctors turned the hospitals into "curing machines," a depersonalization of the patient set in, the profession becoming increasingly absorbed with diseases, while "the sick-man gradually disappeared from the doctor's consciousness."[56] In the asylum, according to Foucault, the director turned into a "medical personage" who sits in perpetual judgment over the inmates.[57] The "liberation" of the insane from their chains may not have given them liberty after all. Jacques Postel and David Allen explore anti-psychiatry later in this book.

An American admirer of Foucault, Jan Goldstein, has recently written an excellent book on *The French Psychiatric Profession in the Nineteenth Century.* Esquirol is the hero of her story. Goldstein designates the so-called moral treatment as the "originative psychiatric paradigm" and argues that Pinel derived this from Pussin and other "concierges" of mental institutions. These men were "charlatans" as defined by the *Encyclopédie*. Pinel's therapeutic method, his essential contribution to psychiatry, according to Goldstein, thus "derived from charlatanistic practice." This derogatory interpretation further strengthens the case for reducing Pinel to a mere chainbreaker.[58]

The myth has thus served to obscure Pinel's real achievements in the field he called mental alienation. More than anyone else, he is responsible for transforming French society's perception of the mad into that of sick and often curable men or women. In his nineteen months at Bicêtre he carefully watched each patient and listened to the story of each life and symptom so he could track the "natural history of the disease" as well as the patient's life history. For he conceived of each illness as the intersection of two ongoing developments, in the disease and in the person. He was also keenly aware of the interaction of psychologic with physical complaints and published three books explicating his nosologic method, his ideas on mental alienation, and his experience at the sickbed. He taught his approach to clinical medicine for thirty years while living at Salpêtrière Hospice among his patients, most of whom were indigent. That message of a humane and patient-centered public medicine conveys the image of Pinel that should replace the myth.

Notes

The research underlying this chapter was undertaken with the help of Grant RO 1 LM 04901 from the National Library of Medicine and a Faculty Research Grant from the UCLA Senate. The work was completed with the support of a Charles E. Culpeper Scholarship in the Medical Humanities. This assistance is here gratefully acknowledged.

1. M. Gourévitch, "Pinel père fondateur, mythes et rélites," *L'évolution psychiatrique*, lvi (1991), 595–602; the citation is on p. 602.

2. There is as yet no modern, critical biography of Pinel in the context of the Revolution. The standard work is R. Semelaigne, *Philippe Pinel et son oeuvre au point de vue de la médecine mentale* (Paris: Imprimeries réunies, 1888). Building blocks for a detailed study can be found in the published articles by G. Bollotte, P. Chabbert, J. Postel, and D. B. Weiner. See the Bio-Bibliographic Note on Pinel in Weiner, "Mind and Body in the Clinic: Philippe Pinel, Alexander Crichton, Dominique Esquirol and the Birth of Psychiatry" in G. Rousseau (ed.), *The Languages of Psyche: Mind and Body in Enlightenment Thought* (Berkeley: University of California Press, 1990), 331–404. For masterful brief sketches of Pinel's importance to psychiatry, see J. Delay, "Philippe Pinel à la Salpêtrière," *Médecine de France*, xcvi (1958), 1–16; and P. Chabbert, "Pinel," in *Dictionary of Scientific Biography, 10*: 611–614. The topic of the myth was recently explored in J. Gortais, "Le rôle du mythe de Pinel dans l'organisation et le fonctionnement de la psychiatrie du 19ème siècle," *Psychiatrie française*, xi (1980), 77–82; and in J. Postel, "Philippe Pinel et le mythe fondateur de la psychiatrie française," *Psychanalyse à l'Université*, iv (1979), 197–244. For the historic context of this story, see D. B. Weiner, *The Citizen-Patient in Revolutionary and Imperial Paris* (Baltimore: Johns Hopkins University Press, 1993), ch. 9.

3. Gladys Swain's work is of fundamental importance in the recent reinterpretation of Pinel's meaning and influence. See G. Swain, *Le sujet de la folie: Naissance de la psychiatrie* (Toulouse: Privat, 1977), especially Part 3, "Les chaînes qu'on enlève;" idem, "La nouveauté du *Traité*

médico-philosophique et ses racines historiques," *Information psychiatrique*, liii (1977), 463–476; idem, "Une logique de l'inclusion: Les infirmes du signe," *Esprit*, v (1982), 61–75; idem, "Du traitement moral: Remarques sur la formation de l'idée contemporaine de psychothérapie," *Confrontations psychiatriques*, xxvi (1986), 19–40.

4. S. Pinel, "'Sur l'abolition des chaînes des aliénés,' par Philippe Pinel, membre de l'Institut, etc.; Note extraite de ses cahiers et communiquée par M. Pinel fils," *Archives générales de médecine*, ii (1823), 15–17.

5. It is curious to discover that Gevingey is a village not far from Géruge where Madame Pinel was born. She may have named the ex-prisoner "Chevingé" when she watched him become her husband's protector and her sons' playmate.

6. S. Pinel, "Bicêtre en 1792. De l'abolition des chaînes," *Mémoires de l'Académie royale de médecine*, v (1836), 31–40.

7. E. Peyriller, "Le geste de Pinel," *Presse médicale*, (1950), no. 59: 1027–1028.

8. These problems are analyzed in D. B. Weiner, "Philippe Pinel, père: Deux générations en conflit," *Perspectives psychiatriques*, xcvi (1984), 100–103; and idem, "Trois moments-clé dans la vie de Philippe Pinel," *Comptes-rendus du 27ème congrès international d'histoire de la médecine* (Barcelona: Acadèmia de Ciencies Médiques de Catalunya i Balears, 1981), I, 154–161.

9. J. E. D. Esquirol, *Des établissements des aliénés en France et des moyens d'améliorer le sort de ces infortunés, mémoire présenté à S. E. le ministre de l'intérieur en septembre 1818* (Paris: Huzard, 1819) reprinted in J. E. D. Esquirol, *Des maladies mentales considérées sous les rapports médical, hygiénique et médico-légal* (Paris: Baillière, 1838) [Reprint, Paris: Editions Frénésie, 1989], 2: 134–150.

10. Ibid., 157.

11. The argument and sources for this interpretation are indebted to Gladys Swain.

12. P. Chabbert, "Les origines familiales de Philippe Pinel," *Histoire des sciences médicales*, xi (1977), 13–18.

13. Personal communication by the abbé Bernard Desprats, archivist of the bishop of Albi, summer 1992.

14. D. B. Weiner, "Philippe Pinel, clerc tonsuré," *Annales de la Société médico-psychologique*, cxlix (1991), 169–173. The article "tonsure" in Diderot's *Encyclopédie*, written at about the time Pinel underwent the procedure, tells us that it had become a mere formality. The abbé Desprats confirmed this view.

15. Georg Wilhelm Friedrich Hegel, *Encyclopedie der philosophischen Wissenschaften im Grundrisse (1830)*, edited by F. Nicolin and O. Poggeler (Hamburg: Meiner, 1969), 338.

16. D. B. Weiner, "Les sources scientifiques de l'aliénisme: L'expertise de Philippe Pinel en histoire naturelle," *Proceedings of the XXXII International Congress for the History of Medicine* (Antwerp, Belgium, 1991), 771–780.

17. P. Pinel, *Nosographie philosophique, ou Méthode de l'analyse appliquée à la médecine* (Paris: Brosson, 1798, 2nd ed., 3 vols., 1802–1803, 3rd. ed., 1807, 4th ed. 1810, 5th ed., 1813, 6th ed., 1818).

18. P. Pinel, *Traité médico-philosophique sur l'aliénation mentale ou la manie* (Paris: Caille et Ravier, 1800). Pinel published a second, much enlarged, edition entitled *Traité médico-philosophique sur l'aliénation mentale* (Paris: Brosson, 1809).

19. P. Pinel, *La médecine clinique rendue plus précise et plus exacte par l'application de l'analyse ou Recueil et résultat d'observations sur les maladies aigües, faites à la Salpêtrière* (Paris: Brosson, Gabon, et Cie., 1802, 2nd ed., 1804, 3rd ed., 1815).

20. L. Castel, *Analyse critique et impartiale de la Nosographie philosophique de Ph. Pinel* (Paris: n.p., An VII [1798–1799]).

21. The other professors demoted to honorary status were the surgeons François Chaussier, Antoine Dubois, A. M. Lallement, and Philippe Joseph Pelletan; the medical inspector Nicolas

René Dufriche Desgenettes; the botanist Antoine Laurent de Jussieu; the pharmacists Nicolas Deyeux, and Nicolas Louis Vauquelin; the former dean Jean Jacques Leroux; and the author and hygienist Moreau de la Sarthe.

22. E. Geoffroy St. Hilaire, "Discours aux funérailles de Philippe Pinel à l'Académie royale des sciences," 27 octobre 1826. Archives, Muséum d'histoire naturelle, b 4143.

23. E. Pariset, "Eloge de Philippe Pinel," lu à la séance du 28 août 1827, *Histoire des membres de l'Académie royale de médecine*, 2 vols. (Paris: Baillère, 1845), I, 209–259.

24. Anon., "Notice" in the *Archives générales de médecine*, xiii (1827), "Variétés," 623–628.

25. G. Dupuytren, "Notice sur Philippe Pinel," *Journal des Débats*, 7 novembre 1826, 14–15.

26. France. Ministère de l'instruction publique. *Procès-verbaux et rapports du comité de mendicité de la Constituante, 1790–1791*, edited by C. Bloch and A. Tuetey (Paris: Imprimerie nationale, 1911), 604.

27. D. B. Weiner, "Philippe Pinel's 'Memoir on Madness' of 11 December 1794: A Fundamental Text of Modern Psychiatry," *American Journal of Psychiatry*, cxlix (1992), 725–732.

28. Pussin writes "Prairial An V" [that is, May–June 1797] in a document in the Archives nationales, 27 A.P. (8), doc. 2. See D. B. Weiner, "The Apprenticeship of Philippe Pinel: A New Document, 'Observations of Citizen Pussin on the Insane,'" *American Journal of Psychiatry*, cxxxvi (1979), 1128–1134.

29. P. Pinel, *Traité médico-philosophique*, 2ème ed. Introduction, xxxi. I believe that the discrepancy between Pussin's and Pinel's dates is due to an error by Pinel: Pussin wrote down the date in the very year of its occurrence, Pinel mentioned it twelve years later.

30. Seine. Conseil général administratif des hôpitaux et hospices civils. *Rapports au conseil général d'administration des hospices civils de Paris sur les objects confiés à sa direction* (Paris: Imprimerie des hôpitaux, An XI), 82, 85.

31. Seine. Conseil général administratif des hôpitaux et hospices civils. *Rapport au conseil général d'administration des hôpitaux et hospices civils de Paris* (Paris: Imprimerie des hôpitaux, 1816), 184.

32. G. L. Bayle, "Considérations sur la nosologie, la médecine d'observation et la médecine pratique" (Paris: Thèse médecine, 1802).

33. This paragraph is indebted to A. Rousseau, "Gaspard Laurent Bayle (1774–1816), le théoricien de l'Ecole de Paris," *Clio medica*, vi (1971), 205–211.

34. See "Gaspard Laurent Bayle" in A. L. J. Bayle and A. J. Thillaye (eds.), *Biographie médicale par ordre chronologique*, 2 vols. (Paris: Delahaye, 1855), 2, 884–899.

35. In 1802, for example, more than 800 students registered for Pinel's course in "internal pathology" at the medical school. AN, France. Affaires culturelles. *Registres d'inscriptions des élèves à l'Ecole de santé*, AJ 16, 6418.

36. F. J. V. Broussais, *Recherches sur la fièvre hectique, considérée comme dépendante d'une lésion d'action des différents systèmes, sans vice organique* (Paris: Thèse médecine), An XI; and idem, *Histoire des phlegmasies ou inflammations chroniques, fondée sur de nouvelles observations de clinique et d'anatomie pathologique: ouvrage présentant un tableau raisonné des variétés et des combinaisons diverses de ces maladies avec leurs différentes méthodes de traitment*, 2 vols. (Paris: Gabon: 1808).

37. E. H. Ackerknecht, *Medicine at the Paris Hospital, 1794–1848* (Baltimore: Johns Hopkins University Press, 1969), 62. See also idem, "Broussais or A Forgotten Medical Revolution," *Bulletin of the History of Medicine*, xxvii (1953), 320–343.

38. A. L. J. Bayle, *Recherches sur les maladies mentales* (Paris: Thèse médecine, 1822).

39. A. L. J. Bayle, *Centenaire de la thèse de Bayle*, 2 vols. (Paris: Masson, 1922), I, 47.

40. Ackerknecht, *Medicine at the Paris Hospital*, 170–171.

41. G. Cuvier, "Eloge historique de Pinel, lu le 11 juin 1827 à l'Académie des sciences,"

Mémoires (Paris: Académie des sciences, 1830), 2nd ser. *9*: ccxxi–cclx. Georges Bollotte has documented the numerous inaccuracies in the materials that Scipion handed to Cuvier, preserved in the archives of the Institut de France. G. Bollotte, "Documents sur Philippe Pinel, recueillis et commentés," *Information psychiatrique*, xliv (1968), 823–841.

42. E. Pariset, "Éloge de Philippe Pinel, lu à la séance du 28 août 1827" in *Histoire des membres de l'Académie royale de médecine*, 2 vols.-in-1 (Paris: Baillière, 1845), *1*: 209–259.

43. I. Violet, *Le myhte de la libération des aliénés de Bicêtre par Philippe Pinel pendant la révolution française* (Paris: UER d'histoire, Paris IV, 1898). For the letter commissioning the painting, see AN F 21 47, 5ème série, dossier 52. These details are given in Violet, *Le mythe*, 103.

44. *Gazette des hôpitaux civils et militaires*, xxii (1849), 459.

45. He may well have chosen the artist, Catherine Sophie Céleste Grandsire (who married François Heussée in 1853). The only thing known about her is that she exhibited two paintings in the Salon of 1845.

46. Seine. Conseil général administratif des hôpitaux et hospices de Paris. *Comptes généraux des hôpitaux et hospices civils, enfants abandonnés, secours à domicile et direction des nourrices de la Ville de Paris. Recette, dépense, population* (Paris: Imprimerie des hôpitaux, An XIII), 194.

47. It is surprising that a learned physician should have written a long and detailed article about laundry. See P. Pinel, "Reflexions sur la buanderie, comme objet d'économie domestique et de salubrité, et application de ces principes à un établissement à l'île du pont de Sève, "*La médecine éclairée par les sciences physiques*, ii (1791), 12–21.

48. Société de médecine de Bruxelles, *Recueil des Observations de Médecine, Chirurgie et Pharmacie, depuis sa réorganisation et dont elle a arrêté l'impression pour l'année 1808 . . .* (Bruxelles, Weissenbruch, 1808), liv.

49. *Les souvenirs du père Richard*, Bibliothèque historique de la Ville de Paris. MS C P 5318, fol. 62–63, quoted in P. Bru, *Histoire de Bicêtre* (Paris: Progrès médical, 1890), 165, n.1. See also L. Boulle, "Bicêtre dans la tourmente révolutionnaire," *Bulletin de la société de l'histoire de Paris et de l'Isle de France*, cxvi (1989), 309–329.

50. Seine. . . . *Comptes généraux*, 194.

51. Designed by A. Spitz and engraved by A. Cottet.

52. "Centenaire de la mort de Pinel et de la naissance de Vulpian," *Annales médico-psychologiques*, lxxxv (1927), and "La condition du malade mental en France, de Pinel à nos jours," Ibid., cxxxiv (1976).

53. T. Gineste and R. Mises, "Le statut fait à l'enfant malade mental, la place de la controverse entre Pinel et Itard," Ibid., 73–81.

54. "Inauguration de la statue de Pinel" in A. Ritti, (ed.), *Histoire des travaux de la Société médico-psychologique et éloges de ses membres*, 2 vols. (Paris: Masson, 1913–1914), I, 425–477.

55. The phrase occurs in a paper on "Bayle and his Critics: The Reception of A. L. J. Bayle's Discovery of General Paresis by French Psychiatry," presented at the 63rd Annual Meeting of the American Association for the History of Medicine, Baltimore, Maryland 10–13 May 1990.

56. See N. J. Jewson, "The Disappearance of the Sick-Man from Medical Cosmology," *Sociology*, x (1976), 225–244.

57. See M. Foucault, *Madness and Civilization: A History of Insanity in the Age of Reason* (New York: Random House, 1973), ch. 9, "Birth of the Asylum."

58. J. Goldstein, *Console and Classify: The French Psychiatric Profession in the Nineteenth Century* (New York: Cambridge University Press, 1987). See especially ch. 3, "The Transformation of Charlatanism, or the Moral Treatment," and especially 72, n. 31.

13

The History of Psychiatry in Italy: A Century of Studies

PATRIZIA GUARNIERI

The Construction of a Past

To establish a real identity it is essential to have a past, a memory. Italian psychiatry has constructed its past while constructing itself: It has tried to emancipate itself—from philosophy, from general medicine, from common sense—and to attain an independent status, in the universities as well as in the asylums where physicians were striving to gain total control.[1]

At first it was only the alienists who began to sketch out their past. A few of them published their memoirs; some commemorated their masters, even sons and grandsons wrote of fathers whose profession they pursued; and when there were no male heirs there were daughters who, if they could not inherit the careers of their fathers, could at least glorify their lives and work, as did Gina and Paola Lombroso.[2] The result was a view of the recent past decidedly hagiographic, though providing useful information, often limited to a few pages in university yearbooks or to obituaries in psychiatric journals. This was not a typical history of psychiatry, but the reflection of academic practices common to all disciplines.

What was instead specific to the psychiatrist-historians were the histories they wrote of the institutions of which they were, or were to become, the directors. Interest in the madhouse of the past was aroused immediately (with Andrea Verga in 1844) in connection with the project for establishing a modern asylum, and was to remain a major interest in Italy from preunification times to the postwar period.[3] This interest was not first triggered by the crusade against the asylums launched in the 1960s and 1970s, as has been suggested by some recent historians. What is significant is precisely how the attitude toward the same subject of research changes, before and after, how strikingly different are the methods and intentions.

From the theoretical viewpoint, with positivism, as well as for the social function it assumed in the unified nation, Italian psychiatry since the midnineteenth century followed an upward path, at least until World War I. The past that was being constructed during this period was designed to glorify a successful journey: *One hundred years and more of conquests (Cento e più anni di conquiste)* was the title of the history proposed in 1920 by the nearly seventy-year-old Enrico Morselli. Splits and dissension had not in fact been lacking; but the official image proposed by these self-satisfied psychiatrists was one of unceasing evolution, in the Comptian sense, "from the errors of the past through current progress and through the reforms still to be enacted." As is apparent in the book by Augusto Tamburini, Giulio Cesare Ferrari, and Giuseppe Antonini entitled *L'assistenza degli alienati in Italia e nelle altre nazioni* (1918), the historical question was viewed in conjunction with analysis of the present, with two main goals: that of supporting a program based on the thesis that the empiricism of asylum techniques should be transcended through growth, both scientific and pertinent to the social role; and that of forging a unitary image of psychiatry on the national level, which was to be sanctioned by the first law on asylums only in 1904, and then only on paper. In composing this unified history, however, the existing wide variety in regional situations, stemming from deeply rooted traditions and influxes from many foreign cultures, would have been poorly representative. As a result, it is still difficult today to unearth knowledge, to discover the significance of many experiences disdained by official psychiatry.

National psychiatry wanted to glorify itself, to show that it had progressed always "through the work of our own men and not merely through importation from lands beyond the Alps." Accordingly, the foreign masters were reappraised or even rejected, although vivid interest was felt in contemporary psychiatry abroad. In various parts of the nation, the presumed Italian pioneers of the legendary French psychiatry were "discovered": Valsalva, Daquin, and Chiarugi, national heroes set above, even in opposition to, Pinel, who was said to have secretly exploited their ideas and usurped their primacy.[4]

If I were asked to name one text from which the history of Italian psychiatry should start, I would choose—for its significance, not for it "objectivity"—an article not restricted to specialists, published by an important daily newspaper in 1864, which dealt expressly with the question of priority between Pinel and Chiarugi. The author was the psychiatrist Carlo Livi.[5] While sustaining the Italian—or better, Tuscan—historical primacy, he simultaneously proclaimed that in his time assistance to the mentally ill in Italy was the most backward in Europe, due to "the indolence and neglect of the governments." Psychiatric reform, Livi declared, could not consist of a gesture or a treatise by a single physician. It must derive from a transformation of society as a whole, such as had taken place in Tuscany in the late eighteenth century, and of which Chiarugi had been only an interpreter in "stripping the chains from the poor madmen and hurling them into the Arno." Thus Livi introduced a new historical perspective, one that was not strictly exclusive to the discipline or to medical institutions. His proposal was to be ignored by subsequent historiography, self-satisfied with the presumed national glories, and although his article was reprinted and discussed, it was for nationalistic purposes only.

Italianizing psychiatry was an undertaking especially apparent in works published during the twenty years of fascism: "We, born of internationalism and, if you wish, of servilism, must react and become more and more Italian," exclaimed Bilancioni in 1923.[6] Some authors shifted attention to the remote past, claiming that modern psychiatry sprang from classic Graeco-Roman, and hence Italian, roots, since "as in all other fields of thought and action, in psychiatry too . . . the Italians have the historical advantage . . . of an unquestionable primacy." This attitude is not surprising for the times, nor was it exclusive to psychiatrists. Nonetheless, the celebration of Italian genius benefited by the contribution of a previous historiographical tradition (that of "great men," "famous scientists") and a certain view of science common to the positivist age; when the subject of science was naturalized as far as possible, the historical dimension was necessarily channeled only through knowledge of that atemporal subject.

In the broad historical overview published by C. Ferrio in 1948, the thought and work of psychiatrists, depicted as continuous progress, were the only possible subjects for the history of psychiatry.[7] The historical subject could not be that of mental illnesses, considered merely as disorders of the brain without social or individual dimensions. Even less could it be the mentally ill themselves, whose life stories were excluded not only from historiography, which in general has given no voice to the weak and oppressed, but primarily from a neuropsychiatry in which they were treated only as the bearers of some organic pathology who were, unlike other sufferers from illness, entirely devoid of the basic human characteristics: the power of reasoning, conscience, and freedom.

With fascism and later, throughout the 1950s, official Italian psychiatry, relegated by academic institutions to a situation of isolation and backwardness, seems to have been entirely overshadowed by neurology. The historiography of this period is equally poor, consisting of a few works offering little more than description, research being nonexistent. The academic portraits of the late masters continued to be produced, with repetitive mention, often eulogizing, of the asylum buildings of the past, but not of what went on inside them. International success, finally attained in 1938 with Cerletti's invention of electroshock treatment, seemed to coincide with an abrupt decline of interest in history on the part of Italian psychiatrists, who had previously viewed it as a means for their own self-aggrandizement. In 1936, it was a lawyer who was to write a superficial work entitled *History of madness (Storia della pazzia)*, which was reprinted in several editions.[8] The need for history was to reemerge during periods of crisis, when it was to act as a stimulus for considering the same subjects from different viewpoints.

Eulogy and Rejection

In the mid-1950s, the introduction of psychotropic drugs aroused great optimism, with the hope that the old asylums packed with chronic cases existing in shameful conditions could be transformed into modern psychiatric hospitals, efficient centers of treatment. The historical studies of this period also focused on the institutions (in 1956, C.I.S.O., a special Italian center for hospital history studies, was established). But in contrast to this, almost as if a sinister history of the past were needed to provide reassurance as to the present, the asylums of former times were portrayed as sites of daily horror, torture, and exploitation, where the poor madmen were turned over "to the hands of jailers."[9] From glorification to rejection: Fluctuation between these two opposite extremes was to continue at length. In Reggio Emilia a competition was held in 1978 to award a contract for setting up a historiographical museum of psychiatry. The examining commission saw that, from the majority of the projects presented, a museum of horrors would be forthcoming, and decided to abandon the idea.[10]

In 1963, four years after the original, the Italian edition of Michel Foucault's *Histoire de la folie à l'âge classique* was published. The thesis of the "great confinement" met with widespread success rather than critical examination, arriving at a moment when the crisis in institutional psychiatry was exploding in Italy, too, where public participation was more intense than elsewhere. The press, the students' movements, the very strong workers' movements, as well as politicians and intellectuals focused on the problems of hospitalized patients, madmen or not, and their families, as the problems of everyone. Drawn out of its isolation and monopolization, the compact image of Italian psychiatry began to splinter into fragments. Formerly marginal trends, such as analytic anthropology and existential phenomenology, Karl Jaspers's and Ludwig Binswanger's ideas, were spreading rapidly; alternative experiences of community and home therapy were becoming more popular. Psychiatry became willingly tainted with philosophy and the human sciences, epistemology, Marxism, the Frankfurt school as well as, in a more controversial manner, the lately introduced psychoanalysis, previously opposed by fascism and by the Church, and viewed by Marxism with indifference up until the sixties (the Italian edition of Freud's *Works* dates from 1967), when a "Freudian-Marxist connubium" began to emerge.[11]

In all this there was a great deal of ideology and flagrant contradictions, but also a remarkable outcry for knowledge, which the university-based medical culture predominating in Italy had been unable even to express. In this climate, the question of history was opened afresh. The Basaglia group called for a history of psychiatry to be written, which Giovanni Jervis and Lucio Schittar were to acclaim in 1967 as the "real history of relations between psychiatrists and the mentally ill."[12] What had seemed "negligible" was now reemerging: for example, even some autobiographical testimony from patients.[13]

That it would be possible to look backward, while going through a profound crisis, was by no means a foregone conclusion. Precisely among those who attacked asylum psychiatry, attempting to strip away its official mask of neutral, progressive science, the temptation to simply deny the past could have prevailed, considering how this past had been falsified or silenced in the heredity that was handed down.[14] There was the risk that, after so much celebration of heroes, a witch-hunt might be launched to discover the sins of the forefathers; the lurking suspicion that the past might hold only something shameful, from which nothing of value could be learned.

Even Foucault's fascinating interpretation gave rise to some paralyzing side effects, among psychiatrists in crisis confronted with the real failure of the asylums and dismayed by the idea that their knowledge was nothing more than an instrument of power of the ruling class. An indirect stimulus to reconsider nineteenth-century Italian psychiatry as compared to that of other European nations arrived with Henri Ellenberger's *The Discovery of the Unconscious* and above all with Klaus Doerner's *Madmen and the Bourgeoisie*, translated in 1975 with an introduction by the psychiatrist Ferruccio Giacanelli, who proclaimed that an Italian history of psychiatry was still entirely to be written, or rewritten.[15]

This negative appraisal met with universal agreement. But, I would like to add, the silence and the inadequate history should be interpreted. The lack of studies was not so much one of quantity as of quality. Some scholars believe that it is merely a question of competence, and opinions differ as to whose competence is involved. The dispute over competence risks becoming a sterile question, especially in Italy, where physicians and historians have no common tradition of mutual exchange of ideas, tending to ignore each other even in their common interest in "the history around us," as admitted by the professor of history of the University of Turin, convinced that "our culture is always, primarily and essentially, notionism."

The representation of a past in which psychiatrists appear as solitary heroes, where their knowledge is presented as a science in constant progress, its practice an increasingly advanced direct application of such knowledge, clashed too sharply with direct experience. Nothing explained the misery hidden behind the walls of the asylum, no voice spoke of the persons who lived there, no prospects were offered for possible change.

It is outside of the academic or official institutions that some historians and psychiatrists have begun to work, occasionally together, with profit. In the last twenty-five years the number of studies carried out in Italy is twice that of those previously produced in an entire century. The quality is higher, enriched by different approaches to a wide range of subjects, accompanied at last by methodological reflection.[16] The inversion of tendency is generally considered to date from 1978. That was the year in which, in Italy, two laws were passed, the 833 and the 180 (known as the Basaglia reform), which called for radical transformation in a psychiatry still anchored to the law of 1904. Changes were made in the role of the physician, the definition of the patient, and the criteria for treatment and the places where it was offered. In this revolution in how psychiatry should be conducted, the final result of a lengthy process, the writing of its history was also to receive new impetus.

The first book to come out after the reform dealt expressly with the past of the institutions that were now supposed to have no future. The *History of the Asylum in Italy from Pre-Unification Times to Today* was written by a judge who repeated the usual theme of the asylum as place for the exercise of social control.[17] Precisely because the law decreed the suppression of the asylums, greater attention was being focused on them by historical research, and there arose the problem of conserving and utilizing their wealth of books, archives, and material, often dispersed. Still today, this problem remains dramatically unsolved.[18] A number of former provincial government and hospital administrations, not the universities, decided to finance the salvaging of sources as well as historical research and centers of study (at Bologna, Naples, Venice, Reggio Emilia, Milan, Turin, Trieste, Arezzo, etc.). Everywhere debates, conferences, and publications were organized. Many of these expressed a rhetorical ideology now outdated and unacceptable. Those who today attempt to view them within their proper context should first of all distinguish between positions. There has not been only one antipsychiatry, just as there has not been only one psychiatry. What emerges, often thanks to research carried out by isolated scholars coming from diverse backgrounds, is an enormous variety. The hundred-year history of the two insane asylums in the south (Aversa and Palermo), ignored up to a few years ago, profoundly changes the unified national image based mainly on the northern institutes (Milan and Reggio Emilia)[19] or deduced from the interpretational models of Klaus Doerner or Michel Foucault or Andrew Scull (translated in 1983), pertinent to different national contexts.

In addition to the concrete need for knowledge, it has been necessary to eliminate ideological simplifications. To do this, much work was required and at last historians, too, have become aware of this.

Historians and Psychiatrists

It was, above all, a conjunction of crises that, in the late 1970s, stimulated historians to discover insanity and psychiatry: crisis in psychiatry, obviously, with all the debate on mental suffering in the family and in society, a debate that was not restricted to an encounter between psychiatrists but became a part of social culture. But also crisis in historiography and in politics, which were closely linked in the Italian scenario of that period. Italian historiography, in fact, which long remained essentially political history and as such retained its cultural primacy, has been seeking, in its disillusion with politics, for other subjects and is more sensitive to the new tendencies coming from abroad (social and quantitative history, anthropology and hermeneutics, etc.).[20]

Some historians, contemporary historians in particular, have begun to work on psychiatric themes as a choice of militant research, politically involved, at times in direct collaboration with some of the ''new psychiatrists'' and magistrates sensitive to the history of social control.[21] They thus show preference for institutional and legislative history and study the former asylums and the criminal lunatics' asylum established in 1876 and surviving even the 1978 reform, as a residue of the past.[22] They propose to describe how the experts in deviant behavior (psychiatrists, as well as anthropologists and criminologists) have played a decisive and ''organic'' role in the constitution of the Italian state.[23] They historicize the nosographic categories and the concepts of ''dangerous individual'' adopted by legal psychiatry;[24] they point out the psychiatrization of prostitutes, or of anarchists, brigands, and other ''primitive rebels'';[25] reveal how psychiatric medicalism masked a socially paradigmatic pathology that is comparable to pellagra, deriving from chronic poverty and malnutrition.[26] While they conduct research on sources never before utilized, these historians are also, of course, strongly attacking the traditional glorification of psychiatry's past. They criticize its presentist or meliorist approach, rejecting its internalistic, scientistic, neutral logic.

Another aspect, in my opinion, is highly interesting and perhaps more original. The Italian historians' ''discovery'' of the history of psychiatry also provides an occasion for self-criticism, for reflecting on widely accepted models and viewpoints. To concern itself with madmen and prostitutes, criminals and vagabonds, Italian Marxist historiography has had to acknowledge that it is responsible for having excluded from history subjects with deviating behavior, insofar as it has always presented ''a sort of implicit glorification of the positive, progressive values of the working classes, of the 'socially conscious' proletariat.''[27] The interest in psychiatric institutions and mental illness has immediately contributed to a less schematic social history, forming a special observation point from which previously explored topics (for example, the war) could be viewed from another angle.[28]

Instead of insisting on the dual theme of administration and ideology, emphasizing the links between social control and psychiatry, ruling classes, and subordinate classes, it is proposed that an identity be given to those interned; according to social order, as is customary, but also according to age and gender, as some women historians are now doing, for example, in regard to hysterics or infanticides.[29] Some researchers are attempting to reconstruct the life stories of the patients, the real experiences of concrete individuals. These are essentially micro-histories of madmen, or those suspected of madness, at the center of legal and psychiatric events; cases rich in mixed documentation (the records of the trial, the medical experts' reports, the press), contribute equally to the history of *mentalités* and the history of the sciences. They are highly suitable for verifying how and which psychiatric theses were applied in practice, not behind the walls of the asylum but openly before public opinion, either in contrast to or agreement with the magistrates' authority.[30]

While the social historians have been concerned mainly with institutions, subordinate classes, and social rejection, the historians of ideas, of culture, and of the sciences have been focusing their attention on psychiatric knowledge, free from any hagiographic concerns.

Since the late 1970s, there has been a growing interest in the history of the culture of positivism, formerly neglected in favor of Hegelism and Marxism and, to an even greater degree, of the philosophical and scientific culture of the modern era, which has long been a major interest of Italian scholars. The scholars of Italian positivism inevitably run up against debates on science and philosophy, on ethical and social issues such as suicide, in which the psychiatrists of the nineteenth and twentieth centuries participated as protagonists, as was, for example, the case of Enrico Morselli, the founder of the *Rivista di filosofia scientifica*, the journal of the Italian positivists.[31]

In a 1984 congress on Italian positivist culture, a special sector was dedicated to psychiatry. Recent research critically compares widely varying sources, does not limit itself to reflecting official sources (proceedings of congresses or psychiatric textbooks), but distinguishes between the fame of some theories or personages and the degree to which they have been truly influential (Italian psychiatry, for instance, is certainly not entirely Lombrosian).[32] The panorama it reveals is complex, consisting of more than a mere accumulation of new knowledge on subjects previously ignored. Italian historians have often applied the stereotyped, deprecating label of "biological" to the psychiatry of positivism as a whole. Recently, however, it has been admitted that this historiographical category is inadequate for representing a complex cultural situation where, for example, along with some official declarations of "biological" nature, there was also experimental research, therapies, and psychiatric-legal expertise based on a psychological approach.

Currently, the demand for knowledge of a historical nature is growing among psychiatric professionals. Some mental health centers are offering courses on this subject. In the Italian university, instead, the history of psychiatry and of insanity is still unrecognized, nor does it find an easy welcome in the existing disciplines where its presence would be legitimate and stimulating, such as the history of medicine and the history of science, the latter having been too long restricted to the so-called strong sciences.

Once more I would like to state that this is not merely a question of extending the field of historical research to psychiatry, nor even less of confining it to a specially reserved area. Precisely due to the difficult identity of psychiatry, a critical knowledge of its past is important. It will help also to renovate certain historiographical and conceptual traditions, to reflect on broader issues, such as the model of scientific thought that has historically prevailed in our culture, the relationship between natural sciences and behavioral sciences, and the controversy between explanation and comprehension first launched by Dilthey and then taken up by Jaspers and Binswanger, a controversy in which the philosophers, but not yet the historians of science and of ideas, have shown interest.

Much still remains to be done. Among the many planned research projects, some have not been carried out, and there has been more criticism than constructive work.

However, the ferment of work among historians has had positive repercussions among the psychiatrists who are writing history, now with greater attention to methodology. It is a very recent innovation that even official psychiatry, often accused of immobility and hostility to new ideas, is declaring an interest in history. In 1986, a national congress on the history of psychiatry was organized at the Faculty of Medicine of the Università Cattolica in Rome. The broad range of subjects of the many papers presented by scholars of widely varying backgrounds gives some idea of the variety (and also of a certain confusion) that distinguishes current historiography.[33] If the reawakened interest in historical studies in the last twenty-five years has taken place, thanks to the more critical psychiatrists who have backed, from various positions, the reform movement (I purposely avoid using the term "anti-psychiatry," as its connotations are too restricted), it is interesting to note that recently some psychiatrists totally opposed to the 1978 reform have also turned to history; occasionally with presentist intentions, and ideological ones again, to condemn a monolithic anti-psychiatry, caricatured as "nothing but a power maneuver, an internecine struggle for power in the Palace, a transferral of psychiatric control from those who possessed medical knowledge to those who possessed socio-political power."[34] This, when Basaglia's former collaboraters are now inviting us, as Jervis has done, to reflect on the recent history of Italian psychiatry, avoiding ideological simplifications in which "psychiatry" and "anti-psychiatry" are counterpoised as if they were two homogeneous camps.[35] Ideological simplification is really the last thing we need, either in writing history or in trying to deal better with the complex problems of mental suffering. At this very moment in Italy, the politicians are discussing a proposed new law for psychiatric assistance. It would be sad, indeed, if future decisions should be made without a thorough critical knowledge of the past.

Notes

For their criticisms to this paper I would like to thank Giovanni Jervis, Roy Porter, and Renzo Villa. For an enlarged version in a volume with an Italian bibliography of the history of psychiatry (1864–1990) including about 820 titles, see Patrizia Guarnieri, *La storia della psichiatria: un secolo di studi in Italia* (Florence: Olschki, 1991).

1. In 1874, psychiatry was first organized into a national association, *the Società Italiana di Freniatria*, with a journal of its own, the *Rivista sperimentale di freniatria e di medicina legale*, founded in 1875 by Carlo Livi; for the proceedings of the Società italiana di freniatria, since 1874, see also the *Archivio Italiano per le Malattie Nervose e più particolarmente per le Alienazioni Mentali*.

2. Gina Lombroso and Paola Lombroso, *Cesare Lombroso: appunti sulla vita* (Turin: Bocca, 1906); Gina Lombroso Ferrero, *Cesare Lombroso. Storia della vita e delle opere narrata dalla figlia* (Turin: Bocca, 1915). Also, Giuseppe Vidoni, *Giacomo Vidoni e il manicomio di S. Daniele nel Friuli* (Messina: La Sicilia, 1924); Biagio Miraglia, Jr., "Un grande frenologo italiano: Biagio Miraglia," *Bollettino dell'Istituto storico italiano di arte sanitaria*, ix (1929), 217–243; Biagio Miraglia, *Un alienista patriota: B. Miraglia nel cinquantenario della sua morte* (Milan: Scuola tip. Villa Russo, 1936); Enrico Morselli, "La mente di Carlo Livi," *Rivista sperimentale di freniatria*, v (1879), 1–47; and Augusto Tamburini, "La mente di Carlo Livi," *Rivista sperimentale di freniatria*, vi (1880) i–xxxiii; articles on Biffi by Giuseppe Antonini, A. Raggi, A. Ratti, and Augusto Tamburini in Serafino Biffi, *Opere complete* (Milan: Hoepli, 1902) rispetti-

vamente lxiii–lxxi, xliv–lxi, xxv–xli, and xiii–xxiv. Among the autobiographies: Clodimiro Bonfigli, "Sulla vita scientifica e professionale del Dott. Prof. Comm. Clodimiro Bonfigli," *Giornale di psichiatria clinica e tecnica manicomiale*, xxv (1907), 151–188; Enrico Morselli, "Enrico Morselli" in Onofrio Roux (ed.), *Infanzia e giovinezza di Illustri Italiani contemporanei*, vol. 3 (Florence: Bemporad, 1910), 315–363; Francesco De Sarlo, *Esame di coscienza. Quarant'anni dopo la laurea* (Florence: stab. Bardellini, 1928); Corrado Tumiati, *I tetti rossi. Ricordi di un manicomio* (Milan: Treves, 1931).

3. Andrea Verga, "Cenni storici sugli stabilimenti dei pazzi in Lombardia," *Gazzetta medica di Milano*, iii (1844), 342 ff., repr. in *Studi anatomici sul cranio e sull'encefalo psicologici e freniatrici*, vol. 3 (Milan: Manini-Wiget, 1897), 455–481; and Serafino Biffi, "Sui manicomi," *Rendiconti R. Istituto Lombardo di scienze e lettere* (Milan: Vallardi, 1876), repr. in *Opere complete*, 423–455. For the long list of historical writings on madhouses, see "Bibliografia italiana di storia della psichiatria," in Patrizia Guarnieri, *La storia della psichiatria*; but here at least compare the earlier essays of this kind, such as Alfredo Alvisi, *L'antico ospedale dei pazzi in Bologna* (Bologna: tip. Fava e Garagnani, 1881), Antonio Marro, *Le condizioni passate e presenti del R. Manicomio di Torino* (Turin, 1893), Vincenzo Grasselli, *L'ospedale di S. Lazzaro presso Reggio nell'Emilia* (Reggio Emilia: Calderini, 1897), Ferdinando Ugolotti, *L'assistenza degli alienati e i loro ospedali di ricovero in quel di Parma* (Parma: tip. Operaia, 1907), Luigi Scabia, *Il frenocomio di San Girolamo in Volterra* (Volterra: stab. Carneri, 1910), F. Cascella, *Il manicomio di Aversa nel I centenario della fondazione* (Aversa: Noviello, 1913).

4. See G. Bilancioni, "Un grande precursore di Pinel: Valsalva," *Rivista di storia critica delle scienze mediche e naturali*, iv (1913), 75–79; Arturo Castiglioni, "I precursori italiani di Filippo Pinel," *Rassegna clinico-scientifica*, v (1927), 366–369; Emilio Padovani, "Pinel e il rinnovamento dell'assistenza agli alienati. I suoi precursori," *Giornale di psichiatria clinica e tecnica manicomiale*, lv (1927), 68–124.

5. Carlo Livi, "Pinel o Chiarugi? Lettera al celebre Dott. A. Brierre de Boismont," *La Nazione*, 18, 19, 20 Sept. 1864, repr. in *Gazzetta del manicomio di Macerata*, iii (1879); see also Antonio D'Ormea, "Pagine di storia. Pinel o Chiarugi," *Rassegna di studi psichiatrici*, xvi (1927), 213–233; and Carlo Ferrio, *La psiche e i nervi. Introduzione storica* (Turin: Utet, 1948), 306–318.

6. G. Bilancioni, "La figura e l'opera di Valsalva," *Rivista di storia delle scienze mediche e naturali*, xiv (1923), 319–340. The quotation is from Marco Levi Bianchini, "Contributo alla storia della stampa psichiatrica e neurologica in Italia dalla origine (fine del secolo xviii) all'epoca attuale," *Archivio generale di neurologia, psichiatria e psicoanalisi*, xviii (1937), 5–20. Typical P. Capparoni, "La riforma Pinel nel trattamento degli alienati preconizzata in Italia dal Valsalva, Daquin e Chiarugi non è che un ritorno agli antichi precetti dei medici greci e romani," *Il Sanitario di Puglia, Basilicata e Calabria*, vii, 1927, 11–22; also see the collected essays by Lorenzo Gualino, *Saggi di medicina storica* (Turin: Minerva Medica, 1930).

7. See Ferrio, *La psiche e i nervi*.

8. See Bruno Cassinelli, *Storia della pazzia* (Milan: Corbaccio, 1936), translated into French in 1939. The most useful contributions of that time concerned the Italian psychiatric press, see Levi Bianchini, "Contributo alla storia," and Giorgio Padovani, *La stampa periodica italiana di neuropsichiatria e scienze affini nel primo centenario di sua vita (1843–1943)* (Milan: Hoepli, 1946).

9. See, among the contributions presented at the 1st Italian Congress of C.I.S.O., Piero Benassi, "I più antichi ospedali psichiatrici italiani," and Emilio Padovani, "Appunti di storia dell'assistenza ospedaliera degli infermi di mente," both in *Atti del Primo congresso italiano di storia ospitaliera (14–17 giugno 1956)* (Reggio Emilia: A.G.E., 1957), 41–50 and 523–536.

10. But see some of the collected materials "Per un museo storiografico della psichiatria. Atti del 'Concorso pubblico di idee,' " *Rivista sperimentale di freniatria*, ciii (1979), suppl. 667–855 and 1089–1317, and the catalogue of the exhibition, Maurizio Bergomi et al. (eds.), *Il cerchio*

del contagio. Il S. Lazzaro tra lebbra, povertà e follia 1178–1980 (Reggio Emilia: Ist. Neuropsichiatrici S. Lazzaro, 1980).

11. The first book on the difficult story of Freudian ideas in Italy is by the French scholar Michel David, *La psicoanalisi nella cultura italiana* (Turin: Boringhieri, 1966), rev. and enlarged ed. 1990; and cf. Aldo Carotenuto, *Jung e la cultura italiana* (Rome: Astrolabio, 1976).

12. Giovanni Jervis and Lucio Schittar, "Storia e politica in psichiatria: alcune proposte di studio" in Franco Basaglia (ed.), *Che cos'è la psichiatria* (Parma: Amministrazione Provinciale, 1967, repr. Turin: Einaudi, 1973), 171–202.

13. See the autobiography of a woman inmate of the asylum in Arezzo for forty years, Adalgisa Conti, *Manicomio 1914, Gentilissimo sig. dottore questa è la mia vita*, edited by Luciano Della Mea (Milan: Mazzotta, 1978); and a collection of letters by inmates of the asylum in Volterra that had been censored by the directors, Carmelo Pellicanò et al. (eds.), *Corrispondenza negata. Epistolario della nave dei folli (1889–1974)* (Pisa: Pacini, 1983). Also, Giuliana Morandini (ed.), *E allora mi hanno rinchiusa. Testimonianze dal manicomio femminile* (Milan: Bompiani, 1977).

14. Thus not by chance one preferred to look elsewhere: Reading Laing and Cooper suggested that Conolly should be reevaluated in place of Pinel, whose importance has been reduced; see Agostino Pirella, "Introduzione" in John Conolly, *Trattamento del malato di mente senza metodi costrittivi* (Turin: Einaudi, 1976), vii–xxxvii.

15. Ferruccio Giacanelli, "Appunti per una storia della psichiatria in Italia," in Klaus Doerner, *Il borghese e il folle. Storia sociale della psichiatria* (Rome-Bari: Laterza, 1975), v–xxxii.

16. It was precisely to problems of methodology that the C.I.S.O. Congress of 1975 was dedicated, with the participation of, among others, Franco Basaglia and Paolo Conti, Stefano Bianchi, Fabrizio Asioli, Ferruccio Giacanelli, and Hrayr Terzian; see *Storia della sanità in Italia. Metodo e indicazioni di ricerca* (Rome: Il pensiero scientifico, 1978).

17. See Romano Canosa, *Storia del manicomio in Italia dall'Unità ad oggi* (Milan: Feltrinelli, 1979). Among other historical research on specific asylums, see also Fabio Stok, *L'officina dell'intelletto: Alle origini dell'istituzione psichiatrica in Toscana* (Rome: Il pensiero scientifico, 1983); Stok, "Luigi Scabia e l'ospedale psichiatrico di Volterra," extr. *Neopsichiatria*, i–iv (1983); Paolo Giovannini, *Il manicomio di S. Benedetto di Pesaro. Follia, psichiatria e sanità (1829–1914)* (Urbino: Montefeltro ed. 1983); Valeria Pezzi, "Il S. Lazzaro negli anni del regime (1920–1945)," in *Regime e società civile a Reggio Emilia* (Reggio Emilia: Bibl. Municipale A. Panizzi, 1986), 385–596.

18. A first incomplete attempt to give a map of the sources existing in the national archives is by Gino Badini, "Archivi e psichiatria. Primi risultati per una ricerca delle fonti documentarie negli Archivi di stato italiani," in *L'emarginazione psichiatrica nella storia e nella società. Atti del convegno nazionale*, suppl. *Rivista sperimentale di freniatria*, 1980, 1281–1302. But some specific archives have been ordered and evaluated; for a discussion on this, see Mario Galzigna (ed.), *La follia, la norma, l'archivio. Prospettive storiografiche e orientamenti archivistici* (Venice: Marsilio, 1984).

19. On these better-known institutions, consult Francesco De Peri, "Il medico e il folle: istituzione psichiatrica, sapere scientifico e pensiero medico tra otto e Novecento" in Franco Della Peruta (ed.), *Storia d'Italia. Annali 7: Malattia e Medicina* (Turin: Einaudi, 1984), 679–704. On the southern asylums, see at least, Vittorio Donato Catapano, *Le Reali Case de' Matti nel Regno di Napoli* (Naples: Liguori, 1986), Germana Agnetti and Angelo Barbato, *Il barone Pisani e la Real Casa de' Matti* (Palermo: Sellerio, 1987).

20. For the analysis of Italian historiography and its crisis, see Tommaso Detti, Nicola Gallerano, and Tim Mason (eds.), the special issue on "Storia contemporanea oggi. Per una discussione," *Movimento operaio e socialista*, x (1987), no. 1–2, especially Nicola Gallerano, "Fine del caso italiano? La storia politica tra 'politicità' e 'scienza,' " 5–26 and Paola Di Cori, "Soggettività e pratica storica," 77–90.

21. This is the case of Alberto De Bernardi, Francesco De Peri, Laura Panzeri, *Tempo e catene. Manicomio, psichiatria e classi subalterne. Il caso milanese* (Milan: F. Angeli, 1980) and of many among the contributers to a congress (Milan, April 1980) of which see Alberto De Bernardi (ed.), *Follia, psichiatria e società. Istituzioni manicomiali, scienza psichiatrica e classi sociali nell'età moderna e contemporanea* (Milan: F. Angeli, 1982). At the same time, there was the congress on *L'emarginazione psichiatrica*, (Reggio Emilia, April 1980).

22. See Alberto Manacorda, *Il manicomio giudiziario. Cultura psichiatrica e scienza giuridica nella storia di un'istituzione totale* (Bari: De Donato, 1982) and S. Gadioli, M. Lescovelli, S. Panizza, V. Micheletti, "Origine dottrinaria e storica del manicomio criminale," *Rivista sperimentale di freniatria*, cvi (1982), 742–766 and "Il problema del manicomio giudiziario dal dopoguerra a oggi," *ivi*, 767–783; Francesco Degl'Innocenti, "La funzione del manicomio criminale in Italia 1872–1891," *ivi*, cxiii (1989), 1218–1235.

23. For example, Ferruccio Giacanelli, "Un nuovo quadro professionale della borghesia nel secolo XIX: il passaggio dello psichiatra fra filantropia medica e controllo sociale," in *L'emarginazione psichiatrica*, 915–928; Valeria Paola Babini et al., *Tra sapere e potere. La psichiatria italiana nella seconda metà dell'Ottocento* (Bologna: il Mulino, 1982), exp. Maurizia Cotti, "L'istituzione manicomiale nel nuovo stato unitario," *ivi*, 199–246 and Fernanda Minuz, "Gli psichiatri italiani e l'immagine della loro scienza 1860–1875," 27–76; Minuz, "Le sedi dell'apprendimento della pratica psichiatrica. Psichiatria nazionale e psichiatria negli Stati pontifici," *Sanità, scienza e storia*, i (1985), 109–138. For the criminological aspects, see the catalogue of the exhibition in Turin, Umberto Levra (ed.), *La scienza e la colpa. Crimini, criminali, criminologi: un volto dell'Ottocento* (Milan: Electa, 1985).

24. Raffaele Castiglioni, "Malattia mentale e pericolosità. Osservazioni sul concetto di pericolosità," *Rivista sperimentale di freniatria*, cviii (1984), 1280–1298, 1633–1648; Ugo Fornari, "Monomania e pazzia morale. Il contributo della psichiatria italiana," *Criminologia*, viii (1986), 3–49; Fornari, "Nozione di malattia, valore di malattia, vizio di mente e problemi nel trattamento dell'autore del reato," *Rivista sperimentale di freniatria*, cxi (1987), 1043–1063; Fornari, "Improvviso furore, coscienza e volontà dell'atto: storia di un concetto," *ivi*, 1325–1351; Fornari, "Irresistibile impulso e responsabilità penale," *ivi*, cxii (1988), 43–85; Fornari and Rossana Rosso, "Libertà morale, infermità di mente e forza irresistibile," *Rivista italiana di medicina legale*, x (1988), 1139–1174; Rossana Rosso, "Piromania e disturbo del controllo degli impulsi", *ivi*, xi (1989), 899–937.

25. Cf. Sergio Mellina, "L'emigrante alienato di fine Ottocento" in F. M. Ferro et al. (eds.), *Passioni della mente e della storia* (Milan: Vita e pensiero, 1989), 409–420; Renzo Villa, "Davide Lazzaretti e il monte Amiata" in *Protesta sociale e rinnovamento religioso*, edited by Carlo Pazzagli (Florence: Nuova Guaraldi, 1981), 340–353; Roberto Cappuccio, Ellena Pioli, "Dementi, gettatelli, mendicanti, devianti," *Studi Lunigianesi*, xiv–xv (1984–85), 39–70; and Cappuccio and Pioli: "Affermazione del modello di intervento psichiatrico in una realtà territoriale circoscritta," *Psichiatria e territorio*, vi (1989), 143–80.

26. Alberto De Bernardi, *Il mal della rosa. Denutrizione e pellagra nelle campagne italiane fra Ottocento e Novecento* (Milan: F. Angeli, 1984); on more studies about this topic, see the review by Paolo Sorcinelli, "Per una storia della malattia in Italia," *Sanità, scienza e storia*, ii (1984), 64–100.

27. Antonio Gibelli, "Emarginati e classi lavoratrici. le ragioni di un nodo storiografico," *Movimento operaio e socialista*, iii (1980), 361–367; it is the self-critical preface by the editor of the journal to a special issue on "Crimine e follia" including articles by Antonio Gibelli, Luigi Ganapini, Paola Lanzavecchia, Piero Lingua, Giuseppe Sinigaglia, Massimo Quaini, and Renzo Villa.

28. In the 1980s some additional historical journals dealt with the history of the mentally ill and criminals, such as *Rivista di storia contemporanea*, xi (1982), no.3, 337–398); *Società e storia*; and *Sanità, scienza e storia*, founded in 1984.

29. Among women historians' studies, see C. Cacciari, R. Lamberti, "Moebius, Weininger. La donna come meno, la donna come nulla," *Nuova Dwf*, xvi (1981), suppl., 56–72; Mariapina Colazzo, "Quale donna turba il cervello dell'alienista? Ipotesi di lavoro alla ricerca del paradigma della follia declinata al femminile," in *Follia, psichiatria*, 414–425; Maria A. Trasforini, "Corpo isterico e sguardo medico. Storie di vita e storie di sguardi," *Aut aut*, clxxxvii–clxxxviii (1982), 175–206; AnnaMaria Tagliavini, "Il fondo oscuro dell'anima femminile" in Valeria Paola Babini et al. (eds.), *La donna nelle scienze dell'uomo* (Milan: F. Angeli, 1986), 78–113; Sabina Cremonini, "Un'arpa senza concerto. Il caso di Clelia, un'isterica nel manicomio di Reggio Emilia" in Alessandro Pastore and Paolo Sorcinelli (eds.), *Sanità e società*, vol. II (Udine: Casamassima-Fidia, 1987), 351–370. But the majority deal with criminological and anthropological aspects; see on infanticide, mainly on legal aspects, Rossella Selmini, *Profili di uno studio storico sull'infanticidio. Esame di 31 processi per infanticidio giudicati dalla Corte di Assise di Bologna dal 1880 al 1913* (Milan: Giuffré, 1987) and the bibliography of the special issue on "Donne devianza e controllo sociale," *Dei delitti e delle pene*, i (1983).

30. Patrizia Guarnieri, *L'ammazzabambini. Legge e scienza in un processo toscano di fine Ottocento* (Turin: Einaudi, 1988, "microstorie"); Eng. trans., *A Case of Child Murder*, Polity Press, 1993); Paolo Sorcinelli, *La repressione ambigua. Il caso giudiziario e psichiatrico di un finto frate agli inizi del '900* (Milan: F. Angeli, 1989).

31. Patrizia Guarnieri, *Individualità difformi. La psichiatria antropologica di Enrico Morselli* (Milan: F. Angeli, 1986); and on the positivistic journal founded by Morselli, cf. Guarnieri, "La volpe e l'uva'. Cultura scientifica e filosofia nel positivismo italiano," *Physis*, xxv (1983), 601–636. A collection of Morselli's writings is edited by Lino Rossi, "Enrico Morselli e le scienze dell'uomo nell'età del positivismo," *Rivista sperimentale di freniatria*, suppl. no.6, 1984.

32. Among his several essays on Lombroso, see the book by Renzo Villa, *Il deviante e i suoi segni. Lombroso e la nascita dell'antropologia criminale* (Milan: F. Angeli, 1985) and cf. with the useful but traditional biography by Luigi Bulferetti, *Cesare Lombroso* (Turin: Utet, 1975). In the context of social Darwinism and the crisis of Italian positivism, Lombroso is seen by Giuliano Pancaldi, *Darwin in Italia. Impresa scientifica e frontiere culturali* (Bologna: il Mulino, 1983), 379–391 and Luisa Mangoni, *Una crisi di fine secolo. La cultura italiana e la Francia fra Otto e Novecento* (Turin: Einaudi, 1985).

33. See *Passioni della mente e della storia* (note 25)

34. Luciano Del Pistoia, Luciano Canova, "Pinel, Chiarugi, Lucca: origine e senso del trattamento morale" in Luciano Del Pistoia and Franco Bellato (eds.), *Curare e ideologia del curare* (Lucca: Pacini-Fazzi, 1981), 54–69, quote p. 68.

35. Giovanni Jervis, "L'antipsichiatria fra innovazione e settarismo," paper at the congress on "Psichiatria a confronto" (Rome: 28 June 1985), *Mondoperaio*, xxxix (1986), 125–28, repr. *Lavoro neuropsichiatrico*, i (1986), 55–61. For the experiences of Italian psychiatry during the last forty-five years told by one of its protagonists, see Sergio Piro, *Cronache psichiatriche. Appunti per una storia della psichiatria italiana dal 1945* (Naples: Edizioni scientifiche italiane, 1988).

14

The History of the Asylum Revisited: Personal Reflections

GERALD N. GROB

More than thirty years ago a colleague asked me a seemingly innocuous question about the history of psychiatry and the mentally ill. Intellectual curiosity then led me on a scholarly odyssey that began with a study of a single hospital and state, and concluded with a three-volume work that attempted to provide a comprehensive narrative of the ways in which American society managed the human, social, and economic problems associated with mental illnesses. At the time there was virtually no indication that the subject would become the focal point of a rich and controversial debate that served to act as a catalyst for research and a means of illuminating relationships between social structures and individual behavior. In this essay I should like to recount and to evaluate—employing both historiographical and autobiographical perspectives—the transformation of a marginal subject into one that has engaged historians, physicians, social and behavioral scientists, policy analysts, and public officials.

Before 1960 the study of mental illnesses and asylums was a relatively insignificant subject virtually lacking controversy. Many works dealing with the history of psychiatry were written by psychiatrists. Their celebratory tone indicated a desire to demonstrate the march of progress in their specialty. Gregory Zilboorg's well-known volume, which traced the evolution of psychiatric thought, was written with an inevitable Whig and historicist bias. To Zilboorg the history of psychiatry represented a secularizing movement from superstition to medical science. Nor was his approach unique. The volume of essays edited by J. K. Hall—the one-time president of the American Psychiatric Association—celebrated the centennial of the organization and embodied a similar theme, though in a somewhat more muted form. That these works had a Whiggish bias is not to suggest that they were bereft of value. On the contrary, they provided valuable information about a subject all too often ignored by mainstream academic historians. Nevertheless, the underlying commitment to study the history of psychiatry, institutions, and the mentally ill in terms of progress tended to make these works somewhat insensitive to contradictions, paradoxes, and the role of social, cultural, and intellectual factors.[1]

The most significant work on American psychiatry written within the Whig tradition was Albert Deutsch's classic *The Mentally Ill in America*. Paradoxically, Deutsch was not a physician. The son of Jewish immigrants, he grew up in harsh poverty and always identified with the poor and downtrodden. Although he never attended college, he was a voracious reader. While working on a project in the early 1930s that involved the collection of documents on the New York State Department of Welfare, he became fascinated with historical sources pertaining to the mentally ill. With verve and imagination, he persuaded Clifford W. Beers and the National Committee for Mental Hygiene to subsidize the research and writing of his book. When the completed manuscript was sent out for review to some prominent psychiatrists, profound differences emerged. The committee staff took the position that the manuscript was owned by the organization, which had final authority to make changes. In the end the differences were resolved, and the book appeared in 1937. Deutsch subsequently coauthored a history of public welfare in New York State, and during the 1940s and 1950s became the preeminent psychiatric and medical journalist of his generation. Indeed, his political liberalism and activist stance made him persona non grata to such AMA figures as Morris Fishbein, who regarded Deutsch as an exponent of Communist and Marxian ideology.[2]

The Mentally Ill in America was, in many ways, a tour de force. It reflected admirably the prevailing progressive ethos that dominated the writing of American history from the early twentieth century through World War II.[3] Written at a time when interest in or knowledge about the history of psychiatry and the mentally ill was nil, the work was based on primary sources that heretofore had not been used. Starting from scratch, Deutsch created an imposing historical framework that began with the travails of the mentally ill in colonial America when "punishment, repression and indifference" were characteristic. He then detailed the creation of mental hospitals in the early nineteenth century and their subsequent checkered development. Deutsch ranged widely over a variety of topics: concepts of mental illnesses, mental hygiene, and public policy. Committed to a historical tradition that emphasized progress, he nevertheless concluded that prevailing practices and policies still left much to be desired. Responsibility for existing shortcomings, he averred, rested with American society, which had failed to provide sufficient resources to meet the needs of the mentally ill. Even in his devastating exposés of public mental hospitals first published in the columns of the liberal newspaper *PM* in the mid-1940s and issued in book from in 1948, Deutsch did not despair about the future of institutional care and treatment. The "Ideal State Hospital," he insisted, was not a utopian dream, and he issued a clarion call for the public and their elected representatives to provide the needed resources.[4] In all of his work Deutsch combined historical analysis and a commitment to liberal reform, thus avoiding the extremes of either defending the status quo or rejecting psychiatry.

For more than a generation *The Mentally Ill in America* remained the definitive work on the subject even though few followed Deutsch's impressive beginning. Aside from some isolated doctoral dissertations, American historians manifested virtually no interest in the subject. They continued to emphasize political, military, and diplomatic topics. Even those who wrote about cultural and intellectual trends or reform movements rarely mentioned the mentally ill except in passing. Historians who helped to create the consensus school of American history after 1945—a school that minimized class divisions and emphasized the elements that united Americans—largely ignored the mentally ill as well as other dependent and socially marginal groups that remained outside the mainstream.

During and after the 1960s, however, profound changes occurred in the writing of history. The general unrest arising out of war, racism, and poverty stimulated interest in these perennial problems. The growing popularity of the idea that all scholarship inevitably reflected ideological assumptions and commitments, moreover, led to an emphasis on the role of class and gender, and a proliferation of studies of "inarticulate" groups. Fascination with quantification and the influence of the social and behavioral sciences likewise reinforced interest in social structure—an approach that had already enjoyed a renaissance in Europe because of the influence of the French *Annales* school. Under the leadership of Lucien Febvre and Marc Bloch, members of this school attempted to obliterate traditional disciplinary boundaries in the hope of developing a more unified way of studying the experience of entire societies. The new social history, as it was often called, represented a peculiar amalgamation of scholarship, ideology, and activism. In the hands of some practitioners it became a surrogate for social if not revolutionary, change; in the hands of others it led to truly innovative scholarship.

Another source of change came from developments within the social and behavioral sciences. The rapprochement between psychiatry and the social and behavioral sciences, begun by Harry Stack Sullivan in the 1930s, continued after World War II. In the postwar decades the rise of the subdiscipline of medical sociology stimulated additional interest in mental illnesses and the role of psychiatry in America. That many historians were attracted to the subject was hardly surprising, given the fact that scholarly disciplines do not exist in an intellectual and cultural vacuum.

Out of this ferment came a distinctly different approach to the history of medicine. New social historians of medicine began to ask novel questions and explore hitherto neglected problems: the relationship between medicine and society; the interplay of popular and professional concepts of health and disease; the role of environmental and socioeconomic variables in changing morbidity and mortality patterns; the rise of new institutional forms and systems of treatment and care; and the ways in which medical interventions and technologies were actually employed. In so doing, they appreciably weakened the older commitment to Whiggish history and historicism. Less concerned with celebrating the progress of medicine, the new scholarship sought to understand the sources of change, the ways in which health care systems worked, and the uses to which such systems and technologies were put.[5]

Paradoxically, the greatest stimulus to research into the history of mental illnesses and psychiatry came not from historians but from social and psychiatric critics, including Michel Foucault, Thomas Szasz, Erving Goffman, and R. D. Laing. Save for their hostility to traditional forms of psychiatry, these individuals had little in common. Foucault flourished in a postwar revolutionary Parisian environment that had altered traditional forms of discourse and synthesized insights from Marx and Freud. Szasz was committed to a nineteenth-century classical libertarian ideology. Goffman was preoccupied with the overriding importance of personal autonomy. Laing's critique of psychiatry drew heavily on the social activism and political radicalism of the 1960s. Whatever their differences, these and other like-minded individuals adopted a hostile stance toward psychiatry. Their work exerted a powerful influence on new social historians seeking to explain the origins of institutions dealing with deviancy.

In 1961 Foucault published his famous *Histoire de la folie* (translated into English a few years later in truncated form). This provocative and idiosyncratic book sought to describe the changing inner meaning of madness from the late middle ages to the birth of the asylum in the eighteenth century. Unlike liberal scholars who saw the asylum as a symbol of progress, Foucault had a quite different interpretation of this ubiquitous institution. The creation of asylums, he averred, represented an attempt to conquer madness by imposing a new system designed to enforce conformity. In Pinel's hands, he wrote, the asylum became "an instrument of moral conformity and of social denunciation." The new understanding of insanity required that madpersons assume responsibility for their own condition. Nor was moral therapy a synonym for kind and humane treatment; it was rather an effort to force insane persons to develop an understanding of their own moral transgressions and then to alter their behavior by internalizing the values of their keepers. The physician thus became the "essential figure of the asylum." His authority, however, did not derive from science, but rather from the moral and social order associated with bourgeois society and its values. Foucault's writings tended to demythologize psychiatry because of his insistence that the specialty's appeal was to be found not in its contribution to an understanding of human behavior, but in its relationships to the sources of power and domination.[6]

Ever-changing and often obscure, Foucault's writings became one of the pillars of dissenting and counterculture thought during and after the 1960s. His work seemed to strip away the melioristic and idealistic veneer of an alleged medical specialty and presumably benevolent institutions and lay bare their role in enforcing a universal conformity. By the late 1960s Foucault was one of the patron saints of a group of historians and social scientists determined to discredit the older idea that mental hospitals represented progress. Their scholarly studies often emphasized the social control functions of psychiatry and mental hospitals, the abuses inherent in institutionalization, and the demands generated by a capitalist social order that insisted on conformity to a unitary standard of citizenship and behavior.

Szasz, in contrast, was a practicing psychiatrist critical of most of his colleagues. Unlike Foucault, he was committed to a nineteenth-century liberalism that made individual liberty the paramount value. His work emphasized two distinct but interrelated themes: the "myth of mental illness," and the role of psychiatry in suppressing nonconformity. In his eyes there were fundamental distinctions between the concepts of mental illness and conventional (i.e., organic) illnesses. Defined in conventional medical terminology, mental illness was a form of social labeling that had dramatic and drastic consequences for individuals. Indeed, psychiatry was little more than a pseudoscience. Its nosology lacked reliability and validity and embodied a set of value judgments that imposed a particular view of bourgeois reality (with all of its vested interests) upon a minority. Commitment laws, ostensibly intended to promote the welfare of patients, actually enhanced what Szasz called the "Therapeutic State." Psychiatry, therefore, was merely an instrument of social control. As such, it constituted a threat to individual liberty in a free society precisely because of its rejection of such values as personal autonomy, volition, liberty, and responsibility. By the close of the decade Szasz's attack on the specialty had grown even more vituperative. "To maintain that a social institution suffers from certain 'abuses,' " he wrote in an ostensibly historical work, "is to imply that it has certain other desirable or good uses. This, in my opinion, has been the fatal weakness of the countless exposés—old and recent, literary and professional—of private and public mental hospitals. My thesis is quite different: Simply put, it is that there are, and can be, no abuses *of* Institutional Psychiatry, because Institutional Psychiatry *is*, itself, an abuse.''[7]

If Szasz attacked orthodox psychiatry because of his commitment to principles derived from nineteenth-century laissez-faire liberalism, figures such as R. D. Laing in England developed an equally powerful critique more compatible with the social activism and political radicalism of that decade. Laing, a practicing psychiatrist, was concerned with making intelligible the thoughts and feelings of schizophrenics, and subsequently with understanding their behavior within the context of disturbed interpersonal relationships in the family. Laing did not deny madness; he merely insisted that it was not incomprehensible. The basic difference between sanity and insanity was one of adaptation to social and cultural norms; those who refused to adapt were labeled insane. More importantly, Laing insisted that the concept of sanity was based on a statistical statement of normality. Those who defined insanity in such terms failed to question or to criticize dominant cultural values and therefore accepted an unsatisfactory status quo. ''There is no such 'condition' as 'schizophrenia,' '' he wrote in 1967, ''but the label is a social fact and the social fact a *political event*.''[8]

Goffman, on the other hand, was trained in sociology and wrote within the social interactionist tradition of George Herbert Mead. Given his belief in the overriding importance of personal autonomy, it was not surprising that he was most concerned with the impact of institutions such as mental hospitals upon the personality and behavior of patients. As a visiting scientist at the National Institute of Mental Health in Bethesda in the mid-1950s, he undertook field work at St. Elizabeth Hospital, a very large federal institution serving the District of Columbia. Out of his experiences came the publication of his famous *Asylums*. In this book he identified a ''total institution''— ''a place of residence and work where a large number of like-situated individuals, cut off from the wider society for an appreciable period of time, together lead an enclosed, formally administered round of life.'' Goffman's concept of the total institution was by no means unique. Bruno Bettelheim's study of Nazi concentration camps (published in 1943) had already emphasized the ways in which extreme situations could shape and mold the collective behavior of inmates—a theme that resonated through some of the sociological and historical literature of the 1950s.

Goffman's own portrait of mental institutions was devastating; he described the ways in which a humiliating institutionalization stripped individuals of their self-identity and esteem and induced deviant responses. Expressions of hostility toward hospitals by patients were regarded as evidence that their commitment was proper and that they had not sufficiently recovered to be released. Mental hospitals, Goffman insisted, were staffed and administered in order to affirm the legitimacy of a medical service model. A paradox then followed. ''To get out of the hospital, or to ease their life within it, they [patients] must show acceptance of the place accorded them, and the place accorded them is to support the occupational role of those who appear to force this bargain.''[9]

Asylums was the product of a gifted and perceptive observer. Its literary and intellectual qualities were striking, and often overshadowed the methodological difficulties inherent in relying solely on personal observations. The book proved immensely popular among social activists, intellectuals, academics, and counterculture figures, many of whom were persuaded that established institutions served only the rich and powerful. Curiously enough, Goffman's commitment to individual autonomy and a kind of eccentricity ensured that he would be far removed from many public issues. Nor did he offer any prescriptions for better and more effective ways of dealing with individuals designated as mental patients, and even conceded that the closing of all hospitals would "raise a clamor for new ones" by relatives and public authorities. His work, nevertheless, was absorbed into both popular and professional thought and became one of the most significant anti-institutionalist works of the 1960s.[10]

At about the same time that Goffman's critique appeared, others were developing themes that were implicitly or explicitly critical of psychiatry. During the 1950s sociologists by and large accepted the medical model of mental disorders; they were concerned with identifying etiological mechanisms, the extent of pathology in large populations, and the social response to pathology. A decade later epidemiological research was accompanied by an examination of the underlying concepts that shaped psychiatric thought and practice. In developing what became known as "labeling" (or societal reaction) theory, a number of sociologists called into question the very validity of the medical model of mental illnesses and, by indirection, the legitimacy of psychiatry as a whole.

Labeling theory did not emerge in an intellectual vacuum; sociological interest in the ways in which society identified deviant behavior had been longstanding. During the 1960s, however, labeling theory assumed new prominence, partly because it could be used as a form of social criticism. Thomas J. Scheff, a sociologist who helped to popularize labeling theory, argued that psychiatric diagnoses were merely convenient labels attached to individuals who had violated conventional behavioral norms. The breaking of norms, he emphasized, was common. Many violations, however, could not be placed within commonly recognized deviant categories (e.g., criminal, homosexual, vandal, etc.); mental illnesses therefore served as a residual category. Persons placed within this category in turn stimulated a response by agents representing dominant social groups. A label of mental illness, therefore, led to commitment to a mental hospital. In turn, the process of institutionalization altered self-conceptions and created a form of secondary deviance in which behavior reflected a new deviant self-image. The labeling or stigmatizing of individuals as mentally ill produced disturbed behavior. A diagnosis of mental illness, in other words, said less about the individual patient and more about the social system itself, the reaction of others to unconventional behavior, and the official agencies of control and treatment.[11]

The implications of labeling theory were obvious. Concepts of mental illnesses were not "neutral, value-free, [or] scientifically precise terms." They were, rather, as Scheff observed, "the leading edge of an ideology embedded in the historical and cultural present of the white middle class of Western societies." The real use of psychiatric labels such as schizophrenia was to reify and legitimate the existing social order. Psychiatrists were in reality fulfilling a social control rather than a medical purpose. Labeling theory was especially attractive to those who were critical of psychiatry and persuaded that fundamental social change was long overdue. Indeed, labeling theory proved appealing to a variety of activists, including civil rights advocates, feminists, and radicals of all persuasions.[12]

The powerful critiques developed by Foucault and others influenced historical scholarship. During the 1960s and 1970s a group of American historians (who constituted only a small minority) were especially receptive to approaches that placed American, if not all of Western society, in a negative light. The emphasis on the persistence of racism, sexism, and poverty, when added to the controversy generated by the American involvement in Vietnam, quickly transformed the writing of history. The rise of the new social history, which was preoccupied with inarticulate groups, strengthened the conviction that its practitioners could play important roles in a forthcoming social transformation. By revealing the fundamental flaws in the American past, historians would prepare the foundation for the creation of a society in which inequality in all of its protean forms no longer existed.

The initial focus of new social historians was on race, gender, and class, which in turn stimulated interest in the history of welfare, dependency, and medicine. The emergence of the social history of medicine as a subspecialty in its own right was accompanied by a parallel interest in the history of mental illness and psychiatry. Yet the best-known work representing this new tradition—*The Discovery of the Asylum*—was not written by a social historian of medicine, but by David J. Rothman, a scholar whose initial interests lay in late nineteenth-century American politics. To be sure, Rothman was familiar with the field because his wife was a psychiatric social worker and their circle of friends included some psychiatrists. Nevertheless, his initial interest was with psychoanalysis; he hoped to pursue William L. Langer's call to apply psychoanalytic concepts to historical problems. Oscar Handlin, Rothman's mentor at Harvard, was less than enthusiastic. Discussions with Handlin in 1964 led Rothman to consider the possibility of studying the origins and rise of the asylum as an alternative to psychoanalytic history. During the early stages of his research, he quickly broadened his focus to include penal and welfare institutions that had some of the same characteristics as asylums.[13]

The Discovery of the Asylum, published in 1971, was a widely read and influential work focused on the origins of institutions of confinement in nineteenth-century America. Cognizant of his debt to Goffman in particular, Rothman developed a unique analysis that placed mental hospitals, prisons, and other institutions in a new light. The book embodied several related but distinct themes. In the early nineteenth century, according to Rothman, the stable society of colonial America was transformed. Economic and demographic changes in particular heightened concern with the social problems related to poverty, crime, indolence, and disease. Concerned with the need to restore social cohesion and obsessed with deviant and dependent behavior, Americans ultimately came to the conclusion that "to comprehend and control abnormal behavior promised to be the first step in establishing a new system for stabilizing the community, for binding citizens together." The solution, according to Rothman, involved the creation of the "asylum"—a unique institution designed to reform criminals, juvenile delinquents, poor and indigent groups, mentally ill persons, and all other deviants whose abnormal behavior threatened community stability and safety.[14]

Rothman, however, went beyond a study of origins. He presented a theory of the asylum that gave it a constant if not eternal character. Specifically, he insisted that the *character* of the asylum—its emphasis on authority, obedience, regularity, and discipline—ensured that it could never serve its intended purpose. Abuse, neglect, and inmate powerlessness were inherent in its very structure and organization. Indeed, Rothman seemed to imply that the development of the asylum followed an inexorable and predetermined pattern that mandated its custodial character for socially marginal groups.

That the book was written with a didactic purpose in mind was evident in its author's closing peroration, which both reflected and anticipated what sometimes is referred to as "deinstitutionalization."

> The history of the discovery of the asylum is not without a relevance that may be more liberating than stifling for us. . . . We tend to forget that they were the invention of one generation to serve very special needs, not the only possible reaction to social problems. . . . In this sense the story of the origins of the asylum is liberating. We need not remain trapped in inherited answers.[15]

The radicalism and anti-institutional ethos in certain intellectual circles during these years was also conducive to quasi-Marxian ideas. Andrew Scull—a sociologist by training who worked largely, if not exclusively, with historical data and materials—employed a quasi-Marxian analysis to delineate the functions and character of mental hospitals and psychiatry. Scottish-born, Scull grew up in a household committed to the Labor Party and left-wing politics. After graduating from Oxford, he came to Princeton to pursue graduate study; his interests lay in political sociology and particularly French politics. Since the Princeton sociology department had no specialist in that field, Scull enrolled in a seminar dealing with deviance and social control, and was introduced to Foucault and Rothman. His attention then shifted to mental illnesses, and he decided to undertake a dissertation that dealt with the origins of the asylum in England. Although focusing primarily on the English experience, he was attracted to a comparative approach. His articles and books offered a coherent, detailed, and logical history of the emergence of the asylum and the specialty of psychiatry.[16]

The origins of the asylum, according to Scull, lay in a series of "historically specific and closely interrelated changes." Specifically, an authentic shift in moral consciousness occurred. In the seventeenth century madness was equated with bestiality and a suspension of all rational faculties. Consequently, external discipline and compulsion were required to break the will of madpeople and to subjugate them. By the early nineteenth century, by contrast, madness had been domesticated. Lunatics were no longer perceived as beasts who lacked moral understanding; they were now perceived as having the same sensibilities as normal human beings. Hence they were receptive to appeals to reason and self-esteem. There was a shift, therefore, from external controls designed to enforce outward conformity toward an emphasis on the internalization of moral standards.

Such a change, Scull insisted, led unerringly to the creation of the ubiquitous asylum and the rise in the nineteenth century of what was known as moral treatment. This novel form of therapy was not an outgrowth of humanitarian sentiment; rather it was intended to transform lunatics and to remodel them "into something approximating the bourgeois ideal of the rational individual." Most important, the profound transformation in the perception and treatment of lunacy was a function of the rise of capitalism. "Just as those who formed the new industrial work force were to be taught the 'rational' self-interest essential if the market system were to work, the lunatics, too, were to be made over in the image of bourgeois rationality: defective human mechanisms were to be repaired so that they could once more compete in the marketplace."[17]

According to Scull, the rise of the asylum was also accompanied by the medicalizing of insanity and the emergence of the specialty of psychiatry. This development mirrored a larger social trend whereby elites rationalized and legitimated their control over deviant and troublesome groups by assigning them to the authority of experts. The actual consequences of the medicalization of insanity and rise of the asylum, of course, were quite different. In short, asylums failed to live up to their promise and "remained a convenient place to get rid of inconvenient people."[18]

Scull's interpretation of recent developments in Anglo-American psychiatry followed along similar lines. Just as the asylum was the product of capitalism, so was deinstitutionalization. This new policy, which came into vogue during and after the 1950s, measured success by the decline in mental hospital inpatient populations and lengths of stay. Although its supporters idealized community care and treatment, reality was quite different. In practice, deinstitutionalization meant the transfer of aged mentally ill persons from hospitals to nursing homes, a policy that benefited entrepreneurs concerned with profits. Those who promoted community care, moreover, ignored "the reality of the increasingly segmented, isolated and atomized existence characteristic of late capitalist societies." In other words, just as capitalism had created the ubiquitous mental hospital in the nineteenth century, so, too, it abandoned its own creation after World War II.[19]

The heightened interest in psychiatry and the mentally ill paralleled the social and intellectual ferment of the 1960s and 1970s. During these years institutions and policies came under close scrutiny by scholars and activists, some of whom were critical of the ways in which public policies sometimes diminished individual and group rights. Demands for empowering those who were deemed disadvantaged also grew in significance. That historians would turn their attention to the roots of inequality and powerlessness was not unexpected. Equally understandable was the appearance of a body of historical literature critical of psychiatry and mental hospitals.

It was precisely at the beginning of the 1960s that I became involved with the history of psychiatry and the mentally ill. To have remained oblivious to the rich and stimulating scholarly controversies dealing with the origins and functions of asylums, the role of psychiatry, and the nature of the mentally ill population was inconceivable. Much of my own work, therefore, was inextricably bound up with the historiographical and policy debates of these years. Yet my original interest and involvement in this subject had somewhat different origins. This is not to suggest that I was able to transcend the influences that shaped other scholars. It is simply to assert that the forces that conditioned both my approach to and understanding of history were somewhat different.

Like many other American historians, I shared in the liberal ethos that dominated the discipline through World War II. I was born in 1931 at the beginning of the Great Depression. My parents were Polish Jews who migrated to the United States in 1922 and 1923 to escape a hostile environment. Married in 1929, they lacked any formal education. Nevertheless, they instilled in my sister and myself an almost naive faith in the redemptive authority of education quite apart from its role in enhancing career opportunities. Their Judaism, poverty, and liberal outlook made them staunch supporters of Franklin Delano Roosevelt and the New Deal. I can even recall when Roosevelt visited the Bronx on a rainy day during his reelection campaign in 1944, the thousands that lined the streets to pay him homage.

My commitment to the social democratic Left was strengthened during my years at the City College of New York. In the late 1940s City College remained a bastion of liberal if not radical thinking. A substantial part of its overwhelmingly Jewish student body would have voted for Wallace in 1948 if they possessed the franchise (at that time those under the age of twenty-one years could not vote). The student body included many committed to Marxist and Communist ideals, which in their eyes provided an alternative to what appeared to be a rapacious capitalism already committed to a Cold War diplomacy. Although I was not unsympathetic to campus Marxists, their single-mindedness and hostility to alternative ideas proved unacceptable. My allegiances, therefore, remained with the liberal and social democratic Left.

My faith in a liberal political ideology and the promise of a better world, nevertheless, was always tempered by a recognition that human beings were neither completely rational nor moral. Too young to serve in World War II, I was increasingly aware of the horrors of nazism and the Holocaust. Not all members of my family had left Poland. With but a single exception, those who remained—including my grandfather—were murdered by the Nazis. The Holocaust left me with an abiding sense of tragedy and a recognition of human frailty. My approach to history, then, reflected a number of contradictory tendencies: a commitment to social democratic principles; a belief in the fallibility of human nature; a faith in the ability of individuals to make genuine choices that were in part independent of the forces operating upon them; and a hostility to any overarching historical explanations that bordered on determinism. Nor was I persuaded that all phenomena were linked or that it was possible to apply all-encompassing theories to human behavior and society. When introduced to the writings of Reinhold Niebuhr in the early 1950s, I immediately felt an affinity for the ways in which he combined conservative theology and radical politics while simultaneously warning of the dangers and pitfalls presented by the possession of power. Neibuhr employed irony and paradox without sanctifying or legitimating the claims of both the extreme Left and Right.

After graduating from City College in 1951, I briefly attended Columbia University. Receiving my MA in 1952, I left Columbia because I did not care for the factorylike atmosphere characteristic of its approach to graduate education. Through a circuitous route, I ended up at Northwestern University and received my Ph.D. in 1958. My dissertation dealt with late-nineteenth-century American trade unionism, a subject that had interested me since my undergraduate years at City College.

After two years of military service in the mid-1950s, I accepted my first teaching position at Clark University in Worcester, Massachusetts, in 1957. After my dissertation was accepted for publication, I began to search for a new research problem because I realized that my first book represented an institutional approach that was already dated.[20] Clark was then a very small school but one with a rich intellectual tradition. With a total faculty of no more than seventy, friendships transcended disciplinary affiliation. A colleague in psychology with extraordinarily broad interests suggested that I set a graduate student to work on the history of an old state mental hospital in Worcester. Quite ignorant about the subject, I nevertheless agreed to familiarize myself with the institution's past. Much to my surprise, I found that Worcester State Hospital had played an important role in the history of the care and treatment of the mentally ill. I also found that a large mass of manuscript material had survived, including every single patient case history since its formal opening in 1833 (which by the 1960s exceeded 70,000). I decided, therefore, to undertake myself a study of the history of the institution.

In retrospect, my decision to pursue research on the history of psychiatry and mental illnesses was somewhat presumptuous. My knowledge of both was nil, nor was I even remotely familiar with a large social and behavioral science literature on the subject. Ignorance and fear of the unknown, however, did not prevail over what only can be described as a youthful hubris. I decided that with some work I could surmount my lack of knowledge, background, and training.

At the outset I pursued two related strategies. First, I began a systematic reading program in both psychiatry and the social and behavioral sciences. This proved an imposing experience, if only because of the unfamiliar terminology. Some of the figures who dealt with mental illnesses and psychiatry had a remarkable if misplaced affinity for dense and complex language and obscure terms. With a reasonable amount of hard work, however, I was able to familiarize myself with its underlying concepts (which often proved much more manageable than the language in which they were expressed). My second strategy, however, proved even more significant. In the early 1960s I attended on a fairly regular basis the training sessions offered to residents at the Worcester hospital in order to familiarize myself with clinical cases and institutional life. The experiences of being in contact with severely and chronically mentally ill patients led me to reject many of the social control and deviance theories and reflexive anti-psychiatric thinking that was just then emerging and becoming so prevalent.

Other elements also influenced my thinking at this time. I was not enamored with the ideology of the New Left and other activists that became so important for many scholars. Nor was I much influenced by some of the prevailing anti-institutional ideologies of these years. As far as the Vietnam War was concerned, I was a staunch opponent of American involvement as early as 1964 and signed one of the first anti-war advertisements in early 1965 that appeared in the *New York Times*. Nevertheless, I was quite disillusioned by what I felt was a partial abrogation of critical and careful thinking about social problems generally.

Consequently, I did not share the view that institutions—including mental hospitals—were inherently repressive (even though many in fact had such a character). My experience at Worcester State Hospital, of course, posed the risk of accepting conventional psychiatric claims at face value, but my reluctance to become involved in the ongoing policy debates dealing with the mentally ill helped me to retain at least a partial distance. The difficult and sometimes intractable nature of mental illnesses, moreover, led me to conclude that easy solutions were not readily available, and that most policy choices had at best ambiguous consequences. In this respect I was influenced both by Niebuhr's emphasis on human fallibility and Rene Dubos's attack on the illusion of medical utopias or disease-free societies.[21]

My book on Worcester State Hospital and public policy in Massachusetts was completed in 1965 and published the following year. At that time I was working in a partial historiographical vacuum. With the exception of Deutsch's classic work, relatively few scholars had worked on the history of psychiatry. Norman Dain's important study of early American psychiatric thought, completed as a doctoral dissertation in 1961, was not published until 1964.[22] The few institutional histories that had been published were written in filiopietistic terms. By the time I read Foucault's *Madness and Civilization* (which did not appear in translation until 1965), my book was largely finished. More important, I found Foucault's use of primary sources misleading and his writing extraordinarily dense and obscure. Although fascinated by many of his shrewd insights, I found the book to be neither logical nor coherent. Ultimately I came to the conclusion that

Foucault had to be read as a social critic rather than as a historian. Consequently, I was literally forced to create my own conceptual framework.

The writing of *The State and the Mentally Ill* presented formidable problems. I was determined not to write a purely local institutional history. Fortunately, the very process of research suggested some alternatives. While going through the hospital's own records, I became increasingly aware that its evolution and character were shaped in part by broader external considerations. This, in turn, led me to an examination of a category of sources all too often neglected, namely, Massachusetts state government records. The state, after all, was responsible for both the formulation and implementation of public policy. In the end I made a conscious decision to write what was in some respects a disjointed book that attempted to integrate the history of the hospital, the evolution of state policy, as well as an analysis of relevant external psychiatric, medical, social, and intellectual factors. My overriding concern, therefore, was with historical context and the ways in which seemingly disparate elements interacted. Moreover, I wanted to avoid the temptation of explaining events in purely logical terms. There is an important distinction, after all, between intentions and outcomes; to infer the former from a knowledge of the latter represents a form of ahistorical thinking.

A preoccupation with context, however, did not resolve complex interpretive issues; I found it virtually impossible to subsume institutional history within a one-dimensional framework. Institutional character and patient outcomes, for example, were by no means constant. Ethnicity and class, the process of professionalization, and ever-shifting state policies all interacted in subtle ways to give rise to unanticipated consequences. Well before Foucault, Rothman, and Scull published their works, I had already decided that the consequences of institutional care and treatment had varied sharply over time, and that it was all but impossible to assess the legacy of institutional care and treatment in simplistic or stark terms. The character of both individuals and institutions, I concluded, could not

> be easily portrayed or sharply delineated, for both contain elements of good and evil, white and black. This is particularly true for the history of psychiatry in general and mental hospitals in particular. Horace Mann and the other humanitarian reformers whose labors had resulted in the creation of Worcester State Hospital had envisaged a utopia of sorts, where an evil malady had once and for all been eradicated. Instead they found that for every problem solved and every obstacle overcome, two more had risen in their place. Like other institutions, the hospital had been influenced by prevailing social, economic, and intellectual forces; what had seemed worthy at one time had become less than ideal at another. . . . Perhaps the hospital had not accomplished all that its founders had hoped for, but surely it had done some things of value. By this standard the dreams of Mann and other reformers had not been in vain.[23]

The State and the Mentally Ill, though a narrow study, shaped virtually all of my subsequent thinking about the institutional history of American psychiatry. Even before its completion, I had decided to undertake a national study. In 1965 I had no indication that it would take more than twenty-five years and three volumes to complete the work. Nor did I envision the project as a response to the anti-psychiatry movement or to the subsequent writings of such scholars as Rothman and Scull. There is, I believe, a risk in writing within a prevailing historiographical tradition; to do so permits the work of others to have an overly decisive role. Equally significant, I was concerned with process and change, and felt that many of the interpretations that were current were ahistorical in character. Moreover, the quest for overarching generalizations tended to homogenize the past and blur important changes over time.

I also felt that the process of research should play the primary role in shaping the questions ultimately asked by the historian. In emphasizing the significance of research in often obscure primary sources in shaping the evolution of my thinking, I do not mean to imply that the work of other scholars had no influence. Indeed, the historical and policy debates about the nature of institutions, the relative merits of institutional or community policies, and the role of psychiatry have always served as an indispensable intellectual stimulus. Yet a preoccupation with interpretive issues can lead to a neglect of sources that in turn suggest novel ways of dealing with familiar problems.

Let me offer several examples of how the process of research can assist in framing novel conclusions. Much of the scholarly and policy literature of the post–World War II era was based on the presumption that asylums functioned almost exclusively as custodial institutions; their therapeutic claims were dismissed as exaggerations if not overt falsifications. From this it was but a short step to emphasize the dehumanizing aspects of institutionalization on the personality and behavior of their inmates.

My research on the nature of the institutionalized population, however, led me to question formulations that made custodialism an inherent and seemingly eternal characteristic. I found, for example, that chronicity was not characteristic of hospital populations before 1890, when the typical length of stay (with some notable exceptions) was between three and nine months. The dramatic rise in the number of long-stay chronic patients began only in the 1890s. This finding directed my research in a new direction, namely, to identify the circumstances that transformed the nature of the institutionalized population.

Data from a variety of primary sources provided the basis for new kinds of formulations. I found that after 1890 aged senile patients (in addition to those whose abnormal behavioral characteristics had a somatic etiology) tended to be sent to mental hospitals instead of almshouses (which in the nineteenth century served as the old-age homes of that era). The transfer of aged patients grew out of a redefinition of senility in psychiatric terms by local government officials who took advantage of the passage of state care acts to shift fiscal responsibility for the aged from the local community to the state. As mental hospitals accepted ever-larger numbers of individuals over the age of sixty-five, their therapeutic functions declined correspondingly and internal environments changed sharply in less than positive ways. In an ideal world, of course, such a development would not have occurred. But in the real world, mental hospitals assumed a critical function—not necessarily willingly—of providing care and shelter for aged senile patients. Many of these individuals lacked access to basic care; some had no families and others had families who were unable or unwilling to assume responsibility. That other and perhaps better alternatives could have been found is besides the point; from a historical point of view it is important to recognize that reality does not always follow ideal patterns.[24]

Similarly, my research on the decades since World War II yielded some surprising findings. I found that the word generally used to describe these years–*deinstitutionalization*–was inappropriate if not misleading. Once again complexity, not simplicity, was characteristic. The dissolution of the prevailing consensus around the wisdom of an institutionally oriented policy had a variety of sources. First, there was a shift in psychiatric thinking toward a psychodynamic and psychoanalytic model emphasizing the importance of prior life experiences as well as the role of socioenvironmental factors. Second, the experiences of World War II appeared to demonstrate the efficacy of community and outpatient treatment of disturbed persons. Third, the belief that early intervention in the community would be effective in preventing subsequent hospitalization became popular. Fourth, a faith developed that psychiatry could promote prevention by contributing toward the amelioration of social problems that allegedly fostered mental diseases. Fifth, the introduction of psychological and somatic therapies (including, but not limited to, psychotropic drugs) held out the promise of a more normal existence for patients outside of institutions. Finally, an enhanced social welfare role for the federal government not only began to diminish the authority of state governments, but also hastened the transition from an institution-based to a community-oriented policy. Throughout the postwar decades the rhetoric of community care and treatment and the alleged efficacy of various psychotherapies and, by implication, the obsolescence of mental hospitals, shaped public debates and agendas. That many of the rhetorical claims had little basis in fact was all but ignored by professionals, public officials, and especially the larger public.

My analysis of post–World War II developments, therefore, was framed in terms that did not break with the conceptual framework employed in *The State and the Mentally Ill*. The consequences of the innovations that transformed the mental health system, I wrote—like those of all human activities—were at best mixed. When the emphasis on treatment in the community was combined with an expansion of services to new groups, the result was a policy that often overlooked the need to provide supportive services for the seriously and chronically mentally ill. In this sense mental health activists all but ignored what their nineteenth-century predecessors had perhaps instinctively grasped, namely, that care and treatment, though conceptually separate, were not mutually exclusive. Thus the driving force of the postwar decades—antipathy toward traditional mental hospitals and a faith in community-oriented policies and institutions—gave rise to a bifurcated system with weak institutional linkages or mechanisms to ensure continuity and coordination of services. Severely and chronically mentally ill persons were released from public mental hospitals after brief lengths of stay into communities without adequate support mechanisms. The implications of the absence of longitudinal responsibility for meeting some of their basic needs in the community—including housing, medical care, welfare, and social support services—became painfully evident when the contraction of public welfare and housing programs exacerbated an already difficult situation.

In 1960 the history of psychiatry and mental illnesses as a subspecialty was virtually nonexistent. In ensuing decades a remarkable transformation took place. Within historical studies as well as the social and behavioral sciences, mental illnesses had become the focus of numerous and sustained inquiries. Interest in the subject, moreover, was not limited to scholarly discourse. The emphasis on civil rights fostered both a concern for the rights of the mentally ill and an interest in gender and class differences in the definition, identification, and treatment of mental disorders. The result was a lively, enlightening, if not fierce controversy.[25] Nor was the dialogue esoteric, if only because particular historical interpretations were in turn employed to justify and to legitimate particular policies. To avoid involvement in these controversies was neither possible nor desirable; I was concerned that facile and attractive but inadequate historical explanations might become a justification for novel policies that promised more than it was possible to deliver. This is not to suggest that historical knowledge ought to have no role in policy debates. It is merely to insist upon the need to expose policymakers to the complexities and ambiguities of the past as well as to conflicting explanations. During the past two decades, for example, arguably questionable historical claims about mental hospitals were used to justify the alleged superiority of community-oriented policies.[26]

That I would find shortcomings in the work of other scholars was hardly surprising. Some lacked a firm empirical base; some rested on faulty logic; and others employed an overarching determinism that used the history of asylums and psychiatry to shed light on Western society. Above all, part of the historical literature was designed to undermine institutional care and psychiatric legitimacy or to provide a hostile critique of a capitalist social order. To be sure, no historian writes from a purely objective vantage point; basic assumptions and personal beliefs play a significant part in the manner in which reality is perceived and interpreted. To argue in this vein, however, is not to engage in reductionist thinking that rejects both the possibility of degrees of objectivity or insists that evidence matters but little.

Consider, for example, the controversy over the very definition of the "mental illnesses." Figures such as Szasz and Scheff emphasized the inability to identify physiological causes of mental disorders. From this they concluded that individuals designated as insane were in fact stigmatized and punished for their violation of conventional social norms. Foucault and Scull (who accepts the reality of mental disorders) went even further; they interpreted institutionalization as a way of disciplining idleness and nonproductivity. Within such a framework mental hospitals naturally assume an unyielding and eternal custodial and penal character; they merely symbolize the reactions of a bourgeois society committed to the ideals of rational production.

To equate psychiatric categories with stigmatization and deviance is understandable and perhaps to a certain extent logical. Yet to do so reduces psychiatric classifications to appendages of social, cultural, and intellectual factors. Admittedly, classification systems are neither inherently self-evident nor given. On the contrary, they emerge from the crucible of human experience; change and variability, not immutability, are characteristic. Indeed, the ways in which data are organized at various times reflect specific historical circumstances. Empirical data, after all, can be presented and analyzed in a variety of ways.[27]

To concede the arbitrary nature of classification, however, is not to maintain that psychiatrists were serving as agents of bourgeois capitalism by stigmatizing deviant and unproductive individuals. On the contrary, the evolution of psychiatric nosology involved the interplay of complex and subtle factors. Before the articulation of the specific germ theory of disease in the late nineteenth century, all physicians—psychiatrists or generalists—defined pathological states by describing them in terms of external signs and symptoms. This process was perhaps inevitable, if only because neither prevailing technology nor theory could establish a relationship between biological mechanisms and external and visible signs. Admittedly, a classification system based on external signs created formidable intellectual and scientific difficulties; the midnineteenth century preoccupation with differentiating among various fevers was but one striking example of the problems faced by all physicians, general as well as psychiatric. Although disagreements on the diagnosis of signs and symptoms were common, few physicians questioned this approach, if only because other alternatives were largely absent. Nor was there any tendency to argue that individuals with a high fever were social deviants because their immediate condition (mental as well as physical) differed significantly from the population at large. Indeed, it is quite common at present to define pathological states even when patients appear to be in good health.

The psychiatric and medical definition of disease, moreover, was virtually identical; the inability of patients to function, combined with severe behavioral signs, was sufficient evidence to infer the presence of pathology. An explanation of disease often led to a rationale for treatment. In a certain sense psychiatrists were meeting a perhaps universal human need for explanations of unexpected or abnormal phenomena. Had they rejected this role, they could have fatally impaired their legitimacy.[28]

The theme of social control also resonates through part of the historical literature dealing with deviance and mental illnesses. The concept of social control has a long and somewhat checkered past since coming into vogue at the turn of the twentieth century. In 1901 E. A. Ross, an eminent sociologist, emphasized the tension between the behavior of individuals and the common interests and general welfare of society at large. In premodern societies, primary groups—family, church, local community—socialized and controlled the behavior of individuals. The progressive weakening of the authority of primary groups created a need for new forms of controls. Social control—the term Ross used to distinguish between premodern and modern societies—was a synonym for social welfare and implied that there had to be a balance between the desire for unregulated individual freedom and the needs of society for order and justice. As late as the 1930s Helen Everett identified social control with social planning and a rejection of laissez faire. By the mid-twentieth century, however, social control had acquired a new meaning; it now referred to the means employed by elites to perpetuate their hegemony and authority.[29]

Rothman's influential work owed much to social control theorists. In his view the invention of the asylum in the United States was a response to a perceived fear that hitherto stable social relationships were becoming unstable and thus posing a threat of social disorder. The asylum, paradoxically, sought to restore an older and presumably integrated community. If Rothman denied (somewhat unconvincingly) that his interpretation implied social control, Scull made this concept his central organizing theme. Thus the nineteenth-century emphasis on moral management "proved highly efficacious as a repressive instrument for controlling large numbers of people." In the twentieth century "the rise of the therapeutic state constituted a potentially massive expansion of psychiatry's role in the processes of social control." Indeed, psychiatry's "explanatory schema locates the source of pathology it identifies in intra-individual forces, and in principle can allow the redefinition of all protest and deviation from the dominant social order in individualistic and pathological terms."[30]

"Social control," of course, has a variety of meanings. That institutions and organizations control behavior is self-evident, if only in definitional terms. But is control the primary motive or is it a necessary by-product or concomitant? Surely it is evident that asylums restricted the freedom of patients. Yet asylums also served some of their patients in beneficial ways. Like most institutions, they included a variety of features.

What historians such as Rothman and Scull have done is to conflate intent and outcome. Implicit in their work is the belief that asylums were established to control deviant behavior and hence were the immoral products of a particular social system. To my way of thinking, social control is a given; it is inherent in the very definition of society. To use it in a pejorative way is to render the term all but meaningless.[31]

Equally important, asylums were hardly monolithic. The harsh, even terrifying, descriptions provided by Foucault, Rothman, and Scull tend to rest on a selective use of evidence; all data to the contrary are vigorously excluded. Rothman, for example, quotes early nineteenth-century asylum physicians to demonstrate the rigid, authoritarian, and repressive nature of moral treatment. To prove his point he italicizes key words in quotations such as *"perfect precision . . . neatness . . . orderly . . . systematic . . . regular."* What this does is to alter in a subtle way the context of these remarks. What justification exists for such emphasis? Had physicians desired to single out these words, surely they would have done so (especially in light of the fact that italicization was very common in the midnineteenth century). Rothman could have just as easily italicized such words as *humane* and *kind*, but this would have contradicted his thesis. Scull uses evidence in much the same manner. And Foucault's use of data is so idiosyncratic as to make it virtually impossible to judge his work by normal historical standards. Moreover, these scholars make little or no use of patient correspondence, a source that provides a far more complex and ambiguous portrait of institutional life.

Nor do historical critics of asylums and psychiatry ever refer to outcome data. That the evaluation of institutionalization is extremely difficult is obvious. Nevertheless, admittedly imperfect data suggest that some individuals—whatever the reasons—were discharged from asylums in better condition than they entered. One late nineteenth-century study that followed about 1,000 patients discharged as recovered until they died found that about fifty-eight percent were never again hospitalized. Similarly, recent studies of nineteenth-century institutional outcomes by Nancy Tomes, Ellen Dwyer, and Constance McGovern—all based on a careful evaluation of surviving sources—demonstrated that institutions were hardly monolithic either in their internal character or outcomes. Twentieth-century data offer an equally variegated and ambiguous pattern. In an analysis of more than 15,000 patient cohorts admitted to Warren State Hospital between 1916 and 1950, Morton Kramer (a key figure in the collection and evaluation of psychiatric statistics) and his colleagues found large numbers of chronic and aged patients who remained institutionalized for long periods of time. But the study also found that the probability of release of first admissions of functional psychotics within twelve months increased from forty-two to sixty-two percent between 1919/1925 and 1946/1950. Such findings suggested that a high proportion of chronic and aged patients in public institutions led many to overlook the reality that substantial numbers of patients were admitted, treated, and discharged in less than a year.[32]

Other data also call into question the validity of historical interpretations that attribute to asylums and psychiatry invidious characteristics. If hospitals were agencies of social control, why were the majority of commitments initiated by families and not public authorities, including the police? Commitment, as a number of recent scholars have demonstrated, was overwhelmingly a family affair. In early twentieth-century San Francisco, for example, fifty-seven percent of commitments were inaugurated by relatives, twenty-one percent by physicians, and only eight percent by the police. The experiences of the Utica State Hospital and Pennsylvania Hospital for the Insane in the nineteenth century were much the same. The familial decision to commit, Tomes noted in her study, generally came "after a prolonged crisis of escalating tension and desperation culminated in a crisis." Only when the very integrity of the family was threatened did its members consider hospitalization, a decision that was made with considerable ambivalence and reluctance.[33]

Equally significant, historical critics rarely refer to the nature of the institutionalized population. Between 1890 and 1950, a large proportion of patients in mental hospitals had somatic diagnoses, including senility, cerebral arteriosclerosis, general paresis, cerebral syphilis, Huntington's disease, pellagra, or various brain diseases. Many of these patients required total care. Lacking other alternatives, it was understandable (even if undesirable) that mental hospitals assumed a caring or custodial function. Moreover, institutional character was not merely shaped by asylum physicians or elites; the natures of patients were an important determinant of internal environments. The hegemonic arguments of Foucault, Rothman, and Scull often neglect or overlook such evidence. Thus they write about *the* asylum as though differences were of no consequence whatsoever. If historians of American higher education were to write a history of *the* college and university, they would immediately come under criticism for their failure to distinguish between very different types of institutions. Why then should we accept a one-dimensional view of mental hospitals that ignores significant temporal and regional variations. Indeed, the very concept of a monolithic eternal asylum is akin to an "ahistorical history"!

Admittedly, the coherence and symmetry of these reductionist interpretations are alluring. There are no inconsistencies; individual and collective behavior are explainable in rational terms; human volition, chance, and accident are largely absent; and the merging of historical data with social and behavioral science insights creates an all-encompassing structure capable of comprehending all of the details that constitute an approximation of social reality. The entire universe is linked within a unitary system that can be both understood and explained. Within this system all phenomena are linked in causal ways. The asylum and psychiatry are either shaped by an impersonal economic system and a commitment to productivity and the internalization of controls or by inexorable laws that govern all institutions.

Some years ago J. H. Plumb drew a sharp distinction between the past and history. History, he insisted, is not the past, even though they share common elements. History represents an effort "to see things as they actually were, and from this study to formulate processes of social change which are acceptable on historical grounds and none other." The past, on the other hand, has always been "a created ideology with a purpose, designed to control individuals, or motivate societies, or inspire classes."[34] Plumb's distinction is particularly applicable to part of the scholarship pertaining to the history of the asylum and psychiatry, which is designed to rationalize the need for presumably fundamental social and economic change. The result is a scholarship that is partly distorted because of its didactic qualities. Fortunately, younger scholars writing about mental illnesses and psychiatry have moved away from the rigid ideological traditions so characteristic of the 1960s and 1970s.

In concluding, I would be less than honest if I did not concede that my own experiences and assumptions played a role in the ways in which I have written about asylums and psychiatry. I remain skeptical of the modern faith that human beings can mold and control their world in predetermined and predictable ways. This is not to suggest that we are totally powerless to control our destiny. It is only to insist upon both our fallibility and our inability to predict all of the consequences of our actions. Nor do I believe that human behavior can be reduced to a set of deterministic or quasi-deterministic laws or generalizations, or that solutions are readily available for all problems. Tragedy is a recurring theme in human history and defines the parameters of our existence.

Historians must also be cognizant of the inherent dangers of arguing that the answers to contemporary problems resides in historical analysis. For if this were true, then surely our society should be governed not by Plato's proverbial philosophers or Lester Frank Ward's sociologists but by historians. A *historiocracy* (to coin a new word) would in all likelihood be no wiser than a sociocracy or aristocracy! In so arguing I do not mean to suggest that the study of history is of no value or importance. That historical knowledge shapes and is shaped by contemporary attitudes and behavior is to some degree obvious. All human beings employ history in one form or another to mold, validate, and justify their prescriptions for the present and future. The issue, then, is not whether historical knowledge will be used, but what kind of history.

Above all, those of us who write about the past must avoid, insofar as is possible, the seductive temptation to judge past events without at least a small measure of compassion and understanding as well as a frank recognition that we are not omniscient. If we fail to do so, our successors will be justified in judging our own generation in equally harsh terms.

Notes

1. Gregory Zilboorg, *A History of Medical Psychology* (New York: Norton, 1941) and *The Medical Man and Witch during the Renaissance* (Baltimore: Johns Hopkins Press, 1935); J. K. Hall (ed.), *One Hundred Years of American Psychiatry* (New York: Columbia University Press, 1944). Many standard works fell within this tradition, including *The Institutional Care of the Insane in the United States and Canada*, 4 vols. edited by Henry M. Hurd (Baltimore, Johns Hopkins Press, 1916–1917), William L. Russell's *The New York Hospital: A History of the Psychiatric Service 1771–1936* (New York: Columbia University Press, 1945), and Earl D. Bond's *Dr. Kirkbride and His Mental Hospital* (Philadelphia: J. B. Lippincott, 1947).

2. Jeanne L. Brand, "Albert Deutsch: The Historian as Social Reformer," *Journal of the History of Medicine and Allied Sciences*, xviii (1963), 149–157; Deutsch, *The Mentally Ill in America: A History of Their Care and Treatment from Colonial Times* (Garden City, New York: Doubleday Doran, 1937); David M. Schneider and Albert Deutsch, *The History of Public Welfare in New York State 1867–1940* (Chicago: University of Chicago Press, 1941); George Mora, "Three American Historians of Psychiatry: Albert Deutsch, Gregory Zilboorg, George Rosen" in *Essays in the History of Psychiatry*, edited by Edwin R. Wallace and Lucius C. Pressley (Columbia, South Carolina: William S. Hall Psychiatric Institute, 1980), 1–21. The American Foundation for Mental Health Papers at the Archives of Psychiatry, New York Hospital-Cornell Medical Center, New York, NY, contain correspondence between Beers, Edmund Bullis, and Deutsch over the issue of organizational censorship.

3. For an analysis of what has been termed the Progressive School of American Historiography, see John Higham, *History* (Englewood Cliffs, New Jersey: Prentice-Hall, 1965).

4. Deutsch, *Mentally Ill in America* and *The Shame of the States* (New York: Harcourt, Brace, 1948).

5. Cf. Gerald N. Grob, "The Social History of Medicine and Disease in America: Problems and Possibilities," *Journal of Social History*, x (1977), 391–409.

6. Foucault's numerous books include *Madness and Civilization: A History of Insanity in the Age of Reason* (New York: Pantheon, 1965), quote from p. 259, originally issued as *Folie et deraison, Histoire de la folie à l'âge classique* (Paris: Union generale d'editions, 1961); *The Order of Things: An Archaeology of the Human Sciences* (New York: Pantheon, 1970); *The Archaeology of Knowledge and the Discourse on Language* (New York: Pantheon, 1972); *The Birth of the Clinic: An Archaeology of Medical Perception* (New York: Pantheon, 1973); *Discipline and Punish: The Birth of the Prison* (New York: Pantheon, 1977).

7. Space precludes a complete listing of Szasz's numerous articles and books. For some representative writings in the late 1950s see "Commitment of the Mentally Ill: 'Treatment' or Social Restraint?" *Journal of Nervous and Mental Disease*, cxxv (1957), 293–307, and "The Classification of 'Mental Illness,' " *Psychiatric Quarterly*, xxxiii (1959), 77–101. His most controversial books published during the 1960s include *The Myth of Mental Illness: Foundations of a Theory of Personal Conduct* (New York: Hoeber-Harper, 1961); *Law, Liberty, and Psychiatry: An Inquiry Into the Social Uses of Mental Health Practices* (New York: Macmillan, 1963); *Psychiatric Justice* (New York: Macmillan, 1965); and *The Manufacture of Madness: A Comparative Study of the Inquisition and the Mental Health Movement* (New York: Harper & Row, 1970), quotes from pp. xix–xxv.

8. R. D. Laing, *The Politics of Experience and the Bird of Paradise* (London: Penguin Books 1967), 100; *The Divided Self: An Existential Study in Sanity and Madness* (London: Penguin, 1960), and (with A. Esterson) *Sanity, Madness, and the Family* (London: Tavistock, 1964).

9. Erving Goffman, *Asylums: Essays on the Social Situation of Mental Patients and other Inmates* (Garden City, New York: Doubleday, 1961), xiii, 385–386. See also Bruno Bettelheim, "Individual and Mass Behavior in Extreme Situations," *Journal of Abnormal and Social Psychology*, xxxviii (1943), 417–452, Gresham M. Sykes, *The Society of Captives: A Study of a Maximum Security Prison* (Princeton: Princeton University Press, 1958), and Stanley M. Elkins, *Slavery: A Problem in American Institutional and Intellectual Life* (Chicago: University of Chicago Press, 1959).

10. Goffman, *Asylums*, 384. The social and behavioral science and counterculture literature of the 1960s and early 1970s are replete with references to Goffman's work. For subsequent critical evaluations of Goffman's methodology and interpretations see Roger Peele, P. V. Luisada, M. Jo Lucas, D. Russell, and D. Taylor, "*Asylums* Revisited," *American Journal of Psychiatry*, cxxxiv (1977), 1077–1081; Peter Sedgwick, *Psycho-Politics* (New York: Harper & Row, 1982); and David Mechanic, "Medical Sociology: Some Tensions Among Theory, Method, and Substance," *Journal of Health and Social Behavior*, xxx (1989), 147–150.

11. Thomas J. Scheff's *Being Mentally Ill: A Sociological Theory* (Chicago: Aldine Publishing Co., 1966) was the classic statement of labeling theory. The concept, however, set off a heated and controversial debate among sociologists. See, for example, Walter R. Gove, "Societal Reaction as an Explanation of Mental Illness: An Evaluation," *American Sociological Review*, xxxv (1970), 873–884 (and the comments in ibid., xxxvii [1972], 487–490); Gove and Patrick Howell, "Individual Resources and Mental Hospitalization: A Comparison and Evaluation of the Societal Reaction and Psychiatric Perspectives," ibid., xxxix (1974), 86–100; and Scheff, "The Labelling Theory of Mental Illness," ibid., 444–452.

12. Scheff, "Schizophrenia as Ideology," *Schizophrenia Bulletin*, no. 2 (Fall 1970), 15–19.

13. David J. Rothman, *Politics and Power: The United States Senate, 1869–1901* (Cambridge: Harvard University Press, 1966). Biographical details from a conversation with Rothman on 2 April, 1992. William L. Langer's call for a psychoanalytic history was the theme of his presidential address at the American Historical Association in December 1957. It was published as "The Next Assignment," *American Historical Review*, lxiii (1958), 283–304.

14. David J. Rothman, *The Discovery of the Asylum: Social Order and Disorder in the New*

Republic (Boston: Little, Brown, 1971), 58–59. His sequel volume, *Conscience and Convenience: The Asylum and Its Alternatives in Progressive America* (Boston: Little, Brown, 1980), drew far less attention.

15. Rothman, *Discovery of the Asylum*, 295.

16. Scull's books include *Museums of Madness: The Social Organization of Insanity in Nineteenth Century England* (New York: St. Martin's Press, 1979) and *Decarceration: Community Treatment and the Deviant—A Radical View* (Englewood Cliffs, New Jersey: Prentice-Hall, 1977). Many of his articles are collected in his *Social Order/Mental Disorder: Anglo-American Psychiatry in Historical Perspective* (Berkeley: University of California Press, 1989). Biographical details were provided by Scull in a conversation on 1 April 1992.

17. Scull, *Social Order/Mental Disorder*, 43, 89, 94.

18. Ibid., 231, 305, 307.

19. Ibid., 314, 322–323, 327. For an extended treatment see also Scull's *Decarceration*. Although concerned largely with indigency and dependency, Michael Katz also developed an interpretation of the asylum in the United States somewhat similar to that of Scull. Katz's most incisive interpretation appeared in his article "Origins of the Institutional State," *Marxist Perspectives*, i (1978), 6–22.

20. My dissertation appeared as *Workers and Utopia: A Study of Ideological Conflict in the American Labor Movement, 1865–1900* (Evanston: Northwestern University Press, 1961).

21. I was especially taken with Reinhold Niebuhr's *The Children of Light and the Children of Darkness* (New York: Scribner, 1944), although I had also read *Moral Man and Immoral Society* (New York: Scribner, 1932), *The Nature and Destiny of Man*, 2 vols. (New York: Scribner, 1942), and *The Irony of American History* (New York: Scribner, 1952). René Dubos's *Mirage of Health: Utopias, Progress, and Biological Change* (New York: Harper, 1959) was also crucial to my thinking; his subsequent book *Man Adapting* (New Haven: Yale University Press, 1965) filled in many details.

22. Norman Dain, *Concepts of Insanity in the United States 1789–1865* (New Brunswick: Rutgers University Press, 1964). Examples of older institutional histories included Hurd, *Institutional Care of the Insane* and Russell's *New York Hospital*. The essays in Hall, *One Hundred Years of American Psychiatry*, were of some value.

23. Grob, *The State and the Mentally Ill: A History of Worcester State Hospital in Massachusetts, 1830–1920* (Chapel Hill: University of North Carolina Press, 1966), 363.

24. Grob, *Mental Institutions in America: Social Policy to 1875* (New York: Free Press, 1973), *Mental Illness and American Society 1875–1940* (Princeton: Princeton University Press, 1983), and *From Asylum to Community: Mental Health Policy in Modern America* (Princeton: Princeton University Press, 1991). The delay in completing the second volume was due to the fact that I spent several years in completing a biography (*Edward Jarvis and the Medical World of Nineteenth-Century America* [Knoxville: University of Tennessee Press, 1978]).

25. See, for example, Phyllis Chesler, *Women and Madness* (New York: Doubleday, 1972), and Elaine Showalter, *The Female Malady: Women, Madness, and English Culture, 1830–1980* (New York: Pantheon, 1985). For an insightful review see Nancy Tomes, "Historical Perspectives on Women and Mental Illness" in *Women, Health, and Medicine in America: A Historical Handbook*, edited by Rima D. Apple (New York: Garland Publishing Co., 1990), 143–171.

26. My contributions to the debate were the following articles: "Welfare and Poverty in American History," *Reviews in American History*, i (1973), 43–52; "Reflections on the History of Social Policy in America," ibid., vii (1979), 293–306; "Doing Good and Getting Worse: The Dilemma of Social Policy," *Michigan Law Review*, lxxvii (1979), 761–783; "Rediscovering Asylums: The Unhistorical History of the Mental Hospital" in *The Therapeutic Revolution: Essays in the Social History of American Medicine*, edited by Morris Vogel and Charles E. Rosenberg (Philadelphia: University of Pennsylvania Press, 1979), 135–157; "Marxian Analysis and Mental Illness," *History of Psychiatry*, i (1990), 223–232.

27. See Grob, "The Origins of American Psychiatric Epidemiology," *American Journal of Public Health*, lxxv (1985), 229–236, and "Origins of DSM-I: A Study in Appearance and Reality," *American Journal of Psychiatry*, cxxxxviii (1991): 421–431.

28. To maintain that psychiatric and medical nosologies are not fundamentally dissimilar is not to reject the view that the concept of disease is in part socially constructed and hence dependent in part on nonscientific and external variables. With the possible exception of a number of infectious diseases, most pathological states are still described in terms of symptoms rather than etiology. Admittedly, there is a difference between defining disease in terms of behavioral signs, on the one hand, and physiological symptoms, on the other. But that difference may not be of fundamental significance, particularly if little or no distinction is made between behavior and physiological processes. In fact, knowledge about "mental illnesses" is still extremely limited. Moreover, in many cases it is still not feasible to establish the validity of psychiatric disease categories. Schizophrenia, for example, may be, in fact, what "fever" was before 1870—a general inclusive category that comprehends a multiplicity of diseases. Assertions about the existence or nonexistence of mental illnesses represent, in part, acts of faith, which in turn reflect commitments to particular explanations and interventions.

29. E. A. Ross, *Social Control: A Survey of the Foundations of Social Order* (New York: Macmillan, 1901), and Helen Everett, "Control, Social" in *Encyclopedia of the Social Sciences*, vol. 4 (New York: Macmillan, 1930–1935), 344—both cited in James Leiby, "Social Control and Historical Explanation: Historians View the Piven and Cloward Thesis" in *Social Welfare or Social Control? Some Historical Reflections on Regulating the Poor*, edited by Walter I. Trattner (Knoxville: University of Tennessee Press, 1983), 97–98.

30. Rothman, *Discovery of the Asylum*, "Introduction to the 1990 Edition," xxxviff.; Scull, "Psychiatry and Social Control in the Nineteenth and Twentieth Centuries," *History of Psychiatry*, ii (1991), 159–169.

31. For sophisticated and nonpejorative uses of the concept of social control see Morris Janowitz, "Sociological Theory and Social Control," *American Journal of Sociology*, lxxxi (1975), 82–108; idem, *On Social Organization and Social Control* (Chicago: University of Chicago Press, 1991); and Jack P. Gibbs, *Control: Sociology's Central Notion* (Urbana: University of Illinois Press, 1989).

32. Grob, *The State and the Mentally Ill*, 252–255; Nancy Tomes, *A Generous Confidence: Thomas Story Kirkbride and the Art of Asylum-keeping, 1840–1883* (New York: Cambridge University Press, 1984); Ellen Dwyer, *Homes for the Mad: Life Inside Two Nineteenth-Century Asylums* (New Brunswick: Rutgers University Press, 1987); Constance M. McGovern, "The Myths of Social Control and Custodial Oppression: Patterns of Psychiatric Medicine in Late Nineteenth-Century Institutions," *Journal of Social History*, xx (1986), 3–23; Morton Kramer et al., *A Historical Study of First Admissions to a State Mental Hospital: Experience of the Warren State Hospital during the Period 1916–50* (Washington, D. C.: Government Printing Office, 1955), 12.

33. Dwyer, *Homes for the Mad*, 86ff.; Richard W. Fox, *So Far Disordered in Mind: Insanity in California, 1870—1930* (Berkeley: University of California Press, 1978), 84ff.; Tomes, *A Generous Confidence*, 109.

34. J. H. Plumb, *The Death of the Past* (Boston: Houghton Mifflin, 1970), 13, 17.

15

German Psychiatry, Psychotherapy, and Psychoanalysis during the Nazi Period: Historiographical Reflections

GEOFFREY COCKS

In 1949 Alexander Mitscherlich, a lecturer in psychiatry, and Fred Mielke, a medical student, published *Wissenschaft ohne Menschlichkeit*, a book for a research commission formed by the West German Physicians Chambers that documented the recent "doctors' trial" at Nuremberg. The foreword, by the members of the working group that sent the commission to Nuremberg, observed that of the 90,000 doctors active in wartime Germany, only about 350 had committed medical crimes. This observation was echoed by Mitscherlich and Mielke in the preface, but at the same time they pointed to a larger moral crisis among German doctors as a whole.[1] That this book was largely ignored by the medical profession in Germany indicates the tensions and disagreements existing among physicians regarding their profession's conduct under Hitler.[2]

Wissenschaft ohne Menschlichkeit includes a chapter on the sterilization and murder of mental patients, but in following the trials, the book concentrates on bureaucrats and medical experiments rather than on the role of psychiatrists in the so-called T 4 program. Mitscherlich, who with his wife, Margarete, would become a leading psychoanalytic critic of the postwar German denial of the Nazi past,[3] was himself entangled in the skeins of history and memory regarding his own profession's immediate past. This is evident in the small flier included with *Wissenschaft ohne Menschlichkeit* advertising *Psyche*, a new journal for depth psychology founded by Mitscherlich, who had wintered the Nazi regime in Heidelberg. The flier claims that *Psyche* is the only German publication carrying on the tradition of earlier journals that had been forced to cease publication by the Nazis. Yet this version of the Year Zero argument for a new beginning after 1945 ignores the fact of significant developments in the field of depth psychology in Germany between 1933 and 1945, developments that carried over into the postwar period. Although *Psyche*, in the words of its subtitle, was transformed in 1966 from *A Journal for Depth Psychology and Anthropology in Research and Praxis (Eine Zeitschrift für Tiefenpsychologie und Menschenkunde in Forschung und Praxis)* to one for *Psychoanalysis and Its Applications (Zeitschrift für Psychoanalyse und ihre Anwendungen)*, its original aim as described in 1949 was to provide a forum for all schools of "*grosse Psychotherapie.*" This represented a continuation of the work of the so-called Göring Institute, which, alongside and in line with its stated Nazi goal of establishing a "new German psychotherapy," from 1936 to 1945 attempted to unite the various schools of psychotherapeutic thought, chiefly the Jungian, Adlerian, and Freudian factions. Of the twenty-nine contributors listed in the flier, eight had been members of the Göring Institute, including one who was director of the outpatient clinic and another who was a member of the Nazi party, as well as at least two others who had trained at or had otherwise been associated with the institute.

It is within this context of institutional and personal continuities between the postwar Germanies and the Nazi era that an analysis of the phenomenon of "missed resistance" among psychiatrists, psychotherapists, and psychoanalysts must be conducted. This is especially the case with the professions in general, because between 1933 and 1945 a number of professions displayed "a significant degree of functional unity"[4] in defending, advancing, and sacrificing their interests in service to the Nazi regime. The Nazi era also witnessed a process of "deprofessionalization" insofar as the regime imposed political control over the professions, damaged the educational system, and trampled professional ethics.[5] Physicians, for example, achieved recognition as a profession in 1935, but they paid dearly for this status through the imposition of government control and the erosion of professional ethics. Individual professionals took advantage of the situation by joining the Nazi party (forty-five percent of all physicians did) or by benefiting from the exclusion of Jewish competitors. And disciplines like psychology and psychotherapy exploited specific conditions created by the Nazi seizure of power to achieve for the first time a significant degree of professionalization.[6] Psychiatrists, psychotherapists, and psychoanalysts all to one degree or another sought professional advantage in competition with one another during the Third Reich, an instance of what in connection with the Holocaust has been called "the nature of modern sin, the withdrawal of moral concerns from public roles in our lives."[7] As historian Hans Mommsen rightly observes, there are specific reasons why German elites did not resist Hitler,[8] as much of it having to do with greed, ambition, and power as with obedience, fear, and cowardice. Thus reflections on the missed resistance on the part of psychiatrists, psychotherapists, and psychoanalysts themselves have taken place (or not) in the context of a continuum of morally ambiguous professional development, general German culpability, and more general features of the evolution of modern European society.[9]

There are three senses in which the term *missed resistance* can be used to illuminate the ways in which German psychiatrists, psychotherapists, and psychoanalysts have avoided as well as confronted the history and memory of the Third Reich. The first sense is that of the missed opportunity for resistance embodied in the accusations of collaboration made by young Germans in the 1960s. They confronted elders who during the "economic miracle" of the 1950s had lied or remained silent about their actions and inactions under nazism. The second sense of missed resistance is that of regret/empathy and longing: regret over and empathy with the conditions that rendered resistance problematic as well as regret over the moral derelictions of their own professional ancestors; and longing for a legacy of resistance as redemption of the past and for moral commitment in the present. The third sense constitutes overlooking the nonheroic tradition of quotidian resistance mixed with compromise and even collaboration. As historian David Large points out, heroism almost by definition describes actions that are too late; while concentrating on heroism devalues "low-level" civil disobedience that if not preempting evil can mitigate it.[10] This is not to celebrate those many who went along at the expense of those few who did not. There is, as historian Klemens von Klemperer argues, great importance in the example of an individual resister (*Einzel-kämpfer*) like psychoanalyst John Rittmeister.[11] But even Rittmeister's life contains instructive ambiguities in terms of his profession: Alongside resistance, Rittmeister noted in his prison diary, was enthusiasm for much of his work at the Göring Institute, where he was director of the outpatient clinic.[12] And a post hoc fixation on resistance heroes can substitute a wish-fulfilling "ego-ideal" for historical inquiry, obscuring lines of continuity between past and present. As we shall see, the figure of Rittmeister has been used in just such a way for conscious political purposes by groups of psycho-therapists and psychoanalysts in both postwar German states.

Psychiatrists, psychotherapists, and psychoanalysts have shared in the gradual recapturing of memory after 1945, which went through three distinct stages in West Germany before 1990. First, there was the repression characteristic of the 1950s; second, the angry generational confrontations of the 1960s; and, third, the more complicated and thoroughgoing recollections of the 1970s and 1980s. To be sure, all three styles have overlapped to some degree, and both the criticism and the excesses that arose from the social crises and youth rebellions of the late 1960s and early 1970s largely laid the basis for subsequent professional critiques and self-examinations. And while it is difficult to generalize about the respective ages and generational experiences of the two groups, the "protest cohort" of the 1980s necessarily has engaged in a more specific and sobering critique of predecessors to whom it is linked by profession. But just as important is the fact that avoidance of and confrontation with the past have taken different forms for each discipline. This is so for two reasons. First, the three disciplines have grown increasingly distinct during the twentieth century, especially since 1933; and, second, the experience of each in the Third Reich differed in crucial respects.

Psychiatrists have displayed an almost seamless repression of the field's activities under Hitler, so much so that instances of genuine resistance as well as collaboration were ignored in the silent assertion of general innocence.[13] But recent research has shown the wide extent to which psychiatrists were involved in Nazi campaigns to sterilize and murder mental patients.[14] This collaboration began with the Law for the Prevention of Genetically Diseased Offspring of July 14, 1933. This law mandated the sterilization of those individuals suffering from a wide range of illnesses that, in keeping with Nazi racial theory and the physicalist views of most psychiatrists, were defined as hereditary. These included schizophrenia, manic-depressive insanity, and alcoholism, among others. One of the three chief authors of the expert commentary on the law was the prominent psychiatrist Ernst Rüdin.[15] So-called genetic health courts (*Erbgesund-heitsgerichte*) were set up to evaluate such cases. Approximately 400,000 men and women were sterilized under this law,[16] about ninety-five percent of these before the outbreak of World War II in 1939. The radical decline in the number of compulsory sterilizations after 1939 was due to a number of factors, but the most significant was the establishment in that year of the even more radical "euthanasia" program. Under this program, by August 1941 more than 70,000 mental patients had been gassed. Public outrage brought an end to this centrally administered campaign, but the killings went on in asyla and hospitals by means of injections, poisonings, and starvation right up to the end of the war. Psychiatrists and doctors assumed the task of murdering mentally ill men, women, and children. In all, over 300,000 people died in this manner. It is important to note that the original act did not order doctors to murder these patients, it only empowered them to do so. There was significant support for this program among psychiatrists while prewar propaganda emphasizing the financial burden placed on society by hordes of mental patients created a significant degree of popular support for the medically supervised termination of "lives not worth living."

In the years immediately following the war, however, only a very few psychiatrists were prosecuted for their roles in this program of involuntary sterilization and murder. Some were even absolved of guilt because German courts ruled that they had acted in the belief that the program was legally constituted.[17] Moreover, there existed a significant demand for medical expertise in rebuilding a devastated society and therefore a distinct carryover of medical personnel from the Third Reich into the postwar republics.[18] So even though the reputation of traditional university psychiatry suffered in Germany both during and after the war because of its involvement with the destructive racial policy of the Nazis, many of its representatives, as well as their students, continued on in positions of authority after 1945. The continuities were not only personal but conceptual. The psychiatric preoccupation with the hereditary determinants of mental illness had been easily exploited by the Nazis. And apart from the authoritarian social and political views commonly held in the German professoriate often linked with this hereditarianism, psychiatrists, like physicians in general, were also heavily influenced by the eugenic thought, social Darwinism, and racism endemic to Germany during the late nineteenth and early twentieth centuries.[19] The persistence of this way of thinking into the postwar era is evident in the West German disposition of compensation cases for psychic damage caused by Nazi persecution. A number of these claims were rejected on the basis of psychiatric evaluations that declared that these individuals' difficulties were due to hereditary predisposition (*Anlage*), decisions that produced vigorous dissent from psychoanalysts and psychotherapists.[20]

A systematic confrontation with psychiatry's past did not occur until the 1980s. At first, this critique was part of a larger critical "history of the everyday" (*Alltagsgeschichte*) directed "from below" by students and citizens against the silent bastions of academic and political authority. These campaigns took the form of conferences and the collection, exhibition, and publication of documents, recollections, and studies concerning the activities of individuals, communities, and groups under National Socialism. Some of these concentrated on the medical profession, including psychiatry, and constituted criticism primarily from outside the profession from sociologists, pedagogues, historians, theologians, and the like.[21] Much of this critical work has been neo-Marxist or structuralist in orientation and sees Nazi medicine as a culmination of the Western bourgeois trend toward "social control" and eugenic engineering. Especially since the fall of communism in the Soviet Union and Eastern Europe, however, there has also been a greater willingness to confront the abuse of psychiatry by totalitarian socialist regimes.

Only recently have members of the psychiatric community begun to question their collective past. And instead of seeking distance between themselves and their compromised predecessors, as was characteristic of the radical confrontation of the late 1960s with "fascism" at home and abroad, these inquiries have focused with some humility on those processes and structures for dealing with the mentally ill that contribute *now as then* to inhumanity. This does not constitute a facile equation of contemporary society with Nazi Germany but, rather, an attempt to deal with those tendencies toward categorization and evaluation within psychiatry that can stigmatize mental patients as especially disruptive of society and the economy.

Klaus Doerner, one of the very few psychiatrists to address the subject relatively early on,[22] has more lately expressed concern that he had only intellectualized the subject rather than confronting it emotionally and that such an emotional confrontation involved for him an effort to work with relatives of mental patients killed by the Nazis who were denied compensation under the Federal Compensation Law. This effort, Doerner says, has brought him face to face with a continuity of attitude and issue between the Nazi period and the present.[23] Moreover, according to Doerner, such continuity extends back into the late eighteenth century. He has characterized modern European psychiatry as an exercise in "therapeutic idealism" by which "industrial-capitalist bourgeois society" could "deal with those who, by its gauge of rationality, it deems irrational."[24] The coercive social effects of this tyranny of reason ushered in by the Enlightenment and the Industrial Revolution were aggravated in Germany by Prussian authoritarianism. The Nazi period represented the extremity of both of these traditions.[25] In line with this thinking, most recently Doerner's was a strong voice raised in protest against Peter Singer's argument for euthanasia of severely handicapped newborns.[26]

A similar ethic pervades the documentation by a group of young mental health care workers of the operations of the asylum at Wittenau in Berlin between 1933 and 1945. The authors ask why they failed during the 1960s to take their teachers to task for their collaboration with the Nazis. The answer, they feel, lies in their own desire to divorce themselves from the horrors of the Nazi era by broadening and thus diluting their criticism into a radical condemnation of society in general and fascism in particular. What they found in scouring the archives at Wittenau was that the procedures and judgments involved in the sterilization and murder of mental patients under Nazi direction blended in rather smoothly with the workings of what up until 1933 had been an institution renowned for its progressive treatment of the mentally ill. This continuity of operation is the reason why documents detailing these measures were found in the archives while documents dealing with Jewish patients had long since disappeared.[27] Investigations and attitudes such as these are in keeping with the second sense of missed resistance, a regret for failure in the past and the congruent need for commitment in the present.

This is not to say, however, that there are no professional, political, or ideological agendas involved in these efforts at confronting psychiatry's past. Most of the criticism still comes from various left-of-center segments of the German polity who, with considerable justification, see distinct continuities in professional attitudes among psychiatrists before and after 1945. These critiques have most often been part of a general rejection of the conservative West German establishment embodied principally by the Christian Democratic Union, which has dominated political life since 1945. Moreover, while this confrontation has, to a great extent, been between generations, with the postwar young challenging the wartime old, the more recent concern with the moral ambiguities inherent in the social place of the mentally ill carries with it an implicit critique of professionalization, which can be applied to all practitioners, particularly those of the postwar generations who are advancing professionally in a prosperous Germany. At the same time, the unification of Germany has injected a great deal of Marxist-inspired research into the relationships between fascism and capitalism in the

Third Reich.[28] Two basic moral positions have evolved out of this combination of Western and Eastern scholarship, which pose questions relevant to the debate over the role of psychiatry in Nazi Germany. The first maintains that moral choice is obviated by membership in historically determined collectivities; the second emphasizes individual choices between good and evil that can and must be made: Which is it more important to change, structures or people? Which are more susceptible to change?

While psychotherapists and psychoanalysts have not had to confront direct participation in Nazi atrocities, their history displays some disturbing lines of professional continuity extending through the Nazi years. Under the Nazis this meant some specific as well as general violations of professional ethics, but it also fed into a longer-term and morally ambiguous trend toward adjustment of individuals to the demands of society. Agencies of the Nazi regime, such as the Labor Front, the SS, and the Luftwaffe, funded the Göring Institute generously in their mobilization of expertise to assist in rearmament and war. Between 1936 and 1945 a significant number of the men and women who would constitute the postwar psychotherapeutic movement in both German states were members or trainees of Matthias Heinrich Göring's German Institute for Psychological Research and Psychotherapy in Berlin or at its branches in several other cities. It was in this way that those physicians and lay practitioners in Germany who conceived of mental illness principally in psychological rather than physical terms established themselves as competitors to the dominant university psychiatrists. Some of the impetus for the critical examination of the history of German psychotherapy and psychoanalysis stems from concern over the resultant social identity, role, and responsibility of the field, a concern that also often obstructs understanding of the past.

Psychotherapists have largely ignored their recent professional past, in part because they were busy first surviving the difficult years after the war and then exploiting their newly professionalized position to meet a growing demand for psychological services in both the Federal and the Democratic Republic. It is also true that time is necessary for historical perspective and that psychotherapists, like psychiatrists and psychoanalysts, are not professional historians, but a distinct unwillingness to deal with the legacy of the Nazi years also marks their treatments of the past. The accepted professional view in West Germany was that the "political events following 1933 pushed German psychotherapy . . . into the background for a long time."[29] In 1977, on the occasion of the fiftieth anniversary of the founding of the General Medical Society for Psychotherapy, its president observed that the only significance of the psychotherapeutic institute in Nazi Germany was the degree of protection and enforced cooperation it provided for those psychotherapists who had not emigrated.[30]

In East Germany, an even greater distance was put between postwar psychotherapy and its precedents under German fascism, even though in the socialist republic there was a similar emphasis placed on expert service to the state and a reliance on the short-term methods pioneered in Germany by, among others, Johannes Heinrich Schultz, deputy director of the Göring Institute.[31] Former East German psychotherapists and psychiatrists now face the task of confronting a likewise compromised association with the late Communist regime. The difficulty of this task is compounded by the fact that former East Germans in general never had to confront questions of collaboration with the Nazis, since by official German Democratic Republic definition all former Nazis lived in the Federal Republic. On the other hand, the infamy and incompetence that prompted the collapse of the Communist regime may combine with the relatively advanced state in the West of confrontation with the Nazi past to produce an easier and quicker coming to terms with this even more recent compromised past. And whatever the psychiatric and psychotherapeutic injustices perpetrated by the East German government in aping its big Soviet brother, they, of course, pale in comparison to collaboration with the much more evil Nazi regime.

Challenges to the assertion of professional innocence among psychotherapists first came across disciplinary boundaries in West Germany as a result of the professional competition sharpened and even created under National Socialism. In 1960 the director of the German Society for Psychology responded to charges of Nazi collaboration among psychologists by arguing that psychotherapists had compromised themselves to a much greater degree.[32] This type of counterattack, however, raised defenses and not curiosity or consciousness. As a result, the first study of the history of psychotherapy in Nazi Germany came from abroad in the 1970s.[33] By the 1980s, some additional work was being done by historians of medicine at the University of Leipzig, but its thematic comprehensiveness is limited by a Marxist-Leninist approach emphasizing a top-down nazification of psychotherapy.[34] By this time as well, research in the West had integrated the history of psychotherapy in the Third Reich into the study of professions and professionalization in Germany.[35] This work has had little discernible effect on psychotherapists in Germany, at least partly because the course of their profession's development has scattered them throughout several disciplines and the nature of their practice has oriented them toward issues of application rather than of introspection.

It was the good fortune of this author to have been the first historian to have stumbled onto the subject of psychotherapy in the Third Reich. My major field as a graduate student at the University of California in Los Angeles was German history and one of my minor fields was in psychohistory, which is the application of psychoanalytic methods to history. As a result, I became interested in the history of psychoanalysis in Germany. In searching for a topic for my dissertation I quite by accident came across some bound volumes of the *Zentralblatt für Psychotherapie*. Upon noticing that the volumes covered the years from 1928 to 1939, I immediately assumed that the journal was Austrian or Swiss, because I already knew that psychoanalysis had been banned in Germany in 1933 and that therefore anything like psychotherapy certainly could not have survived there. I was wrong. The journal was that of the General Medical Society for Psychotherapy, it was published in Leipzig, and the editors included the Swiss Carl Jung and a man I had never heard of, Matthias Heinrich Göring. It turned out that Göring's cousin was Reich Marshal Hermann Göring and I immediately understood that the fortunes of psychotherapy in the Third Reich were bound up with the family relations of the second most powerful Nazi in Germany. And I noticed that while there were shrill denunciations of "Jewish" psychoanalysis in the pages of the journal after 1933, there were also articles that incorporated psychoanalytic points of view. So I talked with some psychoanalysts in nearby Beverly Hills who had fled Nazi Germany and they confirmed that some of their non-Jewish colleagues had stayed in Germany and had continued working in the field during the Nazi period.

A year in West Germany conducting interviews with former members of the institute and scouring archives and libraries produced the first history of the Göring Institute. Early in my research abroad I found myself disliking the people whom I was interviewing and about whom I was reading. At the time I had not found evidence that any of the members of the Göring Institute had been involved in atrocities, but I was bothered by an understandable desire on the part of the people I was interviewing to justify and defend their activities in Nazi Germany, including their acquiescence, or (possibly) worse, in the purging of Jewish colleagues and patients. But I decided that I should take advantage of the fact that I was a foreigner who had no other purpose than to describe accurately and dispassionately the history of this group of aspiring professionals. The wrestling with the moral consequences could be and has been more successfully carried out by professional descendants in Germany. This did not mean that I would not evaluate the social and moral consequences of the professionalization of psychotherapy in Germany between 1933 and 1945. Rather it meant that I would strive to relate all the relevant information I could about psychotherapy in the Third Reich so that as many historical connections as possible could be made by me and by subsequent researchers. It was just about that time that historians of the period were beginning to shift the focus away from the agencies and personalities of Nazi aggression and oppression and toward the broader topic of German society under nazism in order to understand more fully the ways in which everyday "normal" life was part of the environment that allowed Auschwitz to happen. Psychotherapists in the Third Reich, as part of a large set of evolving social and historical conditions, had their own (increasingly professional) agendas that accepted and advanced various interests of the Nazi order while also providing space for occasional individual and collective friction.

I was struck most of all by the amazing success the psychotherapists and psychoanalysts had in the face of opposition from the powerful psychiatric establishment in the universities, in the government, and in the military. Clearly association with the name Göring helped more than association with the name Freud hurt. And, given the protection and visibility afforded the psychotherapists by Göring, it was also the case that psychotherapists were able to make a significant case for the practical applications of their craft. I was also willing to accept the fact that there were wide ranges and degrees of collaboration with the Nazis and many levels of culpability. But, unlike the psychiatrists, whose collaboration meant the maiming and murder of "racial enemies," psychotherapists had the luxury of working for the enhancement of "racial comrades." This meant that what they were doing as professionals was closer to what professionals in easier and better times usually do. The ethical violations of the psychotherapists as a group were largely indirect, that is, more than anything else they helped an immoral regime exploit the capacities of its people for a war of conquest and extermination. As a result, their experience suggests *in extremis* some of the problematic ethical dimensions of professionalization in modern industrial and postindustrial societies. For example, psychotherapists' and psychoanalysts' efforts in Nazi Germany to "cure" homosexuals represented (1) an attempt to enhance professional status; (2) a desire to "help" the "sick;" (3) support for the regime's insistence on a productive populace; (4) an alternative to the policies of punishment, imprisonment, castration, and extermination carried out by psychiatrists, the SS, and the military; and (5) a resulting absence of resistance to overall Nazi persecution of homosexuals and thus degrees of participation in an inhumane system.

Unlike the psychotherapists, psychoanalysts in West Germany (psychoanalysis was officially discouraged in the East) have of late confronted their past. This has to do with the distinct history as well as the distinct nature of psychoanalysis. Two versions of the history of psychoanalysis in Nazi Germany were literally institutionalized in the immediate postwar period. The German Psychoanalytic Society (DPG), which had been founded in 1910 and dissolved in 1938, was reestablished in 1946 but was divided between orthodox Freudians and "neo-analysts" influenced by other schools of psychotherapeutic thought within the Göring Institute. By 1951 the orthodox Freudians had seceded to form the German Psychoanalytic Union (DPV), which in that year was recognized by the International Psycho-Analytical Association (IPA). The "official" position of the DPG with regard to psychoanalysis in the Third Reich has been that it had been "saved" by the Freudian members of the Göring Institute.[36] The DPV argued that psychoanalysis had simply been suppressed by the Nazis.[37]

These positions remained unaltered and largely unnoticed until the 1970s when psychoanalytic candidates began questioning these orthodoxies. Chief among them was Regine Lockot, who in 1985 published a comprehensive critical study of the Göring Institute. By relying on extensive documentary evidence, Lockot demonstrated that psychoanalysis was neither merely suppressed nor simply saved during the Third Reich; rather, it was used, compromised, abused, and perverted. On the one hand, Lockot sought to follow what she labeled the *realpolitisch* perspective of the earlier historical work I had done and, on the other, to utilize a psychoanalytic point of view to begin the process of what Freud in 1914 called "working through" (*Durcharbeiten*). Freud had argued that what "distinguishes analytic treatment from any kind of treatment by suggestion"[38] is the process by which the patient *works through* resistances to an understanding of the repressed content behind neurotic symptoms. This didactic aim is furthered by transference, whereby the patient reexperiences feelings toward parents in the relationship with the analyst, and countertransference, whereby the analyst through the emotions created by the relationship with the patient comes to understand the patient's unconscious. Lockot argues that psychoanalysts in particular must work through the repression of their own past and by means of countertransference come to understand not only their history but themselves as well.[39] The alternative is neurotic repetition of actions in place of self-understanding. Lockot argues that this neurotic pattern of behavior was displayed immediately after the war by leading members of the DPG as they struggled with the emotional consequences of a psychoanalytic identity damaged by compromise and collaboration under National Socialism.[40]

It is this psychoanalytic emphasis on repression that in particular characterizes the challenge that young psychoanalysts have raised against their professional elders. All three senses of the missed resistance have been present in this challenge: confrontation, regret/empathy, and a tendency to overlook resistance for Resistance. This challenge manifested itself first at a conference in Bamberg in 1980 and was developed by analysts and nonanalysts in the pages of *Psyche* between 1982 and 1986. Perhaps predictably for a discipline concerned so much with individual cases and characterized organizationally and emotionally by issues of authority between teacher and student, much of the heat (if less of the light) was generated in a controversy over Göring Institute psychoanalyst Carl Müller-Braunschweig.[41] More recently, the Berlin Forum for the History of Psychoanalysis has begun efforts to deposit documents at the Federal Archives in Coblenz pertaining to the history of psychoanalysis in Germany.

The debate within the DPV has overshadowed the discussions within the DPG, such as those held at DPG conferences in West Berlin in 1985[42] and in Bad Soden in 1989. Young DPV critics see their organization's prior treatment of its past as especially objectionable for two reasons: first, because the notion of the complete suppression of psychoanalysis by the Nazis constitutes silence on the subject; and, second, because collaboration meant forsaking not only the many Jewish colleagues victimized by the Nazi campaign against "Jewish science" but also the ideals embodied in psychoanalytic thought.[43] The DPG, originally displaying the eclecticism in theory and practice that was promoted by the Göring Institute, had been willing to discuss the saving of psychoanalysis but until recently was less willing to examine critically the negative aspects of such salvation. But of late the DPG has been moving away from the somewhat idiosyncratic "neo-Freudian" position established chiefly by the Göring Institute's Harald Schultz-Hencke toward the general Freudian tradition represented by the DPV and IPA. This movement has been encouraged by increasing contacts among newer members of both groups not divided by traditional rivalries as well as by the growing influence of the DPV both at home and abroad.[44]

Both the DPG and the DPV have attempted to capitalize on the figure of John Rittmeister, the Freudian member of the Göring Institute who was executed by the Nazis in 1943 on charges of having spied for the Soviet Union. There is in this memorialization a distinct sense of "our Rittmeister." For former colleagues at the Göring Institute it is a matter of innocence by association.[45] For younger members of the DPV he has been the counterexample they hold up to their professional elders and from whom they draw inspiration.[46] And Rittmeister's involvement with the Communist resistance to Hitler prompted the East German Society for Medical Psychotherapy to create an award in his name in 1979. While Rittmeister is certainly worthy of admiration, concentration on him to the exclusion of the other particulars of the history of psychoanalysis and psychotherapy in the Third Reich has been part of the process of denial and repression characteristic of these groups' perceptions of their collective past until recently. Surely it is a relevant irony that some who lived ethically compromised lives as members of the Göring Institute could at the time and later rationalize their behavior because of small acts of courage and compassion while contemporary critics cannot *do* anything either against the Nazis or for their victims except remember for the sake of memory, their contemporaries, and the future. Under such circumstances the figure of a hero provides a certain degree of vicarious satisfaction and emotional nourishment.

German psychoanalysts have thus been somewhat successful in confronting their history. Psychoanalysis, unlike psychiatry or psychotherapy in general, is based on detailed excavation of the past. Their patients have included those whose lives were directly or indirectly affected by the horrors of the Third Reich, even if for a long time the topic was largely taboo in analytic sessions.[47] Moreover, the DPV in particular is the inheritor of an intellectual tradition that is largely Jewish in origin and many of whose practitioners were persecuted by the Nazis. German psychoanalysts were reminded of this in 1977 when at the Jerusalem meeting of the IPA a proposal to meet in Berlin was turned down. Yet in 1985 the IPA did meet in Hamburg and devoted a day to discussion of "identification and its vicissitudes in relation to the Nazi phenomenon."[48] In conjunction with the congress, a group of young German analysts set up an exhibition on the history of psychoanalysis in Germany, highlighting the activities of psychoanalysts at the Göring Institute, a history that they see as still being repressed and not worked through by the West German psychoanalytic leadership.[49] But although the DPV has been quite willing to benefit from the international success of the Hamburg exhibition, the IPA has not encouraged confrontation with the discipline's German past, preferring at Hamburg as before to concentrate on technical issues of psychoanalytic theory and practice. This neutral "scientific" posture constituted the original response of the IPA to the depredations of nazism in the 1930s.[50]

The Germans make up the second largest national contingent of psychoanalysts in the IPA, behind only the Americans, a position that certainly will be further consolidated through the unification of Germany. But the popularity of psychoanalysis in West Germany is also due to its being "a Jewish heritage in the German language" uncontaminated by the Nazi past that has served, in the eyes of some, to blind the DPV in particular to its compromised past.[51] Moreover, it can be argued that the introspection inherent in psychoanalysis carries a particular appeal for the German Romantic cultural tradition and that such self-absorption can be a means of avoiding rational confrontation with unpleasant truths. Left-wing psychoanalysts such as the Siegfried Bernfeld Group, who wish to realize what they see as the radical social and political implications of psychoanalysis, see contemporary German conservatism in social, political, environmental, and military affairs reflected in the authoritarian practices of psychoanalytic institutes and in the ongoing failure to work through the Nazi past.[52] From this standpoint, the integration of psychoanalysis into the state health care system only aggravated inherent tendencies toward political and social quiescence.[53] Finally, it is anything but clear that Germans in general have laid to rest the legacy of anti-Semitism, particularly with regard to feelings about health and illness.[54]

As with psychiatrists and psychotherapists, psychoanalysts too have tended to concentrate on the actions of individuals independent of the broader context of institutional and professional history, a limitation manifested as well in the anecdotal tendencies of *Alltagsgeschichte*. But in the second sense of missed resistance, that of regret/empathy, for whose exercise the analytic emphasis on intra- and interpersonal psychodynamics is peculiarly suited, German psychoanalysts have also had to deal with the structural continuities in the history of their discipline to, through, and beyond the Third Reich. Such continuities raise the disturbing question of the ethical problems inherent in a professionalizing society. For all three disciplines, therefore, there exists the task of working through the present as well as the past.

Notes

1. Alexander Mitscherlich and Fred Mielke, *Wissenschaft ohne Menschlichkeit. Medizinische und Eugenische Irrwege unter Diktatur, Burokratie und Krieg* (Heidelberg: Verlag Lambert Schneider, 1949), v, 6. (Other editions appeared in 1947 and 1962 and an English translation by Heinz Norden, *Doctors of Infamy*, in 1949.) Michael Kater, *Doctors under Hitler* (Chapel Hill: University of North Carolina Press, 1989), 12, 267, fixes the number of wartime doctors in Germany at around 79,000.

2. Robert N. Proctor, *Racial Hygiene: Medicine under the Nazis* (Cambridge: Harvard University Press, 1988), 309.

3. Alexander and Margarete Mitscherlich, *The Inability to Mourn: Principles of Collective Behavior* [1967], trans. Beverley R. Placzek (New York: Grove Press, 1975).

4. Geoffrey Cocks, "The Professionalization of Psychotherapy in Germany, 1928–1949" in Geoffrey Cocks and Konrad Jarausch (eds.), *German Professions, 1800–1950* (New York: Oxford University Press, 1990), 311.

5. Konrad Jarausch, *The Unfree Professions: German Lawyers, Teachers, and Engineers, 1900–1950* (New York: Oxford University Press, 1990).

6. Ulfried Geuter, *Die Professionalisierung der deutschen Psychologie im Nationalsozialismus* [1984], 2nd ed. (Frankfurt am Main: Suhrkamp Verlag, 1988); Cocks, "Professionalization of Psychotherapy in Germany."

7. Rainer C. Baum, *The Holocaust and the German Elite* (Lanham, Maryland: Rowman & Littlefield, 1981), 266.

8. Hans Mommsen, "Resistance in Germany and the Restoration of Politics," *Journal of Modern History*, lxiv, suppl. (December 1992), S112–S127.

9. Rolf Vogt, "Warum sprechen die Deutschen nicht?" *Psyche*, xl (1986), 896–897. On the dynamic relationship between resistance and collaboration within the shifting and persisting institutional continuities of German and European society in the modern period, see Michael Geyer, "Resistance as Ongoing Project: Visions of Order, Obligations to Strangers, Struggles for Civil Society," *Journal of Modern History*, lxiv, suppl. (December 1992), S217–S241.

10. David Large, " 'A Beacon in the German Darkness': The Anti-Nazi Resistance Legacy in Politics," *Journal of Modern History*, lxiv, suppl. (December 1992), S173–S186.

11. Klemens von Klemperer, " 'What is the Law that Lies Behind these Words?' Antigone's Question and the German Resistance," *Journal of Modern History*, lxiv, suppl. (December 1992), S102–S111.

12. "Tagebuchblätter aus dem Gefängnis von Dr. med. John Rittmeister," pp. 3, 4, 15, 19, 23. Nds 721 Acc 69/76 Lüneburg, vol. 10, pp. 126–157; Niedersächsisches Hauptstaatsarchiv, Hanover. For a critical evaluation of historian Martin Broszat's concepts of *Resistenz* and *Widerstand*, see Saul Friedländer, "Some Reflections on the Historization of National Socialism," *Tel Aviver Jahrbuch für deutsche Geschichte*, xvi (1987), 310–324.

13. Dirk Blasius, "Psychiatrischer Alltag im Nationalsozialismus" in Detlev Peukert and Jürgen Reulecke (eds.), *Die Reihen fest geschlossen. Beiträge zur Geschichte des Alltags unterm Nationalsozialismus* (Wuppertal: Peter Hammer Verlag, 1981), 367–380.

14. Hans-Walter Schmuhl, *Rassenhygiene, Nationalsozialismus, Euthanasie. Von der Verhütung zur Vernichtung "lebensunwerten Lebens," 1890–1945* (Göttingen: Vandenhoeck & Ruprecht, 1987).

15. Arthur Gütt, Ernst Rüdin, and Falk Ruttke, *Gesetz zur Verhütung erbkranken Nachwuchses* (Munich: J. F. Lehmanns, 1934).

16. Gisela Bock, *Zwangssterilisation im Nationalsozialismus* (Opladen: Westdeutscher Verlag, 1986), 230–246.

17. Ernst Klee, *"Euthanasie" im NS-Staat. Die "Vernichtung lebensunwerten Lebens"* (Frankfurt am Main: Fischer Verlag, 1985), 384–386.

18. Kater, *Doctors under Hitler*, 223–224.

19. Paul Weindling, *Health, Race and German Politics Between National Unification and Nazism, 1870–1945* (Cambridge: Cambridge University Press, 1989).

20. Klaus D. Hoppe, "The Emotional Reactions of Psychiatrists when Confronting Survivors of Persecution," *Psychoanalytic Forum*, i (1966), 187–196.

21. Gerhard Baader and Ulrich Schultz (eds.), *Medizin und Nationalsozialismus. Tabuisierte Vergangenheit—Ungebrochene Tradition?* (Berlin: Verlagsgesellschaft Gesundheit mbH, 1980); Projektgruppe "Volk und Gesundheit" (eds.), *Volk und Gesundheit. Heilen und Vernichten im Nationalsozialismus* (Tübingen: Tübinger Vereinigung für Volkskunde, 1982); Kölnische Gesellschaft für Christlich-Jüdische Zusammenarbeit (eds.), *Heilen und Vernichten im Nationalsozialismus* (Cologne: Kölnische Gesellschaft für Christlich-Jüdische Zusammenarbeit, 1985). See also Benno Müller-Hill, *Murderous Science: Elimination by Scientific Selection of Jews, Gypsies, and Others, Germany, 1933–1945* [1984], trans. George R. Fraser (Oxford: Oxford University Press, 1988).

22. Klaus Doerner, "Nationalsozialismus und Lebensvernichtung," *Vierteljahreshefte für Zeitgeschichte*, xv (1967), 121–152.

23. Gerhard Baader et al., "Podiumsdiskussion" in Baader and Schultz (eds.), *Medizin und Nationalsozialismus*, 23–24. Such emotional confrontation, however, allowed Doerner to buttress his original continuity thesis.

24. Klaus Doerner, *Madmen and the Bourgeoisie: A Social History of Insanity and Psychiatry*, trans. Joachim Neugroschel and Jean Steinberg (Oxford: Basil Blackwell, 1981), 218, 291. Cf. Robert Brown, "The Institutions of Insanity," *Times Literary Supplement*, 8 January 1982, 24. Brown criticizes Doerner's thesis as lacking in evidence.

25. Doerner, *Madmen and the Bourgeosie*, 216–217, 329, n. 157.

26. Johann S. Ach and Andreas Gaidt, "Kein Diskurs über Abtreibung und 'Euthanasie'?" Zur Rechtfertigung der Singer-Debatte," *Das Argument*, xxxii (1990), 769–776. Doerner argues that Singer's view represents a mentality concerning expendable life which replaces or disguises earlier eugenic arguments based on social cost with arguments based on sympathy for severely handicapped newborns. Any discussion of such ideas, Doerner says, provides them with a valuation they do not deserve. Of course, one can support Singer's arguments without espousing nazism, just as one can distinguish between nazism and "bourgeois society."

27. Arbeitsgruppe zur Erforschung der Geschichte der Karl-Bonhoeffer-Nervenklinik (eds.), *Totgeschwiegen 1933–1945. Die Geschichte der Karl-Bonhoeffer-Nervenklinik* (Berlin: Edition Hentrich, 1988). See also Tilmann Moser, "Die Unfähigkeit zu trauern: Hält die These einer Überprüfung stand? Zur psychischen Verarbeitung des Holocaust" in idem, *Vorsicht Berührung. Über Sexualisierung, Spaltung, NS-Erbe und Stasi-Angst* (Frankfurt am Main: Suhrkamp Verlag, 1992), 203–220.

28. V. R. Berghahn, "Big Business in the Third Reich," *European History Quarterly*, xxi (1991), 97–108.

29. Walter Theodor Winkler, "The Present Status of Psychotherapy in Germany" in Frieda Fromm-Reichmann and J. L. Moreno (eds.), *Progress in Psychotherapy 1956* (New York: Grune & Stratton, 1956), 288.

30. Walter Theodor Winkler, "50 Jahre AAeGP—ein Rückblick," *Zeitschrift für Psychotherapie und medizinische Psychologie*, xxvii (1977), 79.

31. Kurt Höck, *Psychotherapie in der DDR* (n.p., 1979), 7, 14; Dietfried Müller-Hegemann, "Psychotherapy in the German Democratic Republic" in Ari Kiev (ed.), *Psychiatry in the Communist World* (New York: Science House, 1968), 51–70.

32. Albert Wellek, "Deutsche Psychologie und Nationalsozialismus," *Psychologie und Praxis*, iv (1960), 177–182.

33. Geoffrey Campbell Cocks, "Psyche and Swastika: *Neue deutsche Seelenheilkunde*, 1933–1945" (Ph.D. diss., University of California, Los Angeles, 1975).

34. Christine Schröder, "Programm und Wirksamkeit der 'Neuen deutschen Seelenheilkunde' " in Achim Thom and Genadij Ivanovič Caregorodcev (eds.), *Medizin unterm Hakenkreuz* (Berlin: VEB Verlag Volk und Gesundheit, 1989), 283–306.

35. Geoffrey C. Cocks, "Psychoanalyse, Psychotherapie und Nationalsozialismus," *Psyche*, xxxvii (1983), 1057–1106; idem, *Psychotherapy in the Third Reich: The Göring Institute* (New York: Oxford University Press, 1985); and idem "Professionalization of Psychotherapy in Germany."

36. Franz Baumeyer, "Zur Geschichte der Psychoanalyse in Deutschland. 60 Jahre Deutsche Psychoanalytische Gesellschaft," *Zeitschrift für psychosomatische Medizin und Psychoanalyse*, xvii (1971), 203–240; Rose Spiegel, Gerard Chrzanowski, Arthur Feiner, "On Psychoanalysis in the Third Reich," *Contemporary Psychoanalysis*, xi (1975), 477–510.

37. Gerhard Maetze, "Psychoanalyse in Deutschland" in Dieter Eicke (ed.), *Die Psychologie des 20. Jahrhunderts. Freud und die Folgen* (Zurich: Kindler Verlag, 1976), 1145–1179; Gudrun

Zapp, "Psychoanalyse und Nationalsozialismus. Untersuchungen zum Verhältnis Medizin/Psychoanalyse während des Nationalsozialismus" (Inaug. diss., University of Kiel, 1980).

38. Sigmund Freud, "Remembering, Repeating and Working Through (Further Recommendations on the Technique of Psycho-Analysis II)" in James Strachey (ed. & trans.), *The Standard Edition of the Complete Psychological Works of Sigmund Freud* (London: Hogarth Press, 1958), 155–156.

39. Regine Lockot, *Erinnern und Durcharbeiten. Zur Geschichte der Psychoanalyse und Psychotherapie im Nationalsozialismus* (Frankfurt am Main: Fischer Verlag, 1985), 17–38. See also Wolfgang Huber, *Psychoanalyse in Oesterreich seit 1933* (Vienna: Geyer, 1977).

40. Regine Lockot, "Wiederholen oder Neubeginn: Skizzen zur Geschichte der 'Deutschen Psychoanalytischen Gesellschaft' von 1945–1950," *Jahrbuch der Psychoanalyse*, xxii (1988), 218–235.

41. Hans-Martin Lohmann (ed.), *Psychoanalyse und Nationalsozialismus. Beiträge zur Bearbeitung eines unbewältigten Traumas* (Frankfurt am Main: Fischer Verlag, 1984), 109–136; "Dokumentation des DPV-Vorstands zum Briefwechsel Ehebald/Dahmer" (DPV, September 1984, typescript); Hans Müller-Braunschweig, "Fünfzig Jahre danach. Stellungnahme zu den in PSYCHE 11/1982 zitierten Aeusserungen von Carl-Müller-Braunschweig," *Psyche*, xxxvii (1983), 1140–1145; and Ernst Federn, "Weitere Bemerkungen zum Problemkreis 'Psychoanalyse und Politik,' " *Psyche*, xxxix (1985), 367–374.

42. Friedrich Beese, "Psychoanalyse in Deutschland. Rückblick und Perspektiven" in Gerd Rudolf et al. (eds.), *Psychoanalyse der Gegenwart. Eine kritische Bestandsaufnahme 75 Jahre nach der Gründung der Deutschen Psychoanalytischen Gesellschaft* (Göttingen: Vandenhoeck & Ruprecht, 1987), 15–29; Geoffrey Cocks, "Psychoanalyse und Psychotherapie im Dritten Reich" in Rudolf et al. (eds.), 30–43.

43. Volker Friedrich, "Psychoanalyse im Nationalsozialismus. Vom Widerspruch zur Gleichschaltung," *Jahrbuch der Psychoanalyse*, xx (1987), 207–233.

44. Bernd Nitschke, "La Psychanalyse considérée comme une science 'a'-politique," *Revue internationale d'histoire de la psychanalyse*, v (1992), 169–182; Volker Friedrich, "From Psychoanalysis to the 'Great Treatment': Psychoanalysts under National Socialism," *Political Psychology*, x (1989), 3–26.

45. Werner Kemper, "John F. Rittmeister zum Gedächtnis," *Zeitschrift für psychosomatische Medizin und Psychoanalyse*, xiv (1968), 147–149.

46. Ludger M. Hermanns, "John F. Rittmeister und C. G. Jung," *Psyche*, xxxvi (1982), 1022–1031.

47. Lutz Rosenkötter, "Schatten der Zeitgeschichte auf psychoanalytischen Behandlungen," *Psyche*, xxxiii (1979), 1024–1038.

48. Edith Kurzweil, "The Freudians Meet in Germany," *Partisan Review*, lii (1985), 337–347. See also Kurzweil, "The (Freudian) Congress of Vienna," *Commentary*, lii (1971), 80–83; and Kurzweil, *The Freudians: A Comparative Perspective* (New Haven: Yale University Press, 1989), 231–236, 294–298, 313–315.

49. Karen Brecht et al., *"Hier geht das Leben auf eine sehr merkwürdige Weise weiter . . ." Zur Geschichte der Psychoanalyse in Deutschland* (Hamburg: Verlag Michael Kellner, 1985).

50. Edward Glover, "Report of the Thirteenth International Psycho-Analytical Congress," *International Journal of Psycho-Analysis*, xv (1934), 485–488; Richard F. Sterba, *Reminiscences of a Viennese Psychoanalyst* (Detroit: Wayne State University Press, 1982), 163.

51. Hermann Beland et al., "Podiumsdiskussion: Psychoanalyse unter Hitler—Psychoanalyse heute," *Psyche*, xl (1986), 425; Hans Keilson, "Psychoanalyse und Nationalsozialismus," *Jahrbuch der Psychoanalyse*, xxv (1989), 23; and Robert S. Wallerstein, "Psychoanalysis in Nazi Germany: Historical and Psychoanalytic Lessons," *Psychoanalysis and Contemporary Thought*, xi (1988), 360.

52. Janice Haaken, "The Siegfried Bernfeld Conference: Uncovering the Psychoanalytic Political Unconscious," *American Journal of Psychoanalysis*, l (1990), 289–304.

53. Paul Parin, "Warum die Psychoanalytiker so ungern zu brennenden Zeitproblemen Stellung nehmen," *Psyche*, xxxii (1978), 385–399.

54. Geoffrey Cocks, "Partners and Pariahs: Jews and Medicine in Modern German Society," *Leo Baeck Institute Yearbook*, xxxvi (1991), 192–205.

16

Heroes and Non-Heroes:
Recurring Themes in the Historiography
of Russian-Soviet Psychiatry

JULIE V. BROWN

Even more than in many other countries the history of psychiatry in Russia and the Soviet Union has been written by members of the nation's psychiatric profession. As a consequence, the historical account not only reflects the medical perspective of its authors but also the concerns of that particular group of medical professionals. The assumption that mental disorders are diseases of the brain, which are at least in principle completely explainable and treatable by medical science, is taken for granted in this view of history, as is the position that psychiatric medicine represents a cognitively and a morally superior approach to the problem of mental disturbances.

The construction of the history of psychiatry in Russia and the Soviet Union has also been profoundly influenced both by the internal composition of the psychiatric profession and by those protean forces in the power structure of the larger society with which psychiatrists have continually been compelled to try to come to terms. Ironically, the dramatic changes in ruling elites and ideologies, which have characterized Russia since the first psychiatric histories were written in the late nineteenth century, have been accompanied by an equally significant, albeit remarkably constant, intraprofessional dynamic.

The net effect of these diverse influences has been a psychiatric history in which heroic figures occupy center stage. The aim of this brief account is to chronicle some of the factors that have contributed to the dominance of the Great Man tradition in Russian-Soviet psychiatric history as well as to analyze the social construction of psychiatric heroes in this historiographical tradition.[1] The focus on heroes is, of course, hardly unique to Russian-Soviet psychiatry. Indeed, it is a typical feature of histories written by those convinced of the reality and even the inevitability of medical progress. Given these assumptions, writing the history of medicine is readily viewed as an exercise designed to chronicle the progress already made and confer credit where credit is perceived to be due.

In Russia and later the Soviet Union this tradition in medical history writing has been reinforced by political problems faced by members of the psychiatric profession.

Competing versions of the history of the profession have been used repeatedly as weapons in an enduring intraprofessional dispute. Simultaneously, psychiatric heroes have been both created and forsaken in the effort to establish the ideological legitimacy of the profession to powerful and potentially hostile external audiences.

Intraprofessional Dissension and the Writing of Psychiatric History

Prior to the middle of the nineteenth century there were only a few isolated physicians in Russia who considered themselves specialists in the care of the mentally disturbed. The emergence of a self-conscious community of psychiatric professionals occurred primarily as a result of reforms in medical education that were initiated by the tsarist government immediately after the Crimean War. The government's goal with respect to psychiatry was to produce a native cadre of technical experts with whom it could staff the new mental institutions it planned to build throughout the empire. In other words, the Russian psychiatric profession was more or less a creation of the state, and many of its early leaders were intimately involved in the elaboration of state policies with respect to the mentally disturbed.

The world of this first generation of psychiatrists was centered in St. Petersburg, the imperial capital. The prestigious Military-Medical Academy in that city was the locus of training for most of Russia's earliest psychiatrists. Until the 1890s the St. Petersburg Society of Psychiatrists, the majority of whose leaders were academy faculty, remained the unchallenged voice of the profession as a whole. Local government (*zemstvo*) organizations and universities alike sought the recommendation of the leaders of the St. Petersburg psychiatric community when they were building or renovating asylums or when they were seeking professionally trained psychiatric physicians with whom to staff those institutions.

The earliest histories of psychiatry in Russia reflect the dominant role of St. Petersburg. By the early twentieth century monograph-length works as well as numerous shorter pieces chronicled the theoretical and practical achievements of leading St. Petersburg psychiatrists.[2] I. M. Balinskii, the first head of the Department of Psychiatry at the Military-Medical Academy, was enshrined in this initial version of Russian psychiatric history as the "Father of Russian Psychiatry." A pediatrician by training, Balinskii had been drafted in 1857 for the psychiatric post by the academy's president. His early biographers lauded his level of commitment to this new assignment and credited him with greatly enhancing the status of the profession within the medical world and in the view of the government. They asserted that his charismatic personality and dynamic teaching techniques had attracted a growing number of top students to the field and that his organizational abilities and humanitarian impulses had revolutionized the treatment of the insane in Russia. One of these historians summed up Balinskii's role in the following glowing terms: "Balinskii was the first in Russia to advocate humane attitudes toward the insane and a rational approach to their care. He truly deserves recognition as the 'Russian Pinel.' His students . . . were the first psychiatrists in Russia to eliminate completely the use of [physical] restraints on patients."[3] The respect with which Balinskii was regarded in governmental circles, the historians continued, had also resulted in an increased role for psychiatrists in policy-making in general and particularly in the tsarist legal system, developments that in their view benefited both patients and the profession.

As Balinskii's students (and those of his successor, I. P. Merzheevskii, who took over the headship in 1876) settled into their posts in the new asylums that were popping up across European Russia in the late nineteenth century, these provincial practitioners became discontented with their working situations. Many were convinced that the problems they encountered in the remote areas of the empire were poorly understood and even less appreciated by their senior colleagues and former teachers who worked in the "ivory tower" conditions of the capital. The fact that the names of those esteemed professors were on more than one occasion associated with bureaucratic regulations emanating from the central medical administration in St. Petersburg merely reinforced their sense of separateness.[4]

These rising levels of frustration in combination with the emergence of a professionally ambitious school of psychiatry in St. Petersburg's historical rival city, Moscow, set the stage for the first attempt to rewrite the history of Russian psychiatry. The new version proffered by the fledgling "Moscow school of psychiatry" claimed for a Muscovite instead of for Balinskii the role of initiator of psychiatric reform in Russia.

Given Moscow's importance as Russia's second major city, the development of psychiatry there proceeded at a surprisingly slow pace. The region's institutional facilities for the insane were widely acknowledged to be among the worst in the empire, and shamefully inadequate for an area of such economic importance and with so dense a population.

Psychiatry was slow to take root at Moscow University as well. A. I. Kozhevnikov was assigned in 1867 to teach both psychiatry and neurology. Although he was an active propagandist for improved care for the insane, Kozhevnikov's primary interest was in neurological research. As a result, psychiatric instruction at Moscow University long remained a low priority. Indeed, Moscow University was not the second but the fifth university in Russia to establish an independent department of psychiatry.

Kozhevnikov increasingly delegated responsibility for psychiatric instruction to his student, S. S. Korsakov, and when the university at long last authorized the creation of a separate Department of Psychiatry in 1887, Korsakov was named its head. Like Balinskii, Korsakov was clearly a dynamic personage: a charismatic teacher, creative researcher, and innovative in his approach to the treatment of mental patients.

By the early 1890s an active rivalry had developed between the psychiatric centers in Moscow and St. Petersburg. At least in the initial stages the most vocal partner in the polemics was indisputably the junior one. The Muscovites went to great lengths to emphasize the distinctiveness of their approach to psychiatry and to stress their close ties to the progressive forces within *zemstvo* medicine and the society at large. Repeatedly, they emphasized their sympathetic understanding of the problems of the provincial practitioners. Their commentary invariably contrasted their own "progressive" tendencies with St. Petersburg's myriad associations with "conservative" forces in the central government bureaucracy.[5]

The charges of ideological conservatism hurled at St. Petersburg from Moscow were closely bound to accusations of theoretical and therapeutic conservatism. The Muscovites charged their St. Petersburg colleagues with forgetting the patient and focusing instead solely on the disease. Their own approach, they argued, was more holistic, emphasizing the importance of both the individual and the social environment.[6]

The issue upon which the Moscow psychiatrists chose to focus one of their most enduring public campaigns was a particularly controversial and ultimately political one, the use of physical restraints on institutionalized patients. The Muscovites repeatedly accused St. Petersburg not only of continuing to employ physical restraints on patients but of actually advocating their use. To accuse late nineteenth-century psychiatrists of favoring the use of straitjackets or chains on mental patients was tantamount to associating them with practices from the dark ages in the care of the insane. The modern era in psychiatry to which all late nineteenth-century psychiatrists considered themselves heirs had begun a century earlier with the removal of the chains confining the insane. Associated temporally with the French Revolution, this event symbolized for many the recognition that the mentally disturbed were no less human than their sane counterparts and should be accorded respect as well as those fundamental human rights in support of which the Revolution had presumably been waged.

A more controversial doctrine of absolute nonrestraint of patients developed in England during the second quarter of the nineteenth century. The viability of a mental institution with no mechanical means of controlling patients remained a subject of international controversy through much of the second half of the nineteenth century. The first paper on the subject of "no restraint" in Russia was delivered at the First Conference of Russian Psychiatrists in 1887. The author was S. S. Korsakov, who reported his success in eliminating mechanical restraints at a small private asylum in Moscow. While he urged the broader implementation of the principle, Korsakov neither claimed to be the first to have introduced "no restraint" into a Russian asylum nor did he condemn those psychiatrists who occasionally resorted to the use of mechanical restraints. On the contrary, he argued strongly for professional autonomy for individual practitioners: "the strait jacket is a medical remedy and in that sense it can be utilized. We should not take that right away from the doctor. I don't see that as possible. We cannot completely do away with restraints."[7]

The discussion that followed Korsakov's presentation included psychiatrists from Moscow, St. Petersburg, and a number of provincial cities. Although they disagreed on minor points, all discussants shared essentially the same view: The notion of absolute nonrestraint was a commendable one; however, given the particularly poor conditions in Russia's asylums and the inferior caliber of the nonprofessional staff, it remained an unattainable ideal.

That apparent convergence of opinion notwithstanding, presumed differences in the views of the psychiatric communities of Moscow and St. Petersburg on the issue of "no restraint" subsequently became both a subject of controversy and a means of invective. Central to this dispute was disagreement over the historical matter of who properly deserved credit for initiating psychiatric reform in Russia. Establishing the legitimacy of each school's claim to moral and professional hegemony clearly was perceived as dependent upon the historic role played by individual members of the respective psychiatric communities in the introduction of a modern, humane approach to psychiatry in Russia.

The polemics escalated with the untimely death of Korsakov in 1900. His successors were determined to secure for their mentor, and by extension for their school, the preeminent position in the history of Russian psychiatry. They touted Korsakov's scientific accomplishments, especially the international recognition he had received for his work on alcohol-induced psychoses (Korsakov's Syndrome). They also credited Korsakov with the idea of establishing a psychiatric professional organization in Russia. As that organization, the Russian Union of Neuropathologists and Psychiatrists, began to take shape, they insisted that it should bear his name, both to reward his organizational initiative and to memorialize his contributions to the field as a whole.

This version of events was challenged by the St. Petersburg Psychiatrists and especially by V. M. Bekhterev, who had become the head of the Department of Psychiatry at the Military-Medical Academy in 1893. Bekhterev had been present at the initial planning sessions of the professional society in the 1890s. Supported by the rest of the St. Petersburg group, he insisted that no single individual deserved sole credit for the idea, but that if the name of the Russian Union of Neuropathologists and Psychiatrists was to immortalize a seminal figure in the development of Russian psychiatry, the most appropriate individual would be I. M. Balinskii.[8]

The feuding parties were finally able, in 1905, to reach a compromise on the issue of a name for their professional organization. However, the broader issue of which psychiatric school had made the more significant historical contribution to psychiatric progress in Russia remained highly contentious. St. Petersburg continued to claim paternity rights to modern Russian psychiatry for Balinskii. The Muscovites, by contrast, sought to claim that status for Korsakov. Korsakov's successor as head of Moscow University's Department of Psychiatry, V. P. Serbskii, was particularly vociferous in his insistence that his mentor had been the first to introduce the concept of "no restraint" to Russia and by extension was singlehandedly responsible for the revolutionary changes that had presumably occurred in the care of the insane in Russia's asylums.[9]

These claims that genuine psychiatric reform in Russia began in Moscow were accompanied by accusations that psychiatrists in the capital city continued to adhere to outdated and cruel forms of patient care, particularly the use of physical restraints on patients. This issue was a compelling one in the context of late imperial Russia, as it linked therapeutic and political ideologies in a particularly potent fashion. Accusing colleagues of failing to remove physical restraints from mental patients (and even of advocating their use) not only implied scientific backwardness but a moral and political stance that was unacceptable to most Russian medical practitioners during that era. "No restraint" as a strategy for treating the mentally disturbed was easily presented as analogous to the elimination of corporal punishment in the larger society, a campaign that engaged much of the Russian medical profession at the time.[10]

This effort on the part of the Moscow psychiatric community to elevate its favorite native son into the preeminent position in the pantheon of Russian psychiatric heroes continued unabated throughout the prerevolutionary era. However, so long as the center of political power remained in St. Petersburg, neither Moscow's attempt to modify the dominant historical interpretation nor its campaign to end St. Petersburg's hegemony over the profession was particularly successful.

The Bolshevik Revolution of 1917 changed that situation dramatically. The Revolution not only transformed the power structure of the larger society, but it altered the balance of power within the psychiatric profession as well. Psychiatrists were one of the first groups of professionals to offer their support to the new regime, and many of the profession's leading figures quickly stepped into positions of power in its newly created medical administration.[11] With the move of the capital to Moscow, the psychiatric community in that city found itself closer to the center of power. It was also somewhat less ideologically suspect in part because of its longstanding antagonisms with the St. Petersburg bureaucracy.

After the dust had settled following the chaos of the immediate postrevolutionary period, it was clear that the Muscovites had assumed the leadership of the profession. Not only did many of them occupy important policy-making positions, but they had much greater access to the professional media. Of the numerous psychiatric journals that had been published during the prerevolutionary era, the one that emerged as the official journal of the profession after the Revolution was neither the oldest nor the most widely circulated of the preexisting periodicals. Rather, it was the journal that had been established by the Moscow psychiatric community in 1901 shortly after Korsakov's death and named in his memory, *Zhurnal nevropatologii i psikhiatrii im. S. S. Korsakova* [Korsakov Journal of Neuropathology and Psychiatry].

The Muscovites' closer relationship to the central medical administration of the new regime also increased their access to other publication outlets as well. The psychiatric histories that have been published as monographs since 1917 have almost all been written by individuals affiliated with the Moscow school of psychiatry, a fact that is clearly evident in their interpretation of events.[12] The Moscow version of the history of Russia's psychiatric profession has also made its way into most of the textbooks used in medical education throughout the USSR, and it has been reproduced in English language accounts of the history of Russian psychiatry.[13]

This "official" history continues to emphasize the role of particular individuals in advancing the science and practice of psychiatry in Russia. While a variety of figures appear in this Hall of Fame, the most prominent position belongs to S. S. Korsakov. Although he is not credited with the paternity of the Russian psychiatric profession as a whole, usually no one else is either. Nor is the type of language with which Korsakov is portrayed used with respect to any other historical figure. The number of words devoted to Korsakov's contributions to Russian psychiatry invariably supersedes the number allocated to any other individual. In addition, he is universally described in superlatives. Both his personal and his professional persona are apparently beyond reproach.[14] An "outstanding scientist, physician, and public figure," Korsakov is variously characterized as the "Russian Pinel" and the "Russian Conolly."[15] According to one very typical account, "His prestige helped to introduce the system of no-restraint in all mental hospitals. Thanks to him, this system encountered in Russia much less resistance than in Germany or in France."[16] Korsakov is not only credited with revolutionizing the practice of psychiatry in Russia but psychiatric science as well. His research, the historians contend, introduced "a new nosological trend in psychiatry."

Other significant personages are accorded a place in this dominant historical perspective, yet the shortcomings of most are noted along with their contributions. A very few of the most generous portrayals of Balinskii still accord him the status of "father of scientific psychiatry in Russia"; however, more commonly, he is merely credited with heading the first university Department of Psychiatry or with siring the St. Petersburg school of psychiatry. His pedagogical and organizational accomplishments tend to be juxtaposed against his allegedly meager research accomplishments.

Balinskii's successors at the Military-Medical Academy are also credited with advancing the field; however, less attention is given to their work, and the accounts usually include subtle references to personal or ideological imperfections. While Korsakov is praised as a "convinced materialist," Merzheevskii is more likely to be described as a "naive materialist," while Bekhterev's work is said to suffer from "eclecticism" or "errors of mechanistic materialism."

The "official" psychiatric histories have also often overlooked or minimized the significance of "progressive" actions on the part of St. Petersburg psychiatrists. One suspects that these would have been regarded quite differently had the individual involved been a Muscovite. A striking example of this is the relative inattention in this history to the role of V. M. Bekhterev in the infamous Beilis affair. Beilis, a Jew, was accused in 1913 of the ritual murder of a Gentile. His Kiev trial attracted international attention because of its anti-Semitic character. It also brought down the wrath of the international psychiatric community on the Russian profession because of the testimony of a prominent psychiatrist, Professor I. A. Sikorskii of Kiev University, on behalf of the prosecution.[17] Despite his many earlier contributions to Russian psychiatry, Sikorskii has since been virtually expunged from the history of the profession because of his association with this distasteful episode. One of the few historians who does mention Sikorskii describes him not only as a "militant idealist" but also as a representative of the St. Petersburg school of psychiatry.[18] Largely unnoted in this history, however, has been the role of V. M. Bekhterev, who jeopardized his professional career by testifying for the defense.[19] Bekhterev's role in the Beilis affair has been discussed in several popular biographies of the internationally recognized scientist, but the serious psychiatric histories in the USSR have been consistently silent on the issue.[20]

The Moscow perspective on Russian psychiatric history, while clearly dominant, has not been the only version to appear in printed form. The heirs to the St. Petersburg psychiatric community (especially those at the Psychoneurological Institute founded by Bekhterev in the early twentieth century) have attempted to fill in some of the gaps in the "official" history. Not surprisingly, one of their goals has been to present more thorough and more balanced accounts of the careers and contributions of the leading figures in St. Petersburg's prerevolutionary psychiatric community.[21] Some of this work has involved quite serious scholarship (as evidenced by extensive use of unpublished archival records and careful documentation of findings), a characteristic that distinguishes it from most of the "official" histories.[22] Nonetheless, this research has been published primarily in the form of brief articles in professional journals and chapters in edited collections. The result has been that, while it is accessible to serious students of psychiatric history, this scholarship has had virtually no impact on the more widely distributed Muscovite version of Russian psychiatric history.

The Psychiatrist as Revolutionary Hero

In addition to the effort they have devoted to their intraprofessional relationships, Russian psychiatrists have consistently expended a great deal of energy negotiating a satisfactory relationship with state authorities. Because of the nature of their work, psychiatrists in most societies have tended to have very complicated relationships with governments. The character of psychiatric institutions (not to mention many of the profession's clients) has made them especially dependent on the support of state authorities. Simultaneously, psychiatrists' identity as professional medical experts mandates autonomy in the conduct of their work. Balancing these potentially conflicting pressures has often proved a difficult task. In Russia and the Soviet Union, establishing a mutually satisfactory working relationship between the profession and the state has been especially complex for psychiatrists because of the governments' (tsarist and Soviet alike) reluctance to delegate authority to professional groups in general and its wariness of psychiatry in particular.

In consequence, Russian and Soviet psychiatrists have expended a great deal of energy attempting to demonstrate their political reliability, on the one hand, and the sophistication of their medical expertise, on the other. Particularly in the postrevolutionary era, historical analyses of the development of the profession have played an important role in this endeavor. As in the case of the resort to history as a weapon in intraprofessional disputes, the emphasis has been upon the role of concrete individuals. However, this aspect of historical biography construction has focused on the political dimensions in individuals' careers. Demonstrating ideological prescience has been one goal of this historiographical work; documenting involvement in "progressive" (especially revolutionary) social and political activities another.[23]

This task would have been relatively simple had most psychiatrists before 1917 been committed Bolsheviks working underground in the revolutionary struggle at the same time that they carried on scientifically productive and therapeutically progressive professional lives. Such was not the case. There were a few early Bolsheviks in the profession, but there were also a few equally fervent supporters of the traditional autocratic order. The political leanings of most members of the profession, although left of center, were somewhat less radical. Their unsatisfactory dealings with the tsarist government in the final years of the empire inclined an increasing number of them toward the oppositionist camps, and as indicated earlier, psychiatrists were quick to offer their support to the new Soviet government. Nonetheless, the historians who have sought revolutionary heroes among their professional forebears have faced a sometimes daunting task. This has especially been true in those epochs when the standards of ideological and practical purity have been particularly strict.[24]

Those individuals whose prerevolutionary careers included radical political activity have been accorded special attention by the profession's historians even when their contributions to psychiatry have otherwise been relatively insignificant. A typical example is P. P. Tutyshkin, whose career included a stint at the provincial psychiatric hospital in Khar'kov during the troubled 1905 era. Tutyshkin's biographers credit him with using the institution to hide revolutionaries from the tsarist police and as a base for organizing local Bolsheviks and publishing radical literature.[25]

One of the aims of the profession's historians has been to ensure that the political credentials of leading figures in the profession are beyond reproach. This has sometimes involved selectively ignoring or explaining away ideological or behavioral lapses. It has also entailed the accentuation of activities and ideas that could in any way be interpreted as "progressive" or which resulted in some degree of repression by prerevolutionary authorities. Thus, for example, there is very little attention paid in the official histories to the patently anti-democratic actions taken by V. P. Serbskii, Korsakov's successor, in the Moscow University psychiatric clinic in 1906. The progressive forces within the profession in this era were enthusiastically advocating collegial administration of the empire's psychiatric institutions. However, when his subordinates proposed restructuring the administration of their clinic, Serbskii not only refused to cooperate but began instead to fire the perpetrators.

This episode has rarely been mentioned in biographical accounts. The one author who dealt with it in some detail reported it in the context of his praise for one of Serbskii's students, who was on the other side of the barricades. Even so, the biographer went to great lengths to explain Serbskii's lapse, to stress that it was temporary, and to emphasize both Serbskii's long-lasting regret over his actions and his rapid return to politically correct behavior.[26]

In conclusion, the historiography of Russian and Soviet psychiatry clearly illustrates the extent to which the social construction of history is influenced by extraneous factors. In this particular case many of the most palpable influences have been political. However, as this brief and necessarily selective account has attempted to demonstrate, the internal politics of the profession have influenced the writing of psychiatric history in Russia and the Soviet Union at least as much as the more dramatic governmental transformations experienced by that society during the twentieth century.

Notes

1. These heroic figures were almost exclusively male. There were a few women among them, but their numbers were quite small. One of the figures elevated to hero status for a while in Soviet psychiatry was a nonpsychiatrist, I. P. Pavlov. The role of Pavlovian ideas in Soviet psychiatry and psychology has been thoroughly discussed elsewhere and for that reason will not be included in this account. See, for example, David Joravsky, *Russian Psychology: A Critical History* (Cambridge: Basil Blackwell, 1989).

2. See, for example, F. S. Tekut'ev, *Istoricheskii ocherk kafedry i kliniki dushevnykh i nervnykh boleznei pri imperatorskoi voenno-meditsinskoi akademii* [A Historical Sketch of the Department and Clinic of Mental and Nervous Diseases] (St. Petersburg, 1898) and S. D. Vladychko, *Otchet o deiatel'nosti obshchestva psikhiatrov (1862–1912)* [An Account of the Activities of the Society of Psychiatrists (1862–1912)] (St. Petersburg, 1912).

3. S. D. Vladychko, 8.

4. One of the best examples of this was the so-called Balinskii-Shtrom asylum plan, a model design for a provincial *zemstvo* asylum that was developed in the early 1880s at the behest of the Ministry of Internal Affairs by Professor Balinskii with the assistance of the architect Shtrom. Provincial psychiatrists and their employers complained that the government insisted on rigid adherence to this plan, ignoring local conditions.

5. This was, not surprisingly, an oversimplification of the range and distribution of political opinion within the profession. While there were staunch supporters of the autocracy among St. Petersburg's psychiatrists, there were numerous critics as well (some of them quite radical). By the same token there were committed advocates of the autocracy and central government control who were employed by *zemstvo* psychiatric institutions.

6. As John Hutchinson has pointed out, this portrayal of the respective sympathies of Moscow and St. Petersburg was not unique to psychiatry. See Hutchinson, *Politics and Public Health in Revolutionary Russia: 1890–1918* (Baltimore: Johns Hopkins University Press, 1990), ch. 1.

7. S. S. Korsakov, "K voprosu o nestesnenii (No restraint) [On the question of no restraint]," *Trudy 1887*, 397–436, and discussion, 439.

8. The two groups fought heatedly about this issue, delaying the creation of the organization by several years. See Julie V. Brown, "The Professionalization of Russian Psychiatrists: 1857–1911" (Ph.D. diss., University of Pennsylvania, 1981).

9. See, for example V. P. Serbskii, "Russkii soiuz psikhiatrov i nevropatologov i S. S.

Korsakov,'' *Trudy pervago s'ezda russkago soiuza psikhiatrov i nevropatologov* [''The Russian Union of Psychiatrists and Neuropathologists,'' *Report of the First Congress of the Russian Union of Psychiatrists and Neuropathologists*] (Moscow, 1914), 64–83, and discussion in Brown, ''The Professionalization of Russian Psychiatrists,'' ch. IV.

10. The peasantry was the only segment of the population still subject to this form of punishment and outlawing it became a cause celebre for physicians around the turn of the century. As Nancy Frieden has demonstrated, doctors not only regarded corporal punishment as a violation of the peasantry's fundamental civil rights, but they vehemently objected to the requirement that they participate in the procedure. Nancy M. Frieden, *Russian Physicians in an Era of Reform and Revolution, 1856–1905* (Princeton: Princeton University Press, 1981), 185–192.

11. S. I. Mitskevich, *Zapiski vracha-obshchestvennika (1888–1918)* [Notes of a Physician-Activist] (Moscow, 1969).

12. These include A. O. Edel'shtein, *Psikhiatricheskie s'ezdy i obschestva za polveka (1887–1936)* [Psychiatric conferences and societies for a half-century (1887–1936] (Moscow, 1948); D. D. Fedotov, *Ocherki po istorii otechestvennoi psikhiatrii* [Notes on the History of Native Psychiatry] (Moscow, 1957); T. I. Iudin, *Ocherki istorii otechestvennoi psikhiatrii* [Notes on the History of Native Psychiatry] (Moscow, 1951); Iu. V. Kannabikh, *Istoriia psikhiatrii* [The History of Psychiatry] (Moscow, 1929); and G. V. Morozov et al., *Osnovnye etapy razvitiia otechestvennoi sudebnoi psikhiatrii* [Fundamental Stages in the Development of Native Forensic Psychiatry] (Moscow, 1976). A rare exception to this pattern is V. F. Kruglianskii, *Psikhiatriia: istoriia, problemy, perspektivy* [Psychiatry: History, Problems, Perspectives] (Minsk, 1979).

13. Very few of these English-language accounts have been based on primary research. They are either translations of histories written by Soviet psychiatrists or they rely exclusively on histories published in the USSR since the mid-1920s. See, for example, A. G. Galach'yan, ''Soviet Union'' in A. Kiev (ed.), *Psychiatry in the Communist World* (New York: Science House, 1968); Nancy Rollins, *Child Psychiatry in the Soviet Union: Preliminary Observations* (Cambridge: Harvard University Press, 1972); Joseph Wortis, M.D., *Soviet Psychiatry* (Baltimore: Williams & Wilkins, 1950); and Joseph Wortis and A. G. Galach'yan, ''Union of Soviet Socialist Republics'' in John G. Howells (ed.), *World History of Psychiatry* (New York: Brunner/Mazel, 1975), 308–332.

14. Only in the midst of the Stalinist era was reference ever made to one of Korsakov's obvious shortcomings, his lack of involvement in revolutionary activity. Even so, the references tend to be oblique. Upon the centenary of his birth in 1854, for example, many of Korsakov's published works were reissued in a commemorative volume.

In this collection, his biographers describe Korsakov as one of the ''most left'' of the Moscow professoriate. What they neglect to mention is that such a stance was in fact not very far to the left along the political spectrum. S. S. Korsakov, *Izbrannye proizvedeniia* [Collected Works] (Moscow, 1954).

15. The references are to Philippe Pinel, whose name is associated with the removal of the chains from the insane patients at the Bicêtre in Paris during the French Revolution and to John Conolly, the Englishman who popularized the concept of ''nonrestraint.''

16. Edward Babayan, *The Structure of Psychiatry in the Soviet Union*, trans. V. N. Brobov and B. Meerovich (New York: International Universities Press, 1985), 46.

17. Russian representatives at international congresses were publicly excoriated by their Western colleagues on account of this incident, and many of those same individuals boycotted an international psychiatric congress scheduled in Moscow soon afterward.

18. Iudin, *Ocherki istorii* [Notes on the History].

19. The psychiatric press at the time reported these events in detail. See, for example, ''Khronika,'' *Sovremennaia psikhiatriia* [''Chronicle,'' Contemporary Psychiatry], vii (1913), 837–838; ''Khronika,'' *Voprosy psikhiatrii i nevrologii* [''Chronicle,'' Questions of Psychiatry and Neurology], ii (1913), 523–526; ''Khronika'' *Zhurnal nevropatologii i psikhiatrii im. S. S.*

Korsakova ["Chronicle," Korsakov Journal of Neuropathology and Psychiatry], xiii (1913), 618–619.

20. Popular biographies of V. M. Bekhterev include Georgii Bal'dysh, *Bekhterev v Peterburge-Leningrade* [Bekhterev in Petersburg-Leningrad] (Leningrad, 1979); and I. Guberman, *Bekhterev:stranitsy zhizni* [Bekhterev: Pages from his Life] (Moscow, 1977).

21. In addition to Balinskii, this research has focused on the careers of Merzheevskii, Bekhterev, and L. F. Ragozin, a psychiatrist who was the head of the medical department of the Ministry of Internal Affairs in the final years of the nineteenth century. See, for example, D. S. Ozeretskovskii, "Rol' Balinskogo v razvitii ucheniia o psikhopatiakh," [The role of Balinskii in the Development of the Study of Psychopathy] unpub. paper given at a conference commemorating 150th anniversary of the birth of I. M. Balinskii, May 1977; A. A. Portnov and A. M. Shereshevskii, "Nekotorye voprosy istorii peterburgskogo obshchestva psikhiatrov," [Some Questions about the History of the Petersburg Society of Psychiatrists] *Zhurnal nevropatologii i psikhiatrii im. S. S. Korsakova* [Korsakov Journal of Neuropathology and Psychiatry], lxx (1970), 1389–1393; A. M. Shereshevskii and A. V. Dulov, "I. P. Merzheevskii v meditsinskom sovete," [I. P. Merzheevskii in the Medical Council] *Zhurnal nevropatologii i psikhiatrii im. S. S. Korsakova* [Korsakov Journal of Neuropathology and Psychiatry], lix (1959), 360–361; A. M. Shereshevskii, "Organizatorskaia deiatel'nost' L. F. Ragozina i problemy lecheniia psikhicheskikh bol'nykh," [Organizational Activities of L. F. Ragozin and the Problem of Treating the Mentally Ill] in *Lechenie nervynkh i psikhicheskikh zabolevanii* [The Treatment of Nervous and Psychiatric Diseases] (Leningrad, 1976), 389–395; and L. I. Spivak, "I. M. Balinskii: osnovopolozhnik otechestvennoi psikhiatrii," [I. M. Balinskii: Founder of Native Psychiatry] unpub. paper given at a conference commemorating the 150th anniversary of the birth of I. M. Balinskii, May 1977.

22. Among the most prolific have been the professional staff of the Department (*kafedra*) of the History of Psychiatry at the Psychoneurological Institute, especially A. M. Shereshevskii.

23. This became much more prominent after the 1920s. Kannabikh's monograph, *Istoriia psikhiatrii* [The History of Psychiatry], which was published in 1929, pays little attention to such matters. That they were subsequently considered an important component of the profession's presentation of self is suggested not only by the frequency with which political biographies have appeared but also by the response to a comprehensive history of Russian psychiatry, *Ocherki istorii otechestvennoi psikhiatrii* [Notes on the History of Native Psychiatry], which was written by T. I. Iudin and published (posthumously) in Moscow in 1951. Despite a rather extensive discussion of the "progressive" activities of his colleagues in the revolutionary era, Iudin was criticized for devoting too little attention to that issue. He was also chided for underestimating the importance of Pavlov to Soviet psychiatry. See *Zhurnal nevropatologii i psikhiatrii im. S. S. Korsakova* [Korsakov Journal of Neuropathology and Psychiatry], liv (1954), 960–965.

24. This was particularly true in the 1930s and the early 1950s, before the death of Stalin.

25. Tutyshkin spent a short time in prison during this era and was fired from several positions. Present-day biographers tend to attribute his firing to his political activity. See, for example, A. G. Ianovskii, "P. P. Tutyshkin—vrach, uchenyi, revoliutsioner, [P. P. Tutyshkin—Physician, Scientist, Revolutionary]" *Zhurnal nevropatologii i psikhiatrii im. S. S. Korsakova* [Korsakov Journal of Neuropathology and Psychiatry], lxxiv (1974), 1411–1415. His contemporaries, on the other hand, while acknowledging that his political activities were a factor in those actions, also attributed the firings to other behaviors, e.g., they accused him of devoting too much time to his private practice and lecturing and of publicly insulting a hospital director.

26. A. G. Gerish, *P. B. Gannushkin* (Moscow, 1975), 24–28.

V

CRITICS OF PSYCHIATRY

17

The Rhetorical Paradigm in Psychiatric History: Thomas Szasz and the Myth of Mental Illness

RICHARD E. VATZ and LEE S. WEINBERG

As even his critics acknowledge, psychiatrist Thomas Szasz is the preeminent and most prolific critic of psychiatric theory, practice, and participation in public policy and the law.[1] Born in Budapest, Szasz and his family escaped Nazi Europe when Szasz was in his teens. While forsaking his original interest in internal medicine to specialize in psychiatry, Szasz was always skeptical of the medical pretensions of psychiatry, especially insofar as psychiatric hospitals were represented to be authentic medical hospitals. Instructed by his new department chair at the University of Chicago, where he did his residency, to spend a year of training at a state mental hospital, Szasz refused, saying ''I won't go because I don't believe in it.''[2] Szasz had acquired early on an appreciation of the effects of language and metaphor on perceived reality, which led to skepticism and disbelief of psychiatric orthodoxy. After publishing a number of articles critical of psychiatric concepts and practice, in 1961 Thomas Szasz wrote his seminal work, *The Myth of Mental Illness: Foundations of a Theory of Personal Conduct*, a book that challenged the medical identity of psychiatry.[3] This medical identity has constituted the dominant paradigm of madness since the inception of modern medicine in classical Greece, and continues as the dominant paradigm of American psychiatry, though ''it has waxed and waned''[4] since the institutionalization of the concept of mental illness in America by the ''father of psychiatry,'' Benjamin Rush, in the late eighteenth century, who certified madness as a medical concept in his 1812 publication, *Medical Inquiries and Observations Upon the Disease of Mind*, the first psychiatric textbook.[5] Most histories of psychiatry, E. Fuller Torrey has argued, are typified by Gregory Zilboorg's history of medical psychology in that they ''are written by physicians with the assumption of the medical model as 'truth.' The history is chosen and synthesized to show how everything leads up to the contemporary physician-psychiatrist, 'treating' irrational behavior as mental 'illness.' ''[6]

The historic role and potential consequences of Szasz's revolutionary reconceptualization of the field of psychiatry can best be characterized as a major paradigm change. Thomas Kuhn's groundbreaking theory of paradigmatic change in scientific inquiry offers an illuminating framework for understanding the significance of Thomas Szasz in the evolution of psychiatry as well as some basis for speculation about how Szasz's work will influence future developments in the field.[7] Such an assessment requires an examination of the nature of Szasz's alternative paradigm, its implications for the extant psychiatric paradigm and its practitioners, and the prospect for bringing about a scientific or intellectual revolution.

Thomas Kuhn's Theory of Paradigm Change

In his landmark *Structure of Scientific Revolutions*, Kuhn argued that scientific disciplines operate through agreed-upon paradigms, which constitute the "methods, problem-field, and standards of solution accepted by any mature scientific community at any given time."[8] Crises occur when sufficiently penetrating anomalies, or dashings of "paradigm-induced expectations" make the accepted *modus operandi* of the scientific discipline untenable.[9] The success of an emerging paradigm, which Kuhn terms a "scientific revolution," requires the overcoming—through persuasion—of the presumption that adheres to the status quo. Moreover, the established paradigm can be replaced only "if an alternative candidate is available to take its place."[10]

While Kuhn's concept of paradigm focuses on the competition among paradigms within *scientific* disciplines, Szasz's proposed paradigm differs in that it rejects the validity of psychiatric-enterprise-as-science itself. Consequently, while the progression of Szasz's major paradigm change should follow Kuhn's descriptions of the progression of paradigm change, it should do so more intensely. Kuhn postulates the generation of genuine problem-solving accomplishments as the necessary criterion that distinguishes an enterprise as a "science."[11] Yet, as elaborated below, Thomas Szasz's assertion that psychiatry has produced no genuine problem-solving accomplishment—no progress, in Kuhn's terminology—implicitly places psychiatry in a preparadigmatic stage, in which problems are created rather than solved.

For Kuhn, science involves the solving of puzzles, "that special category of problems that can serve to test ingenuity or skill in solution," and "the assured existence of a solution" is a "criterion for a puzzle."[12] But not all problems are puzzles. Indeed, in Szasz's new paradigm—which we will call a rhetorical paradigm—psychiatry has no clear puzzle to solve. Szasz's rhetorical paradigm implies that the deviant behaviors that constitute psychiatry's "puzzle" are, at least potentially, understandable, if not sensible or commendable, as game-playing and symbolic action strategically chosen as responses to varying social situations. Moreover, in Szasz's view, deviant behavior is not inherently problematic (unlike cancer, for example), and when it is most arguably problematic, as in behavior likely to harm others or oneself, it is not a puzzle because, first, as in Kuhn's example of "a lasting peace," deviant behavior "may not have any solution," and, second, because, in any event, it is potentially understandable as goal-seeking.[13]

To Kuhn, an analysis of problem-solving capability is particularly revealing of the power of prevailing paradigms in a scientific community. For the practice of the traditional endeavors of a scientific enterprise, what Kuhn calls "normal science," the location of problems and determination of their solutions present an often self-validating and circular system, which militates against the production of "major novelties, conceptual or phenomenal."[14] The instrumental value of the dominant paradigm is that it provides a "criterion for choosing problems that ... can be assumed to have solutions."[15]

In his rhetorical attack on the medical paradigm of psychiatry, Szasz was not only arguing for an alternative paradigm, but was explicitly saying that psychiatry was a "pseudoscience," comparable to astrology, two "instances of defining a science by specifying the subject matter of study ... completely disregard[ing] method and ... based on false substantives."[16] Thus, the attack on the "normal science" of psychiatry—what here will be termed the "medical model"—constituted a more damning and disqualifying recommendation for change than is observed in the prototypical scientific revolution described by Kuhn. During scientific revolution, Kuhn finds the theoretical possibility of the new paradigm being practiced by practitioners of the old paradigm, despite the tell-tale paradigmatic creation of a "different world" or new *Weltanschauung*.[17]

But such accommodation to the rhetorical paradigm is quite unlikely. As described herein, the rhetorical paradigm represents so drastic a change—indeed a repudiation of psychiatry-as-scientific-enterprise—that the vocabularies of the two paradigms are completely different and incompatible, a degree of difference Kuhn maintains is not typical in paradigm change. Often, Szasz's use of rhetorical terminology to analyze the behavioral subject matter of psychiatry is dismissed ironically as a type of rhetorical legerdemain, or as one prominent critic called it, "word magic."[18]

As a further illustration of this frequent reaction, we are reminded of the audience reaction to a speech given by Szasz over a decade ago to the Pennsylvania Mental Health Association wherein we observed that few understood what he was talking about, let alone considered adaptation of their current methods to his proposed paradigm. In fact, Szasz's ideas of rhetorically created reality and the symbolic communication perspective of what is considered "mental illness" evoked reactions of confusion and embarrassed humor comparable to what one might witness from conventional theists listening to an evangelist speaking in tongues.

Thomas Szasz's Rhetorical Paradigm

In Szasz's view the subject matter, method, and promotion of psychiatry constitute a rhetorical enterprise masquerading as a medical/scientific one. Human behavior—deviant and conventional—consists of freely chosen, symbol-using, goal-oriented actions or games, in contradistinction to the psychiatric view of human behavior as determined motion. Psychiatry, in this view, functions rhetorically to accredit socially valued behaviors and discredit socially disvalued behaviors, ostensibly through medical analysis and cure, but in reality through the medical rhetoric of "diagnosis" and "treatment" of "mental illness" or "mental disorders."[19] In doing so, Szasz argues, "psychotherapists are [base] rhetoricians," rhetoricians who, in Richard Weaver's terms, use language to deprive people of their autonomy, as in the psychiatric efforts to prevent suicide, while simultaneously increasing their "own power [and producing] converts to [their] own cause."[20] Nowhere is this latter motive more evident than in psychiatrists' writing of "psychohistory," wherein social and political preference masquerades as disinterested scientific analysis. Szasz describes such work as nothing but "[t]he vilification of hated, and glorification of loved, historical figures—presented as the products of impartial psychiatric-historical research."[21] Psychiatry's hidden social and political agenda, among other things, disqualifies it from its claim of being in the category of a scientific enterprise.

For Szasz, psychiatry effects social control through the rhetorical imposing of definitions, but the "problems" it solves are more reasonably viewed as political. The alleged medical/scientific *discovery* of such "problems" amounts to no more than the rhetorical *creation* of problems through strategic defining, the "impos[ing of] their reality on each other and everyone else."[22] As Szasz argues in his epigrammatic book, *The Second Sin*, "The struggle for definition is veritably the struggle for life itself. . . . In ordinary life, the struggle is [for symbols] . . . whoever first defines the situation is the victor; his adversary, the victim. For example in the family, husband and wife, mother and child do not get along; who defines whom as troublesome or mentally sick? . . . In short, he who first seizes the word imposes reality on the other."[23]

Szasz's rhetorical paradigm suggests that deviance has always been subjected to some sort of rhetorically justified forms of social control. As with the medical/scientific pretensions of psychiatry today, such control always succeeds through mystification, which legitimizes it. From Szasz's conception of the "Age of Reason," postulated by him to extend from the end of the Thirty Years' War (1648) to the present (as opposed to the conventional view of historians that the seventeenth and eighteenth centuries were the Age of Reason) the "dominant ideology of the West . . . has been scientific," whereas it had previously been Christian.[24] Moreover, Szasz sees this period also as the "Age of Madness," wherein social control is effected not through theological mystification, but by the "scientific jargon" of psychiatric rhetoric. Thus, as science replaced theology, the concept of mental illness replaced evil, and forcible "therapy" replaced forcible conversion of heretics. Particularly in the Age of Reason, justificatory rhetoric was and is necessary to reconcile the resorting to punishment for those who commit the heresy of rejecting the *Zeitgeist*: "Man has always found it necessary to employ various methods for dealing with interpersonal and social antagonisms. All such methods [include] the use of force. However, [unlike animals, men] must also explain and justify it."[25] The history of psychiatry and the Age of Madness is a history of the use of its armamentarium rhetorically to justify social control through involuntary "therapy" (e.g., mental hospitalization) or the "expulsion from the social order" of those who violate the precepts of mental health, or both, just as in the Age of Faith, rejection of the precepts of God was punished or discredited.[26]

Szasz argues that to understand both the behaviors called "mental illness" and the practices called "psychotherapy," one must understand not medicine but rhetoric and metaphor: "Psychiatry, using the methods of communication analysis, has much in common with the sciences concerned with the study of languages and communicative behavior. In spite of this connection between psychiatry and such disciplines as symbolic logic, semiotic, and sociology, problems of mental health continue to be cast in the traditional framework of medicine."[27] Psychiatry is, therefore, ultimately a linguistic enterprise closely related in the tradition of Aristotle, to ethics and politics and having as its end moral suasion rather than medical cures.[28] Szasz states, "What people now call mental illnesses are, for the most part, communications expressing unacceptable ideas, often framed in an unusual idiom."[29] Only if psychiatry is understood as rhetoric and persuasion rather than medicine can one begin to understand, for example, why:

psychiatrists are seen as medical practitioners even though they don't practice medicine; people are seen as patients despite the fact they have no demonstrable illness; and psychiatrists' nonscientific and nonmedical opinions are seen as scientifically and medically based.

In Szasz's paradigm "mental illness" is a myth; that is, one cannot have a disease of the mind, since the mind is not an organ; it is an "abstraction" or a construct without physical referent. "Mental illness" is a literalized metaphor. Usually, literalized metaphors are recognized as such and may be amusing, such as when a movie alien literally flies a kite when dismissively told to "go fly a kite." This central category error leads psychiatry into a wealth of category errors, which create a pseudoscientific method of problem solving wherein "we use language metaphorically and rhetorically and speak like the poet or the politician, not like the physician or scientist. Accordingly, the psychotherapist does not 'treat' mental illness, but relates to and communicates with a fellow human being."[30]

The prototype of the basic method of psychiatric treatment, Freudian psychoanalysis, is thus "communicat[ing] with patients by means of language, nonverbal signs and rules," as well as "analyz[ing], by means of verbal symbols, the communicative interactions which they observe and in which they themselves engage."[31] But, Szasz says, psychiatrists "talk as though they were physicians, physiologists, biologists, or even physicists."[32] Szasz sees in this not a scientific or medical method of healing, as Freud claimed, but rhetorical skills "in understand[ing] and decod[ing] the patient's communications."[33] To be authentic medical science, however, Szasz maintains that psychiatry would have to deal with its "core concept of disease" medically, not rhetorically, but that foredooms it to failure since "man's sign-using behavior . . . does not seems to lend itself to exploration and understanding in these terms."[34] Thus, psychiatry's "normal science" uses a self-ennobling, but inappropriate, language of medical science, despite "using the methods of communications analysis [which have] much in common with the sciences concerned with the study of languages and communicative behavior."[35]

As exemplified in his analysis of the "establishing [of] hysteria as a medically legitimate illness,"[36] Szasz views the history of psychiatry largely as a series of invalid, unscientific, and nonmedical assertions by physicians seeking to convince others "to view almost any disability—and particularly one such as hysteria that looked so much like a disorder of the body—as illness."[37] These claims, Szasz asserts, have then been repeated, selectively interpreted, and largely accepted by psychiatrists, who cite them as authorities whose earlier work justifies current psychiatric practices. Szasz points to Jean-Martin Charcot's "invention" of "hysteria" and its subsequent acceptance by Freud and others as the prototype for the creation of the concept of "mental illness." Szasz argues that Charcot, a physician specializing in diseases of the nervous system, simply "decided by fiat that, in contrast to organic neurological disease, these people had 'functional nervous illnesses.' "[38] As Szasz reads psychiatric history, Charcot's prestige as a neurologist allowed him to persuade medical and nonmedical people alike that he could distinguish malingering from "hysteria," and thus he transformed hysterics into patients suffering from "illness" and enfranchised doctors to exercise control over their patients' lives. Subsequently, Freud and others built on Charcot's claim to be able to identify "hysterics." As Freud wrote, "Charcot had thrown the whole weight of his authority on the side of the reality and objectivity of hysterical phenomena."[39]

By contrast, for Szasz, an "illness" is exclusively "a condition of the body . . . I define illness as the pathologist defines it—as a structural or functional abnormality of cells, tissues, organs or bodies."[40] The elasticity of the definition of disease allows the subject matter and involvement of psychiatry to be nearly boundless. With its medical/scientific ethos, psychiatry engages in endeavors ranging from accrediting or discrediting witnesses in court to involuntary psychiatric hospitalization, thereby regularly and systematically violating the "ideal" of the Szaszian paradigm: "to change patients only as they desire change."[41] Szasz maintains that the medicalization of personal and social problems simply "invites the use of medical rhetoric [to justify] resorts to coercive interventions to solve vexing social problems."[42]

Psychiatry's Promotion of the Medical/Scientific Paradigm

To Szasz, psychiatry has successfully, but inappropriately, claimed for itself special expertise concerning "man's journey through life" to the extent that "today, particularly in the affluent West, all of the difficulties and problems of living are considered psychiatric diseases." The identity of psychiatry as a medical science of behavior is engineered through the use of "the logic, the imagery and the rhetoric of science, and especially medicine."[43] Regardless of its authenticity, the promoting of psychiatry as science has long been critical to its economic and professional viability, though such a claim is not unique to psychiatry. Since at least the 1950s, Szasz notes, "every contemporary profession, unless based on art, is said to be based on science."[44]

Consistent claims by psychiatrists that psychiatry is a medical specialty are further belied by the fact that there is relatively little medical practice *qua* medical practice in psychiatry. As neurologist Richard Restak noted as recently as 1983, "Fewer than one percent of the nation's psychiatrists claim that their principal method is organic or biological. Only 213 psychiatrists in the United States have completed residency training in neurology."[45] The same article reported that "a 1977 study by C. W. Patterson revealed that 81% of psychiatrists do not refer their patients to other physicians for such examinations. One third of those surveyed in another study admitted that they no longer knew how to perform a physical examination."[46] That psychiatry is not a science is evident in Karl Popper's observation of the impossibility of falsification of its claims; that is, as Szasz notes, psychiatry "cannot be proven wrong."[47] Moreover, conceptually, when viewed through a rhetorical framework, there can *by definition* be no medical or scientific authenticity to a field that focuses on nonmedical and nonscientific matters: the human mind and human behavior.[48] Szasz argues further that use of the medical term "therapy" to describe the clearly nonmedical techniques of psychotherapy betrays the inauthenticity of any medical identity. Szasz concludes, if mental "illnesses" are real illnesses, how could nonmedical approaches be justified, and, if such "illnesses" are not really diseases, "then it makes no sense to adopt a medical approach to [them]."[49] As Szasz said to us in a 1991 conversation, "Would one speak of the 'medical model' of any real disease?"

From *The Myth of Mental Illness* to the present, Szasz insists on a new paradigm for thinking about what he calls the "problems in living" experienced by many or most people and about psychiatric practices aimed at helping people dissatisfied with aspects of their lives to "learn about themselves, others, and life."[50] But to Szasz, psychiatry, which in its modern version constitutes nothing more than a form of strategic or persuasive communication, is a subtopic of rhetoric, not medicine and not science. Szasz treats psychiatry as a rhetorical phenomenon, critiques it from a rhetorical point of view, and frequently resorts to a rhetorical vocabulary, a vocabulary often completely beyond the understanding of psychiatrists.

The Incompatibility of the Rhetorical Paradigm and the Normal Science of Psychiatry

The Szaszian paradigm has brought about only a gradual change in the normal science of psychiatry. One explanation for this may be that it is not in the interest—economic, social, or existential—of psychiatrists to fully adopt the rhetorical model. But another explanation, which Szasz considers, is that a paradigm based on communication and metaphor is too radical a change for those socialized into the medical paradigm. In fact, Szasz notes, many physicians do not even know what a metaphor is. In one interaction wherein Szasz asked a group of medical students to define "metaphor," one said he knew but could not give an example. Szasz suggested he try to give an example. He replied, "My mind is a blank . . . and not a single student laughed."[51]

It is through the persuasive and mystifying literalization of metaphor, Szasz maintains, that institutional psychiatry exerts social control and enjoys tremendous social power. This is illustrated in the position for which Szasz is best known: his opposition to involuntary psychiatric hospitalization. Szasz argues that such forced imprisonment is not generally seen as such because of the therapeutic metaphors by which it is described. When psychiatrists support involuntary psychiatric hospitalization, it is incompatible with the ethics of medicine, says Szasz, which include the right of a patient to refuse service: "So intimate are the connections between psychiatry and coercion . . . [that] noncoercive psychiatry . . . is an oxymoron."[52]

This focus on persuasive language in Szasz's rhetorical paradigm has significant ethical implications for both psychiatrists and mental patients. In rhetorical theory, language inescapably is linked to responsibility, and, Szasz argues, the "entire psychiatric enterprise hinges on [the notion] that human beings diagnosed as 'mentally ill' have a brain disease that deprives them of free will."[53] Szasz's rhetorical paradigm, however, portrays these behaviors as freely chosen and transforms "victims" propelled by their neurobiological environment into free agents, perpetrators of actions for which they are fully responsible.

Rhetorical theorists further maintain that behavior can be seen as "agent" or "scenic," with the former implying free will and the latter implying determinism. The "scenic" approach dominates psychiatry, which even its defenders portray as an essentially deterministic enterprise, wherein patients are seen as not responsible for their behavior.[54] Szasz sees this determinism in the "historicism" of psychoanalytic theory wherein "antecedent historical events [serve] as alleged *determinants* of subsequent behavior . . . [and thus] preclude explanations of valuation, choice, and responsibility in human affairs."[55] The exculpating rhetoric of forensic psychiatry in the insanity plea is illustrative of such rhetorical denial of responsibility. In Szasz's paradigm such a plea denies the responsibility of, say, a brutal murderer, through medical mystification and the consequential rhetorical redefinition that invalidly portrays the perpetrator as lacking the ability to control his behavior.

Just as Szasz insists that psychiatric patients are moral agents, he similarly sees psychiatrists as moral agents. The medical paradigm implicitly argues that psychiatrists are not morally culpable for the consequences of their psychiatric practice. In the rhetorical paradigm the psychiatrist who deprives people of their autonomy would be seen as a consciously imprisoning agent, not merely a doctor providing "therapy," language that insulates psychiatrists from the moral responsibility for their acts. As rhetorical theorist Kenneth Burke points out, "One may deflect attention from the criticism of personal motives by deriving an act or attitude not from the traits of the [person] but from the nature of the situation."[56]

Szasz's rhetorical paradigm denies psychiatry's claim to be a scientific enterprise and, equally significantly, transforms its practitioners from problem-solvers to problem-creators. If deviant behavior is only "disease" through rhetorical creation, then there can be no justification for undesired psychiatric intervention in people's lives. The rhetorical paradigm represents a significant threat to institutional psychiatry, for not only is Szasz arguing that psychiatry is nonscientific, and not only is the language inherent in the rhetorical paradigm foreign and unadaptable to psychiatrists practicing the "normal science," but without the medical model for protection, psychiatry becomes little more than a vehicle for social control—and a primary violator of individual freedom and autonomy—made acceptable by the medical cloak.

In this vein Szasz describes some psychiatric practices—including forced hospitalization, electroshock therapy, and drugging—on involuntary victims (if they are not "patients," they are victims) as simply unethical.[57] Elsewhere, and often, Szasz argues that such involuntary interventions are no less than criminal, violent, and terroristic actions and enslavement. *The Myth of Mental Illness* is written without the polemics of some of Szasz's later work, yet this first major book, according to Harvard psychiatrist Alan Stone, "earned the lasting enmity of his profession."[58]

In sum, Szasz's paradigmatic challenge represents an unusual type of paradigm exchange, one that by replacing the original paradigm would invalidate the existing paradigm without opportunity or provision for new tools to provide similar status and remuneration for the current practitioners. The rhetorical paradigm is simply too different—involving as it does semiotic and rhetoric, especially the defining of "mental illness" as semantics and symbolic action—to assure current practitioners any clear role in its implementation.

The Significance of Biological Psychiatry for the Normal Science

Psychiatrists have often depicted the domain of psychiatry as John Hanley, professor of psychiatry at UCLA, did in the *American Medical News* in 1985, as "the brain and its system therein."[59] Thus, it has been a potential problem when psychiatric puzzle solving has been unable to point to neurobiological correlates specific to "mental illnesses." In Szasz's view this constitutes psychiatry's "unredeemed promissory note" of more than a century's duration.[60]

Kuhn argues that crisis in "normal science" can be stayed "so long as the tools a paradigm supplies continue to prove capable to solving the problem it defines; science moves fastest and penetrates most deeply through confident employment of those tools."[61] In Szasz's depiction, however, psychiatry lacks these tools, or "special instruments," to qualify it as a science. Thus, in the 1970s and 1980s psychiatry experienced the type of crises that Kuhn sees as the "necessary precondition for the emergence of novel theories."[62] Biological psychiatry, which assumes the neurobiological basis of mental disorders and is accompanied by an emphasis on drug therapy, offered a rescue of psychiatry's medical paradigm that Szasz anticipated: "Whatever might be the effects of modern psychopharmacologicals on the so-called mentally ill patients, the effects on the psychiatrists who use them are clear and unquestionably 'beneficial': they restore to the psychiatrist what he has been in grave danger of losing—namely, his *medical identity.*"[63] Psychiatrists often grant this point themselves. Keith Russell Ablow, chief resident in psychiatry at New England Medical Center in Boston, states "The burgeoning growth of biological psychiatry . . . [testifies] to how anxious we are to translate what we know about the human mind into something resembling objective science."[64]

Thus to Szasz the rise of biological psychiatry since the 1970s offers not a new paradigm but an attempt at proof or authentication of the already existing medical paradigm. As one prominent practitioner put it, "The recognition that mental illnesses are diseases affecting the brain is the basis of the biological revolution in psychiatry."[65]

In the Szaszian paradigm, biological psychiatry has not and cannot resolve the conceptual crisis of psychiatry. Biological psychiatry cannot rescue the conceptual bind of focusing on a concept, the "mind." Moreover, any finding that some behaviors are entirely caused by brain disease "would destroy psychiatry's *raison d'être* as a medical specialty distinct and separate from neurology."[66] Yet, in the persuasion used by some supporters of biological psychiatry, there has been an effort to transfer the widespread acceptance of a limited number of "mental illnesses" as bona fide brain diseases to an acceptance that *all* so-called mental illnesses constitute proven brain disease.[67] But for the great preponderance of the wide range of behaviors called "mental illness," there is no comparable proof offered.

In addition, institutional psychiatry identifies a large plurality of Americans as mentally ill, only a tiny percentage of whom demonstrate the behaviors for which biological psychiatry claims to have found neurobiological correlates.[68] The National Institute of Mental Health (NIMH) determined a few years ago through nonmedical interviews by "lay interviewers" that up to twenty-three percent of adults in America have at least one "psychiatric disorder" and that up to thirty-eight percent experience mental disorders at some point in their life.[69] Yale psychiatry professor Jay Katz conceded several years ago, "If you look at [the diagnostic manual], you can classify all of us under one rubric or another of mental disorder."[70]

Recognition of this conceptual bind is not hard to find, even in the establishment journals of psychiatry. An article discussing "conundrums" facing the APA's Task Force on the proposed newest revision of psychiatry's diagnostic manual (*DSM-IV*), authored by several members of the Task Force, admits that "unfortunately, in most instances, biological tests can not be used even as diagnostic indicators" since such tests are not specific to particular "mental disorders."[71]

The same article reports that there has been heavy lobbying of the Task Force to influence its revisions for *DSM-IV* ("The zeal . . . is extraordinary"), and the lobbying is largely based on financial and ideological motives.[72] Financially, there is no more salient issue in mental health than insurance costs. While health costs are rising generally, the Employee Benefit Research Institute reports that the rise in mental health costs is over forty percent higher than the rise in health costs in general. There is grave concern among mental health practitioners as a result of restrictions on mental health coverage through managed care and increased restrictions on mental health care in employers' health plans. In the past several years the APA's newsletter, scholarly articles on the revisions for *DSM-IV*, and the speeches of the APA's leadership are replete with discussions of concerns regarding insurance and reimbursement issues.

The link between psychiatry's definition of "illness" and the financial concerns attending its recognition through health insurance is inextricable. At the 144th annual meeting of the American Psychiatric Association, then-president Elissa Benedek warned that the threat of rising medical costs coupled with new restrictions on health-care insurance provisions for psychiatric care make "many feel that . . . the very future of psychiatry [is] in doubt."[73] The insurance reimbursement issue also is linked to the issue of whether "mental illnesses" are real illnesses. The Task Force wrote that "there are those who want some or all mental disorders designated as diseases in order to protect reimbursement and research funding."[74] The Task Force allows only that changes in *DSM-IV* "cannot be overly influenced by such considerations."[75]

Resistance to the Rhetorical Paradigm

From Kuhn's perspective on scientific revolutions, the intense resistance to Szasz can be understood as an attempt to wean defenders of the "normal science" of psychiatry "whose productive careers have committed them to an older tradition . . . [and who are assured] that the older paradigm will ultimately solve all its problems."[76] Inasmuch as Szasz's proposed rhetorical paradigm constitutes a major paradigm change, Kuhn's theory leads us to anticipate and to find an even greater degree of animosity and resistance from traditionalists of the dominant paradigm.

Criticism of Szasz, for example, has gone well beyond scholarly debate. As Szasz recalls in his second edition of *The Myth of Mental Illness: Foundations of a Theory of Personal Conduct*, "Within a year of the [the publication of the first edition], the Commissioner of the New York State Department of Mental Hygiene demanded, in a letter citing specifically *The Myth of Mental Illness*, that I be dismissed from my university position because I did not 'believe in mental illness.' "[77] Szasz's ideas met with considerable political resistance as well where he was teaching at the Health Science Center in the Department of Psychiatric and Behavioral Sciences. There, his job was threatened—and some of his supporters, who unlike Szasz lacked tenure, were terminated—because of Szasz's rejection of the normal science of psychiatry and his attacks on the ethics of psychiatry and psychiatrists.[78]

Among scholars the opposition to Szasz sometimes appears to ignore what he actually has written, perhaps because, as rhetorical theorist Richard Weaver notes, "Nothing is more feared by [the base rhetorician] than a true dialectic."[79] In fact, Szasz has written that Sigmund Freud was the ultimate "base" rhetorician who used "language to increase his own power, to produce converts to his own cause, and to create loyal followers of his own person."[80] Following Weaver, therefore, Szasz would not expect to find most psychiatrists engaging him in constructive dialogue. Some of the difficulty psychiatrists have with Szasz's paradigm may be due to confusion about his claims. As psychiatrist/columnist Charles Krauthammer notes, "Szasz is the kind of author no one reads but everyone knows about."[81] It is not surprising, therefore, that from its inception the rhetorical paradigm has been met with resistance and misunderstanding.

A frequently repeated criticism of Szasz rests on basic misunderstanding of his position to the effect that, as C. G. Schoenfeld argues, he "fails to offer his readers detailed descriptions, case histories, and the like of a representative cross section of persons whom psychiatrists usually judge to be neurotic or psychotic, but whom he has interviewed or examined as a psychiatrist, and whom he has demonstrated to be completely normal."[82] In one form or another many critics voice this objection. However, in offering such a criticism, Schoenfeld and others who make similar objections demonstrate a lack of understanding of the fundamental assertion of Szasz that the very use of the language of medicine—"neurotic or psychotic" versus "completely normal"— constitutes a type of category error. Schoenfeld's demands make perfect sense *within* the existing paradigm, but no sense whatever from *outside* that paradigm. Viewing behavior from his paradigm, Szasz cannot possibly demonstrate "normality" anymore than he believes psychiatrists can demonstrate "mental illness."

Some of the initial response to *The Myth of Mental Illness* evidenced resistance to the proposed paradigm change but denied that it represented a revolutionary challenge. Writing in *The American Journal of Psychiatry*, Eugen Kahn observed, "[Despite that] this book is the work of a doubtless brilliant mind . . . [I]t damages this book that the author with a few terms of his own pretends to change psychiatry revolutionarily and fundamentally."[83]

But more frequently, the early critics of Szasz misinterpreted and rejected his claims, but did not dispute their revolutionary nature. Jurgen Ruesch's 1962 review of *The Myth of Mental Illness* sounded a familiar critical note: "Mental illness is not a myth to those who have experienced it,"[84] a point that is still frequently made, but that erroneously infers Szasz's denial of the existence of the behaviors called "mental illness" (see below). Ruesch adds, "In an essentially new contribution, Dr. Szasz gives us a brilliant review of the ways of communication that hysterical persons employ" and concludes that this attack on psychiatric conceptions of hysteria may demonstrate the myth of "a mental illness," a conclusion that misses Szasz's point, which was to use hysteria as a prototype for "mental illness" in general.[85] At least one reviewer who did understand Szasz's intent concluded, "The reviewer knows of no psychiatrist who agrees with him, and is sorry to consider his book a total waste of time."[86] Not all response was marked by rejection, however. Very prevalent was the nonconcessionary allowance—and variations of it—that Szasz had raised important and provocative questions, but none with the potential to wholly vitiate the normal science of psychiatry.[87]

Interestingly, reactions to Szasz's 1987 work, *Insanity*, a work Szasz (and we) consider his best, and a work wherein Szasz refines his arguments and engages his critics, received positive, but muted, response: "[Szasz] does an excellent job of answering all of the arguments against his position."[88] There were some positive reviews in the elite popular press.[89] For the most part, however, it was—and is—ignored within (and without) the psychiatric community. Perhaps because of the new language presented by the rhetorical paradigm, Szasz has been consistently misinterpreted in the most elementary way as if he were denying the existence of the behaviors that are labeled "mental illness" despite his unambiguously stating "While I maintain that 'mental illnesses' do not exist, I obviously do not imply or mean that the social and psychological occurrences to which this label is attached also do not exist."[90]

Such misunderstanding or misrepresentation of this basic tenet of Szasz's position remains prevalent both within and outside of psychiatry. In a 1989 interview, Harvard law professor Alan Dershowitz said that while "Szasz has had an enormous impact on psychiatry and the law . . . If you've seen somebody who is . . . troubled, you can't believe Szasz's arguments that there's no such thing as mental illness."[91] One well-regarded text recently attributed to Szasz's *Myth of Mental Illness* (1961) the view that "mental illness did not exist at all but was the product of hospitalization."[92] In a recent issue of the APA's newsletter, *Psychiatric News*, one psychiatrist wrote that if Dr. Szasz "doesn't believe that drug addiction and abuse is a disease, he should go visit with some of the addicts on the street."[93]

Szasz and Anti-Psychiatry

There are significant critiques of psychiatry, known as anti-psychiatry, but as E. Fuller Torrey points out, such critiques represent a wide variety of viewpoints.[94] Most prominent among the anti-psychiatrists has been R. D. Laing.[95] Szasz has often been mislabeled by supporters and practitioners of the "normal science" of psychiatry as belonging to the anti-psychiatry school of thought, whose views Szasz has expressly repudiated.[96] Indeed, Szasz's rhetorical model sees anti-psychiatry as similar to normal psychiatry in its rhetorical structure in which "the struggle over definitions is much the same" and most significantly in its use of "base rhetoric" in that "one cannot reason or argue with any of [the Laingian anti-psychiatrists]." Like normal psychiatry, anti-psychiatry, although "occasionally say[ing] almost exactly what I say about schizophrenia," often uses the same language as psychiatry (e.g., "madness") to glorify or vilify behavior, albeit in anti-psychiatry, the heroes and villains are inverted, in that anti-psychiatry finds the cause of "madness" in "the family and society instead of the patient and his disease."[97] Szasz also maintains that both psychiatry and anti-psychiatry have overriding political agendas, and therefore neither can be truly scientific.

Thus, while Szasz concedes some general similarities in his and anti-psychiatrists' "oppos[ing of] certain aspects of psychiatry," Szasz's rhetorical paradigm is neither intellectually similar, nor even literally anti-psychiatric.[98] The rhetorical paradigm implies the libertarian political grounding wherein the individual must be free to make behavioral decisions and whose unimpeded decisions must be seen as freely made. In contrast, much of anti-psychiatry (like psychiatry itself) utilizes a rhetorically scenic approach, wherein the mad or mentally ill are victims—and often portrayed as heroic *because* of their victimization—of outside social forces. Thus, anti-psychiatrists, such as Laing and Foucault, use mental illness rhetorically to promote a political agenda—usually leftist. The rhetorical paradigm implies that "just as, in psychiatry, the literalized metaphor of schizophrenia as illness leads to and justifies its management by means of doctors, hospitals and drugs, so in antipsychiatry, the literalized metaphor of schizophrenia as journey leads to and justifies its management by means of guides, hostels and first aid."[99]

Finally, from Szasz's perspective, anti-psychiatry's paternalistic rhetoric celebrates the mentally ill as morally superior, but often helpless victims, and therefore, like psychiatry, effectively robs those seen as mentally ill of their autonomy, which includes the right to choose to engage in psychiatric therapy. Thus, Szasz rejects the term *anti-psychiatry* as applied to his views despite agreeing that the medical model is invalid. He does not in fact oppose the practice of psychiatry, except as it is practiced on people involuntarily.[96]

Szasz's rhetorical paradigm, in further contrast to both the medical model and critiques of anti-psychiatry, provides for a contractual relationship to replace the coercive model in saying that those who do wish to talk with psychiatrists should not be prevented from doing so any more than those who do not wish to talk with psychiatrists should be forced to do so. On this point, he differs from both supporters and opponents of traditional institutional psychiatry: "Supporters of the medical model . . . [act] like pediatricians, who must convince parents that their child is sick before they can treat the child—and having convinced the parents, can treat the child regardless of whether or not the child wants to be treated. . . . Opponents of the medical model—typically anti-psychiatrists—[also] act like pediatricians, who, if they can convince parents that their child is not sick, can prevent the child from being treated, whether or not the child wants to be treated.[101] Szasz's contractual psychiatrist is a "private entrepreneur" who, absent medical mystification, "offers himself to his patients, who must pay him, must want to be his patients, and are free to reject his help."[102] In Szasz's rhetorical paradigm, the client (not "patient") is seen as the agent responsible for defining what is a problem, and involuntary psychiatry—but only *involuntary* psychiatry—and third party subsidization are eliminated.

The Future of the Rhetorical Paradigm

Kuhn theorizes that the success of any paradigm conversion ultimately rests on persuasion,[103] a concept that forms the cornerstone of the discipline of rhetoric.[104] But the persuasive process is often a lengthy one and, in the current example, has engendered an acrimonious struggle in both the popular and academic press.

Despite claims by some that the debate over whether "mental illnesses" are diseases is over and that the medical paradigm has won, there is evidence of a slowly increasing skepticism regarding much of the "normal science" of psychiatry.

Of potential significance is ambivalence regarding the key concept of normal psychiatry—"mental illness" itself. The *Diagnostic Manual of Psychiatry* uses the terms *disorder* rather than *illness*, although this is rarely, if ever, discussed in the popular press or public forum.[105] The omission of the term mental *illness* is further evidence within the normal science of some doubt as to its validity, despite the claim that the use of the term *disorder* "by no means implies that mental disorders are unrelated to physical or biological factors or processes."[106] The mental health professionals revising the diagnostic manual (the APA Task Force on *DSM-IV*) demonstrate further erosion of confidence in the concept of mental disorder, even while claiming that such conceptual problems do not put the enterprise outside of science and medicine: "The concept of mental disorder is like other concepts in medicine and science in failing to have a clear and consistent definition. . . . The implicit definition of mental disorders and medical disorders—'that which clinicians treat'—is tautological, but other more abstract concepts consistently fail to provide greater explanatory power.'' This ''tautological'' bind may be increasingly seen by some even within psychiatry's normal science as constituting the previously mentioned Kuhnian concept of a ''self-validating and circular system,'' which militates against the production of ''major novelties, conceptual or phenomenal'' critical to the evolution of problem solving.[107]

Despite their own apparent doubts, mental health interests do not take external criticism of the existing paradigm without significant resistance. In *Commentary*, when Carol Iannone, the embattled former nominee to the advisory council of the National Endowment for the Humanities, reviewed William Styron's book describing his suffering from the ''disease'' of depression, she wondered how Styron overcame his depression by, as he claimed, sheer force of will if the depression were truly a disease. In response, one psychiatrist at Columbia University asked, ''How is it possible that, in the year 1990, one can still come across a person of considerable education (and literary erudition) who somehow has not learned that depression (and, most especially, suicidal depression) is a *psychiatric illness*, not primarily a moral dilemma or a mortal sin.''[108]

Despite this resistance, there is an increasing tendency among mental health practitioners to adopt elements—but only some elements—of Szasz's paradigm. Psychiatrists often concede that Szasz has alerted them to the ''abuses of psychiatry.'' Dr. Thomas Detre, head of the University of Pittsburgh's Western Psychiatric Institute and Clinic, wryly noted in the meeting of the Pennsylvania Mental Health Association in the 1970s that Szasz would be disappointed to learn that ''he is not so heretical as he once was.''

Stronger Szasz-like doubts about the current paradigm usually come from outside of psychiatry and curiously seem to ignore Szasz's contribution. A recent popular book condemns ''the diseasing of America,'' but accepts, contrary to the Szaszian paradigm, the reality of addictions.[109] Yet the author cites Szasz but twice. Philosopher Herbert Fingarette, in his work *Heavy Drinking: The Myth of Alcoholism as a Disease* (1988), argues a position clearly prefigured by Szasz's work and written about by him for decades and yet does not even mention him.[110] Doubts about ''behavioral addictions'' abound now in the popular press: a column in *U.S. News and World Report* deplores the ''It's-Not-My-Fault Syndrome''; a Pulitzer Prize–winning feature writer derides ''The Addiction Addiction''; and a magazine cover story questioning the sympathy accorded people with alleged self-destructive disorders was titled ''Don't Blame Me.''[111] A recent example in the popular press questions psychiatrists' tendencies to label abnormality as ''sick.''[112] In none of these is Szasz even mentioned.

More striking is author Charles Sykes who writes in a 1992 work of how America has ''abolished sin'' and ''redefined inappropriate conduct'' by ''medicalizing'' it. Sykes purports to have conceptualized the ''therapeutic culture,''[113] a conceptualization completely subsumed by Szasz's ''Therapeutic State,'' the term he propounded in 1963 to describe the all-pervasive function of ''psychiatry as an institution of social control,''[114] about which Szasz has been writing since then, including a work by that name.[115] In Sykes' book there are but four scant references to Szasz.

Even among some world-renowned psychiatrists, there is new doubt about the medical nature of ''mental illness.'' Just before his death, Karl Menninger wrote, ''[Szasz's] new book, *Insanity*, makes some points that I agree with and have been trying to get across for years.'' In a published letter to Szasz, Menninger spoke with derisive skepticism about psychiatric diagnosis, prognosis, and treatment, and at one point used the term psychiatric "sickness" in quotation marks. He ended his letter with an implicit admission that much psychiatric "treatment" might not be the cause of patients' feeling better: "Long ago I noticed that some of our very sick patients surprised us by getting well even without much of our 'treatment.' "[116] A recent editorial in *Lancet* seems to support the notion that the medical model as transformed into biological psychiatry has not provided promised solutions either. The editorial states, "We seem to be no closer to finding the real, presumed biological, causes of the major psychiatric illnesses."[117]

In the rhetorical paradigm the unfulfilled promises of the discovery of neurobiological correlates specific to particular "mental illness" constitute an irresolvable crisis for psychiatry, and the promises serve only as rhetorical strategies to buy endless forbearance time. Szasz observes, "If psychiatrists had to pay interest on their promise of pathological lesions [to prove "mental illness" as a putative brain disease], as borrowers must to lenders, the interest alone would already have bankrupted them; instead, they keep reissuing the same notes, undaunted by their perfect record of never meeting their obligations."[118]

Szasz's postulation of a rhetorical paradigm holds out the prospect not of simply a new paradigm within psychiatry but of a complete negation of psychiatry as a scientific enterprise. As Szasz has described it, "With the simple but uncompromising idea that mental illness is a metaphor I hoped to inflict a fatal blow, philosophically speaking, on the conceptual foundations of psychiatry."[119]

The new emphasis on biological psychiatry, representing research advancements in pharmacology with no revisions of basic assumptions—the psychiatric paradigm has all along assumed a biochemical basis for behavior—has provoked considerable resistance within the "normal science." In one typical expression, a recent letter to the editor of *Psychiatric News* sees biological psychiatry as a "danger to psychiatry as a specialty simply because one need not be a psychiatrist to prescribe" pharmacological agents.[120] Some textbooks emphasize the new biological paradigm. Most standard texts do not. Moreover, most psychiatric texts do not even mention Szasz at all, including, for example, one published by the American Psychiatric Press that includes chapters on "Psychiatry and the Law" and "Ethics and Psychiatry," topics on which Szasz is a recognized scholar.[121] Kuhn sees textbooks as an index of the more conservative element of a science's normal research, and therefore also a lagging index to the fact and direction of revolutionary change. As Szasz sees it, however, the substitution of a biological paradigm represents, in reality, a last-ditch effort to retain the medical model paradigm, which was always methodologically inauthentic since it never proceeded with the apparatus of medical science. Szasz does not believe that the interim model will in the end bring about any change in the ability of psychiatry to solve "psychiatric" problems. For, as Szasz often points out, the discovery of brain disease in those labeled mentally ill constitutes an advancement in neurology, not psychiatry.[122]

In the end, as Kuhn suggests, "The transfer of allegiance from paradigm to paradigm is a conversion experience that cannot be forced" and successful arguments for a new paradigm typically are "based upon the competitors' comparative ability to solve problems."[123] Szasz's rhetorical paradigm, in its total rejection of medicine and psychiatry in favor of politics and ethics as the proper discourses for addressing human problems, has not been and may not be successful in the short run in convincing either psychiatrists or the public of its "comparative ability to solve problems." For as difficult and protracted as Kuhn finds scientific paradigmatic revolutions to be, the total replacement of a scientific paradigm with a nonscientific political and moral paradigm will require a degree of change that is nearly unprecedented. Moreover, there appears to be no extra-scientific motive for such change, since not only does Kuhn's "different world" await those who adopt Szasz's method but also a substantial drop in financial reward and an end to the critically prestigious medical identity. Whatever the merits of Szasz's paradigm, its emergence as the dominant paradigm, even if successful, will reflect Kuhn's slow revolution whose completion is at least decades away.

Notes

1. C. G. Schoenfeld, "An Analysis of the Views of Thomas S. Szasz," *Journal of Psychiatry and Law*, iv (1976), 245–263; Charles Krauthammer, *Cutting Edges: Making Sense of the 80's* (New York: Random, 1985).

2. Melanie Hirsch, "Home on the Hot Seat," *Post-Standard* (Syracuse), 19 February 1992, A7.

3. Thomas Szasz, *The Myth of Mental Illness: Foundations of a Theory of Personal Conduct* (New York: Hoeber-Harper, 1961).

4. Thomas Szasz, *Insanity: The Idea and Its Consequences* (New York: Wiley, 1987), 69.

5. Peter Conrad and Joseph W. Schneider (eds.), *Deviance and Medicalization: From Badness to Sickness* (St. Louis: C. V. Mosby, 1980), 49.

6. E. Fuller Torrey, *The Death of Psychiatry* (Radnor, Pennsylvania: Chilton, 1974), 6.

7. Thomas Kuhn, *The Structure of Scientific Revolutions*, 2nd ed. (Chicago: University of Chicago Press, 1970). There have been conceptual modifications made by Kuhn in later editions of this work, but as applied to an analysis of Szasz's rhetorical paradigm, the changes are not significant.

8. Ibid., 103.

9. Ibid., 52–53.

10. Ibid., 77.

11. Ibid., 160.

12. Ibid., 36, 37.

13. Ibid.

14. Ibid., 35.

15. Ibid., 77.

16. Szasz, *Myth of Mental Illness*, 1.

17. Kuhn, *The Structure of Scientific Revolutions*, 134, 118.

18. Schoenfeld, "Analysis of the Views of Thomas Szasz."

19. This is also evident, Szasz maintains, in psychiatrists' analysis of deviant behavior in the past, such as Zilboorg's thesis that "witches were diagnosed mental patients." (Szasz, *Myth of Mental Illness*, 206).

20. Szasz, *The Myth of Psychotherapy: Mental Healing as Religion, Rhetoric, and Repression* (Garden City, New York: Anchor, 1978), 20.

21. Szasz, *The Untamed Tongue: A Dissenting Dictionary* (La Salle, Illinois: Open Court, 1990), 165.

22. Szasz, *The Therapeutic State: Psychiatry in the Mirror of Current Events* (Buffalo, New York: Prometheus Books, 1984), 10. There is in rhetorical theory a body of opinion that holds that the major function of rhetoric is to create reality for chosen audiences, thereby engendering competition among competing persuaders. See Richard E. Vatz, "The Myth of the Rhetorical Situation," *Philosophy and Rhetoric*, vi (1973), 154–161; and Barry Brummett, "Some Impli-

cations of 'Process' or 'Intersubjectivity': Postmodern Rhetoric,'' *Philosophy and Rhetoric*, ix (1976), 21–51.

23. Szasz, *The Second Sin* (Garden City: Doubleday, Anchor, 1973), 24–25.

24. Szasz, *The Age of Madness: The History of Involuntary Hospitalization* (Garden City, New York: Anchor/Doubleday, 1973), 2.

25. Szasz, *The Manufacture of Madness*, 293.

26. Szasz, *Age of Madness*, 3; idem, *Manufacture of Madness*.

27. Szasz, *Myth of Mental Illness*, 3.

28. Ibid., 212.

29. Szasz, *Ideology and Insanity*, 19.

30. Szasz, *The Ethics of Psychoanalysis: The Theory and Method of Autonomous Psychotherapy* (New York: Basic, 1965), 30.

31. Szasz, *Myth of Mental Illness*, 3.

32. Ibid.

33. Szasz, *Ethics of Psychoanalysis*, 38.

34. Szasz, *Insanity: The Idea and Its Consequences*, 23; idem, *Myth of Mental Illness*, 3.

35. Ibid., *Myth of Mental Illness*, 3.

36. Thomas Szasz, *The Myth of Mental Illness: Foundations of a Theory of Personal Conduct* (revised edition) (New York: Harper & Row, 1974), 17.

37. Ibid., 24.

38. Ibid., 22.

39. Szasz, *Myth of Mental Illness*, rev. ed. (1974), 17, 22, 24.

40. Szasz, *Insanity: Idea and Its Consequences*, 12.

41. Szasz, *The Ethics of Psychoanalysis*, 45.

42. Szasz, *Insanity: Idea and Its Consequences*, 24.

43. Szasz, *Ideology and Insanity*, 4, 21–22.

44. Szasz, *Ethics of Psychoanalysis*, 32.

45. Richard Restak, ''Psychiatry in America,'' *The Wilson Quarterly*, vii (1983), 114.

46. Ibid.

47. Szasz, *Insanity: Idea and Its Consequences*, 204.

48. Szasz, *Ethics of Psychoanalysis*, 30.

49. Szasz, *Insanity: Idea and Its Consequences*, 87.

50. Szasz, *Myth of Mental Illness*, xvi.

51. Szasz, *Insanity: Idea and Its Consequences*, 135.

52. Szasz, ''Noncoercive Psychiatry: An Oxymoron; Reflections on Law, Liberty, and Psychiatry,'' *Journal of Humanistic Psychology*, xxxi (1991), 117–125.

53. Szasz, ''Diagnoses are not Diseases,'' *Lancet*, cccxxxviii (1991), 1576.

54. American Psychiatric Association, *American Psychiatric Association Statement on the Insanity Plea* (Washington, D. C.: American Psychiatric Association, 1982).

55. Szasz, *Myth of Mental Illness*, 5.

56. Kenneth Burke, *A Grammar of Motives* (Berkeley: University of California Press, 1969), 17.

57. Szasz, *Myth of Mental Illness*, rev. ed. 259–260.

58. Hirsch, ''Home on the Hot Seat,'' A-7.

59. Szasz, *Insanity: Idea and Its Consequences*, 69.

60. Ibid., 51.

61. Kuhn, *The Structure of Scientific Revolutions*, 77.

62. Ibid.

63. Ibid., 222.

64. Keith Russell Ablow, ''A Preoccupation with Image,'' ''Health,'' *The Washington Post* (June 2, 1992) 9.

65. Nancy C. Andreason, *The Broken Brain: The Biological Revolution in Psychiatry* (New York: Harper & Row, 1984), 8.

66. Szasz, *Insanity: Idea and Its Consequences*, 70.

67. Richard E. Vatz and Lee S. Weinberg, "Letter to the Editor," *Commentary*, xcii (1991), 14.

68. Even for these cases, such as schizophrenia, psychiatry's diagnostic manual lists no such correlates as diagnostic criteria. See American Psychiatric Association, *Diagnostic and Statistical Manual of Mental Disorders*, 3rd ed. (Washington, D. C.: American Psychiatric Association, 1987).

69. Jerome Myers et al., "Six-Month Prevalence of Psychiatric Disorders in Three Communities," *Archives of General Psychiatry*, xli (1954), 959–967; Lee Robins et al., "Lifetime Prevalence of Specific Psychiatric Disorders in Three Sites," *Archives of General Psychiatry*, xli (1984), 949–958.

70. Szasz, *Insanity: Idea and Its Consequences*, 57.

71. Allen Frances et al., "An A to Z Guide to DSM-IV Conundrums," *Journal of Abnormal Psychology*, c (1991), 408.

72. Ibid., 411.

73. Elisa Benedek, Presidential Address, "Looking Ahead: New Psychiatry, Old Values," *American Journal of Psychiatry*, cxlviii (1991), 1126.

74. Frances et al., "An A to Z Guide to DSM-VI Conundrums," 409.

75. Ibid., 410.

76. Kuhn, *Structure of Scientific Revolutions* 151.

77. Szasz, *Myth of Mental Illness*, rev. ed. (1974), vii.

78. Hirsch, "Home on the Hot Seat"; Ronald Leifer, "Introduction: The Medical Model as the Ideology of the Therapeutic States" in David Cohen (ed.), *Challenging the Therapeutic State: Critical Perspectives on Psychiatry and the Mental Health System*, special issue of *Journal of Mind and Behavior*, xi (1990), 247–258.

79. Szasz, *Myth of Psychotherapy*, 20.

80. Ibid.

81. Charles Krauthammer, *Cutting Edges: Making Sense of the 80's* (New York: Random, 1985), 70.

82. Schoenfeld, "An Analysis of the Views of Thomas S. Szasz," 246.

83. Eugen Kahn, review of Thomas Szasz, *The Myth of Mental Illness. American Journal of Psychiatry* (1962), 190.

84. Jurgen Ruesch, review of Thomas Szasz, *The Myth of Mental Illness. Journal of the American Medical Association* (13 January 1992), 190.

85. Ibid.

86. *The Psychiatric Quarterly*, xxxvi (1962), 591.

87. Jerome Frank, review of Thomas Szasz, *The Myth of Mental Illness. Annals of Internal Medicine*, lv (1961), 877–888; O. Hobart Mowrer, review of Thomas Szasz, *Myth of Mental Illness. cxxxiv Science* (1961), 1974–1975.

88. Carl C. Bell, review of Thomas Szasz, *Insanity: The Idea and Its Consequences. Journal of the American Medical Association*, (10 July 1987), 269.

89. Dava Sobel, review of Thomas Szasz, *Insanity: The Idea and Its Consequences. New York Times Book Review*, 15 March 1987, 22.

90. Szasz, *Ideology and Insanity*, 21.

91. Owen Shapiro and Lester Friedman, "Thomas Szasz and the Myth of Mental Illness," Syracuse University, film (1989).

92. Jon Gudeman, "The Person with Chronic Mental Illness" in Armand M. Nicholi (ed.), *The New Harvard Guide to Psychiatry* (Cambridge: Harvard University Press, 1988), 715.

93. Mary D. Bublis, "Letter to the Editor," *Psychiatric News*, xxvii, 15 May 1992, 16.

94. Torrey, *The Death of Psychiatry*.

95. Robert Boyers, *R. D. Laing & Anti-Psychiatry* (New York: Harper & Row, 1971); Norman Dain, "American Psychiatry in the 18th Century" in George Kriefman, Robert D. Garner, and D. Alfred Abse (eds.), *American Psychiatry, Past Present and Future* (Charlottesville: University Press of Virginia, 1985). Nevertheless, in the 1970s Laing was a critic of psychiatry hospitable to Szasz. Torrey is now a supporter of biological psychiatry and the medical model, but only as it pertains to "serious mental illnesses" such as schizophrenia and bipolar disorders, such as manic-depression (see Torrey, *Surviving Schizophrenia: A Family Manual*, 1983).

96. Joseph Adelson, "The Ideology of Homelessness," *Commentary*, xcii (1991); Rael Jean Isaac and Virginia C. Armat, *Madness in the Streets: How Psychiatry and the Law Abandoned the Mentally Ill* (New York: Free Press, 1990).

97. Szasz, *Schizophrenia: The Sacred Symbols of Psychiatry* (New York: Basic, 1976), 54, 66, 72, 73.

98. Szasz, *The Therapeutic State*, 4.

99. Ibid., 24–26.

100. Ibid., 25. It is instructive here to note that one area in which Szasz has been misinterpreted and in which he disagrees with some conclusions associated with anti-psychiatry is the issue of deinstitutionalization, the precipitous removal of many patients from state psychiatric hospitals. Szasz has often been accused of being among those favoring such forcible removal, but, in fact, he has consistently opposed such evictions as further subjugation of "patients'" autonomy: "Institutionalizing human beings in the name of psychiatric care was, as now everyone admits, a sham. Deinstitutionalizing them in the name of psychiatric progress is a sham."

101. Szasz, *Insanity: Idea and Its Consequences*, 91.

102. Szasz, *The Manufacture of Madness*, xxiii

103. Kuhn, *Structure of Scientific Revolutions*, 2nd ed., 198–200. See also the analysis of rhetorical strategies inherent in this process in Bruno Latour, *Science in Action* (Cambridge: Harvard University Press, 1987).

104. Lane Cooper (ed), *The Rhetoric of Aristotle* (New York: Appleton Century Crofts Inc., 1960).

105. We could find no example of such reference.

106. American Psychiatric Association, *DSM-III-R*, xxv.

107. On the problems and consequences of lack of conceptual rigor in the case of the alleged mental disorder of alcoholism see Richard E. Vatz and Lee S. Weinberg, "The Conceptual Bind in Defining the Volitional Component of Alcoholism: Consequences for Public Policy and Scientific Research" in David Cohen (ed.), *Challenging the Therapeutic State*, special issue of *Journal of Mind and Behavior*, xi (1990), 531–544.

108. Robert Lloyd Goldstein, "Letter to the Editor," *Commentary*, xcii (March 1991), 14–15.

109. Stanton Peele, *The Diseasing of America: Addiction Treatment Out of Control* (Lexington: Lexington Books, 1989).

110. Herbert Fingarette, *Heavy Drinking: The Myth of Alcoholism as a Disease* (Berkeley: University of California Press, 1988).

111. John Leo, "The It's-Not-My-Fault Syndrome," *U.S. News and World Report*, 18 June 1990, 16; Alice Steinbach, "The Addiction Addiction," *Baltimore Sun*, 20 May 1991; John Taylor, "Don't Blame Me," *New York*, 3 June 1991, 26–34.

112. Erica E. Goode, "Sick, or Just Quirky: Psychiatrists are Labeling More and More Human Behaviors Abnormal," *U.S. News and World Report*, 10 February 1992, 49–50.

113. Charles J. Sykes, *A Nation of Victims: The Decay of the American Character* (New York: St. Martin's Press, 1992)

114. Thomas Szasz, *Law, Liberty, and Psychiatry* (New York: Collier Books, 1963), 212.

115. Szasz, *The Therapeutic State*.

116. *Bulletin of the Menninger Clinic*, liii (1989), 351.

117. Editorial, "British Psychiatry at 50," *Lancet*, cccxxxviii (1991), 785.

118. Szasz, *Insanity: Idea and Its Consequences*, 51.

119. Szasz, "Noncoercive Psychiatry," *Journal of Humanistic Psychology* (1991), 118.

120. Daniel B. Gadish, "Letter to the Editor," *Psychiatric News*, xvii, 7 August 1992, 23.

121. John A. Talbott, Robert E. Hales, and Stuart C. Yudofsky (eds.), *The American Psychiatric Press Textbook of Psychiatry* (Washington, D. C.: American Psychiatric Press, 1988).

122. To keep the appearance of equal participation of psychodynamic psychiatry and biological psychiatry, there has been the creation of and emphasis on a rhetorical amalgamation: "biopsychosocial" psychiatry. (See, for example, Catherine Brown, "Hartmann Urges Colleagues to Practice Psychiatry from Strong Humane, Biopsychosocial Base," *Psychiatric News*, xxvii, 5 June 1992). Other rhetorical accommodations are found throughout normal research, such as a journal, *Psychiatry*, changing its subheading in 1986 from *Journal for the Study of Interpersonal Processes* to *Interpersonal and Biological Processes*.

123. Kuhn, *Structure of Scientific Revolutions*, 2nd ed., (1970), 151, 155.

18

Michel Foucault's *Phänomenologie des Krankengeistes*

GARY GUTTING

"I am not a professional historian; nobody is perfect."

MICHEL FOUCAULT[1]

Foucault among the Historians—Part I

The reactions of professional historians to Foucault's *Histoire de la folie*[2] seem, at first reading, ambivalent, not to say polarized.[3] There are many acknowledgments of its seminal role, beginning with Robert Mandrou's early review in *Annales*, characterizing it as a "beautiful book" that will be "of central importance for our understanding of the Classical period."[4] Twenty years later, Michael MacDonald confirmed Mandrou's prophecy: "Anyone who writes about the history of insanity in early modern Europe must travel in the spreading wake of Michel Foucault's famous book, *Madness and Civilization*."[5] Later endorsements have been even stronger. Jan Goldstein: "For both their empirical content and their powerful theoretical perspectives, the works of Michel Foucault occupy a special and central place in the historiography of psychiatry."[6] Roy Porter: "Time has proved *Madness and Civilization* far the most penetrating work ever written on the history of madness."[7] More specifically, Foucault has recently been heralded as a prophet of "the new cultural history."[8]

But criticism has also been widespread and often bitter. Consider H. C. Eric Midelfort's conclusion from his very influential assessment of Foucault's historical claims: "What we have discovered in looking at *Madness and Civilization* is that many of its arguments fly in the face of empirical evidence and that many of its broadest generalizations are oversimplifications. Indeed, in his quest for the essence of an age, its *episteme*, Foucault seems simply to indulge in a whim for arbitrary and witty assertion so often that one wonders why so much attention and praise continue to fall his way."[9] Many of Midelfort's criticisms, if not always his overall assessment, have been widely endorsed by, for example, Peter Sedgwick, Lawrence Stone, Ian Hacking, and Dominick LaCapra.[10]

From the above juxtaposition of texts, it would seem that historians are sharply split in their views of the value of Foucault's work. But the division pretty much disappears on closer scrutiny. Those who applaud Foucault have in mind primarily what we may call his meta-level claims about how madness should be approached as a historiographical topic. They are impressed by his view of madness as a variable social construct, not an ahistorical scientific given, and of the history of madness as an essential part of the history of reason. These views are now generally accepted by historians of psychiatry,[11] and Foucault was one of the very first to put them forward. In this sense he is a widely and properly revered father of the new history of psychiatry. But on the "object-level" of specific historical facts and interpretations, the consensus of even favorably disposed historians is that Foucault's work is seriously wanting. Andrew Scull, whose own work shares much of the general spirit of Foucault's, nonetheless endorses what he rightly says is "the verdict of most Anglo-American specialists: that *Madness and Civilization* is a provocative and dazzlingly written prose poem, but one resting on the shakiest of scholarly foundations and riddled with errors of fact and interpretation."[12] Similarly, Patricia O'Brien, in an article expressing great enthusiasm for Foucault's work, agrees that "historians who are willing to admit that Foucault was writing history find it bad history, too general, too unsubstantiated, too mechanistic."[13]

Even historians who have a more favorable view of Foucault's specific historical claims are reluctant to accept him as a member of their tribe. Jan Goldstein, after maintaining that "Foucault used historical material to great advantage" and that "his historical sense was extraordinarily acute," goes on to note that "Foucault always considered himself at least as much a philosopher as a historian, whose epistemological and political project required that he challenge the ordinary canons of history writing."[14] Consequently, as she remarks in a review of *Discipline and Punish*, "the usual criteria of historical scholarship cannot be used to assess" Foucault's work.[15] MacDonald is similarly ambivalent: "Much of what Foucault has to say seems to me to be correct, in spite of his rejection of the prevailing standards of historical discourse."[16] Allan Megill goes even further. For him, not only does Foucault's work fall outside the discipline of history, "he is *anti*disciplinary, standing outside all disciplines and drawing from them only in the hope of undermining them."[17]

At least one Foucaultian, Colin Gordon, has opposed this consensus, arguing that historians have rejected Foucault's conclusions because they have not properly understood him. The difficulties of *Histoire de la folie* and especially the greatly abridged nature of its English translation have led to misinformed criticism. "*Histoire de la folie* has been a largely unread or misread book."[18] If, he suggests, we read Foucault's full text with care, we will find most of the standard criticisms to be misplaced and recognize his work as a rich source of detailed historical insight.

We have, then, three suggestions regarding Foucault's history of madness. The consensus of working historians is that it is bad history. To this Colin Gordon responds that it is good history (or, at least, that there is not yet sufficient grounds for thinking it is bad). And questioning the presupposition of both these views is the claim of Goldstein and Megill that it is not history at all.

Gordon is clearly right that many of the standard historical criticisms of *Histoire*

de la folie are misdirected. Midelfort, because of his wide influence, is the best example.
He says:

> Considered as history, Foucault's argument rests on four basic contentions. The first
> . . . is the forceful parallel between the medieval isolation of leprosy and the modern
> isolation of madness. . . . Second is Foucault's contention that in the late Middle
> Ages and early Renaissance the mad led an "easy wandering life," madness having
> been recognized as part of truth. . . . The third major contention . . . is that this
> openness [of the Middle Ages and Renaissance to madness] disappeared in the Age
> of the Great Confinement, beginning in the mid-seventeenth century. . . . The fourth
> and final contention posits a transition to madness as mental illness in which Fou-
> cault examines the work of the reformers, Tuke and Pinel, and concludes that they
> "invented" mental illness.[19]

The reader of Foucault's book is immediately struck by the oddity of claiming that
these are its "basic contentions." Although Foucault explicitly offered a history of
madness in the Classical Age, it seems that three of his four central claims are about
other periods. In fact, neither of the first two contentions is central to Foucault's argument. He begins his book by suggesting that leprosy in the Middle Ages bore some
striking functional parallels to madness in the Classical Age: Both lepers and the mad
were objects of fear and repulsion; both were isolated in houses designed more for
separation from society than for cures; both were used as joint signs of divine justice
and mercy; and in some cases funds and institutions originally meant for lepers came
to be used for the mad. There is, Foucault thinks, a nice parallel between the two
phenomena, a parallel he uses as a rhetorically effective opening of his book. But as
far as historical substance goes, the leprosy discussion is entirely nonessential. Leave
it out and the core of Foucault's argument about the nature of Classical madness and
its relation to modern psychiatry is unaffected.

To some extent, the same is true of the contrast Foucault sets up between the
integration of madness into medieval and Renaissance existence and its exclusion by
the Classical Age. The main point is that exclusion and confinement were distinctive
features of the Classical Age's attitude toward madness. Foucault sketches an ingenious
and provocative story about the medieval and Renaissance viewpoints, but no central
argument depends on this account. The essential point is merely that exclusion and
confinement distinguish the Classical Age in a fundamental way from the preceding
centuries. Beyond this, Foucault's hypotheses as to what went on in the Middle Ages
and the Renaissance are just intriguing marginalia.

In any case, the specific objections Midelfort raises to Foucault's claims about the
pre-Classical period are of little weight. He points out, for example, that the mad were
isolated from society during this period, particularly when they posed a threat to others
or themselves, and that there were special hospitals for the mad in Spain during the
fifteenth century. Here Midelfort mistakes a claim about the fundamental attitude of a
period with a claim about the first introduction of a practice. Finding examples of
confinement that precede the Classical Age does not count against the claim that confinement had a unique role in that period. One could just as well argue against the
secular character of modern society by citing examples of medieval and Renaissance
free-thinking. Midelfort also misunderstands Foucault's position when he urges against

it that "instances of harsh treatment of the mad [during pre-Classical periods] could be multiplied *ad nauseam*."[20] This evidence counts against Foucault's view only on the assumption that the pre-Classical inclusion of madness as part of the "truth of human existence" entailed humane treatment of the mad. But such an assumption makes a travesty of Foucault's account, on which Renaissance madness, for example, is either the critically ironic inverse of reason or a tragic and horrifying encounter with monstrous truths.[21] In either case, madness is an integral but disconcerting aspect of human life, essential but by no means welcomed.[22]

What Midelfort presents as Foucault's fourth basic contention—the "invention" of mental illness by the nineteenth-century reformers—is indeed central. His history of madness in the Classical Age is intended as a basis for showing that madness as mental illness was a social construction foreign to that period and original with the nineteenth century. Midelfort's criticism of this contention, however, is based on fundamental misunderstandings of Foucault's position. He says, for example, that "Foucault frequently implies that prior to the nineteenth century madness was not a medical problem." As he notes, such an "assertion seems deliberately preposterous," but no more so than Midelfort's attribution of it to Foucault, who has frequent and detailed discussions of Classical medical treatments of the mad. Foucault does insist that confinement was not practiced for therapeutic purposes and that the distinctive Classical experience of madness associated with confinement did not see the mad as ill. But he also insists on the ineliminable role of Classical medical treatment of madness and in fact poses the relation between nonmedical confinement and therapy as a major problem for understanding madness in the Classical Age.

As to Foucault's claim that reformers such as Pinel introduced a fundamentally new conception of madness as mental illness, Midelfort responds that "recent scholarship ... documents Pinel's explicit debt to earlier English theoreticians and to classical antiquity. Far from standing in a new environment governed by new rules . . . , Pinel clearly felt himself in continuous dialogue with the Hippocratic-Galenic tradition."[23] But this response is beside the point unless we falsely assume that conceptual innovation requires complete independence from all intellectual influences.[24] The question is whether Pinel transformed the ideas of those to whom he was "indebted" and "in dialogue with" into a fundamentally new conception. Midelfort's pointing out that, like everyone else, Pinel had intellectual ancestors has no bearing on this issue.

Midelfort's critique of Foucault's third contention—about the place of confinement in the Classical Age—is much more to the point. Foucault's claims about confinement are absolutely central to his position. He maintains that the isolation of the mad (along with various other people whose behavior involved a rejection of reason) in houses of internment was a practice that took on central significance during the Classical Age and is essentially connected with the age's fundamental experience of madness. If Foucault is wrong about Classical confinement, then the foundation of his account of madness in the Classical Age is undermined.

Roy Porter has developed this crucial criticism of Foucault in some detail. Foucault, he notes, insists that large-scale confinement was a Western European phenomenon, occurring, if in somewhat different ways and at different rates, in France, Germany, England, Spain, and Italy. But at least for England during the "long eighteenth century" (from the Restoration to the Regency), Porter maintains, Foucault is very much off the mark. Although there was some confinement of the mad and other deviants in work-houses, "the vast majority of the poor and the troublesome were not interned within institutions, remaining at large in society, under the administrative aegis of the Old Poor Law." In particular, studies of the treatment of the mad in certain regions of England show "that lunatics typically remained at large, the responsibility of their family under the eye of the parish."[25] Although some of the mad were confined, the numbers were quite small: perhaps as few as 5,000 and surely no more than 10,000 by the early nineteenth century, compared with the almost 100,000 confined in 1900. Confinement, Porter suggests, was much more a nineteenth-century phenomenon; during Foucault's Classical Age, "the growth in the practice of excluding the mad was gradual, localized, and piecemeal."[26]

Porter also raises important questions about Foucault's claim that in confinement the mad were homogeneously mixed with a wide variety of other sorts of deviants (prostitutes, free-thinkers, vagabonds, etc.) who violated the Classical Age's ideal of reason. "This picture of indiscriminate confinement does not seem accurately to match what actually happened in England. Few lunatics were kept in gaols, and workhouse superintendents resisted their admission." This tendency "not to lump but to split" was, Porter urges, particularly evident in London, where "scrupulous care was taken to reserve Bethlem for lunatics and Bridewell for the disorderly."[27]

Finally, Porter challenges two of Foucault's key claims about the way the Classical Age conceived madness (its "experience" of madness). According to Foucault, mad-ness, like all the varieties of unreason, was rejected in the first instance because it violated the Classical Age's morality of work. The mad, being idle, were a threat to the stability of a bourgeois society in which labor was the central value. Further, Foucault held that, within the category of unreason, the mad were distinctive for their animality, which put them in radical opposition to the human domain of reason. Porter finds both claims dubious in light of the English experience. "I do not," he says, "find prominent in eighteenth-century discourse the couplings Foucault emphasizes between sanity and work, madness and sloth. Less still was there any concerted attempt to put the asylum population to work."[28] As to the animality of the mad, Porter acknowledges it as one central image but maintains that there is a counterimage at least as important that Foucault scarcely recognizes. This is the Lockean view of the mad as not raging animals but people who, through misassociation of ideas, go desperately awry in their reasoning. Porter says that Foucault sees this view of madness as arising only with the moral therapy of Tuke and Pinel in the early nineteenth century, whereas in fact it was a very important dimension of seventeenth- and eighteenth-century conceptions of madness.

If Porter is right, Foucault is fundamentally wrong in his characterization of madness in the Classical Age: Confinement is not a practice definitive of the epoch's attitude toward madness, the exclusion of the mad is not an expression of bourgeois morality, and animality is not the essence of Classical madness. Is he right? Is Foucault's history bad? Or are Porter and other critics misunderstanding Foucault's historical claims? Or, finally, is Foucault up to something other than history? As a basis for answering these questions, I offer a fairly close reading of the section of *Histoire de la folie* (part II, chapters 2–5) in which Foucault develops the fundamentals of his account of madness in the Classical Age. This will provide grounds for drawing some conclusions about the value as history of Foucault's work on madness.

Foucault on Classical Madness

For all its *annalistes* and structuralist affinities, Foucault's history of madness begins from one great *event*: the confinement, within a few years, of a significant portion of the population of Western Europe in special houses of internment. Foucault presents this event as an abrupt and major change. He speaks of it as an "abruptly reached . . . threshold" (66), which occurred "almost overnight" (66; *MC*, 45), and describes it as a "massive phenomenon" (75; *MC*, 46) that, for example, displaced in just six years one percent of the population of Paris (5,000–6,000 people) and similar proportions elsewhere during the Classical Age (59, 66, n.2; *MC*, 38, 49).

Foucault, however, is not interested in the event of confinement for its own sake but in the attitudes toward and perceptions of madness connected with it in what he repeatedly refers to as "the Classical experience of madness." The event of confinement is the sudden manifestation of a long-developing "social sensibility" (66). The goal of his history of madness is to describe exhaustively this experience or sensibility and show how it provided the basis for the modern psychiatric conception of madness as mental illness.

The experience Foucault is tracking is not, he maintains, simply an experience of madness. Rather, the Classical Age saw madness as one division of a wider category, which Foucault calls "unreason" (*déraison*). This corresponds to the fact that not only the mad but a wide variety of other people were confined. Foucault offers successively deeper analyses of just how those confined were perceived.

On the most immediate level, confinement was an economic policy meant to deal with problems of poverty, particularly begging and unemployment. It was a way of getting a large class of idle, potentially disruptive people off the streets and putting them to work in a controlled environment. In purely economic terms, however, confinement was a failure. It hid but did not eliminate poverty, and any gains in employment due to work requirements on those interned were offset by corresponding losses of employment outside the houses of confinement (82).

But, Foucault maintains, the real significance of internment went beyond this economic surface. Far more than an unsuccessful solution to specific economic problems, it represented a new "ethical consciousness of work, in which the difficulties of the economic mechanisms lost their urgency in favor of an affirmation of value" (82; *MC*, 55). Foucault cites Calvin and Bossuet to show the religious basis for the ethical centrality of work: Since the Fall, a refusal to work manifests an absurd pride, which would presume on divine generosity to provide what we need with no effort of our own. "This is why idleness is rebellion—the worst form of all, in a sense: it waits for nature to be generous as in the innocence of Eden, and seeks to constrain a Goodness to which man cannot lay claim since Adam. . . . Labor in the houses of confinement thus assumed its ethical meaning: since sloth had become the absolute form of rebellion, the idle would be forced to work, in the endless leisure of a labor without utility or profit" (84; *MC*, 56–57). On this second level, then, those confined (*les déraisonnés*) were not regarded as the neutral objects of unfortunate economic processes but as moral reprobates worthy of society's condemnation and punishment.

Foucault goes on to maintain that implicit in the Classical condemnation of "unreasoning" behavior was a deep restructuring of moral categories. He considers the three major classes of those, other than the mad, who were interned: sexual offenders, those guilty of religious profanation, and free-thinkers (*les libertins*). In every case, behavior that was previously evaluated in other terms was reduced to a violation of bourgeois morality. For example, those suffering from venereal diseases were at first treated as merely victims of an illness like any other (97–101). But with the beginning of the Classical Age, their afflictions were seen as punishments for their sexual indiscretions. Another, more interesting case is the inverse fates of sodomy and homosexuality (102). Previously, sodomy was violently condemned as a religious profanation and homosexuality tolerated as an amorous equivocation. With the Classical Age, sodomy is treated less severely, being regarded as a mere moral fault, not a religious offense requiring the stake. Conversely, homosexuality is no longer overlooked but treated like other serious offenses against sexual morality. There is a Classical convergence of diverse attitudes toward deviant behavior to the single level of morality.

Foucault further maintains—with particular illustrations from the Classical attitude toward prostitution and debauchery—that the internment of sexual offenders was primarily designed to protect the bourgeois family: "In a sense, internment and the entire 'police' regime that surrounds it serves to oversee [*contrôler*] a certain order in familial structure. . . The family with its demands becomes one of the essential requirements of reason; and it is it that above all demands and obtains internment. . . . This period sees the great confiscation of sexual ethics by the morality of the family" (104).

Similarly, such things as blasphemy, suicide, and magical practices, previously regarded as outrageous profanations of religion, are all reduced to offenses against the monotone morality of the bourgeoisie. Magic, for example, once violently suppressed as an objectively powerful challenge to religion through its evocation of evil powers, now is regarded as merely a personal delusion that threatens the secular social order. In the same way, free-thinking (*libertinage*) is no longer a perverse but rational assault on religion's holy truth. It is merely the pathetic consequence of a licentious way of life.

Foucault's first fundamental thesis about Classical madness, then, is that it is assimilated to the broader category of unreason. This is a very puzzling category to modern thinking, since it strikes us as trying to occupy a nonexistent middle ground between freely chosen criminality and naturally caused illness. If the mad and their partners in unreason have acted freely against the social order, why, we ask, are they merely confined and not punished like other offenders? If they are not sufficiently responsible to merit punishment, why are they not treated like the ill, as innocent victims of natural forces? Foucault acknowledges our difficulty in grasping the conception, but he insists that this is not due to any intrinsic incoherence but to fundamental disparities between Classical and modern modes of experience.

Foucault does not, however, think we can stop with this simple, if puzzling, account of Classical madness. In some ways the mad were not treated just like others who were interned. There were hospitals (e.g., the Hôtel Dieu in Paris, Bethlem in London) where special provision was made for the medical treatment of the mad. True, such provision is the exception, and Foucault emphasizes that the internment of the mad (apart from the special hospitals) had no medical intention. Physicians were assigned to houses of internment only to treat whatever illnesses the inhabitants might come down with, not as part of a program of medical treatment for madness as such. But even though the medical view of madness is the less prominent (there were only eighty madmen in the Hôtel Dieu to the hundreds—perhaps even a thousand—in the Hôpital

Général), it cannot be ignored: "These two experiences each have their own individuality. The experience of madness as illness, as restricted as it is, cannot be denied" (131). The problem is to understand the juxtaposition of these two very different experiences.

Foucault vehemently rejects the Whiggish temptation to see Classical medical treatment of the mad as the first stirrings of progress toward an enlightened realization (fully blooming in the nineteenth century) that madness is mental illness. He notes that in fact a medical approach to madness developed at the end of the Middle Ages, beginning—possibly under Arab influence—in Spain in the early fifteenth century. During this period there are increasing numbers of institutions (or sections of them) specifically reserved for the mad. What is striking about the Classical Age is its relative regression in the recognition of the mad, who became less distinctive and more part of the undifferentiated mass of the interned. In this process, the mad become much less the object of medical attention. Some of them were treated as hospital patients in the Classical Age; but, according to Foucault, this is mainly a holdover from earlier periods. It is internment rather than treatment of the mad that is characteristically Classical. He supports his claim by citing examples of important institutions (e.g., Bethlem) that became more and more mere houses of confinement in the course of the Classical Age. So Foucault by no means claims that medical treatment of the mad (and hospitals designed for this purpose) did not exist in the Classical Age. He does not even claim that the period represents a regression in the medical knowledge of madness: "the medical texts of the 17th and 18th centuries suffice to prove the contrary" (138). Even though the viewpoints of medical therapy and of internment are by no means on a par in the Classical Age, both are present and need to be accounted for. This shows, he says, how "polymorphic and varied the experience of madness could be in the epoch of classicism" (147).

The fact remains that the specifically medical awareness of madness was neither autonomous nor fundamental. Classical madness is, at root, regarded as a disorder of the will, like other forms of unreason. There is, accordingly, "an obscure connection between madness and evil" that passes "through the individual power of man that is his will. Thus, madness is rooted in the moral world" (155).

Even within the realm of unreason, however, madness has a distinctive status. Foucault traces the special status of madness from the striking Classical practice of exhibiting the mad to a curious public. The standard explicit justification of confinement during the Classical Age was the need to avoid scandal. Unreason is hidden away to prevent imitation, to safeguard the reputation of the Church, to preserve the honor of families. But madness is a paradoxical exception: It is precisely during the Classical Age that the practice of displaying the mad to public view (most famously, at Bethlem and Bicêtre) was most prominent.

Foucault finds the explanation of this exception in the peculiar and essential relation of madness to animality in the Classical conception. Like most historians of the period, Foucault does not resist the temptation to cite some of the more vivid reports of how the Classical Age treated the mad like animals. To some extent, he admits, this is just (as the Classical Age would have urged) a matter of security against the violence of the insane. But Foucault thinks that there was a more specific and much deeper Classical meaning to the animality of madness. "The animal in man no longer has any value as the sign of a Beyond [as it did, for example, in the Renaissance]; it has become his madness, without relation to anything but itself: his madness in the state of nature. The animality that rages in madness dispossesses man of what is specifically human in him; not in order to deliver him over to other powers, but simply to establish him at the zero degree of his own nature. For classicism, madness in its ultimate form is man in immediate relation to his animality.'' (166; *MC*, 73–74). The mad are animals in the precise sense that they have totally rejected their human nature, put themselves outside the community of reasonable persons.

But why should the Classical Age see this sort of animality as a legitimate object of spectacle? Foucault thinks the answer lies in the new role of madness in Christian thought. Previously, there was a reverence and awe before madness based on the idea that Christian faith, as a scandal to reason, was a glorified form of madness. With the Classical Age, this idea is abandoned. Christian wisdom is unequivocally on the side of reason; faith involves no sacrifice of the intellect. Madness, with its choice of animality, is mankind's farthest remove from the truth; the mad are those who have reached the lowest human depths. But this is just why madness can function as the unique sign of the extent of divine mercy and the power of grace. The fact that Christ, in taking on human life, allowed himself to be perceived as mad and that his gracious solicitude extended to lunatics shows that salvation is available even to those who have fallen the farthest from the light. Thus, the exhibition of the mad served the dual salutary purpose of reminding men how far they might fall and that God's mercy extended even this far.

Here, then, we have the essence of the Classical experience of madness, as Foucault explicates it in part I of *Histoire de la folie*. There is much more to his story. While part I extracted the Classical experience from the event of confinement, part II provides a complementary account of the experience from the standpoint of Classical medical theory and practice, arguing, however, that the two forms of the experience share the same fundamental structure.[29] The essence of this structure is a paradoxical unity of moral guilt and animal innocence. To us, the Classical Age's interning the mad along with those belonging to other categories of unreason is a confusion, a blurring of the distinctive psychology of madness. But Foucault thinks that there is the positive structure of a perception, not the negativity of confusion. Madness is understood by the Classical Age precisely via its place on the horizon of unreason. At one point, Foucault marks this place by a striking religious metaphor: ''What the Fall is to the diverse forms of sin, madness is to the other faces of unreason'' (176). It is the principle, the model of all the others. More fully, madness ''flows through the entire domain of unreason, connecting its two opposed banks: that of moral choice . . . and that of animal rage. . . . Madness is, gathered into a single point, the whole of unreason: the guilty day and the innocent night'' (176). This is the ''major paradox'' involved in the Classical experience of madness: It is equally connected to the moral evaluation of ethical faults and to the ''monstrous innocence'' of animality. Madness is experienced as ''founded on an ethical choice and, at the same time, thoroughly inclined toward animal fury'' (177). Such an experience is far removed from (Classical and modern) legal definitions of madness, which seek a division of responsibility (fault) and innocence (external determinism), and from (Classical and modern) medical analyses, which treat madness as a natural phenomenon. Nonetheless, this experience is the key to understanding the Classical view of madness in both thought and practice.

Foucault's ultimate goal in writing his history of madness in the Classical Age was to illuminate (or expose) the true nature of modern (nineteenth-century to present) psychiatry. He repeatedly asserts his view that the modern conception of mental illness and the corresponding institution of the asylum have been unknowingly constructed out of elements of the Classical experience of madness.[30] In particular, he maintains that the theme of innocent animality becomes a "theory of mental alienation as pathological mechanism of nature"; and that, by maintaining the practice of internment invented by the Classical Age, psychiatry has preserved (without admitting it) the moral constraint of madness. Both "the positivist psychiatry of the 19th century" and that of our own age "have thought that they speak of madness solely in terms of its pathological objectivity; in spite of themselves, they dealt with a madness still entirely imbued with the ethics of unreason and the scandal of animality" (177). These Classical residues in the modern period are the basis of Foucault's analysis and critique (in part III of *Histoire de la folie*) of modern psychiatry.

Foucault among the Historians—Part II

We are now in a position to appreciate in a deeper way the difficulties that historians find in Foucault's work on madness, to see why Porter, for example, for all his praise of Foucault, says he came away from reading *Madness and Civilization* "bewitched, bothered, and begrudging."[31] The central issue of confinement is a good starting point. Porter, as we have seen, has serious objections to the existence of any "great confinement," at least in England, during the Classical Age. Most of the mad simply were not confined. Those that were, were, contrary to Foucault, carefully separated from other deviants. How should Foucault respond? He has no hope of refuting Porter on the level of the empirical facts. Porter's claim, incorporating numerous careful studies done since Foucault's book, has a decisive advantage here. Foucault might try a tactical retreat: Porter is right for England; but France, in which Foucault is mainly interested is (as even Porter seems to admit)[32] a different story. Perhaps, then, confinement is a French— or even a Continental—phenomenon, with the English, as so often, following a different drummer. But such a retreat puts Foucault into an impossible position, since he purports to be describing not the practices and beliefs of individuals, which might well differ from country to country, but the experience of a culture. He is interested in the fundamental categories in terms of which people perceive, think, and act, not the specific sensations, beliefs, and, actions falling under these categories. To allow that the English experience of madness was informed by a different set of fundamental categories would require viewing English and French (or Continental) culture as radically different to an extent that seems indefensible—and is certainly never defended by Foucault.

But perhaps Foucault's concern with fundamental experiential categories rather than specific perceptions, beliefs, and actions is itself the key to a response to Porter. For, after all, Porter's critique is based on just the sort of specific beliefs and actions that are not Foucault's primary concern. Foucault is not making empirical generalizations about what people in various countries thought or did; he is trying to construct the categorical system that lay behind what was no doubt a very diverse range of beliefs and practices. Confinement, then, is a fact, perhaps most striking in France, but, as Porter admits, also present in England and the rest of Europe. Foucault is concerned with the categorical conditions of possibility for this fact. He wants to know what in the way the Classical Age experienced madness made the sort of confinement it practiced possible. Of course, there were, as Foucault admits and even emphasizes, other dimensions of Classical practice, most notably medical therapy, which involved integration rather than isolation of the mad from the community. In some cases, this may have meant that, as Porter finds for England, the progress of confinement was slow and piecemeal. But such empirical divergences do not refute Foucault's categorical analysis of the Classical experience of madness.

I think the above is a properly Foucaultian response to Porter. But I also think accepting it alters the terms of Foucault's confrontation with historical criticism. The crux is this: Given that Foucault's categorical analysis is not refuted by the empirical deviations Porter points out, just what would refute the analysis and, even more important, what would support it?

Here there is a crucial, though easily ignored, difference between Foucault and standard historians like Porter. At the onset of his study of madness in the long eighteenth century, Porter formulates his project in a way that seems entirely congruous with Foucault's history of madness. He says that he is "attempting principally to recover the internal coherence of now unfamiliar beliefs about the mind and madness, and to set them in their wider frames of meaning."[33] Further, like Foucault's, Porter's book is filled with facts: names, dates, anecdotes, and quotations from primary sources. Nonetheless, the books are poles apart, and the difference is in the way factual details are related to the overall project of understanding how madness was perceived and treated from 1650 to 1800.

On one level, the difference is that for Porter the facts are primarily *supports* for the interpretative schema, whereas for Foucault they are primarily *illustrations* of it. The opening of Foucault's chapter on confinement is a good example. He begins (57–58) with an analysis of Descartes' rejection of madness as grounds for philosophical doubt, from which he extracts his basic idea of a Classical exclusion of madness from the realm of human existence. Surely he does not regard a single passage from one author as proof of an epoch's conception of madness; the passage from Descartes can only be an illustration of his assertion. He then moves to a discussion of confinement as a practical expression of this exclusion. The development of confinement is discussed with some detail for France (59–64); but only two brief paragraphs, one on England, the other on the rest of Europe, are deemed enough to show that confinement had "European dimensions" (64; *MC*, 43). Neither paragraph offers much beyond a list of houses of confinement and the dates of their founding. Foucault says nothing about other ways of treating the mad (though, as we have seen, he later pays considerable attention to medical treatment). Most important, he never (here or elsewhere) discusses the extent of confinement relative to other practices and provides no data establishing his view that confinement is the typical Classical reaction to madness. Porter, as we have seen, has substantial evidence that confinement was relatively uncommon in England and, given the strong influence of the Lockean conception of madness, was by no means the distinctively Classical way of dealing with it.

Foucault's procedure is similar throughout the book. His claim that a religious view about the role of work in our postlapsarian world underlies the Classical moral condemnation of madness is supported by brief citations from Calvin, Bossuet, and Bourdaloue (83–84). He bases his claim that there was a "great confiscation of sexual ethics by the morality of the family" (104) on two cases of internment, a few quotations from Molière, and two citations from Classical legal documents (104–105). His "proof"

(138) that confinement expressed the fundamental Classical experience of madness and that medical treatment was a marginal holdover of previous practices is that, after Bethlem was opened to the nonmad, there was soon no notable difference between it and the French *hôpitaux généraux*; and that St. Luke's included both the mad and the nonmad from its founding in 1751. With regard to his striking claim that the Classical Age saw unreason as the result of a voluntary choice, he admits that "this awareness is obviously not expressed in an explicit manner in the practices of internment or in their justifications" (156). But he maintains that such a choice can be inferred from Descartes' remarks on madness and that the point is entirely explicit in Spinoza (156–158).

Foucault's penchant for using facts as illustration rather than support does not mean that, as Midelfort suggests, he is "simply indulg[ing] in a whim for arbitrary and witty assertion." It is, rather, a sign of what I will call his idealist (as opposed to empiricist) approach to history. A characterization of Foucault's history of madness as idealist is apt for a variety of reasons. It is primarily not a history of events or institutions but of an experience, the experience of madness. Also, this experience is not understood in terms of the perceptions or thoughts of individuals; rather, its subject is the anonymous consciousness of an age. (Foucault himself later criticized *Histoire de la folie* because it "accorded far too great a place, and a very enigmatic one too, to what I called an 'experience,' thus showing to what extent one was still close to admitting an anonymous and general subject of history.")[34] Further, Foucault's history exhibits the tense Hegelian combination of anarchic and totalitarian tendencies: a fascination with conflicting complexities (so that every thought is almost limitlessly qualified and complemented) along with an ultimately triumphant compulsion for unity, so that all the complexity is relentlessly organized. Finally, in typical idealist fashion, the operative justification of Foucault's historical construction is its interpretative coherence rather than its correspondence with independently given external data.

This idealistic cast makes professional historians very uneasy with Foucault's work. They think that, in his insistence on a single unified interpretation, Foucault ignores the messy loose ends that close empirical scrutiny seems to find everywhere in history. David Rothman, for example, complains that "for all the sweep of the analysis, the categories seem rigid (are reason and unreason mutually exclusive?), and there remains too little room for other considerations." He goes on to remark that Foucault's "explanation is so caught up with ideas that their base in events is practically forgotten."[35] Likewise, Ian Dowbiggin, while acknowledging the debt of his account of nineteenth-century psychiatry to Foucault, remarks that "there is a seamless quality to Foucault's model that . . . fits historical reality poorly."[36]

As an idealist historian Foucault could well respond that he is not after an account gerrymandered to fit every recalcitrant fact, an impossible project in any case. What he wants is a comprehensive, unifying interpretation that will give intelligible order to an otherwise meaningless jumble of individual historical truths. The facts are not irrelevant for Foucault, but the primary support for his position is not its demonstrable correspondence with them but its logical and imaginative power to organize them into intelligible configurations. The idea that the Classical Age was one of confinement is an immensely powerful instrument for connecting themes in the theology, literature, philosophy, and medicine of the Classical Age with one another and with that age's political, religious, social, and economic practices. Once we begin to think in terms of confinement as a fundamental category, we are, as Foucault shows, able to develop an extensive and subtle interpretative framework that both raises provocative questions and gives them intriguing answers. Other interpretations may "fit" the facts as well or better than Foucault's, but his provides a perspective with distinctive advantages in unifying power and intellectual fruitfulness. From this standpoint, the facts that illustrate Foucault's claims about confinement are not merely inadequate pieces of empirical evidence. They are also compelling examples of the power of his interpretative framework.

To distinguish between idealist and empiricist history is, of course, only to specify the opposite ends of a continuum. No system of interpretation can have historical significance if it is not supported by some significant body of corresponding facts, and no factual data can be formulated independent of some prior interpretative system. Consequently, even though most standard historical practice is nowadays much closer to the empirical end of the continuum than Foucault's, my characterization of his work as idealist does not mean that it is, as Goldstein and Megill suggest, outside the discipline of history. Every historical study must balance idealist interpretation with empiricist fact-gathering, and Foucault's work does not cease to be history because it is at the currently less favored end of the continuum.

Moreover, the reasons Goldstein and Megill offer for thinking Foucault is not a historian seem unpersuasive. Goldstein says that Foucault is unhistorical because "he questioned the necessary continuity of history."[37] The issue, however, is whether the continuity Goldstein has in mind is essential for history as such or just the defining characteristic of one sort of history. Foucault himself, in responding to Sartrean claims that his approach eliminates history, insisted that he eliminated only that history for which "there is an absolute subject of history, . . . who assures its continuity."[38] That such an elimination is consistent with the historical nature of his enterprise is supported by the fact that Foucault's approach remains firmly rooted in the central historical category of the event.[39] It is also relevant to recall that, whatever the role of discontinuity between historical periods in his subsequent works, *Histoire de la folie* frequently insists on important continuities between Classical and modern conceptions of madness (cf. the passages cited in n. 29).[40]

Megill argues that *Histoire de la folie* lies outside of history (and of all academic disciplines) because it is ambiguous in a way appropriate to literature rather than an academic discipline. "There is something central to the disciplinary project that seems thwarted in Foucault. It is as if, through his love of ambiguity, he has thrown a monkey wrench into the disciplinary machinery."[41] I agree that the anti-disciplinary rhetoric of ambiguity Megill emphasizes is an important element in *Histoire de la folie*. But this shows only that it is not exclusively a historical analysis. What basis is there for thinking that, for example, Foucault's elaborate interpretation of the Classical experience of madness, sketched in the middle section of this essay, is not a historical account, evaluable by the disciplinary canons of history? It may well be that, even if such evaluation resulted in the total rejection of the account as history, there would still be literary (and, perhaps, some sort of philosophical) merit in what Foucault wrote. But the fact remains that, whatever else may be going on, *Histoire de la folie* does offer a very detailed history of madness in the Classical Age. My own view is that the book shows an anti-historical character primarily in Foucault's intermittent efforts to evoke madness as it is experienced by the mad themselves. This experience he tends to present as an absolute transcending the history of changing social constructions of madness. (The theme is most apparent in the preface to the first edition, which Foucault later dropped.) Contrary to Megill, I think this theme is clearly outside the main thrust of the book.[42]

What, then, should we conclude about what we might now, not entirely facetiously, describe as Foucault's *Die Phänomenologie des Krankengeistes*?[43] Granted, as I have just been arguing, that it *is* history, is it good or bad history? The easy answer is that it is good idealist history but bad empiricist history. That, however, is too easy, since a schema of historical interpretation may be so empirically deficient that even its most ingenious and exciting speculations are not worth pursuing. (In the same way, an empirically impeccable account may be so devoid of interpretative interest as to be hardly worth a historian's yawn.)

This, I think, is as far as philosophical kibitzing can take the discussion of Foucault's history of madness. I have argued that there is no good reason to place *Histoire de la folie* entirely outside the domain of history, immune to the critical norms of historiography. I have also maintained that neither of the two most important historical critiques of Foucault shows that his work is bad history. Midelfort's apparently decisive criticisms are mostly based on misunderstandings of Foucault's views. Porter's critique of Foucault's central views on confinement raises an important empirical challenge but does not, in itself, undermine the interpretative power of Foucault's idealist history. So far, there have been no decisive tests of the fruitfulness of Foucault's complex interpretative framework. What is still needed, it seems to me, is an assessment of his overall picture of Classical madness through detailed deployments of its specific interpretative categories. Is, for example, Jan Goldstein right in her suggestion that historians of the Enlightenment should pay more attention to Foucault's idea of a tension in the Classical experience of madness between man as a juridical subject and man as a social being?[44] How much explanatory power is there in his claim that Classical confinement involved a reduction of all sexual offenses to the norms of bourgeois morality? What level of understanding can we reach by developing his account of the religious significance of Classical madness? To what extent is the nature of nineteenth-century psychiatry illuminated by thinking of it as constructed from the polar Classical conceptions of madness as innocent animality and as moral fault? The issue of Foucault's status as a historian of madness should remain open until historians have posed and answered questions such as these.

Notes

1. Comment at the University of Vermont, 27 October 1982, cited by Allan Megill, "The Reception of Foucault by Historians," *Journal of the History of Ideas*, (1987), 117.

2. *Histoire de la folie à l'âge classique* (Paris: Gallimard, 1972), all references will be given in parentheses in the main text. The English translation, *Madness and Civilization*, trans. Richard Howard (New York: Random House, 1965), is of a drastically abridged French edition. Cited passages that appear in *Madness and Civilization* will be given in Howard's version, other passages in my own translation. For more details on various French editions of *Histoire de la folie*, see Gary Gutting, *Michel Foucault's Archaeology of Scientific Reason* (Cambridge: Cambridge University Press, 1989), 70, n.6.

Colin Gordon has rightly emphasized the need to consult the full French text; see "*Histoire de la folie*: An Unknown Book by Michel Foucault," *History of the Human Sciences*, iii (1990), 3–26. Also see the responses to Gordon's article by a variety of writers (*inter alios*, Robert Castel, Roy Porter, Andrew Scull, H. C. Eric Midelfort, Jan Goldstein, Dominick LaCapra, and Alan Megill) and Gordon's reply, "History, Madness and Other Errors: A Response," in the same volume. An English translation of the full French text by Anthony Pugh is scheduled to appear from Routledge.

3. This essay will focus on *Histoire de la folie*, which is Foucault's only full-scale discussion of madness and, so far, the work of his most influential on historians of psychiatry. Mention should also be made of his earlier, mainly nonhistorical, discussions, *Maladie mentale et personnalité* (Paris: PUF, 1954) and the long introduction to a French translation of Ludwig Binswanger's *Traum und Existenz: Le rêve et l'existence*, trans. J. Verdeaux (Bruges: Descleé de Brouwer, 1954); trans. "Dream, Imagination, and Existence," trans. F. Williams, *Review of Existential Psychology and Psychiatry*, 19 (1984–85), 29–78. A second edition of the former work, greatly revised, mostly in accord with the views of *Histoire de la folie*, appeared as *Maladie mentale et psychologie* (Paris: PUF, 1962); trans. *Mental Illness and Psychology*, trans. A. Sheridan, foreword by H. Dreyfus (Berkeley: University of California Press, 1987). For a discussion of these early works and their relation to *Histoire de la folie*, see Gary Gutting, *Michel Foucault's Archaeology of Scientific Reason*, 55–69.

Foucault's later work on the history of the prison (*Discipline and Punish*, trans. Alan Sheridan (New York: Pantheon, 1978) and on nineteenth century sexuality (*The History of Sexuality*, Vol. I: *An Introduction*, trans. Robert Hurley (New York: Pantheon, 1978) have also had an important influence on historians of psychiatry. Their challenging views on the inextricable connections of power and knowledge and on the deep functional similarities of modern institutions such as asylums, prisons, factories, and schools may in the long run be more important for historians of psychiatry than even the *History of Madness*. In this connection, see Robert Nye's *Crime, Madness, and Politics in Modern France* (Princeton: Princeton University Press, 1984).

4. Robert Mandrou, "Trois clefs pour comprendre la folie à l'époque classique," *Annales E. S. C.* (1962), 761–772.

5. Michael MacDonald, *Mystical Bedlam: Madness, Anxiety, and Healing in Seventeenth-Century England* (Cambridge: Cambridge University Press, 1981), xi.

6. Jan Goldstein, *Console and Classify: The French Psychiatric Profession in the Nineteenth Century* (Cambridge: Cambridge University Press, 1987), 396.

7. Roy Porter, "Foucault's Great Confinement," *History of the Human Sciences*, iii (1990), 47.

8. See Patricia O'Brien, "Foucault's History of Culture" in Lynn Hunt (ed.), *The New Cultural History* (Berkeley: University of California Press, 1989), 25–46.

9. H. C. Eric Midelfort, "Madness and Civilization in Early Modern Europe: A Reappraisal of Michel Foucault" in Barbara Malament (ed.), *After the Reformation: Essays in Honor of J. H. Hexter* (Philadelphia: University of Pennsylvania Press, 1989), 259.

10. Peter Sedgwick, *Psycho Politics* (New York: Harper & Row, 1982), 132, n. 22; Lawrence Stone, "Madness," *New York Review of Books*, 16 Dec. 1982, 36ff. (also see Foucault reply, 31 March 1983, 42–44); Ian Hacking, "The Archaeology of Foucault" in David Hoy (ed.), *Foucault: A Critical Reader* (Oxford: Blackwell, 1986), 29; Dominick LaCapra, "Foucault, History, and Madness," *History of the Human Sciences*, iii (1989), 32–34.

11. Cf. for example Roy Porter, *Mind Forg'd Manacles* (Cambridge: Harvard University Press, 1987), xi, 33; Michael MacDonald, *Mystical Bedlam*, 1; Andrew Scull, *Museums of Madness* (New York: St. Martin's Press), 70; and the introduction to W. F. Bynum, Roy Porter, Michael Shepherd (eds.), *The Anatomy of Madness*, vol. I, (London: Tavistock, 1985), 3–4.

12. Andrew Scull, "Michel Foucault's History of Madness," *History of the Human Sciences*, iii (1990), 57.

13. O'Brien, "Foucault's History of Culture," 31.

14. Goldstein, *Console and Classify*, 3.

15. Jan Goldstein, *Journal of Modern History*, li (1979), 117.

16. Michael MacDonald, *Mystical Bedlam*, xi.

17. Megill, "The Reception of Foucault by Historians," 133–134.

18. See Colin Gordon, "History, Madness and Other Errors: A Response," 381.

19. Midelfort, "Madness and Civilization in Early Modern Europe," 249–251.

20. Ibid., 253.

21. As Colin Gordon points out, Midelfort seems to be misled by a mistranslation in *Madness and Civilization*, which has Foucault speaking of the "easy wandering life" of the mad in the Middle Ages and Renaissance. See "*Histoire de la folie*: An Unknown Book by Michel Foucault," 17. For Midelfort's response to Gordon (on this and other points), see "Comments on Colin Gordon," *History of the Human Sciences*, iii (1990), 41–46.

22. I hesitate to add to the already overextended controversy about Midelfort's contention that Foucault is wrong in his belief that the "ships of fools," so prominent in medieval literature and painting, actually existed. Let me say merely that Foucault's use of the ship is almost entirely concerned with its literary and artistic significance and that it is central to his argument only as a striking (and rich) *symbol* of what he thinks was the status of medieval madness. Depriving him of the assumption that such ships actually existed has a nugatory effect on the evidence for his view.

23. Midelfort, "Madness and Civilization in Early Modern Europe," 258–259.

24. Midelfort also takes Foucault to task for accepting as fact the myth of Pinel's liberation of the mad from their chains at Bicêtre. This is a blatant misreading, since Foucault is not only well aware of the lack of factual basis for the anecdote but explicitly treats the story as a myth. For further details, see Colin Gordon, "*Histoire de la folie*: An Unknown Book by Michel Foucault," 15–16.

25. Porter, "Foucault's Great Confinement," 48.

26. Ibid.

27. Ibid., 49

28. Ibid.

29. On the other hand, Foucault's discussion in part II importantly refines and deepens his view, particularly by relating the experience of madness to Classical conceptions of imagination, passion, the mind-body union, and language. For a full analysis of Foucault's view of Classical madness (and of the entire project of *Histoire de la folie*), see chapter 2 of my *Michel Foucault's Archaeology of Scientific Reason*.

30. See, for example, *Histoire de la folie*, 97, 100–101, 103, 116, 139, 146–149, 177.

31. Porter, "Foucault's Great Confinement," 47.

32. Porter, *Mind Forg'd Manacles*, 7.

33. Ibid., x.

34. Foucault, *The Archaeology of Knowledge*, 16, translation modified.

35. David Rothman, *The Discovery of the Asylum* (Boston: Little, Brown, 1971), xviii.

36. Ian Dowbiggin, *Inheriting Madness: Professionalization and Psychiatric Knowledge in Nineteenth-Century France* (Berkeley: University of California Press, 1991), 170.

37. Goldstein, *Console and Classify*, 3.

38. "Michel Foucault explique son dernier livre," interview with J-J. Brochier, *Magazine littéraire*, xxviii (1969), 24.

39. Cf. Foucault's remarks on this point in Colin Gordon (ed.), *Power/Knowledge* (New York: Pantheon, 1980), 114.

40. For more on Foucault's attitude toward continuity, see Robert Nye, *Crime, Madness, and Politics in Modern France*, 11–12, and Patrick Hutton, "The History of Mentalities: The New Map of Cultural History," *History and Theory*, xx (1981), 254.

41. Allan Megill, ''Foucault, Ambiguity, and the Rhetoric of Historiography,'' *History of the Human Sciences*, iii (1990), 358.

42. Cf. ibid., 350–356. For further discussion of Foucault and the experience of madness, see Gutting, *Michel Foucault's Archaeology of Scientific Reason*, 263–265.

43. In comparing Foucault as a historian of madness to Hegel, I am not, of course, saying that Foucault endorsed the metaphysics of the Absolute that underlies Hegel's own histories. Foucault's idealism is much more methodological than metaphysical, and primarily derives from the strong influence of phenomenology on his earlier writings. (This influence is most prominent in the essay on Binswanger cited in note 3.) Foucault's penchant for idealistic as opposed to empirical history decreased over the years, but I would argue that it remains strong at least through *Les mots et les choses* and never entirely disappears from his work. Foucault was well aware of his Hegelian tendencies: ''We have to determine the extent to which our anti-Hegelianism is possibly one of his tricks directed against us, at the end of which he stands, motionless, waiting for us'' (''The Discourse on Language,'' appendix to *The Archaeology of Knowledge*, 235).

44. Jan Goldstein, '' 'The lively sensibility of the Frenchman': Some Reflections on the Place of France in Foucault's *Histoire de la folie*,'' *History of the Human Sciences*, iii (1990), 336.

19

Feminist Histories of Psychiatry

NANCY TOMES

The category of feminist histories of psychiatry considered in this essay is of comparatively recent origin. Its scholarly agenda originated in the "second wave" of modern feminism (as distinguished from the "first wave" of the nineteenth century), which emerged in the United States and Western Europe during the late 1960s and early 1970s. The first attempts to write a feminist history of psychiatry can be found in the founding texts of the modern women's movement, including Simone de Beauvoir's *The Second Sex* and Betty Friedan's *The Feminine Mystique*. Making women aware of the negative consequences of psychiatry's conservative, indeed soul-damaging, influence on their lives was a central goal of the movement's early "consciousness raising" efforts.[1]

The questions that feminists raised about psychiatry's role in restricting women's aspirations moved from the realm of activism to academia in the 1970s and 1980s. As growing numbers of women entered graduate school and acquired faculty positions, "women's issues" and feminist scholarship became legitimate and vital areas of research in both the humanities and the social sciences. Over the next two decades, feminist scholars produced a thoroughgoing critique of the hidden prejudices of a scholarly discourse about women hitherto dominated by men.

That critique had an influence far beyond the ranks of feminists themselves. Feminist scholarship contributed significantly to the intellectual "revisionisms" that swept through fields as diverse as psychology, literary criticism, and history in the past twenty years. Perhaps more than any other single group, feminists helped to make problematic an older scholarly tradition in which concepts such as "man," "progress," and "objectivity" were confidently and unself-consciously invoked.

Directly relevant to the concerns of this volume, feminist concerns sparked new interest in the history of psychiatry. What was once a topic of interest primarily to psychiatrists themselves became required reading for intellectuals in a variety of fields, in large part because it served as a key domain for developing feminist theory. Within the field itself, feminist scholarship contributed to the demise of what Roy Porter and Mark Micale have termed the "presentist, progressivist, and tenaciously internalist" orientation of the "classic" history of medicine and psychiatry.[2] Reevaluating psychiatric conceptions and treatment of women in the light of contemporary feminist theory helped shape the major themes of post-1960 historical revisionism: the social construction of disease, the uses of psychiatry as social control, and the "deconstruction" of scientific claims to objectivity. Thus feminist scholarship has altered the very terms of debate in the history of psychiatry.

Essential to this feminist project has been a critique of an assumption central to medicine and psychiatry for centuries: that the differences between the sexes are biologically or psychodynamically determined. Feminist histories treat the categories of "masculine and feminine" as cultural constructions, not objective facts; they assume that the content of those categories—the particular traits assigned one sex or the other— are not fixed and universal but are determined by specific historical circumstances and subject to constant contestation and renegotiation. For my purposes in writing this essay, what distinguishes a feminist from a nonfeminist history is this perspective on gender as a social construct.

Although feminists share a contested view of gender, they utilize a wide variety of methods and come to a wide variety of conclusions concerning its meaning: hence the use of the plural rather than the singular form of *history* in the title of my essay. Contrary to conservative laments about "political correctness," there is no agreed-upon feminist orthodoxy on any subject, much less one as complex as psychiatry; as will be evident, feminist scholars have disagreed with one another about key points from the very beginning. Their debates illustrate in microcosm the larger shifts in interpretation that have impelled feminist scholarship over the last two decades.

This essay examines the ways in which the feminist conception of gender identity as cultural construction has forced a fundamental reconsideration of psychiatry's history. Rather than summarize all the many debates and findings about the specialty's treatment of women in the past, I focus instead on their basic arguments and assumptions about gender and madness. First, I want to demonstrate how the new feminism made problematic the assumptions of the old Whig history of psychiatry; second, to survey how feminist scholars envisioned alternative lines of research and argument; and third, to suggest how feminist critiques point to some of the unfinished business of the specialty's past.[3]

In illustrating these points, I will necessarily be quite selective in my choice of historical texts for inclusion. A full discussion of all the ways that the subject of gender informs the history of psychiatry would require a book in and of itself. In this essay I limit my discussion in two basic ways: My examples are drawn primarily from the nineteenth and twentieth centuries, and they remain within the geographic bounds of Western Europe and the United States.[4]

A World Without Women: Traditional Histories of Psychiatry

To appreciate what a profound intellectual shift had to take place before women's distinctive experiences, much less the construction of gendered identities, could become a legitimate part of psychiatry's history, it is necessary to sketch the paradigm of historical writing that prevailed prior to the 1960s. The field was primarily the province of psychiatrists themselves, who practiced the historical craft largely out of a need to construct an inspiring scientific past for their specialty. Casting psychiatry's history in that mold predicated certain basic assumptions about disease, modes of scientific inquiry, and the nature of the doctor-patient relationship that effectively excluded women as significant historical actors and ignored gender as a significant category of analysis.[5]

The central problem of this older style of history, which Herbert Butterfield aptly termed "Whig" history, was to explain how and why scientific knowledge and practice had evolved or progressed to its currently "enlightened" state.[6] Whig assumptions about the past were derived from beliefs about the present; in other words, how modern science worked provided the model for studying and judging its historical antecedents. At the core of the Whig narrative of psychiatry's history was a belief in the fixed nature of disease: that its unfolding within the individual followed a course fixed by biological or psychological imperatives (depending on the historian-practitioner's allegiance to the organic or psychodynamic tradition). In the Whig view, medicine progressed as scientific men came to discern the natural laws governing disease through the increasingly rigorous application of the scientific method.

Whig historians assumed that scientific observation and experiment succeeded only to the extent that it eliminated the nonscientific, that is, the social or cultural dimensions of disease. "The first step toward a truly scientific psychiatry," as Emil Kraepelin, the eminent German psychiatrist and one of the specialty's first historians, put it, was "the victory of scientific observation over philosophical and moral meditation."[7] Thus psychiatry's history was presented as a series of clarifications that abstracted the pure scientific "fact" from its cultural milieu. Its heroes were those individuals who comprehended the "true" nature of mental disease more clearly than their contemporaries; in the Whig narrative, they reached this superior understanding of disease only by rejecting the ordinary world of belief, where prejudice and superstition held sway.

Within this overarching set of assumptions, the Whig history of psychiatry provided very little conceptual space for considering the ways women's experiences differed from men's, much less the ways the Whig definition of science reaffirmed the masculinist assumptions of Western culture. Women were very rarely psychiatrists prior to the midtwentieth century, so the chronicle of intellectual discovery was an exclusively male story for most of the specialty's history. The conception of disease as a fixed biological or psychodynamic entity made gender variations in its expression a source of little historical or contemporary interest. Moreover, to the extent that psychiatry's past skirmishes with the "woman question" had drawn it into the unsavory area of popular prejudice, it hardly formed an appropriate chapter in an uplifting narrative of the specialty's scientific "progress."

The two exceptions to the absence of women in early histories of psychiatry only reinforce these general observations. First, Whig histories of psychiatry inevitably included a treatment of the witchcraft "epidemics" of the early modern period as an example of the progressive nature of scientific thinking. Their witchcraft narratives pitted the superior insight of "truly scientific" men such as Johann Weyer against the ignorance of the Church and the laity. From the Whig perspective, the physicians' realization that witches, the vast majority of whom were women, were in fact mentally ill saved them from what medical historian Erwin Ackerknecht referred to as the "barbarous nonsense" of early modern witchcraft beliefs.[8]

The history of psychoanalysis represented another significant exception to the invisibility of gender in prefeminist psychiatric narratives. What few names of women, either as patients or practitioners, appeared in the older histories were associated exclusively with the psychoanalytic tradition. The fact that unlike other psychiatric approaches, psychoanalysis took gender difference as essential to its theory and practice was part of its historical saga from the outset. In his first attempt to compose a historical account of psychoanalysis, written in 1914, Sigmund Freud portrayed his recognition of the link between his female patients' psychosocial repression and their neuroses as his awakening to the truths of psychoanalysis. To highlight his superior scientific sensibilities, he contrasted his own willingness to confront these truths with the medical profession's lack of "objectivity and tolerance" on the subject of female sexuality.

But from Freud's first efforts onward, historical narratives of psychoanalysis invoked female patients' experience or female analysts' theories in service of a highly deterministic theory of psychosexual development. While acknowledging women's sexual desires, psychoanalytic histories featured them in a secondary, supporting role to the male narrative of scientific discovery. Moreover, historians of psychoanalysis exempted the field's founder from the cultural prejudices about women that they so easily detected among his detractors. The more problematic aspects of the "woman question" within psychoanalysis itself were passed over as quickly as possible in the early celebratory volumes devoted to its past.[9]

By and large, then, the assumptions of traditional histories of psychiatry, whether written in service of an organic or a psychodynamic theory of mental illness, assumed the universality of disease processes, reified a fixed and unproblematic sense of male and female difference, and promoted a view of the psychiatrist as a scientist immune from and actively fighting social prejudice and stereotypes. As we shall see, it was precisely those assumptions that early feminists challenged in their critique of the specialty and its historical legacy to women.

Early Feminist Manifestos

The first attempts to craft a feminist alternative to the traditional Whig history of psychiatry can be found embedded in Simone de Beauvoir's *The Second Sex* (1949) and Betty Friedan's *The Feminine Mystique* (1963), two of the central texts of the early women's movement.[10] Their contentions about the pernicious influence of psychiatry were taken up and expanded in the feminist manifestos published as the movement gained momentum in the late 1960s, among them Kate Millett's *Sexual Politics* (1969), Germaine Greer's *The Female Eunuch* (1970), Eva Figes's *Patriarchal Attitudes* (1970), and Shulamith Firestone's *The Dialectic of Sex* (1970).[11]

Many of the ideas developed by feminists in the early 1960s had been around for several decades. De Beauvoir's path-breaking analysis of the "second sex" had emerged out of French existentialism in the late 1940s, while across the English Channel, Viola Klein, a student of sociologist Karl Mannheim, had published *The Feminine Character*, an impressive study of changing cultural views of femininity, in 1946. Yet neither work inspired large groups of women to question their place in society during the conservative 1950s. As Janet Sayers wrote of Klein's work, the wider feminist implications of her arguments went unappreciated in the absence of an organized women's movement.[12]

Historians are only beginning to understand the conditions that brought about the rise of such an organized women's movement in the late 1960s. Long-term changes in family size, women's work force participation, and levels of educational attainment, combined with the short-term upheavals of the civil rights and anti-war movements in the United States, contributed to the genesis of feminism's "second wave."[13] This new generation of feminists expanded their attention from the political and economic dimensions of equal rights, which had hitherto dominated women's organizations, to include a more radical cultural critique of patriarchal society. They were concerned not only with wages and political influence but also with media images, fashion imperatives, and the reign of "expert" authorities in child care and personality development. The considerable cultural authority developed by psychiatry and psychology over the course of the twentieth century made the mental health "establishment" a natural focus for honing a feminist critique of cultural oppression.

That despite the wide difference in their backgrounds and perspectives—Friedan was a journalist, de Beauvoir had formal training in literature and philosophy, Millett and Greer were literary historians, Figes was a novelist, and Firestone was a Marxist theorist—all these early feminist authors included a critique of psychiatry in their analyses of women's oppression is testimony to its status as a cultural authority. Their work shared the belief that for the "second wave" of feminism to avoid the failures of the earlier women's movement, women had to throw off the historical shackles of psychiatry. As Greer wrote, "The revolutionary woman must know her enemy," and doctors and psychiatrists headed her list of those whom feminists must beware.[14]

Using an eclectic mix of theories and writing styles, the early feminist theorists made the same basic points: that science in general and psychiatry and psychology in particular had played a crucial historical role in providing the intellectual justification for female subordination. Science, for so long an exclusively male domain, had taken the male as the norm in its supposedly "objective" measurements of human nature; the woman was portrayed as the "other," a deviant, imperfect, castrated variant on the healthy, fully realized "man." Deeply steeped in patriarchal privilege, psychiatrists assumed what they should have investigated: that biological and psychological differences between the sexes constituted an "essential" female character, which in turn justified separate and unequal gender roles. In their conceptions of what made women succumb to mental illness, psychiatrists endorsed the profoundly conservative view that man was made for the world of work and aspiration, woman for the home and service to others.

When the early feminists castigated the scientific "double standard" applied to the female psyche, their indictments invariably targeted psychoanalysis as the chief villain, a choice that reflected its intellectual dominance in the immediate post–World War II period. In 1949 De Beauvoir observed, "It is among the psychoanalysts in particular that man is defined as a human being and woman as a female—whenever she behaves as a human being she is said to imitate the male." Friedan offered a more explicitly historical explanation for psychoanalysis's constricted view of female potential. "The whole superstructure of Freudian theory rests on the strict determinism that characterized the scientific thinking of the Victorian period," she wrote. Freud mistook for "penis envy" the understandable jealousy that Victorian women felt for their male counterparts' superior educational, political, and occupational opportunities. Subsequently his many popularizers "embedded his core of unrecognized traditional prejudice against women ever deeper in pseudoscientific cement," concluded Friedan.[15]

Firestone and Millett, arguably the two most sophisticated theoreticians of the early women's movement, made an even more important argument about the historical relationship between feminism and Freudianism. Psychoanalysis, in their view, was a critical aspect of the counterrevolution that led to the demise of the "first wave" of nineteenth-century feminism. The feminist challenge to patriarchy had become extremely threatening by the late 1800s; the women's rights movement had made substantial progress in expanding educational, political, legal, and, at least among the avant garde, sexual freedoms for women. Freudianism supplied the ammunition for a counterrevolutionary backlash: It deflected feminism's challenge back on its proponents by labeling them "neurotic" and "maladjusted" and sending them to the analyst's couch.

For both Millett and Firestone, there was a tragic element in psychoanalysis's historical displacement of "first wave" feminism. They portrayed Freud as a keen clinical observer who acquired genuine insight into the psychic constraints, particularly the stifling sexual and social inhibitions, that upper middle-class women suffered during the Victorian era. Yet his masculinist bias led him to betray that insight in his formulations of such reductionist concepts as "penis envy" and the "masculinity complex." As Millett wrote, "Freud had spurned an excellent opportunity to open the door to hundreds of enlightening studies on the effect of male-supremacist culture on the ego development of the young female, preferring instead to sanctify her oppression in terms of the inevitable law of 'biology.' "[16]

While stressing the reactionary influence of early psychoanalytic models of female development, these authors were quick to acknowledge that the counterrevolution only succeeded to the extent that women themselves internalized the new "feminine mystique." Women's overreliance on expert authorities who belittled their own perceptions and weakened their self-esteem set up a vicious cycle: The more women tried to live their lives in accordance with the experts' stifling dictates, the worse they felt. Germaine Greer put it simply: "As far as the woman is concerned, psychiatry is an extraordinary confidence trick: the unsuspecting creature seeks aid because she feels unhappy, anxious and confused, and psychology persuades her to seek the cause in herself."[17]

The end result was legions of women benumbed by drugs, alcohol, shock treatments, and psychotherapy, whose suffering provided feminists with a powerful argument for change. Significantly, it was the pervasiveness of the "problem with no name," a disabling depression often accompanied by alcohol and drug abuse, among the "happy housewife heroines" of the 1950s that led Betty Friedan to begin formulating her critique of the feminine mystique. The widespread extent of women's emotional distress was compelling proof, from the feminist point of view, of the wrongs being done them by sexist society.

The Chesler Thesis

It remained for a feminist psychologist, Phyllis Chesler, to abstract these arguments about psychiatry from general accounts of women's oppression and develop them into a full-blown, radical critique of the specialty's dealings with the "second sex." Her *Women and Madness*, published in 1972, was one of the most widely read and cited feminist works of the decade, and its arguments continue to influence writings about women and mental illness to this day.[18]

Chesler's work is particularly important because she wed the emerging feminist critique of psychiatry with the intellectual wing of the "anti-psychiatry" movement, which had developed independently of it in the late 1950s and early 1960s. What came to be known as the "social labeling" or "social control" school drew upon the work of dissident psychiatrists, such as Thomas Szasz and R. D. Laing, as well as academic sociologists such as Erving Goffman and Thomas Scheff. Its attack on expert authority and scientific objectivity powerfully reinforced and was in turn strengthened by the feminist critique of psychiatry.[19]

The scholars aligned with the anti-psychiatry movement questioned whether mental illness was in fact a disease at all; in contrast to "real" diseases, they argued, the various diagnostic categories of mental illness lacked a clear-cut, verifiable etiology or set of symptoms. In their view, madness was more properly thought of as a form of social deviance, akin to criminality or juvenile delinquency. The mentally ill were simply individuals who violated certain basic norms about rationality and predictability; labeling them as "sick" allowed society more easily to remove their disturbing presence from the community. To justify this process of expulsion, psychiatry had obligingly provided a "medical model" of insanity, which gave its practitioners tremendous power and social rewards. But, in fact, as the labeling theorists were determined to show, the psychiatric "science" of diagnosing and treating mental illness was a thinly disguised form of social control. The patient's psychiatric career did not reflect some fixed physiological course of disease, but rather depended, from start to finish, on societal needs and values.

In *Women and Madness*, Chesler played out the feminist implications of this iconoclastic model of mental illness. Holding a Ph.D. from the innovative New School of Social Research in New York City, she brought to the subject a range of social scientific perspectives on the mental health field that other feminist critics had lacked. Chesler made good use of the new sociological literature on the asylum, population studies of psychiatric epidemiology, and feminist critiques of psychological testing, as well as her own clinical experience with women mental patients. The result was a powerful synthesis of the feminist and social control perspectives.

In *Women and Madness*, Chesler introduced a number of important arguments about women and psychiatry that would inspire subsequent feminist histories of the subject. First, she pioneered the analysis of exemplary "madwomen's" lives as a form of feminist biography. Using the psychiatric careers of four women who spent time in mental hospitals—Elizabeth Packard, Ellen West, Zelda Fitzgerald, and Sylvia Plath—she argued that "for them, madness and confinement were both an expression of female powerlessness and an unsuccessful attempt to reject and overcome this state." Chesler was careful not to propose that madwomen be viewed as revolutionaries; rather, she described madness as "a socially powerless individual's attempts to unite body and feeling." But she did posit that their lives could be exemplary, in that mentally ill women were often attempting, consciously and unconsciously, to escape the terrible "half-life" imposed by conventional female roles.[20]

Second, Chesler argued that the "symptoms" by which society defined mental illness were intimately related to the accepted norms of masculinity and femininity; in other words, the "norm violations" in madness-cum-deviance involved a transgression of the core male/female identity. "What we consider 'madness,' whether it appears in women or in men," Chesler proposed, "is either the acting out of the devalued female role or the total or partial rejection of one's own sex-role stereotype." Although both sexes transgressed their gender stereotypes, women were more likely than men to be labeled sick or insane as a consequence because of what Chesler termed the "double standard" of mental health. Referring to the standards that psychologists used to define a healthy personality, she observed that to be considered a mentally sound adult—that is, independent, autonomous, objective—was to be at odds with the traits considered healthy for a properly "adjusted" woman—namely, dependency, submissiveness, and emotionality. Thus a woman could end up being labeled crazy "whether she accepts or rejects crucial aspects of the female role," whereas men "acting out" the male role were more likely to be labeled "criminal" or "sociopathic." Given this fact, Chesler concluded, it was not surprising that epidemiological studies of hospitalized and non-hospitalized populations showed that women manifested more symptoms of mental "illness" than men.[21]

Chesler located the historical convergence between conceptions of femaleness and madness in the nineteenth century. "By the end of the nineteenth century, and throughout the twentieth, the portraits of madness, executed by both psychiatrists and novelists, were primarily of women," she wrote. Chesler portrayed the mental hospital as an important reflection of this emerging female/insanity nexus. "Madness and asylums generally function as mirror images of the female experience, and as penalties for being 'female,' as well as for desiring or daring not to be." Moreover, mental hospitals, by their rigid routines and ritualized forms of abuse, subjected women to the same "degradation and disenfranchisement of self" that they experienced in their patriarchal families and the larger society.[22]

Although Chesler's analysis was less explicitly historical than Millet's or Firestone's had been, she nonetheless broadened the potential for a feminist history of psychiatry in a far more fundamental way. First, she provided a model for analyzing the lives of women labeled as "mentally ill" to gain insight into the historical experience of female identity and oppression. Second, by expanding her focus to include not only psychoanalysis but institutional psychiatry as well, she implicitly pushed back the origins of the madness/femininity nexus to the era before Freud. Both those lines of analysis were soon taken up by academic historians, who found in the "nervous women" of the nineteenth century an important and revealing subject for the new women's history.

The New Women's History

Just as academic psychology in the United States and Great Britain was producing feminist practitioners such as Phyllis Chesler, history, long a male-dominated profession, was being colonized by feminists in the early 1970s. And much as Chesler had drawn from and expanded new social science methods and insights, these historians drew strength from the emerging discipline of the "new social history." The first works by professional historians in the English-speaking world to reevaluate the relations between nineteenth-century women and their physicians emerged as part of this larger transformation of historical scholarship.

Social history was a self-consciously revisionist movement within a field that had been preoccupied with political and intellectual history for almost two decades. Its leading practitioners came from outside the ranks of white, male Protestants who had long dominated the historical profession; they tended to enter academia fresh from participation in the political tumults of the 1960s and 1970s, including the civil rights, anti–Vietnam War, labor, and women's movements. Given their background and sense of political engagement, the practitioners of the new social history not surprisingly spurned the traditional methods and consensus-oriented approaches of the 1950s. Social history was often described as "history from the bottom up" because it assumed that groups formerly deemed politically and intellectually insignificant, such as slaves, workers, and housewives, were in fact profoundly interesting and influential historical actors.[23]

One of the most powerful motivations behind the development of social history was the determination of feminist historians to "write women into history," a task that required a radically different sense of what kind of historical sources and issues mattered. To this end, they used documents such as diaries and letters, popular advice books, and novels that had previously been of little interest to historians. And whereas earlier historians interested in women's experience had concentrated primarily on their political and economic gains, the "new women's history" was just as curious about the "underside" of women's experience, particularly the arenas of cultural domination that concerned contemporary feminist activists.

The surge of historical interest in nineteenth-century medical and scientific views of women is a case in point. As the women's movement gained momentum in the 1970s, a variety of issues related to women's bodies, including freedom of sexual expression, access to birth control and abortion, and alternative forms of childbirth, became popular causes; the success of the women's health care movement, epitomized by the Boston Women's Health Collective and their manual, *Our Bodies, Ourselves*, testified to the growing determination of feminists to contest and limit traditional medical authority over female bodies and minds. The phenomenal success of Barbara Ehrenreich and Deirdre English's historical pamphlets, *Witches, Midwives and Nurses* and *Complaints and Disorders*, affirmed the importance of feminist efforts to "reclaim" a historical place for women in the health care system.[24]

Neither Ehrenreich nor English were historians by training; the former had a Ph.D. in biology and the latter an MSW. But they clearly recognized that a good historical critique would help legitimate the feminist challenge to the contemporary medical establishment. Later expanded and published in 1978 as *For Her Own Good: One Hundred Years of Experts' Advice to Women*, their historical analysis focused on how women's traditional roles as healers had been usurped by the medical profession. Reversing the usual Whig logic that science had brought nothing but benefit to its recipients, Ehrenreich and English emphasized the negative side of the scientific revolution for women: how the rise of medical authority had robbed them of autonomy and exposed them to deeply sexist ideologies. Much in the spirit of earlier feminist critiques, they devoted several chapters to the role of psychiatry and psychology in promoting a limiting view of women's abilities.[25]

With a less obviously contemporary agenda in mind, professional historians also pursued the topic of women and medicine in the mid-1970s. Of the papers published from the proceedings of the first Berkshire Conference on Women's History, held at Radcliffe College in Cambridge, Massachusetts in 1973, several focused on the medical "construction" of womanhood in nineteenth-century America.[26] The subject of "the lady and her physician" interested prominent early practitioners of women's history for several reasons: First, it offered a means to explore how the larger social forces refiguring nineteenth-century society, such as industrial capitalism, urbanization, and changes in the family structure, affected the daily lives of women; second, it exposed the historical roots of women's dependence on medical "experts."

Ann Douglas's 1973 article, "The Fashionable Diseases: Women's Complaints and Their Treatment in Nineteenth-Century America," represented an influential formulation of these historical problems. A literary historian by training, Douglas used a variety of published sources, including novels, medical texts, and advice books, to interpret the apparent epidemic of nervous diseases among middle-class women in the nineteenth century. Her work illustrates the kind of propositions that initially engaged academic historians interested in the implications of the "cult of true womanhood" for women's mental health.

First, not unlike Betty Friedan's portrait of the 1950s' housewife, Douglas assumed that nineteenth-century middle-class "ladies" lived extremely restricted lives, both mentally and physically, and as a result suffered from a variety of nervous "complaints." Second, she argued that doctors responded to their largely psychosomatic ailments in terms of a highly unscientific, indeed misogynistic ideology. Lacking any "real" knowledge of women's bodies or psyches, physicians' advice and treatment simply reflected the scientific sexism of the day, which interpreted everything women did or felt in terms of their reproductive organs. Third, Douglas emphasized the highly politicized nature of the doctor-patient relationship; in her words, there was "a complicated if unacknowledged psychological warfare . . . being waged between doctors and their patients." She portrayed the rise of the nineteenth-century women's medical movement as in part a feminist impulse to rescue women from a degrading dependence on male physicians. Then as now, she implied, feminists instinctively understood the dangers of trusting male doctors.[27]

But in the same volume, another feminist historian, Regina Morantz, disputed the idea that all medical thinking about women could be explained in terms of unconscious misogyny. She argued that physicians' so-called ignorance affected men and women patients equally, and that the "heroic treatments" they practiced had a long and ancient lineage, quite independent of contemporary male anxieties about feminism or female sexuality. In addition, Morantz challenged the view that women physicians held a more empowering view of women, insisting that they were "very much Victorian women, prisoners of their own time and culture." Distancing herself from the political uses of feminist history, Morantz concluded, "Surely to view the existence of Victorian women solely from the perspective of male domination has become a sterile and tedious line of inquiry."[28]

The Douglas–Morantz debate revealed a faultline in feminist arguments over how to interpret the motivations of the nineteenth-century male physicians who cared for ailing women. The tension between their points of view was evident in their treatment of S. Weir Mitchell, the famous neurologist who developed the "rest cure" and treated a number of prominent late nineteenth-century women, including Charlotte Perkins Gilman and Jane Addams. In Douglas's account, Mitchell was portrayed as the epitome of "a veiled but aggressively hostile male sexuality and superiority." In contrast, Morantz insisted he was a more complex figure, who may have patronized his women patients yet also "conscientiously sought and relished the company of educated, intelligent, strong-minded women."[29]

The work of Carroll Smith-Rosenberg, probably the most talented and influential women's historian of her generation, successfully negotiated between the "woman as victim" and the "woman as just another patient" dichotomy evident in Douglas and Morantz's disagreements. In the early 1970s, Smith-Rosenberg, who combined professional training in both history and psychoanalysis, wrote a series of fine articles on the nineteenth-century woman patient and her physician that became classics of the new women's history.

Smith-Rosenberg, like Douglas, emphasized that the middle decades of the nineteenth century were extremely unsettled and unsettling ones, and that discontinuities in the female role were a source of anxiety and ill-health among American women. Likewise, she elaborated the "ovarian theory" of women's behavior that dominated medicine in the nineteenth century: Physicians conceived of women's reproductive lives as a series of dangerous physiological crises that, if mismanaged, could lead to insanity or death. Medical prescriptions about how women should live their lives in order to remain healthy were deeply conservative; long before Freud, Smith-Rosenberg showed, male physicians had developed biologically based arguments against women's higher education, careers outside the home, and suffrage.[30]

In adopting the "sick role," Smith-Rosenberg argued, the nervous women of the nineteenth century were attempting an escape from the discontinuity between the ideal and the reality of Victorian middle-class womanhood: While the ideal celebrated the virtues of passivity, dependency, and weakness, to live the reality of an adult woman's life required strength and resourcefulness. "Hysteria thus became one way in which conventional women could express—in most cases unconsciously—dissatisfaction with one or several aspects of their lives."[31]

In Smith-Rosenberg's account, the sick woman's relations with her physician were extremely complex and ambivalent. She needed to get his imprimatur for her illness to assume the sick role; but, if he validated her symptoms, he entered into complicity with her efforts to evade her womanly duties. Smith-Rosenberg suggested that this sense of being manipulated by their female patients accounts for the harsh tone and "draconian" measures physicians often advocated for hysterical females. Their views reflected not a position of masculine confidence and strength but, rather, a sense of frustration and defensiveness.

In these early works, feminist historians wrestled long and hard with the implications of interpreting women's nervous conditions as modes of protest against their limited gender roles. The notion of mental illness as a form of "protofeminism" had an obvious appeal. The well-known cases of talented women such as Charlotte Perkins Gilman and Jane Addams who had nervous breakdowns and recovered only by forging unconventional lives for themselves seemed to suggest that feminism and madness were two sides of the same coin. On the other hand, as Smith-Rosenberg suggested, the hysteric made her "escape" from the cult of true womanhood "only at the cost of pain, disability, and an intensification of women's passivity and dependence."[32] The difficulty of reconciling these two interpretations of female madness remained a fundamental ambiguity in feminist portrayals of nineteenth-century psychiatry and its treatment of women.

The Social History of the Asylum

The historical debates over how to interpret nineteenth-century women's mental disorders and the male medical response to them initially revolved around the domains of general medicine, gynecology, and neurology, not psychiatry proper. In the 1980s, attempts to write a new social history of the mental hospital brought similar questions to play in the interpretation of institutional psychiatry, as evidenced in the work of Ellen Dwyer, Constance McGovern, and myself. Unlike Elaine Showalter's 1985 study, *The Female Malady*, which will be discussed shortly, gender was not the exclusive focus of their research; rather these authors attempted to integrate gender into a general social history of the asylum, reflecting a commitment to move women's history into the mainstream of American history.[33]

In the 1970s, the nineteenth century "discovery of the asylum" had figured prominently in the debate over the so-called social control thesis. Historians David Rothman and Gerald Grob and historical sociologist Andrew Scull examined the rise of the mental hospital both as a new form of social control and a vehicle for the professional aspirations of psychiatry. While they explored the ways in which the asylum represented an effort to control a menacing new class of the poor and foreign born, they did not consider gender concerns as an aspect of the emerging institutional order.[34] In contrast, the second, feminist generation of asylum historians tended to recast the social control functions of the mental hospital in more intimate, familial terms. Using detailed institutional records, including correspondence, case records, and ward diaries, they focused on why families committed patients to asylums, what they hoped to gain from treatment, and how patients responded to the institutional experience.[35]

In exploring the influence of gender roles on nineteenth-century asylum practice, the new historians of the asylum had to confront the thesis advanced by Phyllis Chesler and others that the mental hospital played a special role in disciplining iconoclastic women. The chief historical exemplar of that argument was Elizabeth Packard, a woman committed to an Illinois asylum by her clergyman husband, whose story Chesler presented in *Women and Madness* as an unambiguous account of how the new asylums and their medical superintendents served on the frontline of the nineteenth-century war between the sexes. From Chesler's viewpoint, the Packard saga contained all the elements of the classic feminist "social control" view of the asylum: Packard's independence and assertiveness were labeled madness; the patriarchal family cooperated with the patriarchal psychiatrist to confine the woman rebel; she recognized that treatment for the imprisonment it was and, after successfully regaining her freedom, became a crusader for women's rights and asylum reform.[36]

But the first generation of feminist social historians to look closely at the institutional experience of nineteenth-century women patients came up with a different, far more ambiguous account. While agreeing with Chesler's characterization of the links between patriarchy and the asylum, their historical accounts did not validate the core assumption of the Chesler argument: that the mental hospital bore some unique relationship, as symbol or actual punishment, to nineteenth-century women. Instead they tended toward a more symmetrical view of gender and madness: that social disorder and anxiety disturbed the mental balance of both sexes; that although it manifested itself in somewhat different ways, mental illness afflicted roughly equal numbers of men and women; that insanity in both sexes posed a serious threat to the family order; and that the therapeutic regime mirrored the gender roles and patriarchal relations of the era.

The gender symmetry apparent in these analyses of asylum life reflected in part the peculiar nature of their sources. In comparison with the ''nervous women'' studied by previous feminist historians, these scholars confronted a group of women patients suffering from psychoses, not neuroses, who by any standards would be considered gravely impaired. Contemplating the clinical record of their hallucinations, disconnected or obsessional thought patterns, and violent impulses toward the self and others, it proved difficult for these historians to discern the more subtle ways that a ''double standard'' of mental illness might have affected women and men in the past. Moreover, the complex social dynamics revealed in individual case records and family correspondence defied easy categorization along gender lines. The family's response to a woman relative's mental illness was conditioned by all sorts of factors that had little to do with the nature of what Chesler termed ''sex-role violations.''[37] The fact, too, that in contrast to Chesler's contemporary statistics, nineteenth-century American mental hospitals had roughly equal numbers of men and women, and that the asylum doctors themselves portrayed the two sexes as more or less equally liable to the disease, further discouraged the assertion of any special link between femininity and madness.[38]

But while the new historians of the asylum downplayed the nineteenth-century mental hospital's uses as a form of social control for rebellious females, they strongly confirmed the patriarchal nature of its therapeutic rationale, emphasizing the familial metaphor that asylum physicians used to structure their relations to patients and staff alike. The asylum superintendent assumed the role of the Victorian *pater familias*, and meted out medical and psychological treatments that paralleled the ''separate spheres'' assigned to men and women in the larger society.[39]

Still, for all their emphasis on paternalistic ideology, the new historians of the asylum tended to cast both the physicians' motivations and the women patients' experience in a more varied and positive light than the Chesler argument would allow. Although stressing the asylum superintendents' social conservatism, they did not portray them as particularly misogynistic or harsh toward their women patients. Indeed, the new historians of the asylum went so far as to suggest that the paternalistic order of the asylum privileged women over men patients in some important ways. For example, Dwyer and McGovern noted that in the etiological tabulations of the era, men's illnesses were more likely to be assigned morally negative causes, such as overindulgence in alcohol or sexual passion; in contrast, they noted a surprising degree of psychiatric sympathy for working-class wives and their special burdens. Comparing patterns of drug treatment, McGovern noted that violent women patients were more likely to be sedated rather than confined in physical restraints. And all three historians of the asylum found that women were more likely than men to be discharged as ''cured.''[40]

Along similar lines, the new historians of the asylum took issue with the view of women patients as passive victims. Influenced by revisionist accounts of other ''total institutions'' such as plantation slavery, they emphasized the dialectical nature of the doctor-patient relationship. Clearly opposed to portraying patients, male and female alike, as simply objects of psychiatric domination, they instead chose to emphasize the ways women patients exercised choices despite the constraints imposed by their mental condition and their inferior status in society. For example, Dwyer and McGovern offered evidence that individual women actually welcomed asylum treatment as a refuge from overwork or abusive husbands. From these historians' perspective, then, the asylum experience appeared to be a more checkered one for women inmates: Some women hated it, some women seemed little affected by it, and some actually believed that they had been cured by it.[41]

In sum, the new historians of the asylum insisted that the mental hospital had complex uses for families and patients, male and female alike. They eschewed the view of the asylum as a total institution designed primarily or even secondarily to discipline iconoclastic women. While they agreed that nineteenth-century asylum treatment was modeled on the patriarchal family, they concluded that it offered women (and men) its own distinctive brand of mixed blessings. Certainly the treatments it meted out were not designed to resolve the role conflicts Carroll Smith-Rosenberg so astutely described in her portrait of the "hysterical woman": Rather it offered shelter to those who had found those conflicts too difficult to resolve. Considering some of the alternatives— abusive husbands and employers, or incarceration in the almshouse—the new historians of the asylum concluded that it may not have looked as unrelievedly awful to women inmates as contemporary feminists might believe.

Deconstruction, Hysteria, and Feminist Theory

While social historians were working through the implications of gender for a revisionist history of the nineteenth-century asylum, other feminist scholars in the 1980s were in the process of developing a far bolder form of gender analysis. By the late 1970s and early 1980s, many felt that they had reached the limits of trying to incorporate gender issues into the traditional concerns of their disciplines. Studies of women were proliferating in every field, yet they were difficult to synthesize and were all too easily ignored by male scholars. Moreover, the very methods feminists used seemed to reify the concept of male-female difference in ways that contributed to this sense of marginalization. As Joan Scott, one of the leading historian-advocates for theoretical change, urged in an influential 1986 article, feminists had to aspire to gender analysis that would not just address "dominant disciplinary concerns," but also "shake their power and perhaps transform them."[42]

In search of new theoretical perspectives, feminists scholars found inspiration in the work of French scholars, notably the philosopher Michel Foucault, the linguist Jacques Derrida, and the psychoanalyst Jacques Lacan. To put simply a very complex body of work, these French theorists tended to shift attention from specific historical actors and institutions to the larger "discursive formations," that is, the linguistic and symbolic systems, within which they operated. Domination was conceived not as the direct exercise of power, as in a psychiatrist confining a woman patient, but rather as the existence of a widely diffused, all pervasive system of perception and thought in which both doctor and patient acted. Foucault's work was particularly important in breaking down "the notion that social power is unified, coherent, and centralized" and replacing it with a more diffused notion of power "as dispersed constellations of unequal relationships, discursively constituted in social 'fields of force,' " in the words of Joan Scott.[43]

Increasingly, feminist theorists looked to the importance of *language* in constituting those "fields of force." Following Jacques Derrida, they stressed that Western language and symbolic systems had embedded in them binary oppositions of male-female, mind-body, reason-madness. These gendered categories construct, or determine the boundaries, of discourse not only about gender but about all forms of difference and even the exercise of power itself. In this view, the opposition of male to female has been fundamental to the production and use of knowledge at least since the Enlightenment.

The new theoretical project, then, was to demystify or "deconstruct" how these binary oppositions operated: to show that the categories of "male" and "female" represented no fixed, "objective" reality but were culturally constructed and contested fictions. By calling into question one of the allegedly eternal verities of Western science—that the differences between men and women were universal, fixed, and innate—feminist theorists meant to shake its epistemological foundations to the core. As the editors of a special issue on deconstructionist theory for *Feminist Studies* explained, their "project . . . has centrally consisted of exposing the artificial and hierarchical oppositions (man/woman, mind/body) that lie at the heart of Western thought."[44]

The fusion of psychoanalytic and linguistic theory developed by the French psychoanalyst Jacques Lacan and his students, known as the *école Freudienne*, strongly influenced the new deconstructionist strategies. In the post–World War II period, Lacan sought to return to what he saw as the essential mission of psychoanalysis, long since lost by Freud's disciples, namely, the "task of deciphering the ways in which the human subject is constructed—how it comes into being—out of the small human animal," in the words of psychotherapist Juliet Mitchell, who helped introduce English speakers to his work in a widely read 1982 volume she edited with the literary critic Jacqueline Rose. Lacan critiqued the idea that humans had some gendered "identity" that arose from within themselves; rather, that identity was "assigned" them, according to whether or not they possessed a penis, and then internalized within them by a process of engagement with the "general law" of language, which included the fundamental opposition of male and female. Thus gender identity was not a psychodynamic given, as psychoanalytic theory had come to treat it, but "a mirage arising when the subject forms an image of itself by identifying with others' perception of it."[45]

While Lacan's primary goal was to expose how this arbitrary, constructed character of sexual difference had become reified in analytic theory, his feminist followers revised his theory and broadened its implications for a general analysis of culture. All of Western knowledge could be reinterpreted in light of a linguistic/symbolic system in which "the absolute 'Otherness' of the woman . . . serves to secure for the man his own self-knowledge and truth," in the words of Jacqueline Rose. The representations of women in scientific as well as artistic texts provided a natural starting place for this deconstructive mission. In addition, women's writings might be searched for evidence of a "pre-discursive reality," an "archaic" form of expressivity formed outside the dominant linguistic system. Feminist literary critic Mary Poovey described this "recuperative" mission of deconstruction as trying to "imagine some organization of fantasy, language, and reality other than one based on identity and binary oppositions, which is currently the dominant mode and therefore equated with the dominant sex, men."[46]

A prime focus of the recuperative mission was the rediscovery of the female body and its capacity for erotic expression. In seeking to disrupt the patriarchal system of knowledge, feminist theorists took particular aim at the "male gaze" of science and the ways its clinical measurements and markings of women's bodies served to contain male fears of female sexuality. One of the earliest postmodernist exercises was to try to recapture the subversive, disruptive nature of the female body and its "multiple drives and desires."[47]

The first engagement of these new theoretical perspectives with the history of psychiatry involved a rereading of late nineteenth-century hysteria. Some of Lacan's feminist disciples, notably Hélène Cixous and Catherine Clément, used the case of Dora, perhaps Freud's most famous female hysteric, to explore the possibilities of recovering a "pre-discursive reality." In 1975, they published a dialogue on Dora in their book, *La jeune née*, which stimulated feminist interest in the "admirable hysterics." Cixous in particular tried to interpret Dora's symptoms as a protest or subversion of the patriarchal mode of expression: The "globus hystericus" signified the choked-off words of protest, the refusal to speak the "patriarchal" language of the fathers; the contorted and paralyzed limbs used the body to express an anger and a sexual desire forbidden her.[48]

The 1985 collection, *In Dora's Case*, edited by two literary historians, Charles Bernheimer and Claire Kahane, provided a fuller exploration of the feminist rereadings possible of the "admirable hysteric." In addition to reprinting older articles on the case by Jacques Lacan, the psychoanalyst Erik Erikson, and literary critic Steven Marcus, the volume included pieces by a number of feminist literary critics, including Suzanne Gearhart, Jacqueline Rose, Toril Mol, and Jane Gallop. The various authors used the techniques of literary criticism to dissect Freud's narrative strategies and use of language to uncover the "central paradigms" of psychoanalysis itself.[49]

These readings suggested, in the words of Kahane, that "as brilliant as Freud was in constructing a narrative of Dora's desire, he essentially represented his own." The various critics discerned in Freud's obsession with the case, which ended by Dora's terminating her analysis, evidence of his own "powerfully ambivalent countertransference." In Freud's inability to come to terms with his own desire for and identification with Dora, they saw in microcosm the origins of his larger "repudiation of femininity," that is, his wish "not to *be* Dora, the victim of multiple betrayals and subject to everyone's desire but her own," according to Madelon Sprengnether. This repudiation was at the core of Freud's inability to comprehend the female psyche, as expressed in his famous lament to Marie Bonaparte, "What does a woman want?"[50]

Along similar lines, another literary critic, Dianne Hunter, produced a provocative reading of the case of "Anna O.," or Bertha Pappenheim, whose turbulent protoanalysis by Freud's mentor Josef Breuer also involved issues of countertransference. Following the French theorists, Hunter analyzed Pappenheim's hysteric symptoms as a form of "pre-discursive" expression. Her "linguistic discord and conversion symptoms, her use of gibberish and gestures as means of expression, can be seen as a regression from the cultural order represented by her father as an orthodox patriarch," argued Hunter. In Pappenheim's strange mixture of sign language, made-up terms, and foreign words, Hunter perceived "an attempt to re-create the special semiotic babble that exists between an infant and its mother."[51]

The surge of critical interest in Dora and Anna O. highlights the convergence of interest in linguistic analysis, psychoanalysis, and hysteria among feminist literary theorists in the 1980s. As Hunter explained their mutual attraction, both hysteria and psychoanalysis depend on the play of language and symbol in "translation," the former translating forbidden thoughts using the body as a signifier, the latter translating affect into words. Moreover, the women patients analyzed by Breuer and Freud could properly be thought of as "co-authors" of psychoanalytic theory itself. "Psychoanalysis entered the history of consciousness in dialogue with the subjectivity of women," Hunter observed; "Both psychoanalysis and hysteria subvert the reigning cultural order by exploding its linguistic conventions and decomposing its facade of orderly conduct."[52]

These new critical readings of analytic case histories were widely read and admired for their theoretical sophistication and iconoclastic wit, yet their usefulness as forms of *historical*, as opposed to literary-critical, argument was limited. As psychoanalyst-historian Janet Sayers complained, "Lacanian feminism's account of patriarchy remains entirely formal and devoid of detailed historical, social, or clinical specificity." Although feminist literary critics referred in passing to the specific historical situations of late nineteenth-century women, the psychoanalytic explanations they employed to interpret the hysteric symptoms of Dora and Anna O. seemed profoundly ahistorical. Historian Mark Micale shrewdly commented that such retrospective reanalyses "tell us less about any aspect of the history of hysteria than of contemporary feminist theory and literary criticism."[53]

The "Female Malady"

The discipline of "cultural history" arose in part as a response to the problems with historical context evident in such works of feminist literary criticism. As Mary Poovey observed, the deconstructionist goal of recovering "prediscursive realities" was difficult to adapt to historical sources and concerns. Postmodernist methods worked much better for historians bent on demystifying categories such as gender or "nature." To this end, Joan Scott urged feminist historians to use postmodernism's perspectives "to disrupt the notion of fixity, to discover the nature of the debate or repression that leads to the appearance of timeless permanence in binary gender representation." The "new cultural history" that emerged in the late 1980s represented an attempt to historicize the goals of literary deconstructionism in these ways.[54]

The first systematic attempt to make use of both cultural history and literary criticism to rewrite the history of psychiatry came in 1985 with Elaine Showalter's book, *The Female Malady*. Showalter, a literary critic and historian who now teaches at Princeton University, was not herself a deconstructionist; her work belonged in the more pragmatic, literary-historical tradition of Anglo-American feminist criticism.[55] Yet Showalter drew on certain basic themes from the postmodernist critique in her effort to write what she termed "both a feminist history of madness and a cultural history of madness as a female malady." The book was an ambitious attempt to combine readings of art, novels, and scientific texts to explore the female/madness nexus at two different levels: the representation of madness as female, and the actual treatment of madwomen in asylums.[56]

Showalter began with the Derrida-inspired axiom that since the Enlightenment, "women within our dualistic systems of language and representation, are typically situated on the side of irrationality, silence, nature, and body, while men are situated on the side of reason, discourse, culture, and mind." In the early nineteenth century, she argued, there was a significant symbolic shift in cultural representations of madness: The older, "disturbing images of wild, dark, naked men had been replaced by poetic, artistic, and theatrical images of a youthful, beautiful female insanity.'' When nine-teenth-century artists and writers wished to embody madness, they used the stock figures of ''a suicidal Ophelia, a sentimental Crazy Jane, and the violent Lucia.''[57]

Showalter posited that this shift in the representational tradition facilitated and was facilitated by an institutional ''feminization'' of insanity itself. Over the course of the nineteenth century, she argued, psychiatrists came to differentiate ''between an English malady, associated with the intellectual and economic pressures on highly civilized men, and a female malady, associated with the sexuality and essential nature of women. Women were believed to be more vulnerable to insanity than men, to experience it in specifically feminine ways, and to be differently affected by it in the conduct of their lives,'' she wrote. Simultaneously, women came to outnumber men as inmates of mental hospitals. By the late 1800s, Showalter observed, ''women had decisively taken the lead as psychiatric patients, a lead they have retained ever since, and in ever-increasing numbers.'' For both ideological and institutional reasons, then, Showalter suggested that the female variant of insanity came to dominate the psychiatric tradition as it did the cultural tradition.[58]

Along similar lines, Showalter periodized the history of psychiatry into three epochs—Victorianism, Darwinism, and Modernism—to underline ''the continuity between major periods of intellectual and literary culture and the psychiatric views that they produced.'' Moral treatment was paired with the Romantic image of the mad-woman, degeneration theory with the female hysteric, and modernism with the female schizophrenic. For each of these periods, Showalter demonstrated the ways that both psychiatrists and feminists read women's mental maladies as an indictment of their role in their society. Conservative psychiatrists invoked the ''female malady'' as ''proof'' that the broadening of women's roles was unhealthy and unwise; feminists invoked it as ''proof'' that restrictive roles and male mistreatment were driving women crazy.[59]

In striking contrast to the symmetrical gender emphasis of the American social historians writing at the same time, Showalter's literary-historical approach reaffirmed the special relationship between femaleness and madness. In many ways, her book was a literary-historical working out of the themes advanced in Phyllis Chesler's *Women and Madness*. She portrayed psychiatry as a specialty virtually obsessed with ''female insanity,'' regarding women as its ''primary patients'' from the late nineteenth century on. The inclusion of only one chapter on men, an analysis of the shell shock ''epidemic'' of World War I, reflected Showalter's belief that ''The Great War was the first and, so far, the last time in the twentieth century that men and the wrongs of men occupied a central position in the history of madness.''[60]

While admiring her imaginative readings of literature and art, historians of psychi-atry were skeptical of Showalter's generalizations about psychiatric thought and insti-tutions. Andrew Scull, who had written extensively about nineteenth-century English asylums, disputed her argument that their patient populations became significantly fem-inized: ''[A]mong the institutionalized insane,'' he wrote in a review of her book, the gender imbalance did not ''amount to more than a few percent, itself quite possibly attributable to the greater longevity of the 'weaker' sex and to the disposition of the asylum authorities to keep female lunatics institutionalized longer than their male coun-terparts.'' From the ''symmetrical'' perspective of the American social historians, I argued that Showalter had oversimplified nineteenth-century medical arguments about which sex was more liable to insanity, pointing out that Anglo-American psychiatrists had a variety of compelling reasons not to give women precedence over men in this regard.[61]

Subsequent histories of nineteenth-century psychiatry tried to adopt a more "relational" view of gender and madness, one that assumes concepts of "female madness" cannot be studied or understood apart from those of "male madness." In her 1991 book, *'Shattered Nerves': Doctors, Patients, and Depression in Victorian England*, the historian Janet Oppenheimer covered much the same cultural ground as Showalter, *comparing* medical views of depression in men, women, and children. "The fact that shattered frames were just as likely to belong to men as to women caused Victorian psychiatrists no little difficulty in an era when the differences between the sexes were being relentlessly emphasized," she noted. "It is utterly erroneous to assume that Victorian doctors perceived the male half of the human race as paragons of health and vigor, while assigning all forms of weakness to women," concluded Oppenheimer.[62]

An even more elegant argument was made for a relational understanding of gendered categories in psychiatric thought by the historian Mark Micale in his work on hysteria. "No less than nineteenth-century medical commentary on women," Micale argued in a 1991 essay, "Hysteria Male/Hysteria Female," the medical "literatures concerning sick and suffering men reveal normative gender representations, encoded ideals of normal and abnormal masculinity that repay investigation by the social, cultural, and medical historian." By analyzing the French neurologist Jean-Martin Charcot's work on male hysterics in the late nineteenth century, Micale systematically uncovered the ways French neurologists understood sexual difference in the expression of the disease. He found that contrary to what Showalter's argument might suggest, neurological conceptualizations of male and female hysteria were actually *converging* in late nineteenth-century French medical thought. Likewise, he found important national differences in this process of what he termed gender "relativization" or "stigmatized egalitarianism"; the British medical profession, for example, remained relatively uninterested in hysteria in general and its male manifestations in particular. Thus Micale's work pointed to the potential of cultural history not only to illuminate gender difference but also national scientific cultures as well.[63]

Fasting Girls

Forms of mental disease that have a long historical association with women, such as hysteria or anorexia nervosa, pose a peculiarly difficult interpretive problem for feminist historians. These "woman's diseases" invite speculation about the transhistorical dimensions of women's experience, which might be conceived of in cultural, psychodynamic, or biological terms; yet such a line of inquiry can easily lead into the error feminists refer to as "essentialism," that is, assuming that the continuity in women's experience can be "explained" by some immutable biological or psychodynamic aspect of being female. Since essentialist arguments for women's behavior have often been associated with anti-feminism, feminists naturally approach them with considerable wariness. In the last few years, feminist historians have struggled to develop explanations for diseases such as hysteria and anorexia that take account of their long historical identification with women yet do not resort to essentialism.

The interpretive puzzles posed by hysteria are so rich and complex that they have warranted a review essay all to themselves.[64] I will focus my attention here on anorexia nervosa, a subject that has only recently become the subject of intense historical interest. Compared to hysteria, anorexia nervosa has a shorter, more concise medical history: It was defined as a medical syndrome in the early 1870s, regarded exclusively as a disorder of women, chiefly young ones, and presented a relatively more distinct set of symptoms, chief among them food refusal. Moreover, unlike hysteria, it did not "disappear" in the early 1900s but rather increased steadily to reach epidemic proportions in the 1980s.

Indeed, feminists who wanted to emphasize how far the women's movement had yet to go in the 1980s adopted anorexia as the emblematic woman's disease. Despite a decade of feminist agitation, they pointed out, young women were literally starving themselves to death in order to conform to the culture's overwhelming preoccupation with the perfect female body. Food obsessions revealed the contradictions of an age when women presumably "had it all," yet continued to suffer many forms of objectification. Like the late nineteenth-century hysteric, feminist critics argued, anorectics embodied the pathological consequences of society's unrealistic expectations of modern women. Eating disorders, wrote Susie Orbach in her book, *Hunger Strike: The Anorectic's Struggle as a Metaphor for our Age*, were a "protest against the way in which women are regarded in our society as objects of adornment and pleasure." As Orbach's title suggests, popular feminist critics saw a parallel between anorectics and the suffragist hunger strikers of the early 1900s.[65]

The academic historians who took up the study of anorexia produced a far less polemical reading of the "starving disease." In the first place, a pair of works by medieval historians Caroline Walker Bynum and Rudolph Bell suggested that the historical perspective taken by Orbach and others was far too shortsighted. Although anorexia nervosa was a "modern" disease, the historical association between women and fasting was far older. Bynum's book, *Holy Feast and Holy Fast: The Religious Significance of Food to Medieval Women*, showed that forms of "anorexia mirabilis," that is, religiously inspired food asceticism, were particularly congenial to medieval women because of their cultural associations with food preparation and service to others. In contrast, Bell took a psychodynamic approach to the history of anorexia nervosa, identifying certain recurrent familial themes in the lives of holy women such as Saint Catherine of Siena who became celebrated for their food asceticism. More aggressively than did Bynum, Bell argued for the symptomatic continuity between anorexia mirabilis and anorexia nervosa as forms of female resistance to a patriarchal society.[66]

In her 1988 book, *Fasting Girls: The Emergence of Anorexia Nervosa as a Modern Disease*, Joan Jacobs Brumberg attempted to relate the historical and contemporary experiences of anorexia nervosa. Brumberg insisted on the historical specificity of disease concepts, that women may show certain continuities in symptom choice without experiencing exactly the same illness. She objected, for example, to interpretations that "would have us believe that Karen Carpenter and Catherine of Siena suffered from the same disease." Likewise, she refused to read backward from contemporary feminist explanations for anorexia in her efforts to understand its nineteenth-century manifestations. Brumberg emphasized, for example, that anorexia appeared *before* the widespread imperative for women to have slim bodies.[67]

Perhaps most daringly, while emphasizing cultural factors as paramount in her analysis, Brumberg refused to exclude a biological substrate in the disease process. "Despite the emphasis here on culture," she explained in her introduction, "my interpretation does not disallow the possibility of a biomedical component in anorexia nervosa." By using a two-stage model of the disease, involving first a cultural "recruitment" to fasting behavior, followed by an "anorectic career" involving more potent forms of psychological and physiological addiction to food avoidance, Brumberg developed a more complex model for understanding the disease. The difference in the way male and female bodies store and use fat, for example, may give young women a physiological advantage in adopting rituals of semistarvation that serve aesthetic, psychological, and social needs. But what begins as a voluntary refusal of food can become, again for physiological reasons, an involuntary inability to eat.[68]

As a feminist, Brumberg was expressly critical of the tendency among both popular feminist commentators and literary theorists to interpret anorexia nervosa as a form of protofeminism. The feminist tradition of celebrating "admirable hysterics" had limited appeal to her; as she put it, "The madhouse is a somewhat troubling site for establishing a female pantheon." Brumberg warned that "feminist insistence on thinking about anorexia nervosa as cultural protest leads to an interpretation of the disorder that overemphasizes the level of conscious control at the same time that it presents women and girls as hapless victims of an all-powerful medical profession." Much as Carroll Smith-Rosenberg had done in her treatment of the female hysteric a decade earlier, Brumberg concluded that as a feminist she would provide the anorectic historical "sympathy" but not "veneration."[69]

Brumberg's historical periodization in *Fasting Girls* was based not on literary or artistic conventions, such as those Showalter employed, but rather on two cultural processes that she believed deeply altered the way girls and women conceived of themselves and their emotional lives: secularization, which moved the locus for assigning meanings to behavior from a religious to a scientific realm; and popularization, the process by which new scientific explanations for illness became familiar to both women and their physicians. Against this backdrop, Brumberg explored the evolving significance of women's food refusal. What was once a mode of expressing female spirituality became "pathologized" over the course of the late nineteenth century. Neurologists intent upon advancing a materialist view of the human body were determined to show that the claims of the devout, many of them allegedly miraculous "fasting girls," were false; to this end, Brumberg demonstrated, they helped transform the meaning of food refusal "from a legitimate act of personal piety to a symptom of disease."[70]

At the same time, the growing intensity of the bourgeois family made food an increasingly charged topic for parent-child interactions. Young Victorian girls learned to use the "appetite as voice" to express their struggles and anxieties at the parental dinner table. As Brumberg noted, "Anorexia nervosa was an intense form of nonverbal discourse that honored the emotional guidelines governing the middle-class Victorian family"; it allowed girls to make their point while remaining "discreet, quiet, and ladylike." Moreover, she reasoned that "middle-class girls, rather than boys, turned to food as a symbolic language, because the culture made an important connection between food and femininity and because girls' options for self-expression outside the family were limited by parental concern and social convention."[71]

Thus Brumberg's model for explaining anorexia's historical identification with the female adolescent worked at three levels: biological, psychological, and cultural.

Women may have a biological and cultural predisposition to use the appetite as voice, but that tendency would not be developed to a pathological degree had they more healthy outlets for self-expression and more varied sources of self-esteem. "Sadly," Brumberg concluded, "the cult of diet and exercise is the closest thing our secular society offers women in terms of a coherent philosophy of the self."[72]

The Perils of Feminist "Pathography"

As the literature on anorexia nervosa demonstrates, the intensity of feminist interest in specific historical topics has often been driven by concerns about modern women and their emotional problems. While the contemporary relevance of feminist-historical investigations has given the field much of its vibrancy and interest, it also lends it an explosive potential lacking in other, less contested areas of psychiatric history. The interpretive landmines involved in the history of psychiatry have been particularly evident in recent biographies of women writers.

From the 1970s on, feminist literary historians and critics have been drawn to chronicle the stories of creative women whose lives were marred by mental illness, and to use those lives as emblematic of women's experience. That some of the most talented women of the twentieth century suffered total breakdowns and experienced institutionalization, as well as left a record of their anger and anguish in fiction and poetry, was part of what made the woman/madness connection so compelling to feminists. As Elaine Showalter wrote in the *Female Malady*, "In the annals of feminist literary history, Virginia Woolf, Anne Sexton, and Sylvia Plath have become our sisters and our saints."[73]

Although never written to present full-fledged historical explications of psychiatry's treatment of women, the best of these literary biographies offered an intimate look at the meaning of mental illness as experienced by sensitive, highly articulate women. So many of their male contemporaries also suffered from mental illness that biographers had to tread lightly around the "madness as uniquely female" argument. Yet the copious journals, letters, and, most important, artistic productions left by women writers gave ample testimony to the kinds of emotional dilemmas over sexuality, marriage, motherhood, and the constraints of "femaleness" on the creative persona that they encountered. From Woolf's experience as an upper middle-class daughter in Edwardian England to Plath and Sexton's struggles with the "feminine mystique" of the 1950s, the literary biography provides an insight into the emotional landscape inhabited by their less talented sisters.[74]

Diane Wood Middlebrook's recent biography of Anne Sexton, the "mad housewife-turned-poet," is a good example of this genre of biography, as well as the kinds of controversy it may provoke. Middlebrook dealt with the genesis of Sexton's emotional problems in a complex way: She noted that there was a history of mental illness in the family, suggesting a possible genetic element; she implicated, as did the poet herself, the complex psychodynamics of her family, including possible incest experiences. Middlebrook also portrayed Sexton as a casualty of the "happy heroine housewife" mythology of the 1950s. She was raised to believe that marriage and children were the only legitimate source of female self-esteem, yet she did not herself find satisfaction in these roles. As her biographer explained, Sexton's ''irrepressible wish for an authentic social presence that was not wife, lover, or mother'' led her to write poetry.[75]

Middlebrook's biography explores how the personal experience of breakdown and psychiatric treatment was used in the ''confessional poetry'' of the late 1950s and 1960s. She noted that Sexton's teacher, Robert Lowell, who launched the movement, was a manic-depressive who incorporated his sense of a ''discredited masculinity'' into his work; similarly, Sexton and Sylvia Plath made extensive poetic use of their experiences of attempted suicide and mental hospitalization, and ''layered into their poetry . . . a protest against the equation of womanhood with motherhood.'' Beyond simply noting the ''hilarious conversations'' Sexton and Plath used to have ''comparing their suicides and talking about their psychiatrists,'' Middlebrook ventured some interesting observations about the relationship between psychoanalysis and the emerging feminist poetics of the late 1950s. ''The two world wars of the century had definitively reduced the scale in which human heroism could be invoked credibly in art, but psychoanalysis, which focused on the childhood origins of adult behavior, could evoke memories of a time when adults loomed very large,'' Middlebrook wrote; ''The psychoanalytic point of view, paradoxically, legitimized the return, in art, of exorbitant passions and a sense of destiny, understood as an economy of sublimation.''[76]

Despite Middlebrook's obvious effort to avoid sensationalism in her treatment of Sexton's mental illness, the book aroused controversy for two different reasons: First, Middlebrook was granted access to tapes and notes of Sexton's therapy kept by her long-time psychiatrist, Martin Orne. Stating his belief that if Sexton were alive, she would approve of his decision, Orne defended this apparent breach of professional ethics. But many prominent psychotherapists were appalled by Orne's decision and Middlebrook's willingness to use such privileged material, which they felt was a profound violation of doctor-patient confidentiality.[77]

Second, although Middlebrook had the full support of Sexton's immediate family (including her daughter Linda, who had herself suffered from her mother's incestuous advances), other members of the family objected to the book's portrayal of her early life, particularly the discussion of Sexton's incest experiences. Although Middlebrook never accepted Sexton's memories of sexualized encounters with her father and her great-aunt as ''facts,'' Sexton's nieces accused her of presenting their beloved relatives as ''libidinous, perverted beasts.''[78]

The controversies surrounding Middlebrook's work, which has otherwise been widely praised as a well-researched, thoughtful account of a difficult subject, again suggests how hard it is to write dispassionately about highly sensitive topics such as doctor-patient privilege or incest. Middlebrook's experience in writing about Anne Sexton is not an isolated example; the warfare between Sylvia Plath's family and her biographers has if anything been more intense.[79] As in reading their poems, reading the lives of these troubled women to ''explain'' why they became ill or how their illness shaped their work produces multiple and conflicting interpretations. What may seem like a safe generalization about women becomes a hotly contested hypothesis when applied to a well-known woman, especially if she has family and friends still living. Even more so than portraying women's collective experience of madness, individual biographies highlight both the insights and the puzzles presented by the lives of exemplary madwomen.

Mothers of Psychoanalysis

Another popular and less contested area of biography relevant to feminist interpretations of psychiatric history focuses on the lives of women psychoanalysts. Since the publication in 1974 of Juliet Mitchell's work, *Psychoanalysis and Feminism*, feminists have been deeply engaged with psychoanalytic theory; over the course of the 1980s, feminist theory was profoundly influenced not only by the *École Freudienne* discussed earlier, but also the object-relations school exemplified by the work of Nancy Chodorow. But this intellectual engagement has been aimed more at revising psychoanalytic theory than understanding the historical forces that made such a revision possible.[80]

Feminists have tended to assume, as Elaine Showalter wrote in the epilogue of *The Female Malady*, that "in the 1970s, for the first time, women came together to challenge both the psychoanalytic and the medical categories of traditional psychiatry." But a series of recent biographies on the women prominent in the analytical movement before the rebirth of feminism—including Anna Freud, Melanie Klein, Karen Horney, Helene Deutsch, and Marie Bonaparte—suggests that this historical perspective is foreshortened. For the most part, these biographers have confined themselves to straightforward accounts of their subjects' lives and theoretical contributions, at best sorting them into two simplistic camps, the "dutiful daughters" and the "rebels." With one important exception, they do not explore the larger historical question of how and why women analysts contributed to the growing critique of phallocentrism within psychoanalytic theory.[81]

Only Janet Sayers, a psychoanalyst-turned-historian, has advanced a more sweeping proposition about the place of women analysts in the history of psychoanalysis. In her collective biography of Freud, Klein, Horney, and Deutsch, entitled *The Mothers of Psychoanalysis*, Sayers tried to push back the creative engagement of women thinkers with psychoanalysis to the interwar period. Although the four women analysts she chose for her study varied dramatically in their attitudes toward organized feminism, Sayers nonetheless argued that their work all tended toward the same important theoretical end: a "feminization" of psychoanalysis.[82]

In Sayers's view, women analysts played a central role in precipitating the theoretical shift in focus from fathers and the Oedipus complex, to mothers and the "mirroring" dynamics of object-relations. "Once patriarchal and phallocentric," psychoanalysis expressed itself in the language of castration, repression, and resistance; now it is "almost entirely mother-centered," and cast in terms of identification, introjection, and projection. This shift can be attributed in part, Sayers argued, to women analysts, who brought to the discipline their own experiences of being mothered and mothering, a perspective that helped compensate for Freud's theoretical neglect of mothers. Although Sayers fears that analytic theory may now have gone too far in the other direction, to the neglect of paternal influence, she concluded that "women analysts' use of their own and their patients' mothering experience has indeed advanced psychoanalysis a long way from its patriarchal beginnings."[83]

While appreciated for its attempts at synthesis, Sayers's argument was criticized for being somewhat simplistic in its explanations for the shift in psychoanalytic theory. As Phyllis Grosskurth, a biographer of Melanie Klein, commented on Sayers's book, "Not once does Ms. Sayers consider the possibility that many of these women's ideas have been accepted only after being incorporated into the theories of male theorists like

D. W. Winnicott, Otto Kernberg, and Heinz Kohut.'' Sayers's work points to the problems involved in separating "male" theory from "female" theory in historical accounts of intellectual change.[84]

Psychiatry and Female Sexuality

One final area of feminist scholarship that has profound implications for the history of psychiatry is the history of sexuality. In the 1970s and 1980s, as Lisa Duggan noted in a recent review essay, the increasing separation of sexuality from reproduction and the rise of the gay rights movement encouraged historical interest in the construction of sexual identities. The first volume of Michel Foucault's *History of Sexuality*, which appeared in English in 1978, helped undermine assumptions about the "naturalness" of particular forms of sexual desire. The growing influence of postmodernist theory, which emphasized the role of cultural systems in channeling the inchoate, diffuse sexuality of the child into the rigid categories of heterosexuality, further challenged the notion of fixed biological drives.[85]

This work has important implications for feminist histories of psychiatry for several reasons. First, histories of sexuality were among the first to explore systematically the differences among women; sexual ideologies and identities varied so dramatically depending on a woman's class, race, or sexual preference that no unitary category of "female sexuality" sufficed. Second, the evolution of sexuality over the last century clearly placed psychiatric ideas in the service of broader cultural concerns and institutions. Beginning in the late nineteenth century, psychiatrists helped forge new definitions of normal and abnormal sexuality. The "mental hygiene" of sexual development provided a major platform for extending the psychiatrist's "expert advice" beyond the walls of the mental hospital to a much wider audience.

For our purposes here, two strands of the new work on sexuality deserve special emphasis. First, feminist historians examined the ways that the state, aided and abetted by the psychiatric profession, began more aggressively to define and to regulate "deviant" sexuality beginning in the late 1890s and early 1900s. The concept of the sexual sociopath or psychopath—an individual whose psychiatric symptoms consisted primarily of defying middle-class sexual mores—became the basis for new forms of institutional surveillance. For example, Elizabeth Lunbeck's groundbreaking work on the Boston Psychopathic Hospital demonstrated that in the 1910s, the label "sociopath" was assigned to young working-class women who enjoyed frequent and varied sexual encounters with men. Similarly, Estelle Freedman examined the recurrent "sex crime panics" of the years 1935 to 1965, which emphasized the dangers to women and children posed by the male sexual psychopath. The fear of the sexual psychopath not only extended psychiatry's social authority, she argued, but also provided "an extremely powerful tool for mobilizing political support against nonconforming individuals," in this case homosexual men.[86]

A second strand of the new work of sexuality focused on psychiatry's role in "pathologizing" same-sex relationships. Historians such as Carroll Smith-Rosenberg, Lillian Faderman, John D'Emilio, and Estelle Freedman suggested that prior to the late nineteenth century, both men and women were allowed a broad range of physical and emotional relationships with members of their own sex. Beginning in the late 1800s, psychiatrists and other medical authorities helped to stigmatize such relationships as part of a larger effort to define and protect a heterosexual standard of "normality."[87]

Lillian Faderman's influential 1981 study of women's romantic friendships in *Surpassing the Love of Men* argued that late nineteenth-century sexologists such as the German Richard von Kraft-Ebbing and the Englishman Havelock Ellis played a critical role in pathologizing female friendships and giving them what she terms "outlaw status" after World War I. Other historians took issue with Faderman's thesis, pointing out that concerns about female homosexuality long predated the late nineteenth-century sexologists' work. But while they disagreed about its timing and consequences, historians concurred that from the turn of the century on, psychiatrists became more invested in helping to maintain the boundaries of "normal" and "abnormal" sexual behavior and identity. The challenge remained for historians to describe the relationship between these medical experts and the emergent homosexual communities of the twentieth century without using overly simplistic doctor-victim dichotomies.[88]

Using the new methods of cultural history, Jennifer Terry's work on the psychiatric and medical construction of lesbianism in the midtwentieth century suggested strategies for conceptualizing this process in a more complex and satisfying way. In "Lesbians under the Medical Gaze," Terry described the work of the 1935 Committee for the Study of Sex Variants, headed by the American psychiatrist George Henry. By using a battery of physical and psychological tests, the committee tried to locate what Terry terms "remarkable differences" between heterosexual and lesbian women. But their efforts, in her words, "to interpret the bodies and experiences of subjects in terms of the binary system of masculinity and femininity" foundered on the diversity of the lesbian women they surveyed. Confronted with evidence that seemingly "feminine" women felt a "masculine" desire for other women, "the lesbian remained, and, in many ways still remains, a confounding character in a context where an autonomous female sexuality was literally unthinkable," Terry concluded.[89]

Terry's work is also notable for the ways in which she used the literary-critical techniques of cultural history to analyze the personal narratives of lesbian subjects compiled by the committee. In an article called "Theorizing Deviant Historiography," she illustrated how these interviews could be read to illustrate the subjects' resistance to the experts' pathologizing discourse concerning their homosexuality. For example, their detailed, often exuberant accounts of love-making practices challenged the researchers' assumptions about female homosexuality; lesbians who referred to their "remarkable genitals" and their capacity to satisfy female partners aroused in the physician-researchers "a mixture of anxiety, curiosity, terror, and disbelief." The interpretive strategies that Terry used illustrate a "way of reading and understanding history against the grain of heterosexual hegemony" that could profitably be applied to other types of case histories as well.[90]

Directions for the Future

To sum up, one of the most basic tensions evident in feminist histories of psychiatry might be termed the asymmetry/symmetry debate. Feminist historians have consistently differed over whether to accept what Showalter terms as the historic correlation between madness and the "wrongs of woman."[91] For some feminists, the special link between femaleness and madness is of paramount importance and endless fascination. They conceptualize mental illness as a mark of women's oppression in society, and believe madness can be analyzed as a form of protofeminism that yields valuable insights into all women's experiences. Likewise, they see the specialty of psychiatry as having a special interest and investment in constructing and controlling female identity and sexuality.

In contrast, other feminists have adopted what might be thought of as a symmetrical approach. Although they may acknowledge the rich associations between femaleness and madness in the representational tradition, they reject the proposition that madness is a condition that *literally* befalls women more than men. They assume that the cultural constructions of gender are pathogenic for both women and men, and that the psychiatric conceptions of male and female insanity are best studied in relational terms. Similarly, their approach to the psychiatric profession tends to see the construction and maintenance of gendered identities as central to its treatment of *both* sexes.

The tension between the asymmetrical and symmetrical approaches to gender and mental illness is likely to persist in the work to come. But one promising way to move beyond the impasse they present is to pay more attention to the role of gendered language itself. Recent work in the feminist history of science has convincingly demonstrated how important gendered metaphors and language were to the emergence of scientific categories in the eighteenth and nineteenth centuries. Such an approach might well open up new insights into the scientific texts of psychiatry as well.[92]

For example, when revising the Whig narrative of psychiatry's quest to be scientific, feminist historians might want to explore how psychiatry's struggle to be respected as a medical specialty involved challenging the "masculinist" values of science as a whole. Compared to physics or mathematics, medicine has always had to deal with the comparatively "messy" subjects of human bodies and behaviors. Moreover, of the medical specialties that sought to approximate a higher degree of scientific rigor in the nineteenth century, psychiatry had perhaps the most difficult task in crafting a science of the mind. In examining psychiatrists' struggles to establish their scientific authority, historians might profitably reflect on the gendered meanings assigned to the doing of science itself.

Gender concerns informed not only what scientific psychiatry did in the nineteenth century but what it ceased to do, suggesting another important line of investigation. In her book, *The Mind Has No Sex?*, Londa Schiebinger reminds us, "Science is not a cumulative enterprise; the history of science is as much about the loss of traditions as it is about the creation of new ones."[93] As the Whig paradigm of psychiatric history I started with suggests, the rise of psychiatry has inevitably led to the exclusion of women and the values so often associated with them.

One of the most important traditions eclipsed by the rise of psychiatry was that of explaining emotional distress and mental illness in religious terms. The story of this transformation has yet to be told fully, in part because historians, feminist and nonfeminist alike, have had a tendency to project the pervasiveness and persuasiveness of the late twentieth-century "medical model" back in time. Yet over the last century, women's and men's relations to medical, and explicitly psychiatric authority, have changed dramatically. In the midnineteenth century, for example, women drew on a wide range of sources, including older women, clergymen, and general practitioners, for their health care; yet historians have devoted very little attention to what those authorities had to say about emotional distress or mental illness.[94]

Instead, feminist historians have lavished attention on the more easily accessible genre of medical texts with the unreflective assumption that they are the key texts for understanding the construction of femininity and its implications for the definition of madness. Enormous historical energy has been focused on the highly specialized literature written by medical specialists, chiefly neurologists and asylum doctors. To be sure, these two groups, particularly the former, were increasingly important arbiters of popular opinion in the second half of the nineteenth century. But there is still a pressing need to contextualize what these specialists said about femininity and female insanity within a broader framework of other, possibly competing sources of authority, chief among them the Church.

A similar argument might be made for contextualizing the place of psychoanalysis in the twentieth-century history of psychiatry. For a variety of reasons, feminists have focused so exclusively on it that they have neglected the role of gender in another important tradition, namely, organic psychiatry. Historians as yet know little about what consequences the more "ontological" view of disease that gained dominance in the late nineteenth century had for psychiatric conceptions of gender difference. In *The Female Malady*, Showalter raises important questions about why the "active treatments" developed in the 1930s and 1940s, such as lobotomies and electroconvulsive shock treatments, were administered more to women than men.[95]

The growing competition between psychology and psychiatry opens up another critical issue that badly needs attention from historians, namely, the recruitment of growing numbers of women not just into psychoanalysis but into the mental health professions as a whole. Psychology, psychiatric social work, and psychiatric nursing were all fields that developed in the early twentieth century as "helpmeets" of psychiatry; they were also fields, not coincidentally, that were seen as appropriate for women practitioners. What influence their growing presence had on changing conceptions of women's mental health and illness remains to be seen.[96]

Finally, new directions in both recent women's history and medical history suggest the need to move beyond the invocation of terms such as "women" or "doctors" as if they represented unitary categories. Since the mid-1980s, feminist historians have become much more sensitive to exploring differences among women, that is, the ways in which class, race, and sexual orientation cut against the supposed commonality of female experience. Most of the history supposedly written about "women" and madness has in fact been only about white, upper middle-class, heterosexual women and madness. Historians have paid far too little attention to the experiences of working-class, nonwhite, and lesbian women, and how their emotional lives or their institutional experiences may have differed from their affluent, white, straight counterparts.

Likewise, the tendency of historians, particularly those with limited familiarity with medical history, to treat physicians as a monolithic group needs correction. Recent work strongly suggests that different medical specialties constructed the definition of "women's diseases" in significantly different ways. As a result, feminist historians have to take particular care to locate theories such as "reflex insanity" and procedures such as gynecological operations in a larger, comparative perspective. Perhaps most important, historians have to realize that physicians may have stressed a particular view of the female for professional reasons that had little direct relation to the actual treatment of women.[97]

Conclusion

As this essay demonstrates, feminist histories of psychiatry have been intimately related to the late twentieth-century rebirth of feminism as a political and intellectual movement. We might predict, then, that the continued vigor of its contributions will depend on the historical survival of academic feminism itself. Given the conservative attacks on it, such as Allan Bloom's *The Closing of the American Mind*, this survival cannot be taken for granted.[98] Yet it is difficult to see how the intellectual backlash against academic feminism could succeed in expunging all that it has accomplished in the last twenty years.

While certainly perpetuating their share of misconceptions and exaggerations, feminist histories of psychiatry have played a critical role in identifying the historical genesis of what psychiatrist Alan Stone termed psychiatry's "hidden and destructive values" concerning not only women but other groups as well.[99] Exposing the deep historical roots of the psychiatric theories used to limit women's aspirations and to deride feminism helps to ensure that new such theories will be more difficult to formulate in the future. In another sense, feminist scholarship has exposed how the history of psychiatry itself has embodied many hidden and not so hidden biases against the inclusion of women as valid historical subjects. The Whig tradition would seem to have taken a mortal blow, not just from feminism but from the whole panoply of postmodern intellectual currents.

Yet the danger remains that the kinds of historical questions raised by recent works of feminist scholarship will remain marginalized within the history of psychiatry itself. It is not surprising that the vast majority of work discussed in this essay has been done by women scholars. But I would hope that in the future, this asymmetry of interest would begin to disappear. There are hopeful signs that such is the case, not the least of which is the inclusion of this essay in the volume at hand. For so long as the issues discussed here are seen as "woman's work" within the historical profession, they will remain evidence that the very hierarchy of values they identify continues to hobble our historical imaginations.

Notes

1. Simone de Beauvoir, *The Second Sex* (New York: Bantam Books, 1961; reprint of 1952 English translation); Betty Friedan, *The Feminine Mystique* (New York: Norton, 1963).

2. Roy Porter and Mark S. Micale, "Reflections on Psychiatry and Its Histories," this volume, p. 6.

3. For a different kind of review essay, in which I try to summarize the state of knowledge in the field, see my earlier essay, "Historical Perspectives on Women and Mental Illness" in Rima Apple (ed.), *Women, Health, and Medicine in America: A Historical Handbook* (New York: Garland, 1990), 143–171.

4. I regret this narrowness of focus because the work being done on earlier topics is not only extremely interesting but supplies a valuable corrective to historians' tendency to assume that many trends and dilemmas are the product of the Industrial Revolution. In addition to scholars I will cite briefly later in the essay, I would point the reader to the work of Michael MacDonald and Roy Porter as examples of the fascinating work being done on preindustrial society. See Michael MacDonald, *Mystical Bedlam: Madness, Anxiety, and Healing in Seventeenth Century England* (New York: Cambridge University Press, 1981) and Roy Porter, *Mind Forg'd Manacles: A History of Madness in England from the Restoration to the Regency* (London: Athlone Press, 1987). In addition, I anticipate that the field will be profoundly affected once the current interest in colonial or imperial medicine broadens to include the evolution of psychiatric hospitals in non-Western cultures. This sort of work will allow a fruitful comparison of the influence of gender as well as race on psychiatric thinking.

5. The subtitle of this section, "A World Without Women," acknowledges my debt here to the new feminist history of science. See, for example, David Noble, *A World Without Women* (New York: Knopf, 1992) and Londa Schiebinger, *The Mind Has No Sex?* (Cambridge: Harvard University Press, 1989).

6. Herbert Butterfield, *The Whig Interpretation of History*, 1st American ed. (New York: Scribner, 1951).

7. Emil Kraepelin, *One Hundred Years of Psychiatry* (New York: Citadel Press, 1962), 111.

8. Erwin Ackerknecht, *A Short History of Psychiatry*, trans. Sula Wolff, 2nd rev. ed. (New York: Hafner Publishing Company, 1968), 19.

9. Sigmund Freud, *On the History of the Psycho-Analytic Movement*, trans. Joan Riviere, rev. and edited by James Strachey (New York: Norton, 1966), esp. 13–15, 21–22. Quote is from p. 22. For a good example of how gender issues were usually treated in histories of psychoanalysis, see the discussions on Alfred Adler and Karen Horney in Franz G. Alexander and Sheldon T. Selesnick, *The History of Psychiatry* (New York: Harper & Row, 1966), 228–230, 366–367.

10. De Beauvoir and Friedan, cited in note 1.

11. Eva Figes, *Patriarchal Attitudes* (New York; Stein and Day, 1970); Shulamith Firestone, *The Dialectic of Sex* (New York: Bantam Books, 1970); Germaine Greer, *The Female Eunuch* [1970] (New York: Bantam Books, 1971); Kate Millett, *Sexual Politics* (Garden City, New York: Doubleday, 1969).

12. Janet Sayers, introduction to *The Feminine Character: History of an Ideology*, by Viola Klein, 3rd ed. (London: Routledge, 1989), ix–xxxiv. In comparing the two works, it is evident that de Beauvoir was much more willing to acknowledge the radical implications of her argument, whereas Klein tended to mute her feminism. This difference helps explain why in the late 1960s, only the former was hailed as the intellectual forerunner of radical feminism. Perhaps de Beauvoir's comparatively more secure academic and intellectual position within French existentialism allowed her to be more adventuresome than the emigré Klein, who, as Sayers points out, had to struggle to make a living on the margins of English academia.

13. For a contemporary account of the "second wave's" genesis, see Judith Hole and Ellen Levine, *The Rebirth of Feminism* (New York: Quadrangle Books, 1971). For more recent historical and sociological perspectives, see Steven Buechler, *Women's Movements in the United States: Woman Suffrage, Equal Rights, and Beyond* (New Brunswick, New Jersey: Rutgers University Press, 1990), and Leila Rupp and Verta Taylor, *Survival in the Doldrums* (New York: Oxford University Press, 1987).

14. Greer, *The Female Eunuch*, 10.

15. De Beauvoir, *The Second Sex*, 47; Friedan, *The Feminine Mystique*, 120.

16. Millett, *Sexual Politics*, 187.

17. Greer, *The Female Eunuch*, 91.

18. Phyllis Chesler, *Women and Madness* (New York: Avon Books, 1972).

19. On anti-psychiatry, see Peter Sedgwick, *Psycho Politics: Laing, Foucault, Szasz, and the*

Future of Psychiatry (New York: Harper & Row, 1981), and Norman Dain, "Critics and Dissenters: Reflections on Anti-Psychiatry in the United States," *Journal of the History of the Behavioral Sciences* 25 (1989), 3–25.

20. Chesler, *Women and Madness*, 15–16, 56.

21. Ibid., 52, 56.

22. Ibid., 16, 32, 34.

23. For a good overview of the social history "revolution," see Peter Novick, *That Noble Dream: The "Objectivity Question" and the American Historical Profession* (New York: Cambridge University Press, 1988), 415–510.

24. The Boston Women's Health Book Collective, *Our Bodies, Ourselves* (New York: Simon & Schuster, 1973); Barbara Ehrenreich and Deirdre English, *Witches, Midwives, and Nurses* (Old Westbury, New York: The Feminist Press, 1973) and *Complaints and Disorders: The Sexual Politics of Sickness* (Old Westbury, New York: The Feminist Press, 1973). The two authors recount the history of how they came to write and distribute the two pamphlets in Barbara Ehrenreich and Deirdre English, *For Her Own Good: One Hundred Years of the Experts' Advice to Women* (Garden City, New York: Anchor Press, 1978), vii–ix. For a good overview of the women's health care movement, see Sheryl Ruzek, *The Women's Health Movement: Feminist Alternatives to Medical Control* (New York: Praeger, 1978).

25. Ehrenreich and English, *For Her Own Good*, esp. 91–126, 190–239.

26. Mary Hartman and Lois Banner (eds.), *Clio's Consciousness Raised: New Perspectives on the History of Women* (New York: Harper & Row, 1974).

27. Ann Douglas Wood, " 'The Fashionable Diseases': Women's Complaints and Their Treatment in Nineteenth-Century America" in Hartman and Banner (eds.), *Clio's Consciousness Raised*, 1–22. Quote is from p. 6.

28. Regina Morantz, "The Lady and Her Physician" in Hartman and Banner (eds.) *Clio's Consciousness Raised*, 38–53. Quotes are from pp. 50–51.

29. Douglas Wood, 9; Morantz, 42. The "rest cure" and its implications for women have continued to spark interesting interpretations. See, for example, Barbara Sicherman, "The Uses of a Diagnosis: Doctors, Patients, and Neurasthenia," *Journal of the History of Medicine and Allied Sciences*, 32 (1977), 33–55; Suzanne Poirier, "The Weir Mitchell Rest Cure: Doctors and Patients," *Women Studies*, 10 (1983), 15–40; and Ellen L. Bassuk, "The Rest Cure: Repetition or Resolution of Victorian Women's Conflicts?" in Susan Rubin Suleiman (ed.), *The Female Body in Western Culture: Contemporary Perspectives* (Cambridge: Harvard University Press, 1985), 139–151.

30. Carroll Smith-Rosenberg, "The Hysterical Woman," *Social Research*, 39 (1972), 652–678; see also her "From Puberty to Menopause" in Hartman and Banner (eds.), *Clio's Consciousness Raised*, 23–37; with Charles Rosenberg, "The Female Animal," *Journal of American History*, 60 (1973), 332–356.

31. Smith-Rosenberg, "The Hysterical Woman," 672.

32. Ibid., 671.

33. For works of Ellen Dwyer, see her *Homes for the Mad* (New Brunswick, New Jersey: Rutgers University Press, 1988); "A Historical Perspective" in Cathy S. Widom (ed.), *Sex Roles and Psychopathology* (New York: Plenum Press, 1984), 19–48; "The Weaker Vessel" in D. Kelly Weisberg (ed.), *Women and the Law* (Cambridge: Schenckman Publishing Co., 1982), 85–106. For work of Constance McGovern, see "The Myths of Social Control and Custodial Oppression," *Journal of Social History*, 20 (1986), 3–23; and "Doctors or Ladies?" *Bulletin of the History of Medicine*, 55 (1981), 88–107. For work of Nancy Tomes, see *A Generous Confidence* (New York: Cambridge University Press, 1984); "Devils in the Heart: Historical Perspectives on Women and Depression in Nineteenth Century America," *Transactions and Studies of the College of Physicians of Philadelphia*, Series V, 13 (1991), 363–386; and "Women and Depression: A Nineteenth Century Perspective on the Boundaries between Religion and Psychiatry,"

Proceedings of the 16th International Symposium on the Comparative History of Medicine—East and West, forthcoming, 1994.

34. David Rothman, *The Discovery of the Asylum: Social Order and Disorder in the New Republic* (Boston: Little, Brown, 1971); Gerald Grob, *Mental Institutions in America: Social Policy to 1875* (New York: Free Press, 1973); Andrew Scull, *Museums of Madness: The Social Organization of Insanity in Nineteenth Century England* (New York: St. Martin's Press, 1979).

35. See Nancy Tomes, "The Anatomy of Madness: New Directions in the History of Psychiatry," *Social Studies of Science*, 17 (1987), 358–370, for an attempt to put the two generations of asylum historians in perspective.

36. See Chesler, *Women and Madness*, esp. 9–13, for her account of Packard's institutionalization. For fuller accounts of the life and career of Packard, see Myra Himelhock and Arthur Shaffer, "Elizabeth Packard: Nineteenth Century Crusader for the Rights of Mental Patients," *Journal of American Studies*, 13 (1979), 343–375; and Barbara Sapinsley, *The Private War of Mrs. Packard* (New York: Paragon House, 1991).

37. See especially Tomes, *A Generous Confidence*, esp. 96–103; and Dwyer, *Homes for the Mad*, 85–116.

38. I review the evidence about sex ratios in asylum populations and nineteenth-century psychiatric views of female liability to insanity in Tomes, "Historical Perspectives," esp. 157–158, 165–166.

39. See especially Dwyer, "A Historical Perspective," 24–35; Dwyer, *Homes for the Mad*, 133–34; and Tomes, *A Generous Confidence*, 201–203.

40. Dwyer, "A Historical Perspective," 22–23, 39; Dwyer, "A Weaker Vessel," 96; McGovern, "The Myths of Social Control," 11, 13–15; See also the longer summary of these debates in Tomes, "Historical Perspectives," 158–162.

This work suggests that nineteenth-century psychiatrists were less inclined toward the "ovarian theory" of insanity than were other physicians, and rarely performed any gynecological operations on their female patients. In her review of medical writings on women's insanity, Ellen Dwyer reported that asylum superintendents were "less likely than neurologists or gynecologists to lose sight of the role played by environmental stresses in producing insanity."

41. Dwyer, "A Historical Perspective," 25, 39; McGovern, "The Myths of Social Control," 8, 10; Tomes, *A Generous Confidence*, 324, 326.

42. Joan Scott, "Gender: A Useful Category of Historical Analysis," *American Historical Review*, 91 (1986), 1055. This article is an excellent introduction to the recent theoretical debates within feminist scholarship.

43. Scott, "Gender: A Useful Category," 1067. My discussion of deconstructionist theory here is heavily indebted to Scott's excellent summary and the special issue on deconstruction that appeared in *Feminist Studies*, 14:1 (Spring 1988).

44. Judith Newton and Nancy Hoffman, preface to *Feminist Studies*, 14 (1988), 3.

45. Juliet Mitchell, introduction to *Feminine Sexuality: Jacques Lacan and the école freudienne* (London: Macmillan, 1982), 5.

46. Jacqueline Rose, introduction II to *Feminine Sexuality*, 50, 54; Poovey, "Feminism and Deconstruction," 56.

47. For an introduction to the concern with "body politics" in postmodernist theory, see Susan Rubin Suleiman (ed.), *The Female Body in Western Culture*, especially her essay, "(Re)writing the Body: The Politics and Poetics of Female Eroticism," 7–29.

48. Hélène Cixous and Catherine Clément, *La jeune née* (Paris: 10/18, 1975). The dialogue appeared in English as *The Newly Born Woman*, trans. Betsy Wing (Minneapolis: University of Minnesota Press, 1986). Many English-speaking readers got their first introduction to the Cixous-Clément debate by reading Jane Gallop's chapter on it, entitled "Keys to Dora," which appeared in *The Daughter's Seduction* (Ithaca: Cornell University Press, 1982), 132–150.

49. Charles Bernheimer and Claire Kahane (eds.), *In Dora's Case: Freud—Hysteria—Fem-*

inism (New York: Columbia University Press, 1985). The phrase "central paradigms" appears on p. 19.

50. Ibid. Quotes are from pp. 20, 17, and 270–271.

51. Dianne Hunter, "Hysteria, Psychoanalysis, and Feminism: The Case of Anna O.," *Feminist Studies*, 9:3 (Fall 1983), 465–488. Quotes are from pp. 474–475.

52. Ibid, 485, 486.

53. Janet Sayers, *The Mothers of Psychoanalysis* (New York: Norton, 1991), 267; Mark Micale, "Hysteria and Its Historiography: A Review of Past and Present Writings II," in *History of Science*, 27 (1989), 331.

As Micale suggests in his review essay, Dianne Hunter's article is the most historically nuanced of the lot, yet even she succumbs to the tendency to make facile comments about her subject's inner life. For example, she writes of the young Bertha Pappenheimer's attendance on her dying father that it was "a situation that cannot have failed to arouse erotic and aggressive wishes in such a lively and imaginative person." Perhaps Hunter is right, but such unreflective assertions about how individuals may have felt, consciously or unconsciously, in the past, are bound to make historians uncomfortable. See Hunter, "Hysteria, Psychoanalysis, and Feminism," 470.

54. Poovey, 58; Scott, "Gender," 1068. Both these articles give an excellent sense of the evolution from literary-critical deconstructionist approaches to the more historicized concerns of the "new cultural history." See also Lynn A. Hunt, "Introduction: History, Culture, and Text," in Lynn A. Hunt (ed.), *The New Cultural History* (Berkeley: University of California Press, 1989), 1–22.

55. For a good overview of what this distinction entails, see Betsy Draine, "Refusing the Wisdom of Solomon: Some Recent Feminist Literary Theory," *Signs*, 15 (1989), especially 145–148.

56. Elaine Showalter, *The Female Malady* (New York: Pantheon Books, 1985), 5.

57. Ibid., 3–4, 10.

58. Ibid., 7, 52.

59. Ibid., 17.

60. Ibid., 194.

61. Andrew Scull, *Social Order/Mental Disorder* (Berkeley: University of California Press, 1989), 270; Tomes, "Historical Perspectives," 154–158.

62. Showalter, *The Female Malady*, 194; Janet Oppenheimer, *'Shattered Nerves': Doctors, Patients, and Depression in Victorian England* (New York: Oxford University Press, 1991), 141.

63. Mark Micale, "Hysteria Male/Hysteria Female: Reflections on Comparative Gender Construction in Nineteenth-Century France and Britain" in Marina Benjamin (ed.), *Science and Sensibility: Gender and Scientific Enquiry, 1780–1945* (Cambridge: Basil Blackwell, 1991), 200–239 (quote is from p. 202); and "Charcot and the Idea of Hysteria in the Male: Gender, Mental Science, and Medical Diagnosis in Late Nineteenth-Century France," *Medical History*, 34 (1990), 363–411.

64. Micale, "Hysteria and Its Historiography: A Review of Past and Present Writings (I and II)," *History of Science*, 27 (1989), 223–261, 319–351.

65. Susie Orbach, *Hunger Strike: The Anorectic's Struggle as a Metaphor for Our Age* (New York: Norton, 1986), 63. See pp. 33–35.

66. Caroline Walker Bynum, *Holy Feast and Holy Fast: The Religious Significance of Food to Medieval Women* (Berkeley: University of California Press, 1987) and Rudolph Bell, *Holy Anorexia* (Chicago: University of Chicago Press, 1985).

67. Joan Jacobs Brumberg, *Fasting Girls: The Emergence of Anorexia Nervosa as A Modern Disease* (Cambridge: Harvard University Press, 1988), 42.

68. Ibid., 40.

69. Ibid., 35, 36.

70. Ibid., 98.

71. Ibid., 140, 188.

72. Ibid., 269.

73. Showalter, *The Female Malady*, 4.

74. Some early literary biographies that awakened interest in creative "madwomen" include Nancy Milford, *Zelda: A Biography* (New York: Harper & Row, 1970) and Quentin Bell, *Virginia Woolf: A Biography*, 2 vols. (London: Hogarth Press, 1972). The literature on Virginia Woolf is now voluminous. In addition to the Bell biography, historians might find particularly interesting Louise De Salvo, "1897: Virginia Woolf at Fifteen" in Jane Marcus (ed.), *Virginia Woolf: A Feminist Slant* (Lincoln: University of Nebraska Press, 1983), 78–108, 236–253. On Sylvia Plath, see, for example, Anne Stevenson, *Bitter Fame: A Life of Sylvia Plath* (Boston: Houghton Mifflin, 1989) and Jacqueline Rose, *The Haunting of Sylvia Plath* (London: Virago Press, 1991).

Sandra M. Gilbert and Susan Gubar, *The Madwoman in the Attic: The Woman Writer and the Nineteenth-Century Literary Imagination* (New Haven: Yale University Press, 1979) and Shoshana Felman, *Writing and Madness* (Ithaca: Cornell University Press, 1985) dealt with more general literary themes regarding madness and writing.

A notable autobiography by a feminist writer describing her struggles with manic-depression is Kate Millett, *The Loony Bin Trip* (New York: Simon & Schuster, 1991).

75. Diane Wood Middlebrook, *Anne Sexton: A Biography* (Boston: Houghton Mifflin, 1991), 40.

76. Ibid., 111–112.

77. A running account of the Orne–Sexton controversy can be found in the July 1991, pages of the *New York Times*, starting with a front-page article on the controversy that appeared 15 July 1991, pp. A-1, C-13. Orne was censured by spokesmen for the American Academy of Psychoanalysis and the American Psychiatric Association. Interestingly, another major breach of the doctor-patient relationship revealed in the biography itself—that one of Sexton's psychiatrists had had an affair with her—did not much concern them. In her review of the book, the feminist commentator Katha Pollit noted, "The posthumous revealing of Sexton's confidences seems a peccadillo compared to what some of her therapists did to her when she was alive." See the *New York Times Book Review*, 18 August 1991, p. 1.

78. Sexton's nieces, Lisa Taylor Tompson and Mary Gray Ford, made their charges in a letter to the *New York Times Book Review* published 25 August 1991, p. 4. Essentially they argued that Sexton was a very sick woman whose memories of abuse should not be taken seriously because they were products of her diseased mind.

79. Ronald Hayman, *The Death and Life of Sylvia Plath* (Secaucus, New Jersey: Carol Publishing Group, 1991), 198–212 summarizes the battles between Ted Hughes and his sister Olwyn, who control Plath's literary estate, and her various recent biographers. In the preface of her book, *The Haunting of Sylvia Plath*, pp. xi–xiv, Jacqueline Rose recounts her literary and personal disagreements with the Hugheses.

80. Juliet Mitchell, *Feminism and Psychoanalysis* (1974); Nancy Chodorow, *The Reproduction of Mothering* (Berkeley: University of California Press, 1978, and *Feminism and Psychoanalytic Theory* (New Haven: Yale University Press, 1989).

81. Showalter, *The Female Malady*, 249–250. Phyllis Grosskurth, *Melanie Klein: Her World and Her Work* (New York: Knopf, 1986); Elisabeth Young-Bruehl, *Anna Freud* (New York: Summit Books/Simon & Schuster, 1988); Susan Quinn, *A Mind of Her Own: The Life of Karen Horney* (New York: Summit Books, 1987); Paul Roazen, *Helene Deutsch: A Psychoanalyst's Life* (Garden City, New York: Anchor/Doubleday, 1985); Celia Bertin, *Marie Bonaparte: A Life* (New York: Harcourt, Brace, Jovanovich, 1982).

82. Janet Sayers, *Mothers of Psychoanalysis*, cited in note 53.

83. Ibid., 3, 261.

84. Phyllis Grosskurth, in review of *Mothers of Psychoanalysis, New York Times Book Review*, 29 September 1991, p. 11.

85. Lisa Duggan, "Review Essay: From Instincts to Politics: Writing the History of Sexuality in the U.S.," *The Journal of Sex Research*, 27:1 (February 1990), 95–109; Michel Foucault, *The History of Sexuality, Vol. I: An Introduction*, trans. Robert Hurley (New York: Pantheon Books, 1978). Suleiman, *The Female Body in Western Culture*, provides a good introduction to postmodernist concerns with the female body and sexuality. For an excellent overview of the history of sexuality, see John D'Emilio and Estelle B. Freedman, *Intimate Matters* (New York: Harper & Row, 1988).

86. Elizabeth Lunbeck, "A 'New Generation of Women,'" *Feminist Studies*, 13 (1987), 513–543; Estelle Freedman, "'Uncontrolled Desires': The Response to the Sexual Psychopath, 1920–1960," *Journal of American History*, 74:1 (June 1987), 83–106. Quotes are from p. 106.

87. Carroll Smith-Rosenberg, "The Female World of Love and Ritual," *Signs*, 1 (Autumn 1975), 1–29; Lillian Faderman, *Surpassing the Love of Men: Romantic Friendships between Women from the Renaissance to the Present* (New York: Morrow, 1981); John D'Emilio and Estelle Freedman, "Problems Encountered in Writing the History of Sexuality," *Journal of Sex Research*, 27:4 (November 1990), 481–495. Smith-Rosenberg's 1975 article is reprinted, along with other interesting articles on sexuality and gender, in her *Disorderly Conduct: Visions of Gender in Victorian America* (New York: Knopf, 1985).

Nancy Cott's work on early twentieth-century feminism also points to the influence of varied schools of *psychology*, among them behaviorism, in identifying feminism with abnormality in general and lesbianism in particular. See Nancy Cott, *The Grounding of Modern Feminism* (New Haven: Yale University Press, 1987), 149–162.

88. See Lisa Duggan, "Review Essay," 104–105 for a review of the debate over Faderman's argument. In addition to her earlier book cited in the previous note, see also Lillian Faderman, *Twilight Girls and Odd Lovers: A History of Lesbian Life in Twentieth Century America* (New York: Columbia University Press, 1991), esp. 130–138.

89. Jennifer Terry, "Lesbians Under the Medical Gaze: Scientists Search for Remarkable Differences," *The Journal of Sex Research*, 27:3 (August 1990), 317–339. Quotes are from p. 338.

90. Jennifer Terry, "Theorizing Deviant Historiography," *Differences*, 3 (1991), 55–74. Quotes are from pp. 66, 71.

91. Showalter, *The Female Malady*, 10.

92. Schiebinger, *The Mind Has No Sex?*; Cynthia Eagle Russett, *Sexual Science* (Cambridge: Harvard University Press, 1989); David Noble, *A World Without Women* (New York: Knopf, 1992); Marina Benjamin (ed.), *Science and Sensibility: Gender and Scientific Enquiry, 1780–1945* (Cambridge: Basil Blackwell, 1991).

93. Schiebinger, *The Mind Has No Sex?*, 2.

94. I have made a small effort to begin such a project with "Devils in the Heart," cited in note 33.

95. Showalter, *A Female Malady*, 205–210.

96. Nancy Tomes, "The Rise of the Mental Health Professions," unpublished manuscript.

97. The place of the hysteria diagnosis in French psychiatry is a case in point. Jan Goldstein, for example, argues that the centrality of the hysteria diagnosis to French neurologists had much to do with their ongoing power struggle with the Roman Catholic Church. Mark Micale has presented a convincing argument that the hysteria diagnosis "disappeared" in the early twentieth century largely because it ceased to serve the professional purposes of Charcot's disciples. Thus feminist historians have to appreciate that medical theories about all sorts of diseases, including those that afflict women, circulated in an intellectual economy that did not have as its *only* purpose the definition and control of women. See Jan Goldstein, *Console and Classify* (New York: Cam-

bridge University Press, 1987) especially pp. 322–377; Mark Micale, "On the 'Disappearance' of Hysteria: A Study in the Clinical Deconstruction of a Diagnosis," *Isis,* lxxxiv (Autumn, 1993).

98. Allan Bloom, *The Closing of the American Mind* (New York: Simon & Schuster, 1987). See Susan Faludi, *Backlash: The Undeclared War Against American Women* (New York: Crown, 1991) for a journalistic account of the "backlash" phenomena.

99. Alan A. Stone, "Conceptual Ambiguity and Morality in Modern Psychiatry," *The American Journal of Psychiatry*, 137 (1980), 887–891.

20

History and Anti-Psychiatry in France

JACQUES POSTEL and DAVID F. ALLEN

There is a fundamental gap between what is expressed and what is understood, between the signifier and the signified, the "map" and the "terrain." This already complex situation is further complicated by the importing, exporting, and juxtapositioning of ideas. Imported ideas tend to be retranslated during their absorption into the previous historical totality of ideas and praxis. The sociologist and historian S. P. Fullinwider remarked that Americans were Jacksonian first and Freudian second: Freud was rewritten in the United States so as to be translatable—usable—within the American context. The same occurred in France with "anti-psychiatry."

In this chapter we will sketch the historical conflicts preceding the semantic existence of anti-psychiatry to relate the shifting patterns of interplay and juxtaposition constituting the French reinvention of anti-psychiatry; for, as the sociologist J. Gabel wrote: "Ideas tend to break free from their creators just as children break away from parental prejudice in order to lead lives of their own and associate with whom they please."[1] We shall also attempt a historical sketch of the way people related, rightly or wrongly,[2] to anti-psychiatry and used history as a mask to further their aims. This brings us to another methodological problem. As one of us pointed out more than twenty years ago,[3] the word *anti-psychiatry* has a shifting meaning. Doubtless, this word is "over-defined" in A. Korzybski's sense, semantic double-dutch, and, as Wittgenstein says, "if a sign is not necessary, it is meaningless."[4] We must therefore try to unravel the various strands of confusion and mystification and come to terms with the historical forces in action.

The close of the Second World War left France politically and economically devastated. Petainism and the period of collaboration caused scars that have not yet entirely healed. The war changed attitudes between psychiatric patients and staff—in the St. Alban asylum, for example, they had had to live together day in day out, grow food together, in short, form a community. In other institutions, as Max Lafont noted in his remarkable *L'Extermination douce*, many psychotics were allowed to starve because of food shortages; in other words, food was stolen from them.[5] The title, literally "soft extermination," implies that part of the French psychiatric establishment willingly closed its eyes to a few thousand more corpses here and there. We have, in a raw form, a dialectic that reappears in anti-psychiatry. For here we see one of the origins of institutional psychotherapy—born of necessity, perhaps encouraged by those who had been in camps themselves and were therefore unwilling to go back to systems of incarceration. We are also brought up against the perception of psychotics as a persecuted minority, "soft" extermination as opposed to the quantified extermination of the Nazis aided by the collaboration of many French public officials. The shadow of six million dead Jews is there in the very title of Lafont's work. (One could add that David Cooper was of South African origin. He saw the ugliness of the apartheid system, its segregation and double values, as a daily "reality"—is it not possible that the man who coined the expression *anti-psychiatry* was motivated in part by anti-apartheid feelings?) In postwar France those in the institutional psychotherapy movement (F. Tosquelles, R. Gentis, J. Ayme, G. Daumézon, J. Oury) rejected any return to the prison or camplike asylum system. To what extent was this rejection of the worst aspects of the traditional psychiatric hospital shadowed by the rejection of nazism?

The next question is: What ancestors did this movement invent or discover? The critique of the old-style asylums began slowly. In 1957 P. C. Racamier published a vitriolic article in *L'Évolution psychiatrique*, a journal that had refused to appear during the war. He argued, convincingly, that traditional mental hospitals were themselves instruments of alienation. Thus he opposed subjective alienation to institutional alienation, the latter confirming and worsening the former. This long article was also important in that it introduced American sociological references—a taste of things to come. One should bear in mind that Jacques Lacan's "De la causalité psychique" was published in the same journal in 1947. Lacan's thesis (1932) signaled the introduction of Kretschmerian thinking into French circles; it was also marked by the influence of Karl Jaspers, whose major work of psychopathology, *La Psychopathologie générale*, was published by Alcan in 1927.

The anti-psychiatric reading of history must be taken into account; with its tints of young Marx, Hegel, and Foucault's Binswanger-inspired structuralism, it is inseparable from its theoretical, clinical, and philosophical foundations. B. de Freminville posited a historical continuum of violence and false conciousness in the history of psychiatry, and the historian G. Césari looked at delusions within German psychiatry and Nazi ideology. Sartre's role is a further case in point: Not only was he attracted to phenomenology at an early age, but he corrected the proofs of the French edition of Jaspers's book while still studying at the École Normale Supérieure. He was also attracted to a series of left-wing causes, so that when the French translation of *Reason and Violence* appeared, with a fairly warm introduction by Sartre himself, the reader could be forgiven for thinking that there was a visible connection between Sartre, champion of the Left, and of phenomenology and the ideas marching under the dubious banner of anti-psychiatry. E. Minkowski's historical role is fundamental to any understanding of the events in question. His Bergsonian brand of phenomenology provided R. D. Laing (who had wished to study with Jaspers) with a theoretical framework that allowed him to combine the influence of D. W. Winnicott with that of European phenomenology. Winnicott's "fundamental submission" in psychosis gave birth to "ontological insecurity." Laing had effectively introduced schizophrenia into Hegel's master/slave dialectic, and his work on fundamental ontological insecurity was hailed by some in France as extremely significant.[7]

The postwar years in France propelled three great psychiatrists to the fore: Henri Ey, Eugène Minkowski, and Jacques Lacan. Lacan had early written a long review of Minkowski's *Lived Time*,[8] and in later years commented ironically on his former passion for Jaspers.[9] Lacan aimed for a return to Freud and worked on a theory of the subject; having drunk at phenomenology's fountain he moved on. Minkowski's research remained within the phenomenological sphere. Ey was one of the most respected traditional French psychiatrists. He had read almost all the important French and German authors and was widely credited with the introduction of Bleuler's ideas into France, translating part of his 1911 work. All three were members of *L'Évolution psychiatrique*; despite their outstanding intellectual influence, none was able to obtain an official teaching post.

Ey's attitude is of interest because it exemplifies a larger conflict; during the Séminaire de Thuir on schizophrenia, Ey explained why he felt uncomfortable about anti-psychiatry: "Such a conception would lead to the disappearance of schizophrenia."[10] His fundamental misgiving was that if psychiatry became enmeshed in ideological and sociological problems, the question of defining and classifying individual psychopathological problems would be made infinitely more complicated. Laing's point was that Bleulerian psychiatry provides little or no scientific guarantee. His critique of Emil Kraepelin struck a chord in France among psychologists, psychiatrists, and analysts— though not always for the same reasons. The Lacanians might have approved of the critique of Kraepelin because they favored a "clinic of the structure." Ey's seminar on schizophrenia gives another clue to the rejection of anti-psychiatry. An undergraduate (not Ey) delivered a short unforgiving lecture on H. S. Sullivan—he is dismissed, as is Laing, for being inaccurate, not using psychiatric jargon properly. Sadly, the speaker had not bothered to read any of Sullivan's work himself. This is symptomatic of the ahistoric perception of the Laing–Cooper–Esterson axis; one can even see Laing quoted as the inventor of the double-bind hypothesis. Obviously the serious reader would have perceived the Sartre/Minkowski roots—but the trio's references to Sullivan and L. C. Wynne et al. met with little or no response. There are a few notable exceptions: Jean Oury refers to Sullivan;[11] Gisella Pankow, Kretschmer's former assistant, had read Sullivan and quoted him with respect; and she was also responsible for the introduction of the ideas of R. Scott and P. Ashworth (*Soins psychiatriques*, 1981).

Last, R. Gentis translated Sullivan in 1968 for the *Revue de psychothérapie institutionnelle*. He was an important figure: first as a campaigner for institutional reform, and second, for being responsible for a collection of books called "Textes à l'appui" published by a left-wing publisher, F. Maspero. In this capacity he published not only his manifesto for reform, *Les murs de l'asile*, but also Laing's early work, *Sanity, Madness and the Family*. The date is important, for the popularity of anti-psychiatry as a catchword is inextricably bound not only to the gathering malaise within psychiatry but also to the political and economic malaise that temporarily united the student activists of the new universities like Nanterre with certain industrial workers. "Anti" was "in"—anti-war, anti-state, anti-boss, anti-star. The French Left, socialist, Maoist, Trotskyist and Hegelian, found a new *raison d'être* in the Vietnam War, just as in earlier years some of the French Left had been able to unite against the Algerian War. The Stalinist Communist party, though weakened by the events of 1956, was still a formidable force. The Maoists cultivated the myth of "the worker" in cloth cap and overalls exploited and alienated by the bosses; they looked to China or Cuba as an anti-model and sometimes talked of shooting the bourgeoisie, their parents, in other words. The post-Hegelians, with their impressive personal libraries, were the most extreme and the most actively interested in history and psychopathology. Indeed, one notes at least three psychiatric references in Guy Debord's *The Society of the Spectacle*: one to P. Abely's mirror sign, indicative of incipient schizophrenia, another to J. Gabel's work on false consciousness as a common denominator of both ideology and schizophrenia, and one to autism. " 'In clinical schizophrenia,' says J. Gabel, 'the destruction of the dialectic of totality (with its extreme form, dissociation) and the destruction of the dialectic of the becoming (with its extreme form, catatonia) seem to be in solid union.'' The consciousness of the spectator, prisoner of a flattened universe which is narrowed by the screen of the spectacle behind which his own life has been deported, knows only the fictional others who maintain him and speak unilaterally of their commodities and of the politics of their commodities. The spectacle, in all its width and length, is his (the spectator's) mirror sign. Here the stage is being set for a false exit from generalised autism'' (section 218). So it was that many demanded an end to all ideologies. Obviously this subsumes psychiatric ideologies.[12]

All these political groups had an interest in anti-psychiatry. It allowed a curiously flawed aggregation of causes to merge and in turn gave new life to causes marred first by Stalinism and later by the ugly truth behind Maoism. The schizophrenic, along with women, homosexuals, low-paid workers, prisoners, and army conscripts, became part of "the oppressed." The problem of clinical schizophrenia per se tended to be obscured by this global perspective. The slogans tell part of the story: Along with "Neither God nor master" one could read "Never work" and "Schizophrenics are the proletariat." This made sense to young firebrand psychiatrists in state hospitals, for it corresponded to their empirical observations and helps to explain the untranslatable *"psychiatrie = fliciatrie."* The young psychiatrist saw himself as the state's policeman (*flic* means cop). Add this to the political and social agitation of the period from 1965 to 1977 and one understands that anti-psychiatry was welcomed by some (whatever it was, wherever it came from) in that it corresponded to specific political concerns. The ambiguous use of the word *alienation* covered a variety of different meanings. For the Hegelians it was used in the Marxist sense. They were particularly fond of Marx's early period, particularly the 1844 Manuscripts. The worker, Marx argued, because his labor belongs to another, because he is quantified in his production and being, is pushed out of time and into space. It is curious to bear in mind that Minkowski, an outstanding influence on Gabel and Laing, concluded that the schizophrenic was pushed out of time and into space (1933), so that, for some in France, anti-psychiatry meant a dialectical understanding of mental illness that transcended mere classification. To explore anti-psychiatric references, one would be obliged to start with Laing's early work on the Ganser syndrome[13] and his midperiod research on Minkowski. It would be absurd to say that either S. J. M. Ganser or E. Minkowski were anti-psychiatric; they were both, however, anti-Bleulerian. That aspect of anti-psychiatry in France, despite, or because of, the complexities, cannot be ignored.

Other aspects were integral to the debate: The Spanish Civil War, a fundamental reference and experience for those of the institutional psychotherapy movement (Tosquelles, Daumezon, etc); the Second World War, which brought the equation: concentration camp = asylum; the role of psychiatry within German ideology from 1933; the Vichy regime and the death of a significant number of mental hospital inmates (1939–1945); and the demands for change in the asylum system that came after the Liberation. One must also remember that Sartre dominated postwar France, not only as philosopher, writer, and political activist, but also as a beacon for those who could not return to the middle-class values of *Travail, Famille, Patrie* and the "*Prix Cognac*" and who found a rallying point in existentialism, Juliette Gréco, and American jazz in the clubs of St. Germain-des-Prés. Sartre's key concepts, engagement and alienation, reappear in anti-psychiatry. François Dosse argues in his impressive *History of Structuralism*[14] that Foucault and Laing were pushed to the fore by the rebellion or "events" of 1968. According to one of France's great historians of the psychoanalytical movement, E. Roudinesco, Laing and Cooper entered the stage in October 1967, the year of the Tavistock publication of *Psychiatry and Anti-Psychiatry*, and in France the year of *The Society of the Spectacle* by Debord and the *Revolution of Everyday Life* by R. Vaneigem. Says Roudinesco[15] "Cooper and Laing wrote *Reason and Violence* [a decade of Sartre's philosophy] (1964). . . . So that at the very time when French intellectuals were rejecting Sartre's philosophy in favour of . . . structuralism, the English psychiatric movement was using Sartre to reject a structural position that had contributed to the hey-day of humanist psychiatry. And, paradox of paradoxes, it wasn't the Sartrian path that introduced anti-psychiatry to France in 1967, but the Lacanian way"[16] (p. 494).

Concerning the term *anti-psychiatry*, we agree with J. P. Rumen[17] who argued that it is more or less meaningless, open to almost any interpretation; we have therefore concentrated on the various debates that took place around the problems of institutional reform, the nature of madness, and the reaction to the United Kingdom imports—the writings of Laing, Cooper, et al. We have decided to leave to one side the role of Michel Foucault and Thomas Szasz, and the problem of psychoanalysis as anti-psychiatry. We have, however, included elements of debate about institutional psychotherapy and asylum conditions in France. This debate started after World War II and merged with the anti-psychiatry problem. Although we have focused on French aspects of the anti-psychiatry debate, it was impossible to limit our work to French thinkers only. We have therefore tried to work within an international frame of reference and have respected the "spirit" of the words if not the words themselves.

Our definition of the anti-psychiatry question in France is as follows: an ethical and historical debate caught up with and amplified by the ideological instability of post-1968 France in which the ideas of anti-psychiatry—Sullivan, Sartre, Minkowski—collided with those of Foucault, Tosquelles, Daumézon, and Lacan. This debate was stimulated by the need to lay the ghosts of the patients who died in asylums during the war and the period of collaboration. There was agreement about the rejection of "mechanical and police-style psychiatry" (Ey), and the variety of alternative projects mirrored a new conflictual ideological constellation. The rise of structuralism pushed the anti-psychiatry debate into the background, and the focus today in France is to be found in the triangular structural antagonism between biological psychiatrists, members of the International Psychoanalytical Association and the disciples of Lacan. Foucault's work encouraged research in the history of psychopathology; and paradoxically when one asks young French psychologists or psychiatrists what drew them to their profession many will quote the "myth" of St. Alban or *The Divided Self*. Historically, anti-psychiatry (from the UK) was a new synthesis—not new ideas per se—so that the revulsion it met in France was in part an inability to look in the mirror.

The French Anti-Psychiatry Debate: An Overview

Reformism vs. Radicalism: The Role of P. C. Racamier

Paul Claude Racamier's position offers a starting point, as he provides a good example of "centrist" or humanist reformist thinking. In *La Nef* (1971), this respected member of the French branch of the IPA expounded a position that effectively reflects the thinking of the traditional non-Lacanian and non-Hegelian French Freudians. The title and opening paragraphs speak for themselves: "New psychiatry faced with new illusions" (p. 54). "A theoretical and practical movement of radical contestation has emerged in these past years, he argues, under the heading of anti-psychiatry. It contends that the very concept of mental illness is an oppressive and opportunist invention of society and the psychiatrist (the accomplice); the family and society, having rendered certain subjects disturbed, condemns them by declaring them to be ill and reduces them still further by inflicting treatments; in brief, the psychiatrist mistreats [patients] by labeling them 'ill' and treating them as if they were 'ill.' " Racamier's remarks are the result of an interesting historical paradox, for, as we shall show, his own remarkable critique of institutional alienation (1957) probably helped make the bed in which the imported brand of critique would flirt with the Maoist, Lacanian, and Hegelian Left. Psychiatrist and orthodox IPA analyst, Racamier believes in the use of analysts in asylums, but the questioning of the social foundation of psychiatry or the rejection of "ego psychology" cannot correspond to his ideological requirements. This is perhaps reflected in his reading of history. He continues: "It is obvious that an anti-psychiatry either openly or secretly has always existed in the spirit and behavior of some of the public, just as medicine has always known anti-doctors (*anti-médecins*) of several types." The historical subtext evoked here must be discussed. Racamier has introduced a subtle equation in which "anti-psychiatry" is placed in parallel with a collection of charlatans, faith healers, and magnetizers that runs through the history of French psychiatry. The problem became acute during the French Revolution when the medical teaching institutions were closed. Mesmer and Puységur are two cases in point.

These "anti-doctors" developed psychological theories that were of obvious functional value in treating hysteria and may even have led toward the understanding of unconscious mechanisms. By equating anti-psychiatry with pre-Freudian theorists of "hysteria," Racamier is, to some extent, sawing the branch he is sitting on. He is also touching on a raw nerve, as if anti-psychiatry would or could reduce the prestige, salary, and influence of psychiatrists by flooding France with a new breed of "anti-doctors." [18] Racamier has, in fact, fought his way into an epistemological corner—for the "founding myth" of St. Alban is said to have been "staged" by an anti-doctor, Tissot. "Psychiatry today sees the birth of an anti-psychiatry in its own breast." This, Racamier explains, is due to "an increased public interest in psychiatry" and the "mutation crisis" (*crise d'évolution*) that psychiatry was going through. This "crisis" is compared to the adolescent identity crisis. Anti-psychiatry was, in Racamier's eyes, the naughty adolescent who rejected everything. From the height of his orthodox analytic wisdom he explains that anti-psychiatry is a bad, bad boy "doomed to failure" (p. 57). To his lasting credit, the author recognizes that both "new psychiatry" (or institutional psychotherapy and reform) and anti-psychiatry share "a basic image of man and of interpersonal relationships'' (p. 58). These short lines throw a fig leaf over some common historical origins shared by anti-psychiatry and the movement for institutional renewal.

In 1957 Racamier published his much-discussed paper, an ''Introduction to the Sociopathology of Hospitalised Schizophrenics,'' which would surely have found favor with A. Esterson et al. He writes: ''A young psychiatrist learns quickly that he has been given the most remarkable instrument of alienation that one could imagine—I mean a psychiatric ward. Never can we allow ourselves to forget that the psychiatric milieu is a double-edged weapon. It cures or intensifies [symptoms] especially as we know for schizophrenics, the hard core of the insane (aliénés achevés)'' (p. 48). ''The patient is . . . indoctrinated, despite himself, by the group, into a role, which is effectively that of the madman'' (p. 51). The question of Racamier's succinct and somewhat limited historical critique of anti-psychiatry is now less opaque: The bibliography of this remarkable study that introduces the concept of ''critical distance'' to the sphere of schizophrenia is of the very same mettle as that of many so-called anti-psychiatric works. Reluctant to enter into a precise debate as to the ''prehistory'' of anti-psychiatry, Racamier sketches an outline as follows:

> Before any exposé of anti-psychiatry, it is useful to situate it in its historical context in terms of the psychiatry it contests and aims to combat. . . . At the origin of our culture, psychopathological events were considered in a religious perspective; psychological suffering was understood and combatted as a manifestation of evil. Let's not forget that it was the same case for all illness (the doctors of Antiquity, were they not priests?) but psychiatry separated itself [from religion] with more difficulty and much later than [general] medicine.

To understand Racamier's use of history, we require a theory of the narrator. In this case the narrator is in conflict with aspects of his own reflection—he shares the interpersonal perspective that Laing and others promoted, yet is compelled to say that ''although anti-psychiatry understands this, it understands it badly [le comprend mal]''—misunderstands it, in other words. It is difficult to avoid the possibility that the subtexts—the works of H. S. Sullivan and K. S. Weinberg—have been reinterpreted into differing historical totalities. Racamier's position is that of the master; his discourse is that of certitude. His reading of anti-psychiatry as adolescent negativism is perhaps better understood in this perspective. He continues:

> [In] other times ''explained'' as a manifestation of the devil, psychopathological suffering has remained with the hallmark of the redoubtable, the incomprehensible, the inadmissible and the unspeakable. . . . These motives, amongst others, gave a strong rapid push to the development of psychiatry in precise directions: a considerable effort to separate the pathological from the non-pathological; an effort to define clear subdivisions, within that enclosed area [psychopathology], as in medicine.

The conclusion is that psychiatry found itself out of step both with general medicine and society; patients and psychiatrists realized this and psychiatry became and remains a poor relation:

> The prison and madhouse-like (asilaire) condition into which the main body of l'Assistance Publique has silently fallen, and not yet recovered from is no [mere] contingency. It reflects (or translates) an embedded perspective in which mental

illness is much more scandal than suffering. It is true that the scandal is easier to stifle than the suffering. These are [in] simplified [form] the historical sources of the anti-psychiatry movement'' (*La Nef*, 42 [Paris, 1971], 58–60).

Racamier uses two voices, that of enlightened and warm agreement, and that of paternal rebuke. Although he might well have hitched a ride halfway down the road under the sign of ''new'' psychiatry, he is not quite the fellow-traveler that F. Basaglia, M. Mannoni, B. Cuau, D. Zigante, G. Jervis, and others were perceived to be. Something is oddly missing, as if a symphony were being played without violins. Some of the missing historical fragments are to be found in the bibliography of Racamier's pioneering 1957 article, ''Introduction à une sociopathologie des schizophrènes hospitalisés,'' in which we find:

38. Stanton and Schwartz, The mental hospital.
39. Sullivan H. S., Socio-psychiatric research; its implication for the schizophrenia problem. (Translated into French eleven years later [1968] by R. Gentis, who had spent at least five years in St. Alban.)
40. Sullivan H. S., The interpersonal theory of psychiatry.
43. Weinberg S. K., Society and personality disorders.

Racamier was surely in a position to recognize the continuum between the authors he was happy to use in 1957 and those whose influence he now sought to limit in an awkwardly apologetic mood of compromise and dressing-down. In his rapid sketch, the author has wiped out any references to the theoretical origins of anti-psychiatry; they are too close to his own. This act of writing himself out of history skews the debate.

Racamier's task is to maintain the idea that there has always been an anti-psychiatric movement and to distance himself from any leftist stance perceived to be connected to anti-psychiatry. To balance his critique Racamier has to introduce a list of innovations within French psychiatry since Dr. Moreau de Tours. In a way he is formulating an ideology of progress. ''It would be unjust,'' he adds, ''to forget what follows. At almost all times, particularly since the [second world] war, psychiatry has advanced . . . In 1850 Moreau de Tours suggested that the . . . dream be adopted as the fundamental model of psychosis. . . . A great effort of renovation and criticism of psychiatric hospitals has been undertaken since 1946 by psychiatrists themselves'' (*La Nef*, p. 61). This central sentence begs the question. If the various movements toward reform were doing their good work, why did the label *anti-psychiatry* catch on, why was there such an awkward rift between people who may well have had shared sources, why the split between well-meaning reformers and more radical groups? Part of an answer lies in the fact that the Gaullist period had provided economic growth, consumer goods, new universities, a return to the prewar status quo, and boredom and dissatisfaction among students in roughly equal quantities. This meant that the imported works of Laing, Basaglia, Jervis, and others were seen as echoes of an undiscernible request for ''*autre chose*.'' It is significant that Racamier chose to identify anti-psychiatry with the sixties rather than enter the lion's den of the prehistory of anti-psychiatry, which would have meant a return to Tosquelles, Minkowski, Sartre, Binswanger, Ganser, and Sullivan. He writes: ''Anti-psychiatry was born and grew in England just ten years ago.'' The reader is thus left to assume that it rose from nowhere, whereas, after the attempted revolt of May 1968, it was obvious that the movement of social critique that swept through many factories, universities, and asylums had discernible origins in the *hic et nunc* of daily life.

Harold Heyward, himself a psychiatrist, picks up the historical debate where Racamier left off. In 1971, with Mireille Varigas, he published "Une Antipsychiatrie?"— a characteristic document, not only because it was part of the home-grown anti-psychiatric product but also because it gives a confused answer to the question of the meaning of anti-psychiatry.

A Maoist Anti-Psychiatrist

For Heyward, anti-psychiatry meant anti-Kraepelinian and anti-Bleulerian psychiatry. The historical focus is shorter and sharper than Racamier's; the bibliographical references move from Morel's *Traité des maladies mentales* (1860) and *La dégénérescence de l'espèce humaine* (1857) to Laing's *The Divided Self*, published in Paris in 1970. Heyward tried to relate the dementia praecox-schizophrenia problem to the Industrial Revolution and to forms of aborted or crushed individual revolt. Again we find a dialectic that was to subtend many anti-psychiatry works, that the schizophrenic belongs to the logical category of the oppressed (along with badly paid workers, minorities, etc.) rather than to the logical category of the "ill" (along with those who have cancer or brain tumors, etc.). One is tempted to add that such feelings had been expressed, in varying degrees, many years before the anti-psychiatry label appeared. Weinberg "shows" that schizophrenics come mainly from large towns and low-rent-paying groups, whereas the ever-righteous Sullivan puts the blame squarely on religious excess, poor social conditions, and group pathology. This overall perspective is echoed in much French published work: It is the driving force behind Césari's *Psychiatrie et pouvoir* and the remarkable *Critique de la raison délirante*; it also appears in *L'Homme se drogue, l'état se renforce*, a long and extraordinarily well-detailed critique of psychiatric "drug" consumption in France. If nothing else, the word *anti-psychiatry* appears to have encouraged a rejection of what some have called "*l'immobilisme du gaullisme immobilier*" (the stagnation of graft and corruption), so that anti-psychiatry, with its own roots, *raison d'être*, and prehistory, is never quite dealt with as a historical event; rather, defining features are borrowed from it here and there so as to complete other schemes and visions. Heyward's critique of the history of schizophrenia is quite representative: Part one of the book, entitled "Madness or Mental Illness" (*Folie ou maladie mentale*), is a naive outgrowth of Laing's famous (or infamous!) critique of Emil Kraepelin in *The Divided Self*. Laing used the same method of critique in *The Politics of the Family*; understandably Heyward also discusses Morel's understanding of his patients and the ideology that underlies the diagnosis.

To comprehend Heyward's use of history, it is useful to bear in mind Laing's critique of Kraepelin. The case from *The Lectures on Clinical Psychiatry* was extensively commented on and quoted from by both Laing[19] and Heyward[20]. Heyward was obviously seduced by Laing's focus on Kraepelin's attitude to his patient; he argues that what is supposed to be incomprehensible becomes very comprehensible if we focus on the situation as a whole—rather than only on the patient's "incomprehensible" answers out of context. Heyward's target, defined in the introduction, is the medical "model" of madness, the Bleulerian "disease process" or equivalent.

Myth and "Anti"-Myth

> A myth of major importance has existed from Hippocratic times onward which
> affirms that madness is but the consequence of an illness. This is the myth or more
> precisely the hypothesis of mental illness. It is obviously this point that founded
> psychiatry and gives it its historical roots. . . . For us anti-psychiatry is a myth which
> affirms that madness is not due to an illness. As this myth pertains to the same
> ideological domain as that of mental illness, there is no reason to refuse it the same
> quality or value, namely, that of a working hypothesis. . . . In the 19th century there
> was a symmetrical kind of ideology in the field which had never been considered
> an illness before Lombroso and his attempt to "medicalise" crime. Within the
> narrow limits of these definitions we would agree to this study being called . . . anti-
> psychiatric (H. Heyward and M. Varigas, *Une Anti-Psychiatrie*, p. 8).

The semantic options are evident here; Heyward's "anti-psychiatry" means rejection
of the morbid disease process as theorized by Morel, Kraepelin, and Bleuler: To some
extent anti-psychiatry meant anti-Bleulerian psychiatry. Other meanings had been analyzed two years before (1969) by J. Postel, M. Postel, and J. P. Rumen in an article
titled "The Paradoxes of the Anti-Psychiatric Movement." The three authors concentrate on the semantic modifications that may well have contributed to the media success
of anti-psychiatry:

> Over the last few decades the prefix "anti" has undergone semantic modification
> (or displacement). Originally used in military or medical terminology, it signified
> defence against a danger, an enemy (anti-tank-gun), an illness (anti-tetanic). When
> it was added to a word that did not have a pejorative meaning it dragged the word
> down into negative values, like, for example, anti-constitutional, anti-physical or
> anti-poetic, without in any way questioning the opposite term (constitutional, poetic
> etc) as a positive value.[3]

"Anti," in ideology and merchandise alike, had become the desirable value—the
necessary prefix to any fashionable object or discourse. The authors add, "Psychiatry
could not avoid this new semantic avatar; it was on the contrary particularly predisposed
to it by the malaise of the psychiatrists and their therapeutic institutions." The authors
recognize that the main initial thrust of anti-psychiatry was centered on the question of
schizophrenia. This explains their respective need for historical elements of the schizophrenia problem that appear under the subheading "The decay of nosologies: the disappearance of schizophrenia." The authors argue that in Cooper's perspectives:

> the patients will do without psychiatrists all the more easily as they will no longer
> be alienated by the psychiatrists in nosological diagnosis. First of all the death
> certificate of schizophrenia—which bears so many morbid statistics—would have
> to be signed. Born with J. C. Reil, who under the name "Narrheit" described in
> 1808 symptoms which F. Leuret was to identify in his observations of "incoherent
> patients," dementia praecox, so called by Morel in 1834, becomes with Kraepelin
> and his successors the label the psychiatrists will stick on the "madman" every
> time the notion of "manic-depression" can't be made to fit. Bleuler's neologism
> (1908) changed nothing. On the contrary, it is even more bogged down in bio-
> physical causality and forever locks up the "reputed schizophrenics" in the police,
> medical and institutional apparatus that society has designed for them.[3]

Heyward looks at the hidden road of the history of schizophrenia as an ideological and medical concept. Kraepelin's dissatisfied young man, as we know, sets the overall tone: "I find myself pondering the origins of schizophrenia. I know ... that it's a German figure dressed by a great Swiss couturier. ... Where were the schizophrenics before Kraepelin?" Heyward recognizes the historical and clinical consistency of mania "from Areteus to Binswanger," but advances that schizophrenia may have appeared as a "new illness towards the end of the XIXth century."[21] Heyward's questions could be synthesized as follows: Was schizophrenia ever to be used in a purely medical context or was it also a way of removing potential troublemakers from social praxis. He adds that in France, after 1789, "the revolution had happened, no one was afraid of the young ... at least not until the Commune of 1870" (p. 17).

Kraepelin is projected, so to speak, onto a split screen: Other cases from his *Lectures on Clinical Psychiatry* are scrutinized and a central thesis comes into view: Kraepelin the clinician (screen 1) observes "incomprehensible" patients and uses their incomprehensibility to justify the scientific rationale of "dementia praecox"; on screen 2, the Munich professor appears essentially as a producer of ideological discourse, a discourse all the more curious as it is shown to be out of phase or split from what Kraepelin's patients actually say about their position. The ideological distortion, Heyward theorizes, should be noted, for it lays the ground for Césari's later work.

The second relevant aspect of Heyward's short (thirty-six page) history of schizophrenia is the shadow of general paralysis. The tone is informal, as if the author were thinking out loud or chatting to friends in a bar after work.

> Once upon a time there was, sadly, a real mental illness! An intellectual deterioration accompanied by paralysis due to chronic meningitis. Its discovery was, for the most part, due to the work of French alienists and it was called general paralysis. It was always fatal. By 1857 its syphilitic origins were suspected, and largely accepted, mainly by German alienists. This shameful origin was naturally exploited by moral and religious authorities (p.39).

Heyward adds that "it was naturally intolerable [to the post-Bismarck German alienists] that the French revolutionary order had been able to discover a scientifically proven illness. They needed a comparable illness, a German general paralysis" (p.39). So Heyward's reading of "history" leads him to the idea that Kraepelin's dementia praecox was born of an ideological blind spot fueled not only by the moral imperatives of Bismarck's Germany (madmen are crooks, swindlers, pyromaniacs, etc.) but also by a sort of chauvinism. Heyward enjoins his readers to go out and read Kraepelin and make up their own minds. This "return to Kraepelin" was obviously in part due to Laing's remarks in *The Divided Self*, in part perhaps to Kraepelin's role as purveyor of ideological discourse, and in part to his place as founding father of modern psychiatry. Consider J. Postel's opening remarks to the 1970 introduction to Kraepelin's *Leçons cliniques*:

> As the vessel of psychiatric nosology is taking in water port and starboard, it may appear paradoxical to reprint a French translation of the "Leçons cliniques" of its most eminent author. Yet our diagnosis of mental illness is still based on Kraepelin's classification. ... A critique of today's ... nosology cannot overlook this important

oeuvre whose rich clinical precision will have brought a priceless gift to the history
of psychiatry whatever may become of the wreck of its nosology.[22]

Sixteen pages later (p. 23), Postel adds, "Kraepelinian psychiatry, however monumental
it may be, is but a construction for the dead, closed in on itself, that can only function
in an enclosed area that may just as well be called asylum, zoo, botanical garden or
graveyard."[23]

The Lacanians also played a role in this renewed interest in Kraepelin.[24] Their
interest would have been close to anti-psychiatry in that they were anti-Kraepelinian,
anti-Bleulerian, and for the same reasons adamantly opposed to the *D.S.M.-III*. Their
interest in Kraepelin would be to advance the Lacanian "clinic of the structure"; the
elements one perceives here and there are a juxtaposition against a common enemy
rather than an identity of belief, interest, and long-term purpose. The Lacanian critique
of psychiatric nosology was designed to advance the cause of an alternative structural
nosology and, of course, that of the Lacanian cure. Laing and Cooper, despite their oft-
quoted rejection of traditional analysis, were seduced by Lacan's "mirror stage" and
were themselves adopted by some of those who swam the waters of leftism, structuralism, and Maoism. The trick was to be "anti-psychiatric, pro-Mao Tse Tung, anti-
IPA, pro-Lacanian, anti-Stalinist and pro-Fidel Castro"—a caricature, of course, or at
least an aggregation of the various elements. If there was a general agreement around
the critique of Kraepelin, there was an obvious split over what was to replace it. The
analytic community could not afford the nosology it itself used. J. Postel thus defined
the contradiction (1970):

> The Freudian discovery didn't suppress psychiatric nosology. Freud himself didn't
> hesitate to create a new morbid entity like obsessional neurosis. The psychiatrist,
> even if he's an analyst, still needs to use nosological models, if only to clarify his
> therapeutic indications. As long as medical discourse remains inseparable from a
> normative tendency that constantly reappears behind apparent objectivity or "neu-
> trality," nosology will persist even in the spheres most distant from organic med-
> icine.[25]

The gathering malaise in French psychiatry in the late 1960s and early 1970s produced
a variety of positions, alliances, and discourses: In the emerging debates it was obvious
that structural causality (Lacanian) was difficult to integrate into an overall theory of
psychosocial causality and vice versa. The 1967 *"journées de l'enfance aliénée"*
marked a sort of watershed: Cooper arguing social causality of the Sullivan–Weinberg
type claimed that it takes three generations to produce psychosis; Lacan (*discours de
clôture*) agreed with Cooper, but the Lacanian theory of psychosis involves three generations and forced choice within the context of his threefold structure: the "real,"
"symbolic," and "imaginary."

What then explains the crossovers between anti-psychiatry, Lacanism, and the
movement for institutional reform? Lacan's return to Freud had done much to rekindle
interest in analysis and the very nature of neurosis and psychosis. (From 1947 onward
Lacan had probably done more than anyone in France to revitalize the question of
psychic causality in psychosis.) He also used Marx and Hegel as raw materials for his
far-reaching theoretical corpus. This use or reinterpretation would have been recognized
by the post-Hegelians who gravitated around the Marxist philosopher and filmmaker

G. Debord and his publisher Champ Libre (later Les éditions G. Lebovici). M. Mannoni[26] was obviously influenced by Laing's Kingsley Hall project and if the post-
Hegelians (R. Vanegeim) saw structuralism as just another defense of the "bourgeois
state," they could not ignore Lacan's early connections with Breton and the surrealists.
Commenting on this idealism in 1969, we wrote:

> There is in the anti-psychiatric movement a . . . heroic engagement in being posi-
> tioned in the paradox of opposition to an alienating society with all the norms of
> orthodoxy it requires, and this is associated with an identification with the mentally
> ill who would turn out to be the healthy (*sain*) characters facing the so-called sick
> society. That said, it is easier to participate in the patients' revolt than to change
> society. One perceives in that attitude a whiff of adolescence, willingly idealistic
> and poetic. This is perhaps why anti-psychiatric texts are so appealing when read
> for the first time.[27]

The problem is not only that of the psychiatrist, analyst, or therapist in search of a
"good conscience"—it is also the basic problem of who takes what decision: If more
influence is given to psychoanalysis, then conflicts center on who makes the "best"
interpretation, who belongs to which school. The authors were well aware that politics,
clinical psychiatry, and rivalry between psychologists, analysts, and psychiatrists had
merged as if to produce an atmosphere of excited idealism, opportunism, demagogy,
and confusion.

Maoism faded, the lucid scholarship of Simon Leys did much in France to speed
its passing: It died without a funeral, and chairman Mao as an ego ideal was replaced
by other charismatic figures who were nearer to home. Structuralism and semiotics had
now become the hallmarks of intellectual radicalism. The central theme is now clear:
the word *anti-psychiatry* in France was, if nothing else, a symptom (Laing saw himself
as a symptom), a catalyst, and a point of convergence.

Origins—St. Alban—Sectorization

As one of us has argued, myths appear within the field of the history of psychopathology
as a negation of violence. The function of this negation is to project the immediate
present into the past. This "time mastery" is symptomatic of ideological distortion.
The semantics of anti-psychiatry are in themselves indicative of ideological distortion,
in that the theories exposed in the hazy field of anti-psychiatry can very often be found
outside anti-psychiatry in the realm of traditional psychopathology, especially if an
international historical perspective is adopted.

The schizophrenia problem, central to the work of Gentis (*Les murs de l'asile* and
Traité de psychiatrie provisoire) or Cuau and Zigante (*La politique de la folie*), was
certainly not born with anti-psychiatry. As early as 1917 one finds Adolf Meyer tearing
the concept apart in the *Chicago Medical Recorder*. Laing was much criticized for the
idea that schizophrenia was sometimes a period of experience allowing reorganization
of the troubled soul. Surely there is nothing new or anti-psychiatric in this type of
idea—the curious reader will find it in the early work of H. S. Sullivan, A. T. Boisen,
Wier Perry, D. T. Bradford, and even J. L. T. Birley; Pinel himself argued that fits
would cure mania and that the person who tried to prevent curative fits was as mad as
the madman.[28] This incomplete list illustrates the ahistoric perception of anti-psychia-

try—to say that it was born in the United Kingdom in the early sixties is to deny the history of ideas.

In April 1957, the *Évolution psychiatrique* group held its congress at Bonneval on "the schizophrenias." Henri Ey opened the debate with a remarkable paper on "The clinical problems of the schizophrenias." S. Follin followed with a paper on "The psychopathology of the schizophrenic process." Tosquelles (who with Daumezon was one of the founding fathers of institutional psychotherapy in France) intervened in the ensuing debate straight after the remarks of P. Male and A. Green. "We have the proof," Tosquelles said ". . . that schizophrenia is to be found not only at the crossroads of all the problems of psychopathology, but even in the very problem of Mankind itself: tell me how you conceptualize and act towards schizophrenia, and I will tell you what [kind of] psychiatrist and man you are" (p. 267). This oft-quoted sentence is of course a *"detournement"* of the proverb *"Dis-moi qui tu hantes et je te dirai qui tu es"* ("Tell me whom you see and I'll tell you who you are"). The new psychiatric proverb is often quoted by young psychiatrists because it points to a simple "truth": that theory is a function of ideology. Around this simple historical banality one of the focal points of anti-psychiatry crystallizes.

Laing: Sullivan Takes Minkowski Home

The debate continued with Laing's critique of Kallman's and Slater's genetic theories of schizophrenia, which appeared in France in 1979.[29] Laing was already well enough established to have been published by mainstream publishing houses. Esterson's *The Leaves of Spring* (1970) appeared in an excellent translation (Monique Manin) in 1972 with all the advantages of an influential mainstream publisher (Payot, Paris). The pace of translations was accelerating; for example, it took ten years for *The Divided Self* to cross the channel (Stock, Paris, 1970) and seven years for *Sanity, Madness and the Family* (Maspero, Paris, 1971, in the collection directed by R. Gentis and H. Torrubia). By now one would have to have been almost blind[30] not to remark upon the Anglo-American historical roots of the imported brand of anti-psychiatry. On page 11 of the French edition of *The Divided Self* and on page 14 of the 1973 Pelican edition one may read: "Je donne ici une oeuvre subjective, oeuvre cependant qui tend de toutes ses forces vers l'objectivité. E. Minkowski" ("I hereby offer a subjective piece of work that nonetheless reaches toward objectivity with all its might." This quotation is in fact from the 1927 Payot edition of *La Schizophrénie*). This obvious hint was largely confirmed by the bibliography (U.K. edition quoted above, p. 209). There are three entries under Minkowski: The first remarkably lists both editions of Minkowski's *La Schizophrénie*, the Payot edition and the Desclée de Brouwer 1953 edition; this is followed by the original 1933 edition of *Le temps vécu* (Lived Time).

Minkowski was, and remains, one of the pioneers of a dialectical and Bergsonian understanding of schizophrenia: Laing (1963) and Lacan (1936) both wrote studies of his work: Laing concludes his by stating that Minkowski "makes the first serious attempt in psychiatry to reconstruct the other person's lived experience" (p. 207).

Anti-Psychiatry Was French!

Esterson (1970) introduces *The Leaves of Spring* as follows:

This is a report on a family and a possible method of studying families. Family and method have been described to some extent in an earlier work. There, the first eleven of a series of families of diagnosed schizophrenics were presented in some detail. The group described here, the Danzigs, is one of the eleven.

In that report a social, phenomenological method of study was outlined. The method, a synthesis embodying the Sullivan tradition of participant observation of interpersonal relations and the phenomenological tradition in philosophy—particularly the philosophy of Sartre—allowed the clinical method of approaching "schizophrenics" to be depassed, i.e. dissolved and preserved in a wider synthesis. The theory and practice of communications analysis acted as catalyst so to speak. This work is intended as a contribution to dissolving, reconciling, and depassing in a new synthesis the social phenomenology of the earlier work and the psychoanalytic way of studying experience.

The method described is derived from the philosophical tradition of dialectical investigation, particularly as it is embodied in the work of Hegel, Marx, and Sartre, though it is not a direct application of any of these (English edition, p. xi; French edition [1972], p. 9).

The key problem here, one that Gentis echoes, is that of the "intelligibility" of those diagnosed schizophrenic, explaining in part perhaps Laing's and Cooper's use of Minkowski and Sartre. The latter provided the foreword to *Reason and Violence* (Tavistock, 1964); it was not translated in the first edition and reads as follows:

I have read with attention the work [*Reason and Violence*, most probably in ms. form] that you have entrusted me with, and I had the great pleasure of finding a very clear and very exact presentation of my thinking. What attracts me to this book, even more than the perfect understanding of "The Critique of Dialectical Reason" (Laing, Chap. 3), is your constant concern with the completion of an "existential" approach to the mentally ill. I think, as you do, that psychic disorders cannot be understood from the outside, from a positivist determinist position; neither can they be reconstituted from a combination of concepts that remain outside the lived illness (*maladie vécue*).

I also think that one can neither study nor cure a neurosis without a fundamental respect for the person of the patient, without a constant effort to catch the meaning of the basic situation . . . and I hold the opinion, as you do, I think, that mental illness is the result that the free organism, in its total unity, invents in order to live an unbearable situation. For that reason I consider your research to be of the highest value, particularly your study of the family milieu taken as group and series, and I am convinced that your efforts contribute to bringing us closer to the time when psychiatry will finally be human.

Thank you for the trust you have shown in me and I beg you to believe in my very attentive esteem. *November 9th, 1963* Jean-Paul Sartre

St. Alban

Around the central theme—illness as choice—one could assemble a curious group of bedfellows: Kretschmer, Lacan, Laing, Cooper, and obviously Sartre. Tosquelles, has a natural interest in anti-psychiatry that can be deduced from the myth he constructs as the "past" of the institutional therapy movement. In what follows, a series of oral histories published in *La Recherche*, no. 17, 1975, "Histoire de la psychiatrie de secteur ou le secteur impossible," it becomes clear that perhaps the "Front Populaire" and the reaction to the rise of Spanish fascism contributed indirectly but significantly to the impetus behind the movement of institutional therapy. Tosquelles tells his own story thus:

> St Alban was founded by Tissot in 1821. . . . His discourse resembled that of today's (1975) anti-psychiatry in many ways. At the time of the creation of St Alban, Tissot had some partisans, for example two peasants, Gauzi and Rousset; he sent them to Dupuytren in Paris, a guy who was an anti-doctor as we would say today, an anti-psychiatrist, because he fought against blood-letting, baths, the purges, and all those wild therapies that psychiatrists used. And this Tissot sent Gauzi and Rousset, Lozère peasants, to work for a year at Dupuytren's, to learn what could be learnt of therapeutic and clinical value. They were the first two psychiatric nurses of France. Tissot was therefore the anti-psychiatric creator of St Alban's hospital and of 25 others. All this is a strong current that by far preceded the 1838 law, which was already a way of integrating, of recuperating[31] that anti-psychiatry (p. 82).

"When I arrived at Saint-Alban," L. Bonnafé wrote, "Tosquelles was already there and he had played an extraordinary role as a revealer. When I say Popular Front, for us . . . it means the Spanish Civil War. They are one and the same adventure and the discourse of those who lived refers always to the Spanish War. . . . This experience of the war against Franco was our fundamental experience and . . . in the French Resistance, and this is something too often forgotten; the military system was organised and structured on the basis of those who'd fought against Franco's army. All this shows that the course of events or logical thread of Popular Front—Spanish War—Nazi occupation—clandestine combat, etcetera, represents continuity and fidelity" (p. 84). The etcetera, as we shall see, is the struggle to change psychiatric praxis and the perspective in which psychotics were perceived. We are dealing here with oral reports recorded more than thirty years after the events in question. It is, of course, always tempting to take documents at face value. This, however, would be to deny that the history of psychopathology is strewn with myths,[32] half-truths, lies by omission, and outright lies the like of which are found in glossy articles about the magnificent quasi-magical "progress" in mental health. Because of these methodological problems we state clearly that the perception of our actors was that there was a logical ethical continuum between the rejection of Spanish and German fascism and "anti-psychiatry" (institutional psychotherapy). This is our working hypothesis.

"I had crossed the Pyrenees on foot," wrote Tosquelles, "with a small bag in which there was a book of English grammar, Hermann Simon's book[33] and the monthly reports I had to write for the psychiatric service of the republican army. With other colleagues (Pena Sauret and Marin) . . . we established a kind of therapeutic community during the [Spanish Civil] War. I was in charge of the psychiatric section of the army. . . . For example . . . high command would ask me if they should give more leave in such and such a sector or change the soldiers in another sector for psychological reasons. . . . That was sector psychiatry! (*Ca, c'était de la psychiatrie de secteur*)." On that key phrase we must leave St. Alban and our "nun-raping Spanish, red psychiatrist,"[34] who brought German influences and aspects of institutional psychotherapy to France. The idea of institutional change even reached Algeria. In 1954 Tosquelles published a paper with F. Fanon, who in the mid-1950s, during the Algerian war of independence, found himself at the Blida asylum near Algiers. There, Dr. Fanon effectively introduced alternative psychiatry, removing the straitjackets, belts, and leather handcuffs, and teaching his staff that even giving a cigarette to a patient could be therapeutic and that, above all, one should shut up and listen. The same black, French doctor helped the FLN against the French army as if freedom for the mad was a prelude to freedom for the colonized. This logical movement from medical to political engagement and back is central to our debate and explains the reflex quality of much of the reaction to it, and one of the long-term results of the various conflicts from 1945 onward was the introduction of "psychiatrie de secteur" or sectorization.[35]

Sectorization

Robert Castel commented on "the origins and ambiguities of sectorisation" in his paper presented to the Research Committee on Psychiatric Sociology at the VIIIth World Congress of Sociology, Toronto, August 1974, just a year before the publication of the 588-page "*Recherches*" document, which includes contributions by G. Baillon, L. Bonnafé, G. Daumezon, F. Guattari, J. Oury, Ph. Paumelle, and F. Tosquelles. "The policy of sectorisation," says R. Castel, "refers to the total reorganisation of mental health policy in France. The question was to break with asylum isolation by reintroducing psychiatric facilities into the community, in keeping with the wishes of the progressive wing of . . . public hospital psychiatrists" (p. 57). This "break" with the past as government policy dates back to 1960 and to a government document quoted by both Castel and M. Fourré.[36] Castel compares the 1959 UK Mental Health Act, the French *Circulaire sur la sectorisation* (1960), and the Community Mental Health and Centers Act of 1963 (USA) and defines four levels of analysis:

> An institutional modification of the psychiatric hospital . . . towards more diversified institutions, lighter, closer to social life and less rigid. A transformation of the structure of psychiatric professions through increased independence or the creation of new professional and para-professional roles with new power relationships and struggles as a consequence. In terms of theoretical foundations or rationalisations of psychiatric practice [one observes] a fragmentation of the traditional medical scheme of things and of the traditional definition of therapeutic activity. This new pluralism gave rise to frantic competition between old, recent and new schools of thought. In demographic terms one observes a modification of the structure of the population taken in charge by psychiatry. By moving from the traditional asylum to the "sector" or "community" one observes in fact not only a change in the clinical symptoms (for example, the relationship between cases of serious—or chronic—psychosis and cases with lighter symptom-pictures changes) but also in the social, cultural, familial and demographic characteristics of the patients (for example the relationship between rural and urban populations of working and middle-class patients, the socially isolated . . . etc.). It is not only the place of therapeutic activity that changes when it "opens" towards the outside world, it's also its mode and particularly the human material on which it operates by "taking in charge" populations which are in part different from those annexed by the asylums of old.

With sectorization came various innovations—the "maisons de post cure" and the "lieux d'accueil." In the reorganization of power that ensued, analytic references were often used and misused in an attempt to employ psychoanalysis as an ideological discourse valid within the social sphere, so that, in a very perverse sense, psychoanalytic discourse was used as an alternative to or a reinforcement of traditional psychiatry. Rosine Lefort and Robert Lefort[37] give a clear answer to the problem (1990): "Despite Freud's own hopes as to the application of psychoanalysis to pedagogy 'to shape the generation to come,' there are not two types of discourse: that of social praxis does not exist because of its lack of concepts. Social praxis therefore borrows everything from other disciplines, sociology and particularly psychoanalysis; this gives birth to monsters, not very viable at heart, to 'psychoanalytic reeducation,' or worse, to 'reeducative psychoanalysis.' All use of psychoanalysis in a field which is not its own reduces it to a psychology." This kind of alternative to the traditional psychiatric answer to children from "socially deprived" backgrounds was born (or reborn) in the Freudo-Marxist ambitions of 1968 and was coupled with the idea of nature as an idealized value. Many centers sprang up all over France. This was made official after the socialist victory in 1981 by the governmental "circular no. 83-3 of January 27, 1983 relating to the placing of children in non-traditional structures,"[38] which gave a legal and administrative framework for what could be termed a form of anti-psychiatry.

As we move away from the strikes and protests of 1968–1972, the hold of anti-psychiatry fades. Castel explained that "even anti-psychiatry, though very popular in terms of ideological debate, found hardly any practical institutional role comparable to what happened in Italy because its political motivations were rewritten by professionals in terms of Lacanian hyper-orthodoxy" (p. 70). As the problem of psychoanalysis in institutions became central, a number of historical works appeared as if Foucault and anti-psychiatry had stimulated a need for historians of psychopathology. We have limited ourselves to two significant works, leaving Foucault aside because he is dealt with elsewhere in this volume.

The Uses of History: De Freminville and Césari

Violence

"La Raison du plus fort—traiter ou maltraiter les fous?" by B. de Freminville was published by Le Seuil in 1977, in the Combats collection, which had also published D. Cooper, Philip Agee, and Jean Ziegler in 1976. De Freminville—and, to an extent, Cuau and Zigante, who were quick (as was Castel) to realize the significance of Erving Goffman's *Asylums*—uses a critical method that one might use if studying pseudoscience or sects. Pages 63 to 115 are given over to "a small inventory of methods of therapeutics and physical coercion imagined and used by the alienists of the 19th century as an indication of the taking of absolute power over the bodies of patients." As one moves from Esquirol's cold bath shocks to the surprise near-death by drowning favored by Van Helmont, one cannot help feeling that the scientific or psychological knowledge of other times effectively resembles paranoiac (not paranoid) delusions. Consider the following extract from de Freminville's pocket dictionary:

> Castration: Apparently little used by the French authors, quoted by Esquirol (along with "falling on the head, hair cutting, and cataract surgery") as a hit and miss

therapeutic method of hardly any value (1838). Anglo-Saxon authors on the other
hand seemed more decided to use this operation. It was used . . . in 1861 by Dr.
Rooker (of Castelton) on an epileptic "given over to masturbation." During the
eight weeks that followed the operation, "the epilepsy did not reappear, but there
were still (occasional) attempts at masturbation."

The patient became "indolent, fat and lazy," so the surgeon lost all interest in him.
This operation was practiced in the United States on the "mad masturbators" during
almost all of the nineteenth century. De Freminville does not comment on his historical
dictionary, rather he allows information to speak for itself. This method is close to the
one used by Laing and Esterson in *Sanity, Madness and the Family* as if it were no
longer necessary to intervene, comment, explain, or interpret precisely, because the
ideological message—the need to "neutralize" madmen—presents itself in the hand-
tailored combat-dress of medical discourse. This ethical concern is perhaps one of the
common features of anti-psychiatry, and one of the few coherent dictionary definitions
one could offer. "The Second World War," writes de Freminville, "played the role of
revealing what a totalitarian situation could produce. The image of the concentration
camp placed on the asylums was believable enough to bring about the rebellion of a
certain number of psychiatrists. . . . 40,000 hospitalised lunatics, more than a third of
those who found themselves in asylums, had died, mostly of hunger during the war"
("La Raison du plus fort," p. 179).

Nazi Ideology and Psychiatry

The problem of ethics was central to the work of the *Socialistisches Patienten Kollektiv*
(SPK), who organized and published their own critique of psychiatry around Dr. Huber
at the Heidelberg University Clinic in the late 1960s. In chapter 8 of Guy Leverve and
Luc Weibel's French translation, *Faire de la maladie une arme*,[39] we find a chilling
comparison between documents of the Nuremberg trials of doctors who worked with
the Nazis (25 October 1946 to 20 August 1947) and documents about the bureaucratic
methods of university departments at the time of the "liquidation" of the SPK. The
importance of the SPK—perhaps the most direct form of alternative psychiatry (real
sector psychiatry according to Guattari!)—was such that there were at least three publications in France pertaining to it. Here is a brief outline that brings the sterilization-
extermination problem into the Heidelberg perspective:[40]

> During the struggle between patients and the hierarchy of the [Heidelberg] clinic it
> was clear that those responsible for the clinic were in no way blind or unaware of
> the problem [of inhuman conditions], rather they were simply ready to sacrifice the
> patients on the altar of "science." Doctor Blankenburg [head doctor at the Heidel-
> berg University Psychiatric Clinic] expressed himself clearly to the patients in Feb-
> ruary 1970, with the approval of Von Baeyer [director]: "Science demands victims;
> when research and help to patients are in conflict, heads must roll." . . . The con-
> flicts between the clinical authorities and a few doctors who did not comply with
> the anti-patient[41] dictates of their masters, who rather used the needs of the
> patients as starting points for therapy, were used in the selfish interest of career-
> minded colleagues. The doctors who sided with patients rather than profits were
> fired. . . .

> Co-operation between doctors and patients has no place in the dominant [psychiatric] system; . . ., the patient-doctor relationship is defined by distance and mediation. The psychiatrist who habitually considers his patients as cases or as things must learn to stop expressing the ill population in diagnostic terms and start listening to the vital assertions of the reality of the oppressed (pp. 26–27).

In a comparison of documents relating to the Nuremberg trials of doctors and university documents pertaining to the elimination of the SPK (*Faire de la maladie une arme*, p. 121), the dialectic is clarified in no uncertain terms; so that the SPK saw themselves as a refusal of a type of psychiatry still dyed in the colors of German ideology. "A man named Blankenburg explained to us that the Führer had prepared a law on euthanasia. Those who took part in the meeting were absolutely free to provide help. None of the junior doctors had any objections to this programme." This is the declaration under oath of a nurse, P. Kneisler, Doc. No. 863, 1946/47 (*Faire de la maladie une arme*, p. 124). The following testimony confirms, in the eyes of the SPK, that psychiatrists played an active role in the extermination plan: "Each doctor was personally responsible for what he had to do within the measures that led to euthanasia, at the end."

De Freminville, the SPK, and Césari argue continuity: from near-death by drowning to near-death with insulin comas, chains to chemical handcuffs, from the "Gezetz zur Verhütung erbkranken Nachwuchses" (14 July 1933) to the obscene quantification of the final solution. For the three authors it is obvious that the shared ideological ground between nazism and psychiatry has not "disappeared" but rather maintained its praxis, discourse, and mastery. Césari argues that some delusions become historical action and therefore capture the place of reality:

> On January 30, 1933 a cabinet coalition was formed containing members of the National Socialist party. . . . The official publication (Reichsgesetzblatt, No. 86) in Berlin (July 25, 1933) included the text of the law of July 14, 1933, entitled "Law for the Prevention of Children Suffering from Hereditary Illness." This legal text is an important date in the history of German psychiatry. It is very synthetic (little more than two pages of the official publication) and consists of eighteen short paragraphs; it represents the concrete act, the victory even of the biological school of thought, all hues included, under the term "heredity." Based on a scientific falsehood—the very notion of heredity was very vague at the time—this law pointed at medical science to give it full responsibility for its own supposedly scientific basis; [the nazi authorities] were incapable of organising the application [of this law] and left the weight of responsibility to the medical corps.
>
> Paragraph 1 of the law represents one of the most flagrant examples in history of deluded discourse capturing a place in reality (*Critique de la raison délirante*, p. 89).

Césari gives a complete French translation of the law; the essence is that "he who suffers from hereditary illness may be sterilised" if it is probable that his offspring will have physical or mental disorders.[40]

Giorgio Césari's *Critique of Deluded Reason*, along with the works of the SPK[41], F. Basaglia, and G. Jervis, are examples of imported anti-psychiatry—above all Césari's work is an appeal for historicism, for psychiatric theory and practice to be seen as a function of ideology.

Anti Anti-Psychiatry: The Debate Within *L'Évolution psychiatrique*

The Debate

In 1972, the journal *L'Évolution psychiatrique* decided on an open debate, called for anti-psychiatry papers, and finally published an anti-psychiatry poem. These events were preceded by the Colloque de Rozès, 13 June 1971, at St-Lizier. Organized around the theme of anti-psychiatry by Maurel, it was to have been presided over by Henri Ey who in fact fell ill; those invited to give anti-psychiatry viewpoints were also absent, feeling they would not be "heard." Indeed, Maurel's opening remarks set the tone: Anti-psychiatry is a neologism, and every psychiatrist knows that neologisms are indications of psychosis. The tone changes: "The most fruitful theme of anti-psychiatry is its institutional critique. Here anti-psychiatry speaks a coherent language" (p. 78):

> I refuse to admit that I reify patients . . . when I administer psychotropic drugs. My respect for individual experience is great; on that point I consider myself to be a disciple of Laing and Cooper [*sic*].[42] . . . A current of passionate idealism, of mysticism, of prophesising, of romanticism and of pseudo-paranoiac rationalism is circulating in the pathetic "kingdom" of anti-psychiatry.[43]

Within this context, the use of *"idéalisme passionné"* is not a mixture of "idealism" and "passion;" it is rather a psychiatric category that refers to people who complain about or take action against certain working or living conditions. For traditional French psychiatry this is a form of paranoia. Maurel seems to feel that the real problems are not in the camps, asylums, or scientific and ideological delusions of false consciousness but in the psychotic irresponsibility of anti-psychiatry; this from the mouth of a man who does not fear to use "conscious and assumed paternalism," so as to be able to tolerate his "objective superiority over his patients without any anxiety" (p. 80). Henri Ey, who along with Koupernik had absolutely no sympathy for anti-psychiatry, felt obliged to say that:

> If being an anti-psychiatrist means to rebel against the mechanical and police style [of treatment] that psychiatry had locked itself and petrified itself in, then I consider myself to be the most fervent anti-psychiatrist, this is to say he who fights with all the strength of his experience and knowledge against false psychiatry which is but a blueprint of the mosaic of neurological syndromes or fatal constitutional diseases.[44]

This pattern of ambivalent acceptance of some of the basic elements of anti-psychiatry critique was seen by Cuau and Zigante as the method used to weaken and perhaps empty anti-psychiatry of its meaning:

> Within psychiatry the dominant principle is that: to be allowed to speak one must belong to the family and everyone knows that when one belongs to the family one doesn't mention what takes place within the family. We wash our dirty linen together. Together and in secret. It required nothing less than hooligans (*voyous*) like the English anti-psychiatrists to oblige the respectable medical corps, that uni-

formly felt aggressed, to wash its linen in public. But the sooner scores are settled the better.

Then they entitle the next part "refusing, ingesting, vomiting." "On that subject, a simple glimpse at what English anti-psychiatry became in France gives more information than all sorts of discourses. It [antipsychiatry] experienced its relationship to established science according to this immutable ternary rhythm: science, which first refuses the new, then ingests it, so as finally to vomit it. . . . The weak points [within the Laing/Cooper/Esterson framework] are obvious, but the attacks are systematically next to or past the weak points. Everyone can now fish around [in anti-psychiatry] and find what suits them" (p. 48).[45] Then follows a realistic parody of various debates and dinner-party conversations about British anti-psychiatry.[46]

Sztulman's brief history of anti-psychiatry traces it to Foucault, Laing, and Cooper (*Histoire de la folie à l'âge classique* and *The Divided Self*). There is again a blind spot in this kind of "historical" perception, perhaps because the task of working back from Laing and Cooper to Sullivan, Ganser, Sartre, and Minkowski was potentially embarrassing. The lack of any comment on Laing's interest in Minkowski is all the more surprising when one bears in mind that he was one of the founding members of *L'Évolution psychiatrique* itself.

The Breakdown of French Anti-Psychiatry into Three Fractions

Sztulman tries to define three areas of anti-psychiatry, to be able to appropriate some and distance himself from others:

> 1. *Anti psychiatrie d'origine:* mainly Laing and Cooper.
>
> 2. *Anti psychiatrisme rudimentaire:* No known authors—a state of mind (not a theory). "Aggressive, brutal, badly informed and visibly outraged protest . . . of those who disqualify psychiatry because it is part of law and order, reaction and repression. The psychiatrist gives way to brain police or medi-cops (*fliciatres*). These ideas are painted . . . in paranoiac rage."[47, 48]
>
> 3. Politopsychiatry, illustrated by Basaglia's book. "We already knew that we had to treat patients and their institutions. . . . Now the question is the relationships to production; this will bring a chain reaction, change of social (or class) relationships, change of ideology and finally the disappearance of mental illnesses" (p. 94).[49]

According to Cuau and Zigante, politopsychiatry means a position based on Sullivan-type theories of the psychosocial genesis of schizophrenia backed by Marx's early work. The distinctions are of interest in that they signify a path toward the appropriation of aspects of the anti-psychiatry critique as theorized by Cuau and Zigante—in French anti-psychiatry, Basaglia, Foucault, and Laing merge in kaleidoscopic combinations, thus distinctions are but a rearguard action. Relevant also is the fact that anti-psychiatry allowed nurses, psychiatrists, psychologists, and other members of staff to work in the belief that what happened in an asylum was relevant to the outside world. Irène Baloste-Fouletier's *Chronique de l'ordre asilaire*[50] illustrates problems of daily life with psychotic patients in a conservative institutional setting. Her page of international events from France, Vietnam, Cuba, and the United States preceding every chapter of micro-sociopsychiatric events illustrates a need to connect the struggles in the world to those in an asylum.

Waxing and Waning

Anti-psychiatry according to Cuau and Zigante died with Koupernik's articles in *Le Monde*[51] and *Le Nouvel Observateur*,[52] and with alternative attractions, G. Deleuze and F. Guattari's *Anti-Oedipus*, which provided "another year of conversations." It would live according to Delacampagne,[53] who defined it thus: "anti-psychiatry is perhaps first and foremost a state of mind, a language, a way of thinking, that is to say a way of life. It is not an ideal closed in upon itself or an easy to copy model but rather a perpetually renewed incitement to look beyond the appearances and prejudices that social conformism wraps us up in—at things themselves—and that according to Husserl's phenomenology that Sartre transmitted to Laing" (p. 67). But anti-psychiatry had no direct hold on institutions.[54] The strength of the reaction, the curious pattern in which everyone agreed with some of it, was an indication of the force of its impact, an impact so much stronger because it collided with the ideological crisis in France during the late sixties and early seventies. And Guy Baillon was, in our view, correct in arguing that the roots of anti-psychiatry were in part themselves US imports and that the debate that anti-psychiatry caused was in itself long overdue. The crystallization of anti-psychiatry in France was relatively short-lived; it found no lasting place in the French status quo, which could very schematically but accurately be represented by the debate between Henri Ey and Jacques Lacan.

Its clinical prehistory commenced with the problem raised by Ganser of Dresden and with Minkowski's dialectic alternative to Bleuler's schizophrenia. Its use of history (Césari–de Freminville) moved toward an analysis of theory as an ideological function rather than "scientific truth." In that sense, Laing's critique of genetic psychiatry was of fundamental (and overlooked) importance. In France anti-psychiatry was met with, or provoked a curious blind spot, and this is precisely an indication of the ideologization of the debate—the historical equivalent of a "negative hallucination."

We can but agree with J. P. Rumen when he stated that "anti-psychiatry is a word so vague that anyone can put whatever meaning he likes to it."[55] Its popularity reflected the depth of the crisis in France and in the world of mental health professionals. Says Dr. Angelergues (*L'Évolution psychiatrique*, i:1972):

> In France . . . anti-psychiatry provokes the most tumult and whips up the most passion. This is . . . linked to the present state of French psychiatry which is still largely contained in asylum segregation and the university order, shaken here and there—in more and more places—by explosions, which have brought about reforms . . . but neither the repeal of the 1838 law the systematic violation of which is the rule today . . . nor the bringing into being of new principles that would allow modern psychiatry to break with the asylums . . . and to move into the sector or community. In this troubled effervescence that nourishes an unprecedented mutation of minds and habits—in terms of which the symbolic gesture attributed to Pinel may appear derisory—anti-psychiatric models and ideology struck us as progressive fermentation—in theory and practice—as a negativist scandal, as a hope and as an illusion.

Angelergues argued that Pinel's mythical gesture—concocted over the years in the interests of a good conscience—now no longer offered a justification of certain types of praxis. Pinel's so-called gesture as an ideological and mythical guarantee of "psychiatric reason," no longer functioned quite with its usual blind inflexibility. Anti-psychiatry as debate was for Cuau and Zigante a reflection of the confused, contradictory, and chaotic history of the schizophrenia concept, with eyes focused on the etiological theories, so that Koupernik, whose *L'Anti-psychiatrie, sens ou non-sens* was a polite attempt to bury the whole question, wrote an article in the respected newspaper *Le Monde* (9 Feb. 1972, "De la cause au coupable," in "Libres Opinions"). In this article he was to tar with the same brush psychoanalysis, the Palo Alto group, and anti-psychiatry. It contains a remarkable *volte-face*, as if hardline biological psychiatry was desperately trying to wriggle out of the whole problem of the origins of psychotic disorders, as if by changing the definition of etiology from "study of causes of an illness, of an abnormality" to "analysis and discussion of causes that have combined to bring about the events of which history gives a picture"; as if the problem of the historical contradictions within the schizophrenia concept would politely bow out in the manner of an unwanted guest. "Of course that anti-psychiatry story had to finish with a punchline," argue Cuau and Zigante, "and Koupernik had to be the one who made the pun!"[56] Koupernik's recourse to the mass media was indicative of the fact that the May rebellion and Laing, Esterson, Cooper, and Foucault had catalyzed a public debate that also captured some of the interest generated by G. Debord and R. Vanegeim. In the October/December issue of *L'Évolution psychiatrique* (1972)—which announced the death of Minkowski—Harold Heyward contributed an anti-psychiatric poem, which came with an editorial note explaining that it was their "duty to publish it in full."

> (. . .) you have to fight us
> else society will again
> lock up its deviants!
> (. . .) they don't know how
> hard it is to work within anti-psychiatry.
> Have to think hard all the time,
> always on one's guard,
> (. . .)
> One becomes disgusted,
> because we still lock people up
> we still drug them
> and we clash with shrinks
> who sabotage our work with electroshocks
> (. . .)
> But then if [anti-psychiatry] is but
> our expression of the conflict of others
> then admit that that conflict
> before being externalised
> takes place within us
> that we are all psy
> and that anti-psychiatry
> IS WHAT WE ALL DO.

By the end of 1972 the counterattack was well under way with the reorganization of universities, the development of sectorization, changes in medical exam procedures, and a small increase in minimum wages. Those were the moves toward compromise that facilitated a return to a form of stability. Political agitation in French universities continued at Vincennes—which now had a department of psychoanalysis—and elsewhere. Small victories had been won: Vincennes gave official recognition to psycho-analysis as a university subject. The department is now run by J. A. Miller, Lacan's son-in-law, and in its early form this university allowed people who did not have a high school diploma, "Le Bac," as the French say, to study. The idea of sectorization was established slowly along with a network of small institutions—*lieux d'accueil* and *maisons de post-cure*—and also in experimental units like Laborde and Bonneuil.

Reviewing Georget's *De la folie*,[57] the historian Dr. Étienne Trillat argued that "M. Foucault has provoked much irritation . . . but we must recognise his merit in stimulating a taste for old, dusty works mummified in the back of the library; he has opened our eyes to a new way of reading old texts . . . most histories of psychiatry are subtended by an ideology that attributes a progression from obscurity towards the light" (p. 798).

The "ideology of psychiatric progress" was very much weakened, as was the functional value of the Pinel myth, but the Pinel myth cannot die unless the asylums are closed and the patients moved into small institutions. This myth or "adventure story" runs from the United States to Japan, with its lies and half-truths, because it brings comfort and rationalizes a degree of violence that might otherwise be ethically unacceptable. Nineteen seventy-four brought another issue of *L'Évolution psychiatrique* on anti-psychiatry including part of a medical thesis on Laing, and anti-psychiatry was by now food for reformist mainstream psychiatry.

Cuau and Zigante published *The Politics of Madness*, a French synthesis of anti-psychiatry written by two intellectuals who were neither medical doctors nor psychologists. It draws heavily on sources quoted in this chapter (Castel, SPK, Laing, Cooper, Gentis, Marx, Jervis, Foucault, Basaglia), argues for a sociology of mental illness, and introduces American sociological references (just as Racamier had done in 1957); of particular importance is the use of A. B. Hollingshead and F. C. Redlich's *Social Class and Mental Illness*. C. Koupernik published his book *Anti psychiatrie, sens ou non sens*, an interesting thermometer, lacking in any historical analysis of the origins of anti-psychiatry but a confirmation of the rainbow effect of anti-psychiatry as verbal label.

Conclusion

We have tried to connect the evolution of anti-psychiatry to the troubled history of ideas in the France of the past decades. Thus have we come full circle. The Spanish Civil War was closely linked to Tosquelles's experiment at St. Alban. Institutional psychotherapy, reborn in St. Alban, was given a birth certificate by Daumézon in 1952. An ideological foundation was provided by Laing, Esterson, Cooper, and Foucault. The May 1968 rebellion with its questioning of the basic structures of power in a modern society sanctioned the open conflict that was taking place in the psychiatric world. Years of inertia and indecision, backward asylum conditions and laws governing psychiatric practices were included in the general condemnation of modern French society. For some modern intellectuals the Third World offered the hope that it would purify a putrid France. Psychiatric institutions were seen as a kind of Third World of oppression within a France that had given up its former areas of colonization. The Gaullist chapter was closed. Anti-psychiatry had some of its most glorious days at the decline of the French empire with the disappearance of a conservative Gaullist regime. Though its heyday was over, it had accomplished an important role: It had introduced the ideas of Sullivan, Wynne, Bateson, and others into a country in part ready to adopt them as it had realized the limits of its institutional systems. Strangely enough, anti-psychiatry was also a delayed action of ideologies that seemed on the wane: Sartre and Minkowski were perhaps unduly forgotten by French psychiatry, but they hovered over the scene. Laing had grasped Minkowski's contribution to a dialectical understanding of schizophrenia that can never be subsumed by the Maginot line of Kraepelino-Bleulerian reason.

Anti-psychiatry was a plea for historicism in that it appealed for theory to be examined not as an aspect of "scientific truth" but as a function of ideology. Anti-psychiatry was also welcomed even by those who paid only lip-service to it because it pushed the debate about asylums and the nature of psychosis into the open and at the same time revealed a need for a historical perspective that was not sterilized by the ideology of medical "progress" but was nourished by an ocean of contradictory "pataphysics" and the misery of so many practical dead ends. Some French anti-psychiatry authors turned to US thinkers because they saw the sociology of psychosis as an instrument that would give the lie to both the purely organic and the psychogenic visions of madness. The idea that anti-psychiatry came from England in the early sixties is an absurd falsehood, an attempt to duck the issue and bury it. Rather we have tried to indicate that Laing, Cooper, and Esterson borrowed heavily from a plurality of historical perspectives and hence played the role of "unattached intellectuals"—the final synthesis was theirs, not the separate elements they rewrote. For this reason we state clearly that the fear and rejection that anti-psychiatry encountered was not only the mistrust of leftism but also the unwillingness of many to recognize the return of certain elements of French thinking to France often combined with a form of theoretical patriotism.

Anti-psychiatry as a loose set of ideas allowed or encouraged those who worked with psychotics in institutions to function in the belief that their struggles and hopes were meaningful and in some way linked to wars and other political dramas taking place all over the world; therein lies the sense of "politicopsychiatry," a word used by some to signify an ethical position and by others as an insult.

Of course anti-psychiatry is a mere fragment of the history of psychopathology, but it is more than intimately linked to the critique of Kraepelin and the kaleidoscopic history of the schizophrenia concept. To begin to feel the depth of the problem one should bear in mind the closing lines of Dr. Laing's first published paper, "An Instance of the Ganser Syndrome" (1953):

> The paralogia, the regression, the confused disoriented consciousness, the wholesale denial of unpleasant external reality, the hallucinosis, the generalized analgesia, together seem to constitute a peculiar constellation of ego defences which . . . are not perhaps . . . available to every hysteric.
>
> It would seem that this Ganser-like reaction may be understood as a massive, desperate, and temporary defence to a situation fraught with both internal and external danger to the ego. In this case the most intense and immediate danger was intrapsychic.

When one compares Ganser's work on hysteria (1897–1902)[58] to Bleuler's early contributions on schizophrenia (1908–11),[59] one has at least an idea of the history of scientific blind spots that motivated the thinking of R. D. Laing. No one who took a serious interest in Ganser and Minkowski could have taken Bleuler's work at face value or approved of Ellen West as a paradigm of schizophrenia.

Finally, then, anti-psychiatry was the sphere in which scientific and historical deadlocks were exposed to the cold light of day; theory was seen as ideology; Bleulerian "reason" faded and the ideological value of the myth of Pinel, as Angelergues stated, became derisory. Precisely for these reasons, we reject the seductively simple convenience of "anti-psychiatry is dead." Who are we to say that there is no one left in the cave of Adullam, or that the historical and clinical problem of schizophrenia is somehow solved?

Notes

We would like to thank Sylvie Ribes, reader in history at the University of Paris VII, who typed and retyped the manuscript with care and professional intelligence.

1. J. Gabel: "L'Oeuvre d'Eugène Minkowski," *L'Évolution psychiatrique*, lxi–ii (1991), 432.

2. Foucault is an example of the problem; the fact that many sympathizers of the anti-psychiatric movement quote him does not mean that he belongs to such or such a movement. This appears to be the intellectual and historical equivalent of an optical illusion. This illusion was probably reinforced outside of France by the fact that Laing published Foucault in his collection. Lacan and Mannoni published works by David Cooper in the prestigious "Le Champ Freudien" collection. To see them as part of the same thing is nonetheless absurd.

3. J. Postel, M. Postel, J. P. Rumen, "The Paradoxes of the Anti-psychiatric Movement," *Information psychiatrique*, xlv (1969), 1105. Sylvie Faure refers to this work on the problem of the semantics of anti-psychiatry in a double issue of the review *La Nef*, no. 42, January–May 1971, a document entirely devoted to French anti-psychiatry, its meaning and origins. We shall comment more fully on both documents.

4. L. Wittgenstein, *Tractatus Logico-Philosophicus*, 8th ed. (London: Routledge & Kegan Paul, 1960), 57.

5. M. Lafont, *L'Extermination douce* (Nantes: Areppi, 1987).

6. The title may be a nod in Kretschmer's direction; this would not be surprising in that Kretschmer theorizes an invisible psychic choice in Ganser-type hysteria, whereas Lacan argues a "forced choice" in psychosis that would disallow the unity of the real, the symbolic, and the imaginary.

Cf. E. Kretschmer (French trans. Jankelevitch), *Manuel théorique et pratique de psychologie médicale* (Paris: Payot, 1927). (Subheading "La causalité psychique," p. 307.) Lacan quotes this book in his 1932 thesis; cf. p. 373 of the Le François edition (1932), cf. also E. Kretschmer, *Hysteria Reflex and Instinct,* (Eng. trans. V. and W. Baskin) (London: Peter Owen, 1961), 24–29) for Kretschmer's interpretation of the Ganser-type phenomenon.

For Lacan's theory of psychosis see, *Le Séminaire sur les psychoses* (Paris: Le Seuil, 1981), *Écrits: A Selection* (New York: Norton, 1977), his thesis and his "discours de clôture" in *Enfance aliénée* (Paris: Denoël, 1984). The last document is of particular importance for us in that it represents an apparent meeting point between anti-psychiatry and Lacanian thought.

7. G. Amado, *Fondements de la psychopathologie* (Paris: P.U.F., 1982), 264.

8. J. Lacan, in *Recherches Philosophiques* (Paris, v, 1935–1936), 424–431.

9. J. Lacan, *Écrits: A Selection,* trans. Sheridan, 184. Les psychoses, livre III, 163.

10. H. Ey, *La Notion de schizophrénie* (DDB: 1977), 228. (This posthumous homage to Ey cannot be considered as being in any way representative of the depth or scope of Ey's work. See the special issue on Henri Ey, *L'Évolution psychiatrique* (1977) for a bibliography of his publications.

11. J. Oury, *Psychiatrie et psychothérapie institutionnelle* (Paris: Payot, 1976), 57.

12. G. Debord, *The Society of the Spectacle,* section 218 (our trans.). Cf. also Raoul Vaneigem's *The Revolution of Everyday Life,* approved trans. Nicholson Smith (London: Left Bank Books and Rebel Press, 1983). This book was quoted by Cooper in *The Death of the Family* (London: Pelican Books, 1974), 107.

13. R. D. Laing, "An Instance of the Ganser Syndrome." *Journal of the Royal Army Medical Corps,* ic (1953), 169–172.

14. François Dosse, *Histoire du structuralisme,* 2 vols. (Paris: La Découverte, 1991–1992).

15. E. Roudinesco, *La Bataille de cent ans, histoire de la psychanalyse en France (1925– 1985)* (Paris: Seuil), ii, 494–496. (Cf. also the U.S. translation of this volume, 1986.)

16. This was "mischief" according to Roudinesco.

17. J. P. Rumen, *La Nef,* no. 42, January–May 1971, 39.

18. For an account of the historical conflict between state-guaranteed medicine and healers of all sorts, see Dr. Maurice Igert, *Le problème des guérisseurs* (Paris: Vigot, 1931). On page 14, Igert points out the difficulty of having faith healers punished by courts. In 1972 the problem was not so much faith healers—although the problem remained—but the mass production of psychologists by the new universities who, with analytic training, might well "compete" with psychiatrists. For sociological reasons such people would have gravitated to the Left and been more likely to gravitate toward Lacanian thinking. Cf. also G. Lapassade's introduction to Puységur's *Mémoires* (Toulouse: Privat, 1986) and J. Carroy's brilliant study of magnetism, hypnotism and suggestion in nineteenth-century France: *Hypnose, suggestion et psychologie* (Paris: P.U.F., 1991).

19. R. D. Laing, *The Divided Self* (Pelican, 1973), cf. 28–31.

20. H. Heyward and M. Varigas, *Une Anti psychiatrie* (Éditions Universitaires, 1971), cf. 19–33. Cf. also Kraepelin, *Lectures on Clinical Psychiatry,* 3rd ed. (London: Baillière, Tindall and Cox, 1913), 79.

21. See also E. Fuller Torrey, *Schizophrenia and Civilisation* (New York: J. Aronson, 1981) and, of course, Devereux.

22. J. Postel, introduction to the French edition of Kraepelin's *Clinical Psychiatry* (Toulouse: Privat, 1970).

23. Ibid.

24. Navarin published an edition of *Clinical Psychiatry,* and Ornicar published new translations on paranoia.

25. J. Postel, introduction, Kraepelin, *Clinical Psychiatry.*

26. M. Mannoni, *Le Psychiatre, son "fou" et la psychanalyse* (Paris: Le Seuil, 1970).

27. J. Postel, M. Postel, J. P. Rumen, "The paradoxes."

28. See "On Periodic or Intermittent Mania," *History of Psychiatry,* iii, Part 3, no. 11, (1992).

29. Richard Evans, *Rencontres avec Laing* (Paris: Belfond, 1979).

30. According to Gabel, that is blindness to history.

31. Tosquelles uses the verb *récupérer,* which can mean *go and get, to salvage* (as in finding a usable chair in a rubbish dump), or *to be modified ideologically, to sell out to the powers that be.* Tosquelles uses the ideological meaning here. (Tissot was not an MD, but a monk.) Cf. also R. Castel's remarkable *L'Ordre psychiatrique,* ch. 5, for more information on Tissot.

32. It took more than a century and a half to come to terms with the founding myth of French psychiatry, Pinel's "freeing" the lunatics. Cf. Postel, *La Genèse de la psychiatrie* (Paris: Le

Sycomore, 1981). In our view myths appear in the history of psychopathology for ideological reasons, that is, because of an abstraction of history. To that extent the very semantics of anti-psychiatry tend toward myth, to cloud the issues. Giovanni Jervis was quite right to refer to *Le Mythe de l'antipsychiatrie* (Paris: Solin, 1977).

33. H. Simon, *For A More Active Therapeutics in the Psychiatric Hospital.* An English-language edition may well have a different title; this is simply the literal translation of the French title.

34. This is a reference to propaganda used during the Occupation by the Nazis. The idea was to identify the Soviet army as people who raped nuns and thereby encourage French volunteers to fight on the Russian front. The strength of this propaganda is tragically well illustrated in the remarkable historical film *Le chagrin et la pitié.*

35. We have chosen this translation because it has already been used by Martin Gittelman. An alternative would have been geo-psychiatry (Tosquelles). Cf. Gittelman, "Sectorisation: The Quiet Revolution in European Mental Health Cure," *American Journal of Orthopsychiatry*, xlii (1) (January 1972).

36. M. Fourré, *Les lieux d'accueil* (Nice: Z'éditions, 1991).

37. R. Lefort and R. Lefort, preface to M. Fourré, *Les lieux d'accueil* (Nice: Z'éditions, 1991).

38. This document is reproduced *in extenso* in Fourré, *Les lieux d'accueil.* Her book is a critical account of some alternatives to hospitals written from a Lacanian perspective.

39. SPK, *Faire de la maladie une arme* (Paris: Champ Libre, 1973).

40. Eugène Minkowski's daughter Jeannine tells the following story: Before World War II her mother, Dr. Minkowska, went to a congress where she heard a Dr. Rudin speak of sterilization. Dr. Minkowska argued, insulted Rudin, and walked out. During the Occupation the family feared revenge and deportation (personal communication). The family survived but was not allowed out of Paris until 1945.

41. Within the SPK perspective, elements of traditional psychiatry move against the patient, so that *anti-psychiatry* might be taken to mean psychiatry in favor of patient freedom and well-being. The problem is one of ideological choice rather than clinical observation.

42. *L'Évolution psychiatrique* (1972), 79.

43. Ibid., 82.

44. Ibid.

45. B. Cuau and D. Zigante, *La politique de la folie* (Paris: Lutter, Stock 2, 1974).

46. Ibid.

47. *L'Évolution psychiatrique*, op. cit.

48. See also, for example, P. Bernardet, *Les dossiers noirs de l'internement psychiatrique* (Paris: Fayard, 1989).

49. *L'Évolution psychiatrique*, op. cit.

50. Irène Baloste-Fouletier, *Chronique de l'ordre asilaire* (Paris: Maspero, 1973).

51. *Le Monde*, 9 February 1972.

52. *Le Nouvel Observateur*, 21 February 1972.

53. Delacampagne, *Anti-psychiatrie, Les voies du sacré* (Paris: Grasset, 1974).

54. R. Castel, *Sociologie du travail* (Paris: Le Seuil, no., 1, 1975).

55. J. P. Rumen, *La Nef.*

56. Cuau and Zigante, *La politique de la folie*, 79.

57. Georget, *De la folie* (Privat, 1972). Selected articles presented by J. Postel.

58. Cf. the historical presentation of one of his papers in *L'Évolution psychiatrique* 3–4 (1992).

59. See E. Bleuler, *The Clinical Roots of the Schizophrenia Concept* (1908) (Cambridge: Cambridge University Press, 1987) and *Dementia Praecox or the Group of Schizophrenias*, trans. Zinkin (New York: International Universities Press, 1950).

Bibliography

Books

I. Baloste-Fouletier, *Chronique de l'Ordre Asilaire* (Paris: Maspéro, 1973).

P. Bernardet, *Les Dossiers Noirs de l'Internement Psychiatrique* (Paris: Fayard, 1989).

R. Castel, *L'Ordre Psychiatrique* (Paris: Éditions de Minuit, 1976).

G. Césari, *Psychiatrie et Pouvoir* (Paris: Anthropos, 1979).

G. Césari, *Critique de la Raison Délirante* (Paris: Anthropos, 1984).

B. Cuau and D. Zigante, *La Politique de la Folie* (Paris: Stock, 1974).

G. Debord, *La Société du Spectacle* (Paris: Champ Libre, 1983, 1st ed., 1967).

B. De Freminville, *La Raison du plus Fort* (Paris: Seuil, 1977).

C. Delacampagne, *Antipsychiatrie, Les Voies du Sacré* (Paris: Grasset, 1974).

C. Delacampagne, *Figures de l'Opression* (Paris: P.U.F., 1977).

F. Dosse, *Histoire du Structuralisme*, 2 vols. (Paris: La Découverte, 1991–1992).

R. Evans, *Rencontres avec Laing* (Paris: Belfond, 1979).

M. Fourré, *Les lieux d'Accueil* (Nice: Z'éditions, 1991).

E. Fuller Torrey, *Schizophrenia and Civilisation* (New York: Jason Aronson, 1980).

S. Fullinwider, *Technicians of the Finite* (Westport, Connecticut: Greenwood Press, 1982).

R. Gentis, *Les Murs de l'Asile* (Paris: Maspéro, 1971).

R. Gentis, *Traité de Psychiatrie Provisoire* (Paris: Maspéro, 1977).

E. Goffman, *Asylums* (New York: Anchor, 1961; French trans. with presentation by R. Castel, Paris: Éditions de Minuit, 1968).

J. Henry and L. Leger, *Les Hommes se Droguent, l'Etat se Renforce* (Paris: Champ Libre, 1976).

H. Heyward and M. Varigas, *Une Antipsychiatrie* (Paris: Édition Universitaire, 1971).

G. Jervis, *Le Mythe de l'Antipsychiatrie*, trans. de Freminville (Paris: Solin, 1977).

E. Kraepelin, *Leçons Cliniques* (Toulouse: Privat, 1970), presentation and introduction by J. Postel.

J. Lacan, *Écrits* (New York: Norton, 1977).

R. D. Laing and D. Cooper, *Reason and Violence* (London: Tavistock, 1964), foreword by J.-P. Sartre.

R. D. Laing, *Wisdom, Madness and Folly* (London: Macmillan, 1985).

J. Oury, *Psychiatrie et Psychothérapie Institutionnelle* (Paris: Payot, 1976).

J. C. Polack, *La Médecine du Capital* (Paris: Maspéro, 1971).

E. Roudinesco, *Histoire de la Psychanalyse en France*, 2 vols. (Paris: Le Seuil, 1986).

S. P. K., *Faire de la Maladie une Arme* (Paris: Champ Libre, 1973); German edition, *Aus der Krankheit eine Waffe machen* (Munich: Trikant-Verlag, 1972).

S. P. K., *Psychiatrie Politique, l'Affaire de Heidelberg* (Paris: Maspéro, 1973).

R. Vaneigem, *The Revolution of Everyday Life* (Paris: Gallimard, 1967, 1992; London: Left Bank Books and Rebel Press, 1983).

K. S. Weinberg, *Society and Personality Disorders* (New York: Prentice-Hall, 1952).

Articles in Journals

R. Castel, "Genèse et ambiguïtés de la notion de secteur en psychiatrie," *Sociologie du travail* (Paris: Seuil, 1975, I).

P. Fedida, "Psychose et parenté (Naissance de l'Antipsychiatrie)," *Critique*, cclvii (1968), 870–895.

J. Lacan, "Review of Lived Time," *Recherches philosophiques*, v (1935–1936), 424–431.

R. D. Laing, "Minkowski and Schizophrenia," *Review of Existential Psychology*, ix (1963), 195–207.

R. D. Laing, "An Instance of the Ganser Syndrome," *Journal of the Royal Army Medical Corps*, ic (1953), 169–172.

A. Meyer, "Approach to the Investigation of Dementia Praecox," *Chicago Medical Recorder*, xxxiv (1917).

J. Postel, M. Postel, J. P. Rumen, "Les paradoxes du mouvement anti-psychiatrique," *Information psychiatrique*, xlv (1969), 1105.

R. Scott and P. Ashworth, "Closure and the First Schizophrenic Breakdown," *British Journal of Medical Psychology*, xl (1967), 109–145.

Suggested Background Reading and Additional References

J. Cutting and M. Shepherd (eds.), *The Clinical Roots of the Schizophrenia Concept* (Cambridge: Cambridge University Press, 1987).

M. Mannoni, introduction to *Enfance Aliénée* (Denoël, Paris, 1984) (1st ed. *Enfance Aliénée, Recherches*, Sept. 1967, Dec. 1968).

L'Anti-psychiatrie, written roundtable discussion organized by C. Koupernik (Paris: P.U.F., 1974).

Réseau, "Alternative à la Psychiatrie," Collectif International, Union générale d'edition. Collection 10–18, Paris, 1977. A European presentation of anti-psychiatry in its practical evolution. (Castel, Guattari, Cooper, Jervis, Basaglia, Schatzman, Scott et al.). A document of capital importance that shows which elements of anti-psychiatry survived in practice and how various shades of anti-psychiatry combined in a network of alternatives.

La Folie, i–ii (U.G.E.—10.–18.) 1977, (J. Oury, J. C. Polak, A. Esterson, C. Descamps, D. Cooper . . .).

La Violence, i–ii (U.G.E.—10.–18.) 1978, (J. Ayme, Solers, Zizek, Deligny, Benoit . . .). Both edited by A. Verdiglione.

Journals

Recherches, xvii (March 1975), (Paris: Fontenay sous Bois), "History of sectorisation."

L'Évolution psychiatrique: Anti-psychiatry (Angelergues, Ey, Morel, and discussions and reviews of anti-psychiatry texts), i (1972); Anti-psychiatry poem and favorable review of French ed. "Death of the Family" (Cooper), by Davidovitch, iv (1972); "Sociotherapy and Group Psychotherapy," Tosquelles, Daumézon, Ey, iii (1952).

Four articles on anti-psychiatry including part of Layley's medical thesis on Laing, i (1974): "Anti-psychiatry: A Critical Article," Seabra Dinis, iv (1973), 789–805; "Marxism and Psychiatry," iv (1976), 733–786; "The Schizophrenias," a remarkable document. Leclaire presents Lacan's vision of psychosis, doing for preclusion what K. Abraham did for narcissism in 1908, ii–iii (1958); "Schizophrenia and the Family," ii (1975), 339–430.

La Nef, i, no. 42, (1971), (double issue on Anti-psychiatry), 247 pp.

Soins Psychiatriques (Cooper, G. Pankow etc.), 14 Dec. 1981.

"Procès du S.P.K.," *Cahiers de Recherches* (1972/73).

21

Psychiatry and Anti-Psychiatry in the United States

NORMAN DAIN

The growth of anti-psychiatric ideas and activism in the United States during the past thirty years is only the most recent and most extensive upsurge of religious and secular viewpoints largely formulated in the late nineteenth century and played out in different forms thereafter. The nature of anti-psychiatry and its periodic resurgence and decline is the subject of this essay.

Just as there is no widely accepted definition of mental illness and therefore of psychiatry so there is no commonly accepted definition of anti-psychiatry. Anti-psychiatry is an amorphous concept that has never had any fixed meaning. It has changed over time and in connection with religious, legal, political, and social concerns as well as changes in psychiatry and the mental hospital, psychiatry's major venue before the mid-twentieth century. Nor has there ever existed a real anti-psychiatry movement, disagreements among opponents of psychiatry having precluded an attempt to create organized activism with a coherent outlook and recognized leaders. Virtually the only common characteristic exhibited by those one might call anti-psychiatry has been hostility to psychiatry, the medical specialty dealing with mental disorders. (For convenience the terms *psychiatry* and *psychiatrist* will be used for the entire period, from the beginning of the speciality in the eighteenth century to our own time, although the terms first came into use during the late decades of the nineteenth century.) Anti-psychiatry can therefore be defined only as sets of attitudes, opinions, and activities antagonistic to psychiatry, ranging from sharp, serious criticism of psychiatry to absolute denial of its validity and questioning of the concept of mental disorder as a medical entity.

The distinction between anti-psychiatry and criticism of psychiatry is often a distinction without a difference, but anti-psychiatry advocates characteristically differ from critics in their more hostile attitude toward psychiatry. Therefore, although the term *anti-psychiatry* is imprecise and often more confusing than revealing, it remains at present the best term available, for it catches the emotional quality evident among opponents of psychiatry, who were not necessarily skilled logicians, philosophers, or scientists, and whose arguments contained contradictions. The arguments were, however, not thereby pointless or ineffective.

Anti-psychiatry can perhaps best be understood as a variety of groups and individuals who believed that psychiatry was either a vehicle for or an obstacle to attaining certain goals that they valued, goals that often went beyond concern about the plight of mental patients or the faults of psychiatry. Much anti-psychiatry has been primarily interested in the power and influence wielded by the psychiatric profession, not only over the mentally ill but over society as a whole. Opposition to psychiatry has often been part of a larger agenda in which mental patients are of incidental concern.

Both psychiatry and its antithesis, anti-psychiatry, have also been much affected by the singular nature of mental illness as a supposed disorder of the mind, whose "loss" has been seen as a catastrophe, a descent into a nonhuman, even damnable state that can, in its violent or anti-social forms, threaten society. Psychiatry could gain sympathy for the "insane" and status for itself by claiming to restore sick minds, but it could also not help being stigmatized by the common horror and fear of insanity and of institutionalization. And certain of the religious could not help seeing psychiatry as competing with priestly ministration to the insane. Furthermore, psychiatry, concerned as it was with "unhealthy" or pathological human behavior, thought, and feeling, took on to itself a certain authority about what constituted correct—or healthy—behavior, thought, and feeling. Such authority, secular and often nonjudgmental, moved beyond the mental hospital to virtually every aspect of living; as such it could be seen as threatening traditional morality and encroaching upon the realms of religion, law, and social life. Psychiatry dealt with the mind, whose essential nature was a matter of philosophical and religious dispute and whose relation to the body was not scientifically established. Hence psychiatry would be subject to scrutiny—and self-doubt—deeper and sharper than that experienced by other, more unequivocally somatic medical specialties, especially when it failed to make the scientific and therapeutic progress exhibited by those specialties. Psychiatry had many vulnerabilities; anti-psychiatry played upon them and off them.

The so-called mental illnesses have a long history but only relatively recently have physicians played a prominent role in the care and treatment of the mentally ill. In the late eighteenth and early nineteenth centuries Western European and North American physicians first sought to monopolize the care of the insane, through superintending the new asylums built to succor and control them. But in the United States by this time, even before the formal organization of the American psychiatric profession in 1844 into the American Association of Medical Superintendents of Asylums for the Insane (predecessor of the American Psychiatric Association), there was already criticism of the medical profession's role in treating and caring for those called insane, especially among clergymen, jurists, and former mental patients.

For the religious the problem of insanity was of long standing. The tendency of medicine to naturalism had long bedeviled Christian thinkers, most of whom nevertheless made a legitimate place for physicians in the treatment of bodily ills. Insanity or madness, however, was more problematical than the so-called physical illnesses. In traditional Christian thought the mind was closely associated with the soul and assumed to be, like the soul, immortal and impervious to disease. If, on the other hand, insanity was a physical disorder of the brain, as eighteenth-century physicians usually insisted, and the mind simply the brain functioning, as some materialists maintained, then the brain, the mind, and the soul as well were subject to disease and death; therefore the Christian concept of the immortal soul was invalid. Christian religion was hence thought by some theologians to be endangered by the materialism of the developing profession of psychiatry.[1]

For Christians only a miracle could bridge the gap between brain and mind, or soul. But in practical terms Christianity allowed medicine a role in the treatment of insanity by attributing insanity, like illness in general, to punishment for sin for which the sufferers might win God's forgiveness through confession and prayer; only then would medical treatment prove effective. But if the devil or his minions were thought to have invaded an individual, medical ministrations were disallowed. Possession, even if its symptoms resembled or resulted in madness, was a problem for the Church: Its ministry, not physicians, would ultimately decide the nature and disposition of the case. Apparently madness as punishment for sin differed from demonic possession in that in the former case God directly imposed madness while in the latter he gave the devil permission to send evil spirits to possess the sinner. In the first case one sought God's forgiveness after which medicine might be effective. In the latter case religious healers called upon Christ to counteract or expel the devil or his minions as if the cause of the disorder was primarily the devil's independent action; medicine was here inappropriate and ineffective, a view West European and American physicians increasingly contested from the eighteenth century onward.

In practice, mainstream conservative Calvinist ministers such as the eminent Cotton Mather or Jonathan Edwards in seventeenth- and eighteenth-century New England had an ambivalent attitude toward the physician's role in the treatment of insanity. Although in theory sin was commonly considered the cause of insanity, sympathetic individuals who became insane, especially among the clergy, were in Mather's and Edwards's view freed of guilt for their disorder. Mather wondered whether his wife's madness might be caused, if not by sin, by heredity. Edwards saw a charitable clergyman ministering to Native Americans as being attacked by the devil for his good works albeit the clergyman was often melancholic and thereby vulnerable to the evil one, and, one might add, not wholly free from responsibility for his eventual madness because melancholia was often thought to be the consequence of sin.[2] This equivocal position that illness resulted from sin but that nevertheless one might not be condemnable opened the gates for the use of medicine but still allowed some of the religious to denounce the use of medicine as irreligious. At the same time, both Mather and Edwards were attracted to Newtonian science, and near the end of his life Mather wrote a manuscript, "The Angel of Bethesda," in which he gave medicine a major role in the treatment of insanity.[3]

The late seventeenth-century trend among the British upper classes to deprecate religious enthusiasm as dangerous to public order was observable in North America as well. Especially important was the reaction to the Salem witchcraft trials, which contributed toward putting in doubt supernatural explanations for all sorts of phenomena, including insanity. By the mid-eighteenth century medical views of mental disorders, increasingly influential in Britain, won widespread support among the upper classes in several of the North American colonies. The association among the religious of illness with sin as evidence for the existence of the devil and therefore of God was successfully challenged or at least bypassed by an assertive medical profession, some of whose members were now specializing in the study and treatment of insanity.

Most of the mainstream religious leaders about whom we have information accommodated to the new psychiatry, though not always without conflict or cost. This accommodation represented a growing loss of authority over not only the insane but, more importantly, over the interpretation of human nature and the nature of sin and crime, and over modes of rearing and educating children. The secularization of American life strengthened medicine and weakened religious authority, to the point where some psychiatrists in the late eighteenth and early nineteenth centuries were sufficiently sure of themselves to criticize the evangelical preachers whose revival meetings periodically swept the Northeast. Their hellfire sermons, the physicians charged, terrorized people and drove some of them mad. The revivalist leadership denied the charge and insisted that religion and especially revivals protected most persons' mental health, but that in any event the saving of souls was more important than saving mental health. The revivalists viewed secular medical values as secondary; health was not the primary concern of religion nor should it be of society. In effect, revivalists, and indeed most Christian (Protestant) churches before the Civil War, had largely surrendered their healing role to medicine, animal magnetism, and a host of popular nostrums.[4] Increasingly, physicians no longer needed to appeal to the great physician Christ as a precondition for success. Perhaps equally significant, but little noticed, was the admission of revivalist leaders, such as Jonathan Edwards and his nineteenth-century successor Charles Grandison Finney, that saving one's soul might in rare cases endanger one's mental health. The breach between religion's role of saving souls and that of curing human ills meant that a growing medical profession could step in.

Although revivalists continued to preach about damnation for sins, psychiatrists could and sometimes did exclude such preachers from mental hospitals because their sermons terrified patients and undermined physicians' authority. Nevertheless, explicit anti-psychiatry was not a theme in the revivalist movement nor in most established religions; indeed, Quakers played a major role in initiating private mental hospitals. Many clergymen saw psychiatry as a humanitarian movement; they were also intimidated by the successful developments in science and believed, as did Finney, that there was no inherent conflict between science and religion. In contrast to the turmoil in medicine that threatened the authority of the general practitioner in the first half of the nineteenth century, the new profession of psychiatry enjoyed much public prestige. The new mental hospitals, both private and state sponsored, which increasingly came under the direction of medical superintendents, reflected acceptance by laypeople of the importance of establishing asylums to cure madness and to protect society from the insane and the insane from themselves. These institutions advocated and some actually practiced a new, hopeful form of therapy called moral treatment that sought to create a therapeutic, familial environment in which the insane, considered sick rather than sinful, would be treated as much like sane people as possible. Elite religious and secular groups alike initially considered moral treatment highly successful and worthy of public support.

There were condemnations of psychiatry as anti-religious, as materialist, and as a threat to morality, but such charges did not win widespread support until after the Civil War, and then more among nonestablishment churchgoers and ministries than the old, mainstream religions. Anti-psychiatry views gained coherence and energy when new churches were founded with the express purpose of replacing secular medicine with religiously oriented therapy. Such challenges coincided with psychiatry's loss of optimism. By the closing decades of the nineteenth century, mental hospitals, especially the crowded, underfunded state institutions, had become less therapeutic than custodial; moral treatment had not proved to be a panacea, especially for chronic patients, and anyway it was too expensive for state hospitals to maintain; and medicine and psychiatry, influenced by the new science, were becoming more materialist and deterministic.

In part in reaction to the growing influence of science and secularism in American society and to the mainstream churches' accommodation to the new trends, new Christian religions commonly known as the Metaphysical movement arose and gathered force in the late nineteenth century.[5] This occurred at the same time that spiritualism, which sought to create a science dealing with nonmaterial phenomena, was still popular. The Metaphysical movement was, and remains, not an isolated phenomenon but very much in tune with all sorts of popular religious and spiritualist movements that did not necessarily consider themselves anti-medical or anti-science but that dwelled on the so-called nonmaterial aspects of life and tended to be anti-establishment.

The Metaphysical movement differed from most Christian denominations in that, in effect, its adherents believed that the millennium was not to be found in some distant future but had always existed as a creation of God's mind. It offered people everlasting life free of disease if they only accepted and practiced its teachings. Where other Christian religions held medicine in awe and could not but praise or at least respect its efforts on behalf of suffering humanity even while physicians deprecated Christian biblical teachings about miraculous cures, the members of the Metaphysical movement took a definite stand denying the validity of medicine. Of course, even Christians who did not dispute the reality of the material world accepted a higher nonmaterial power: God could work outside the material laws of nature. Philosophically, Christians generally believed that the world was a product of God's thought, as Christian Scientists and other members of the Metaphysical movement claimed. Where they differed was in the Metaphysicalists' belief that human beings could create reality as God did, by thought.

Most visible and authoritarian in organization among the new healing churches was Christian Science, whose founder, Mary Baker Eddy, denied the independent reality of the material world, which, she insisted, was the product of thought. The illnesses that medicine described and treated were of its own creation. Only thought, which created the world, could eliminate illness and death. Eddy's religion aimed to replace traditional medicine with healers who would educate people in right thinking and thus free humankind of disease, suffering, and death.[6] Obviously there was no place for psychiatry and mental hospitals in Christian Science. In fact, however, the matter was not so simple. Eddy believed in malicious animal magnetism, which she greatly feared personally—the idea that one could create an illness or even commit murder by projecting harmful thoughts. This was a conclusion one could draw from Metaphysical religions that stressed mind over matter. Eddy gathered together a number of her supporters, who would, by thought, ward off the evil thoughts of her enemies, that is, those who did not agree with her and whom she feared contested her authority. The power and safety that Eddy and fellow members of the Metaphysical movement believed their religions provided had a dark—and nontherapeutic or anti-therapeutic—side not obvious to most of their supporters or detractors. Furthermore, mind did not always prove itself the master of matter; Christian Scientists and members of the Metaphysical movement did become ill, and some remained immune to Metaphysical healing.

Significant though it was, Christian Science and, for that matter, the Metaphysical movement as a whole did not have as devastating an impact upon psychiatry as the profession feared it might. Even though psychiatrists eventually turned pessimistic about their ability to cure insanity, mental hospitals provided the only extensive system of care and custody for the mentally ill. Discrediting psychiatry's therapeutic effectiveness still left society without an acceptable alternative means of dealing with the insane, whose numbers would increase as the population grew. The movement to build more hospitals to transfer the insane from jails, almshouses, and the community continued. Neither Christian Science nor any other religious movement, with very rare exceptions like the Society of Friends, made provision for those whom they treated but who nevertheless did not recover.

The failures of religious therapy more often than not made their way into public mental hospitals, jails, or the streets and countryside. As long as this situation prevailed, psychiatry had a role to play that provided it with protection from all manner of criticism and rejection. What in part ''saved'' psychiatry as a medical discipline was its practitioners' insistence that effective treatment and the safety, economy, and convenience of society required confinement of the insane in a mental hospital directed by psychiatrists. Psychiatry offered a way to deal with a real social, economic, and personal problem. Furthermore, the new mind cure sects, although they attracted masses of people, tended in the nineteenth century and through most of the twentieth to be marginal, out of the religious mainstream, and not very powerful in the major institutions of American society. And not all the new Christian movements devoted to mental healing were anti-psychiatry. The Emmanuel movement of the early twentieth century sought the support of the psychiatric profession and adopted a policy of sending those they considered psychotic to psychiatrists for treatment.

Psychiatrists themselves were inconsistent in their approach to conditions treated by the religious mind cure practitioners. For example, psychiatrists derisively called persons who had allegedly been cured by the lay healers ''hysterics'' and termed them not truly mentally ill. Their ''cure,'' psychiatrists asserted, was merely consequent to the mental influence of popular or charismatic healers; the truly mentally ill who supposedly suffered from a physical disorder would not respond, except temporarily, to such methods. But when medical men—psychiatrists and the practitioners of the new medical specialty of neurology—did turn their attention to such patients their symptoms were legitimated. The leading American neurologist Weir Mitchell dubbed their affliction *neurasthenia* and subjected neurasthenics to his famous rest cure; Charcot hypnotized them; Freud renamed them neurotics. Once psychiatrists started to treat hysteria, they came to consider it a true mental illness, not just a symptom of the normal state of many weak-willed women.

Even the claim, so derided by psychiatrists, of Eddy and her Metaphysical opponent W. F. Evans that medical means were unnecessary and harmful[7] was in the twentieth century repeated by American psychoanalysts, some of whom preached a secular mind cure. The psychiatric profession had long been conflicted or at least ambivalent in its views about the etiology and proper therapy for the mentally ill and united only in opposition to competitors. Much of anti-psychiatry involved interpreting negatively or from a different perspective ideas and practices that were in dispute or even accepted within psychiatry. The key difference was that the religious view was based on a largely Christian view of humankind: Etiology and cure were ultimately supernatural and in the final analysis not under the unaided control of human beings. Yet a century later an undoubted materialist such as psychiatrist Thomas Szasz, who rejected almost all the assumptions and premises of Christian Scientists and the Metaphysical movement, came to comparable conclusions respecting psychiatry: that mental illness is largely a product of the psychiatric profession's self-interest, that there is really little or no valid role for institutional psychiatry, that psychiatry and mental hospitals are the problem not the solution, and that a change in the public's views on the subject would largely eliminate the so-called problem of insanity. How to account for the similarities? Psychiatry could not establish the etiology of most forms of mental disorder, and psychiatrists could not agree on a unified theory of brain and mind. Consequently, whether opponents started from an immaterialist, dualist, or materialist point of view, they could dismiss the idea of mind as a functioning brain, with no independent existence, and hence deny to psychiatry an unequivocal role as a medical specialty treating what was basically brain pathology.

Psychiatry itself had trouble with this concept of mind-brain unity. The diversity of opinion within the psychiatric profession over the role of medicine as opposed to psychological and social factors in etiology and therapy raised many of the issues dealt with by the religious. From the late eighteenth century to the decline of moral treatment after the Civil War, psychiatrists were ambivalent about the value or relevance of psychiatry as a medical specialty. The initial introduction of moral treatment in England, a system of care that the Society of Friends in Frankford, Pennsylvania (now in Philadelphia) advocated early in the nineteenth century, stressed religious, social, and psychological factors to the neglect and even exclusion of medicine. The psychiatrists who soon came to dominate the new asylums established on principles of moral treatment denied the validity and value of evangelical preaching, in part because of its emotionalism, but were themselves practitioners of a therapy that emphasized moral suasion, that is, they relied largely on the positive effects of emotion and a favorable psychological as well as physical environment. Even the often strict somaticists of a succeeding generation of psychiatrists appealed to patients' emotions through the use of restraint, punishment, and rewards, which were considered essential in disciplining patients and therefore to restoring their sanity. What then separated the emotionalism of revivalism and that of psychiatry? Revivalism gave free rein to open expression of strong emotions and to such extraordinary behavior as swooning, barking, ranting, and the like, in the service of religious conversion. Psychiatrists tried to train patients consciously to subdue, even repress, but above all control emotional expression in the service of mental soundness: Unbridled emotionalism led to illness, self-control, to health.

Dr. Samuel Woodward, for example, the first medical director of the Worcester State Hospital in Massachusetts, established in 1833, considered moral treatment useful but insisted on the necessity for medical therapy since he regarded insanity as a somatic disorder. By the 1840s, however, other medical superintendents accepted moral treatment as the best therapy and deprecated the value of medication. But how then to justify psychiatry as a medical discipline? Where was the somatic disorder that medicine alone was supposedly capable of treating? This was a special problem, since pathological studies in the 1840s failed to reveal a consistent pathology in the brains of those who died while insane.

A compromise was reached that psychiatrists generally found palatable. Before insanity became firmly established in a patient, that is, before somatic pathology took hold and while the disorder was presumably only functional in nature, practices stressing the environment and psychological condition of the patient could restore the individual to health without the use of medicine. Subsequently, when physical pathology was present in the brain or nerves, only medicine, if anything, could work therapeutically. What helped make this compromise and thereby also moral treatment acceptable was the perceived therapeutic success of moral treatment and the view that it could only be applied in medically administered mental hospitals. With the decline in the rates of recovery in mental hospitals after the Civil War, moral treatment's nonmedical aspect resurfaced as a major issue within psychiatry. Influenced by lower recovery rates and ideas of social Darwinism, especially theories of degeneration, psychiatrists increasingly abandoned their theoretical commitment to moral treatment in favor of a more exclusively somatic approach.

The other powerful profession of the nineteenth century, the law, also found psychiatry a significant challenge to its authority on a range of issues over which lawyers and judges had long held largely undisputed sway. By 1843 the British courts had adopted the M'Naghten rule, which was widely accepted as law by state courts in the United States. In essence, under this rule, a defendant could be freed from responsibility for an act if it was proved that he or she could not distinguish right from wrong at the time of the alleged crime or misdemeanor. Psychiatrists, who by this time were being recognized as experts on insanity and called upon as expert witnesses, often objected that the M'Naghten rule relied too exclusively on intellectual understanding. In the psychiatrists' experience, many patients in mental hospitals knew right from wrong but could not control their behavior because their intractable emotions overrode all other considerations. Since there was actually no consistent judicial policy, in some cases the courts, especially juries, did accept psychiatric views not consistent with the usual judicial interpretation of the M'Naghten rule. Nevertheless, jurists usually insisted that in principle psychiatrists did not have the authority to substitute psychiatric criteria for legal criteria as to criminal responsibility.

The most extreme expression of dissatisfaction with psychiatry came in disputes over the so-called moral insanity defense, later called the psychopathic personality defense. In the 1840s Dr. Isaac Ray, author of a classic work on medical jurisprudence, insisted that since science did not know the precise relationship between insanity and a person's failure to abide by the law or act morally, all those declared insane should be freed from responsibility for their behavior. Although other psychiatrists hesitated to advocate this position, many of them did join Ray in advancing the theory that there was a form of insanity evidenced by immoral and illegal acts committed by an essentially rational person. To jurists, along with clergymen, among others, this theory of moral insanity converted all crime to mental disorder: It medicalized crime and hence threatened to undermine the criminal justice system.

As early as the 1840s, one lawyer, John Van Buren, son of President Martin Van Buren, voiced the fears of many lawyers and judges of his day and since about the danger to society of the growing power of psychiatry. If psychiatrists rather than juries were granted the authority to determine sanity or insanity in legal proceedings, then psychiatry would come to dominate society. For example, Van Buren argued, no economic transaction is valid if the individual engaging in it is mentally incompetent, so that allowing psychiatrists to decide such an issue would potentially place in their hands enormous economic power. Another objection was that society had the right and indeed the duty to determine the degree of mental disorder that justified freeing an individual from responsibility. Some prominent psychiatrists argued in effect that human actions were determined and that therefore personal responsibility, as traditionally understood in law, was irrelevant, since where there is no choice there is no freedom and therefore no blame. The English legal system had long held that in criminal cases where there was no evil intent, there could be no blame and therefore no crime or punishment. Critics perceived the criminal justice system to be endangered by such theories as moral insanity and Ray's views about responsibility of the insane. All criminal acts, some jurists, along with clergymen, argued, could be considered the acts of irrational persons. Indeed, in traditional Christian thought, with the fall of Adam all humankind inherited a somewhat defective brain, which could explain why so many people were willing to endanger their immoral souls by disobeying Christ's commandments for some paltry gains during their short stay here on earth. In brief, all people were somewhat mad and innately evil, but that did not absolve them from guilt and sin, as psychiatric deterministic standards would have it.

Psychiatrists insisted that the law accept their "scientific" findings, which must supersede tradition, while jurists held that no scientific findings could replace society's right to protect itself by setting standards for human conduct. New discoveries about human nature or how disease affected responsibility, or questions on whether humans could be considered responsible in the light of deterministic science, were ultimately beside the point. Jurists, in effect, insisted that they must protect society, and they usually saw their professional mission as synonymous with society's interests, which required fixed standards by which to judge human actions. Psychiatry sought to protect the interests of the insane in accord with the uncertain or conditional findings of medicine about human nature, and the needs of psychiatry as a profession. It should be remembered, too, that the insanity defense sometimes involved defendants charged with capital crimes, so that the death sentence was a real option. Psychiatrists, in their view, were saving innocent lives by attempting to prevent the courts from executing madmen.[8]

Since the law did recognize an insanity defense, jurists most commonly demanded from psychiatrists an unambiguous definition of insanity that could be used in determining individual responsibility according to legal criteria; the courts also sought prediction of future behavior to aid judges in sentencing. Instead, psychiatrists gave conflicting definitions of insanity, ambiguous and sometimes contradictory prognostications about future conduct, and contrary opinions on the mental states of defendants. Jurists as a result often objected to granting psychiatrists expert status in court because the discipline of psychiatry had no standard criteria. Any opinion, no matter how outlandish, jurists complained, could find some psychiatrist to support it. None of these issues has been resolved to the present day.

Nineteenth-century psychiatrists believed that they should be able to do much of what jurists asked of them. All would be well if jurists would call as expert witnesses only superintendents of mental hospitals, that is, experienced psychiatrists, and preferably in a nonadversarial setting, rather than physicians who did not specialize in treating the insane. The outcome would be consistent testimony. But prominent psychiatrists also wanted the courts to abandon the M'Naghten rule for one that more closely resembled medical concepts of insanity—rather than knowledge of right from wrong. Psychiatry no less than the law was in a quandary. After all, psychiatrists themselves assumed that their patients had some control over their behavior; otherwise how could moral treatment, which involved reeducation, work? How then could psychiatrists logically ask the courts to accept the view that insane persons who knew right from wrong were nevertheless incapable of controlling their behavior or to abandon the view that punishment or its threat were appropriate deterrents and means of reform? Neither a totally free will view of human conduct nor a determinist position was adequate to the situation that the law and psychiatry faced. What gave passion to the dispute was the fear of jurists that psychiatry was irresponsible, endangering society and the very existence of the criminal justice system, by denying the moral, philosophical, social, and, indeed, Christian values and beliefs.

No anti-psychiatry advocates were more passionate than those who considered themselves the victims of psychiatry—those who were or had been patients in mental hospitals. Until the late twentieth century, only a very minute self-selected group of ex-patients published or in other ways made their dissatisfactions public, and even fewer openly expressed positive feelings about their experiences. The stigma associated with insanity inclined discharged patients either to avoid the subject, except sometimes in personal letters, or to publish their protests with the objective of proving that they were unjustifiably institutionalized or badly treated by hospital personnel, or both. Those who recognized their own madness and believed they had benefited from institutionalization seldom publicized their sentiments except in a very few instances where they sought some sort of reform in the mental hospital system or saw their experience as of potential value to society.

Ex-patients who could express themselves coherently and cogently were, despite the stigma of insanity, very effective critics of psychiatry. The decades before the Civil War witnessed the rise of all sorts of reform movements designed to improve society and right wrongs, including calls for less abusive and more therapeutic care for the insane in the new hospitals constructed for them. When former patients made public complaints that seemed reasonable about being railroaded into mental hospitals and described their mistreatment there, they could win public sympathy. This might happen if the newspapers picked up their cause, which would be likely if the complainants were of "respectable" social and class origins and character, were nonviolent, and had the support of relatives and friends. This public support was for reform, not abolition, of mental hospitals. The ex-patients who argued that they were not insane when institutionalized and that there were many sane people unjustly held in mental hospitals did not deny that some were mad or that mental hospitals, if reformed, could provide helpful care and treatment. Even the famous Elizabeth Packard, institutionalized in 1860 for several years and subsequently able to win legislative support for her demand that a husband no longer be legally able to commit his wife on his unsupported claim that she was insane, never denied the existence of insanity and the need for mental hospitals. The founder of the modern mental health movement, ex-mental patient Clifford Beers, though initially hostile to psychiatrists and playing heavily on mistreatment in mental hospitals, did not question the validity of psychiatry or of mental hospitals per se. Through his famous autobiography, *A Mind That Found Itself*, published in 1908, and his National Committee for Mental Hygiene, formed in 1909 in close collaboration with psychiatrists, Beers campaigned for hospital reform and for public education about mental illness. In the 1920s and 1930s the National Committee was instrumental in the training of psychiatrists and in expanding their role in American society.[9]

The significance for anti-psychiatry of ex-patients' complaints during the late nineteenth and early twentieth centuries involved the ability of such allegations to discredit psychiatry as a helping profession and depict it as bureaucratic, self-serving, and insensitive to patients' needs to the point of permitting and even sometimes participating in mistreating them. Such accusations, and the tendency of public mental hospitals to restrict public access, made psychiatry increasingly suspect, so that over the years the automatic assumption of humane intent and selflessness that initially protected psychiatry and mental hospitals was vitiated.

In the courts, however, suits against medical superintendents (and sometimes also patients' relatives) for false incarceration, as well as for brutality, generally failed, and state legislatures passed laws protecting hospital medical personnel from personal liability. Besides, neither the courts nor legislatures much less the general public were willing to support the closing of mental hospitals or the replacement of psychiatrists with lay people. The only alternative to the mental hospital system being built in nineteenth-century United States was practiced in Gheel, Belgium, where mentally disordered individuals were integrated into an agricultural community that for many years had no hospital facilities or psychiatrists. "Patients" lived in the homes of farmers and performed whatever duties they could and had the freedom to move about the community. A few American medical superintendents—most notably John Minson Galt of the Eastern State Hospital of Williamsburg, Virginia, and Merrick Bemis of Worcester State Hospital—suggested this approach as a supplement to the American hospital system, and reformer Dr. Samuel Gridley Howe proposed it as an alternative, but it never was attempted in the United States. Most psychiatrists, protecting their turf, opposed it, though aspects of the system worked reasonably well in a few communities in Massachusetts, where mental hospital patients were employed on local farms.[10]

More damaging to psychiatrists was the growing perception in the late nineteenth century that psychiatry had lost its primary commitment to the patient and violated the Hippocratic directive to do no harm. This erosion of esteem was abetted by the psychiatric profession's inability to resist state legislative pressures to reduce costs by expanding the size of hospitals, which originally, under moral treatment, were by 1850 to be limited to no more than 150 patients in private institutions and 250 in public institutions. The example of industry's profitable use of efficiencies of scale was now to be applied to mental hospitals, with the widespread result that patients suffered from the anomie encouraged by bigness. Psychiatrists found it difficult if not impossible to counter the argument of efficiency of scale because they were losing their belief in the curability of insanity. Equally important, psychiatrists' class views led to their recommending that hospitals for the nonpaying lower-class patients be permitted to have inferior facilities and to house about twice the patient population as in hospitals housing paying patients, to the point where virtually no limits were applied, and state institutions with many hundreds of patients and, by the twentieth century, even thousands, were established. If custody was the inevitable fate of most mental patients, custodialism at least cost seemed, to state legislatures, the only logical way to go.

Americans have traditionally rejected the tragic view of life: There are no insoluble problems. When psychiatry in the last decades of the nineteenth century accepted the opinion of Luther V. Bell, founding member of the American Association of Medical Superintendents of Asylums for the Insane, who was quoted approvingly by another founder, Pliny Earle, that "when once a man becomes insane, he is about used up for this world,"[11] public attitudes toward psychiatry itself would turn sour and support for therapeutically effective medical hospitals continued to erode. Mental hospitals remained necessary to protect society and patients, but they were no longer the solution to the problem of insanity.

There were attempts in the late nineteenth century to redirect psychiatry by reorienting its growing negative view of the curability of insanity. This was a tall order. Mental hospitals had become overcrowded with chronic patients at the same time as science seemed to justify a hopeless view of human potential in its support for racist and class theories about the inferiority of blacks, Catholics, Jews, the poor, and immigrant working classes. Darwin's theory of evolution was used to justify theories of degeneration that explained all manner of undesirable human activities and characteristics—crime, alcoholism, mental defects, and insanity, to name a few—as the inevitable consequences of undesirable life styles leading to biological degeneration. Darwinian natural selection was converted into a form of the old Lamarckian inheritance of acquired characteristics. From the very beginning, psychiatrists assumed that mode of life significantly influenced the tendency to fall victim to madness.[12] Therefore, they advised the public how to live to maintain good mental health, advice that often far exceeded their knowledge and also reflected their political, religious, and social prejudices. When pessimism about recovery predominated late in the nineteenth century, many leading psychiatrists shifted their attention to advice about eugenics and restricting immigration to protect the fit. This stance not only perpetuated hopelessness about mental illness but vitiated mass public support for psychiatry.

What might be called the first secular anti-psychiatry organization was created by the joint action of members of two new professions, neurology and social work, who formed in New York City in 1880 the National Association for the Protection of the Insane and the Prevention of Insanity. To some extent the issues involved matters of both class and jurisdiction. Neurologists engaged in private office practice condemned medical superintendents and mental hospitals as therapeutically ineffective and even harmful to mental patients. Some prominent neurologists exhibited contempt for state mental hospitals because of the lower-class patients they treated: As Weir Mitchell commented, only poverty and necessity justified entering a state mental hospital, which could never provide the kind of care appropriate to upper-class patients.[13] Hospital leadership, in the hands of medical superintendents, the psychiatrists of their day, excluded the neurologists, who insisted that they were the real scientists, capable of turning mental hospitals into therapeutic institutions devoted to patients' needs and to scientific research that could unravel the mysteries of mental illness. American psychiatrists, they charged, had become so bureaucratized and rigid that they could not adopt new procedures such as nonrestraint, as developed in England; they did not do scientific research; and they relied upon force as their mainstay in custodial care, to the virtual exclusion of therapy. The National Association requested the state legislature of New York to investigate state mental hospitals with a view to replacing their existing leadership—most notably Dr. John P. Gray, head of Utica State Hospital—with real scientists, the neurologists, who would quickly transform these hospitals into true therapeutic institutions.

The social workers in the National Association, including prominent members of elite society, went further to question the value of all medical treatment. The ensuing split between social workers and neurologists combined with a loss of leadership, led to the demise of the reform effort. And when the neurologists failed to win the support of the state legislature, they abandoned their fight to win control of mental hospitals.

A few did eventually achieve medical directorships, especially of private asylums, and joined Clifford Beers's reform effort through work with the National Committee for Mental Hygiene. Despite their bitter and often personal condemnation of psychiatrists, neurologists did not oppose a medical view of insanity. The most critical of them held a marginally anti-psychiatry position in the sense that they regarded psychiatry less as a valid medical or scientific discipline than as a specialized administrative profession. Psychiatry could become genuinely medical and scientific only by accepting the leadership of neurologists, who alone had the requisite scientific knowledge and research training, usually obtained in Germany. This was the first, but not the last, instance in which psychiatrists met opposition from a competing medical discipline or helping profession.

The psychiatrists were in an inherently difficult position, one that could expose them to criticism no matter how hard they worked in behalf of their patients or whatever their theories. State mental hospitals, which came to house the large majority of the insane, characteristically admitted seriously mentally disordered people, who might live on for years and sometimes decades. This problem increased in the late nineteenth century when state mental hospitals also became the institution of last resort for aged ill people with reduced mental capacity, not only the insane. These hospitals served as long-term homes for the chronically ill aged and therefore faced the difficult and expensive task of providing for all the needs of their diverse population. Such institutions were viewed medically as a sign of the therapeutic failure of psychiatry, and state legislatures often begrudged providing adequately for poor and marginal people, especially Irish immigrants, who some medical superintendents believed were unlikely to recover. Almost no provision for mentally ill blacks existed in the North, and segregation into inferior institutions prevailed in the South. Under these circumstances, psychiatrists often uncritically accepted new therapies and, in the hope of winning sufficient financial support, tended to promise more than they could deliver. They were therefore vulnerable to criticism when their promises of effectiveness went unfulfilled. This problem persisted into the twentieth century, despite efforts at reform and especially under the fiscal constraints of the Great Depression and the Second World War. During the 1930s new somatic treatments originating in Europe—insulin therapy, electroshock, and lobotomy—raised hopes among hospital psychiatrists, but the depression and the war placed innovations on hold. It was only much later that fierce protest arose among critics concerned about side effects and the abuse of shock treatments and lobotomies. Meanwhile mental hospitals continued to deteriorate, hospital psychiatry lost professional status, and prominent psychiatrists gravitated toward private practice and the new psychiatric clinics founded in the early twentieth century that focused on short-term care and scientific research.

A new and eventually powerful element in the debates about the nature of psychiatry and in the decline of hospital psychiatry was Freudian theory and psychoanalytical practice, which became influential in the United States in the 1920s and 1930s and most spectacularly after World War II. Although Freud did not deal with psychosis but rather with what he termed the neuroses, some of his American supporters soon claimed his theories applicable to all mental illnesses. A small but growing number of psychiatrists came to believe that in psychoanalysis, psychiatry had finally found an explanation for mental disorders and, contrary to Freud's early view, a therapy for all mental illness, not just the neuroses. The enthusiasm for Freudian ideas among the artistic and literary community helped create a popular view, at least among the sophisticated, that psychoanalysis explained human nature. In a sense, Freud made the public aware of the pervasiveness of emotional disorders and thereby, so to speak, put psychiatry on the map. But among the preponderance of medical practitioners and psychiatrists, the latter before the war still working predominantly in mental hospitals, Freudian ideas met hostility out of all proportion to the limited range of mental disorders that psycho-analysts treated. Neurologists, virtually by definition somatically oriented, were equally antagonistic: Even in the reformist National Committee for Mental Hygiene the neu-rologists were for a number of years able to prevent any official expression of approval of Freud or psychoanalysis.

The primary complaint centered around the "unscientific" or nonmedical nature of Freud's system,[14] but animosity toward Freud, whose theories were quickly American-ized and not always to his liking, arose around other issues than his supposedly non-scientific stress on historical, social, and cultural forces rather than somatic factors in etiology and therapy. Freud's emphasis on the sexual nature of the neuroses, including hysteria, as key to understanding all human actions seemed unverified by evidence and was interpreted as a challenge to a somatic view of mental disorders. To some hospital psychiatrists Freud's theories not only directed psychiatrists away from the central issue of psychoses, they contributed to reorienting granting agencies toward support of pre-ventive psychiatry and neglect of the psychoses. Private-office practice, characteristic of psychoanalysis, and the apparent success of psychoanalysis as therapy also dimin-ished, among the educated public, the significance of psychoses and hospital-based psychiatry and helped thereby to discredit mental hospitals and deny them economic and professional sustenance. At the same time, growing numbers of clinical psychol-ogists, including lay psychoanalysts, battled psychoanalysis and traditional psychiatry to claim their own authority and their right to practice psychotherapy. If the new Freud-ian talk therapy (and its various offshoots) was the answer, why confine it to members of the medical fraternity? Indeed, the psychologists claimed that their training, which concentrated on the psychological, was more thoroughgoing and more sophisticated than that of psychiatrists, who were burdened with irrelevant medical knowledge and ignorant of psychological theory. And social workers, even clergymen, and a variety of other persons, some with rigorous training, some not, hung out their shingles as "therapists." The old mind-body dichotomy reappeared in modern guise, again to challenge or undermine psychiatry as a medical specialty.

One could argue that Freudianism, as interpreted by Americans, encouraged an already existing tendency, derived from disappointing therapeutic results in mental hos-pitals, whereby psychiatry progressively moved away from interest in psychoses to dealing with the neuroses, and finally from neurosis to the "normal" public. After World War II, psychoanalysts, who had achieved great prestige within psychiatry, showed increasing concern with the emotional problems of the "normal," with the pathology of everyday life. All humankind being more or less emotionally disturbed, a truly effective psychiatry would deal with prevention among the entire population. If in traditional Christianity all humankind was somewhat irrational after Adam's fall, with Freud emotional disorder was the price paid for the repressions that civilization necessitated.[15] Just as conversion to Christ promised salvation, so psychoanalysis, through unlocking the secrets of human nature, could enable humankind to mitigate the emotional damage imposed by civilization. Some American psychoanalysts preached that prevention of mental disorder was a step toward "positive" mental health, the elimination of all emotional disorders. An Americanized version of psychoanalysis—totally secular, liberal, and sexually candid—could replace religion as the ultimate explanation and treatment for all human emotional problems.

Freud himself was an atheist who believed that religion deprived people of their ability to understand the material, social, and cultural sources of their emotional problems and inhibited them from accepting psychoanalysis as a means to gain insight and thereby solve or alleviate such problems. Such views brought psychiatry, or, more accurately, psychoanalysis, new enemies among religious groups such as Roman Catholics, who had not been traditionally anti-psychiatry. For all its disagreements with psychiatry's view of possession and exorcism and of sin as the cause of insanity, the Roman Catholic church did not in the nineteenth century oppose psychiatry as a discipline, in part because the public mental hospitals were havens for poor Catholic immigrants who became mentally ill and for whom the church had no facilities. Furthermore, actual cases of demonic possession were considered to be rare, so that insanity could be acknowledged as the province of psychiatry. But psychoanalysis, which was equated with psychiatry, was different—atheistic, anti-religious, immoral. By the 1950s, however, the Roman Catholic Church reached an accommodation with psychoanalysis; the pope made it clear that he did not oppose the practice of psychoanalysis, much less psychiatry, where it did not contradict the tenets of Catholicism, and agreements among the Catholic clergy and sympathetic psychotherapists to cooperate in the treatment of parishioners reflected a shift in both groups' attitudes.[16]

The postwar rise in prestige and power of the psychoanalysts who came to dominate departments of psychiatry in many general teaching hospitals and psychiatric institutes paved the way for unprecedented and eventually successful assaults against the old, traditional institutional power base of psychiatry—mental hospitals. In the process, in which deteriorated hospital conditions, economic considerations, new somatic therapies, ideological and cultural trends, and political activism all played a part, the idea of the mental hospital or asylum, to which psychiatry owed its origins and for so long its influence, was effectively challenged.

During World War II, army psychiatrists, rediscovering what had been learned in World War I, that "battle fatigued" or "shell shocked" soldiers did best when not institutionalized, assumed that the mentally ill among the civilian population at home would benefit equally by being deinstitutionalized. Upon this analogy, and a newfound confidence, was built the view that it was possible to do without mental hospitals. Thus was born a campaign to substitute community mental health centers for mental hospitals.[17] The postwar years witnessed the growth of a psychiatrically led reform movement to reinvest in the decaying mental hospitals, to create therein therapeutic communities, and to supplement the hospitals with community mental health facilities. In this struggle, from about 1945 to the mid-1960s, between those who sought reform and those, led by psychoanalyst Karl Menninger, who wanted to eliminate state mental hospitals in favor of community mental health centers, the latter group, with the help of the National Institute for Mental Health, won the day, although of course only some twenty-five percent of the full 2,000 community mental health centers were ever built. As sociologist Erving Goffman asserted in his influential book, *Asylums*,[18] state-funded mental hospitals were part of the problem rather than its solution: Institutions were by definition vehicles for social control, oppressive and inimical to real therapeutics, and certainly real abuses were rampant there. Economics figured in the situation as well: In response to the pleas of state governments that they could not afford the cost of caring for the mentally ill, federal legislation in the 1960s and early 1970s made it financially advantageous for states to mandate discharge of patients, whom the federal government would support at a higher rate outside than inside public mental hospitals. And the barrage of criticism directed at state hospitals by strongly anti-institutional social activists— charges of patient abuse and neglect, failure to provide adequate treatment, and mistreatment with inappropriate drugs and other misguided therapies—set an ideological climate antithetical to psychiatry. At the same time, advances in psychopharmacology— the new psychotropic drugs like chlorpromazine—would, the public was told, enable patients to control their symptoms sufficiently to allow them to live out in the community.

The advent of these drugs, together with new research into the possible biochemical basis of mental disease, also contributed to the decline of psychoanalysis, whose practitioners had been so active in dismantling mental hospitals. Not only did psychoanalysts have little success in treating hospitalized, psychotic patients, but by the 1960s psychoanalysis became exposed to increasing criticism when its therapeutic claims even in regard to its small select clientele could not be verified. Thus when the new chemical therapies were seen as evidence that mental illness was indeed a somatic disorder, psychoanalysis had no effective response. But the promise of neurobiology was not immediately realized, and the new drugs, along with electroshock and lobotomy—all of which could have quite damaging side effects—raised a storm of protest among a vocal group of patients and ex-patients who won support from various anti-authoritarian liberation movements in the late 1960s and early 1970s. Anti-psychiatry became part of a protest against racism, the Vietnam War, professional authority, and hierarchical distinctions common to "establishment" organizations of all kinds, including state mental hospitals, some of which were "snake pits." The activism included ex-patients organized as never before, to fight against involuntary institutionalization and involuntary treatments and for the empowerment of patients and their civil rights. Also for the first time anti-psychiatry took on a national and international character. Although American psychiatry was always influenced by European developments, earlier outbreaks of anti-psychiatry had remained local phenomena. All this changed in the 1960s and 1970s. Ex-patient anti-psychiatry organizations made contact with like-minded people abroad, and in both the United States and Western Europe persons belonging to prestigious professional organizations—in law, psychiatry, psychology, sociology, and philosophy—and having access to the mass media participated in anti-psychiatry and helped to develop its ideology.[19]

The most influential ideologist of the "new" anti-psychiatry of the 1960s and 1970s was himself a medical psychoanalyst, Thomas Szasz, whose position was a replay of issues raised by moral treatment in the early nineteenth century. Szasz was so attractive to many critics of psychiatry because he rejected the right of psychiatrists forcibly to institutionalize and treat people who he said were as a rule not really mentally ill. Szasz assumed that if mental illness qualified as a medical entity it must be shown to have some sort of somatic etiology, probably in the brain and nervous system. Since such findings were lacking in all but a few forms of insanity such as paresis, Szasz concluded that so-called mental illness was in most cases not a medical disorder; rather, mentally disturbed people had problems in living. He clearly presumed that since medicine had not yet found a somatic basis for many forms of mental illness it never would do so.

In his heyday Szasz proclaimed that psychiatry, having no biological basis, had no moral much less medical justification for forcing treatment upon those it labeled mentally ill. If society eliminated involuntary hospitalization it would remove the primary obstacle to the proper care of the mentally troubled who were, in Szasz's view, merely lazy and irresponsible. This position begged the question of what to do with people who had problems so severe as to make them dysfunctional in society, no matter what their condition is called. To Szasz it was up to the individual to seek and pay for whatever help he or she needed; society had little if any obligation in the matter. Unfortunately for Szasz he put forward his arguments just when medical and biological research was finding evidence for the somatic nature of mental illnesses. His influence was much greater among the lay public, ex-mental patients, and the politically radical Left (whom he disdained and who wanted public funding for mental health facilities) than within the psychiatric community, which for the most part regarded him with disdain.[20]

Another radical critic of psychiatry from within, a counterculture hero of the 1960s, was British psychiatrist R. D. Laing. Initially Laing attributed the origins of schizophrenia, the subject of his primary concern, to the nuclear family, which victimized one of its members and literally drove him or her mad. Then, unable to discover the symptoms characteristic of schizophrenia among mental patients so labeled by psychiatrists, he saw such "patients" as people who were responding sensibly to a genuinely irrational or schizophrenic society. They could even be seen as potentially supernormal, superior beings—the old popular belief in the kinship of madness and genius or madness and divinity. Schizophrenia for Laing became a desirable alternative to sanity, a means of entering a deep inner world from which one would emerge emotionally cleansed and full of keen insights. This radical reversal of the attitude toward psychosis was based on a mystical view antithetical to psychiatry as a medical discipline. Laing took a path that might remove the stigma of psychosis: He viewed schizophrenia not as a clinical category and a disabling condition, but as a normal stage in the growth of some sensitive people, who could be helped by living in a benevolent, supportive group home, not a hospital.[21]

Also contributing to the denial of the so-called medical model of mental illness as well as to the anti-institution mood of the 1960s was Goffman's study of asylums, in which he attributed mental patients' "schizophrenic" characteristics to the hospital rather than the nature of mental illness. The French polymath Michel Foucault, whose ideas became so influential among American intellectuals, postulated that mental illness was a cultural artifact. Asserting, without convincing historical evidence, that the "insane" had once been integrated into society, he suggested reintegrating them but proposed nothing specific to help this supposedly more humane social relationship become established. Then there was labeling theory, championed most prominently by sociologist Thomas Scheff,[22] who, along with certain influential historical writers,[23] saw mental hospitals and psychiatry as forms of social control, as if social control was an all-or-nothing phenomenon and psychiatrists could not also seek the patient's good.

There were also psychiatrists, psychologists, and sociologists who saw learned behavior as an explanation for mental illness; they rejected the relevance of a medical view, that is, a focus on disease, but accepted the concept of mental disorder. Prominent psychologist Hans Eysenck opposed psychoanalysis and psychiatry, arguing that the suffering of the neurotic was a learned response; in such cases there were no "lesions . . . no infection [and] nothing whatever that suggests . . . 'disease.' "[24] In cases where organicity existed, neurologists were the proper therapists; where mere neurosis existed, it had been acquired through some form of learning and was therefore the province of psychologists. Psychiatrists therefore really had no role to play.[25] And psychologist Peter Sedgwick, seeing disease as a social construct, because "*there are no illnesses or diseases in nature,*" also thereby deprecated psychiatry.[26]

These various ideas were taken up by the liberal and leftist anti-psychiatry activists of the 1960s and 1970s, especially the newly vocal and influential organized ex-patients, albeit still a rather small, amorphous group of individualists. The inability of previous anti-psychiatry advocates to offer an acceptable alternative to psychiatry and mental hospitals had always been their Achilles' heel, and the anti-psychiatry religious sects had little influence in urban centers or with most state legislatures. What helped make modern anti-psychiatry much more effective was the existence of an apparent alternative to the mental hospital, the community mental health center, which had originated largely within the psychiatric profession. The new activists, many of them well educated and articulate, operating in urban areas, and supported by an environment of social and cultural change, were impressive witnesses and advocates for reform by state governments of the status and treatment of the mentally ill. Although they did not consider the community mental health centers to be true alternatives to mental hospitals, much less to psychiatry, the idea of such centers could be transformed into new forms of independently established self-help collectives or drop-in centers.[27] To the extent that such patient-run centers succeeded—and most of them eventually died out for lack of money—they tended to serve persons who could function fairly well outside the hospital. As for the mass of newly released patients, there were never enough government-sponsored, "establishment" community mental health centers and outreach workers to take care of them, and such centers never had enough money, especially in the fiscally austere 1980s and 1990s. These centers were in any case not required to make provision for the chronic and seriously mentally ill patients that the hospitals were discharging. The result was that masses of discharged seriously chronically ill but not dangerous persons were transinstitutionalized to old-age homes. Others in that category were left very much on their own, roaming the streets or exploited by boarding house or hotel owners, and, more recently, confined in local jails. The remaining mental hospitals continued to house a declining population of highly deranged, chronic patients and to serve as a short-term last resort for acutely disturbed persons.[28]

Three decades of anti-psychiatry produced a large literature critical of psychiatry but little discussion of the deteriorating condition of the mentally troubled in American society. If anti-psychiatry is not primarily responsible for this situation it is also not blameless. Indeed the lack of centrality of the mental patient is not an oversight but characteristic of and even essential to much anti-psychiatry, past and present, but especially so in the late twentieth century. Many anti-psychiatry advocates were guilty of what they charged psychiatrists—ignoring the needs of seriously ill patients, especially the aged. The long-term commitment of the American public to care for such persons in specialized institutions was being reversed.

Why would ex-patients take such a position? Why not establish facilities that included this class of patients? An obvious answer is that the ex-patients lacked the resources to do so. But more important was the ideological commitment to anti-psychiatry. Psychiatry could not be depicted as so completely evil, irrelevant, and destructive if it dealt with a real social problem with a medical component, no matter how ineffectively. The goal of activist ex-patients was to disallow any valid role to psychiatry by disallowing the existence of insanity as a medical disorder. They could then justify the establishment of self-run nonmedical facilities; ex-patients could and should control their own lives without the interference of psychiatrists or even sympathetic "sane" people. The title of ex-patient leader Judi Chamberlin's influential book put it succinctly: *On Our Own*. Such a separation proved to be impractical, and Chamberlin abandoned this position. But for others the issue became not as at first in the 1970s, capitalism, class, economic status, and gender, but the ex-mental patient versus the "sane" world.

From the beginning of the new ex-patient activism the conceptual justification came from both a Szaszian laissez-faire denial of the existence of insanity and a "Marxist" view of psychiatry as serving the interests of a capitalist, exploitative, ruling class that drove people mad or defined revolutionaries as mad in order to discredit them and confine them in mental hospitals. Both views, which incorporated well-founded claims of abuse of mental patients in hospitals and valid charges of bad side effects of indiscriminate drug prescription, found psychiatry irreconcilable with the needs of the so-called mentally disordered. For the Marxists the only solution was social revolution not reform. At the same time, a growing group of ex-patients sought to gain control over their lives before the victory of socialism. These "reformist" types were more influenced by conservative, libertarian, individualistic Szaszian social views.

Other dilemmas surfaced. Until the 1980s the spokespersons for the organized ex-patients were white, middle class, and largely politically Left in orientation. They sought to run their own facilities and thereby provide for the true needs of the mentally troubled. These facilities, however, needed the assistance of mental hospitals, which acted as an informal backup system to take in clients unable to control themselves sufficiently to function in ex-patient housing. To be on their own, ex-patients also needed substantial financial support from the very society that allegedly produced the conditions that drove people mad or at least labeled them mad and then oppressed them in hospitals and used them as a source of cheap labor. Leftist ex-patients sought the resources to become self-regulating from a government it wished to destroy and then complained when the resources were inadequate or not forthcoming. Other politically Left-oriented ex-patients believed that capitalism of necessity must oppress the "insane" who were in fact, as Laing had taught, often merely sensitive, rebellious individuals. The class struggle was the only way of liberating the "mentally ill," and the struggle against psychiatry was a means of accomplishing that broader goal, the liberation of all the oppressed classes, not just the "mentally ill." But as the more radical Marxists insisted, the only effective way of stopping the exploitation of the masses that produced insanity was to introduce socialism, so that it was a waste of time to fight psychiatry and wrong to accept government funding; the anti-government anarchists agreed.

The radicals tended to reject alliances with their natural allies, such as the National Alliance for the Mentally Ill, an organization of parents with mentally ill children. The ex-patients objected not so much to these parents' opposition to the popular psychiatric view, heavily promoted in the 1970s by Laing and his followers, that schizophrenia was the consequence of dysfunctional family relations—strong mothers and weak fathers. Offensive to the ex-patients was the Alliance's position that insanity existed as a medical entity and that its etiology was somatic, a position that gained strength with the growth of neurobiological psychiatry.[29]

In the mid-1980s the anti-psychiatry ex-patient activism, never a well-organized, unified effort, split into several factions. At issue were its growing middle-class reformist leadership; the need to fund mental health centers by the only agencies having sufficient resources—government and private philanthropies; and the failure of radical politics significantly to empower the ex-patient activists. There were also theoretical differences. Among the leadership a critical view of psychiatry still prevailed, but some had come not absolutely to disclaim the reality of mental disorders or reject possible cooperation with psychiatry. Even before then, anti-psychiatry advocates among left-wing intellectuals, psychiatrists, and political activists had admitted that their expectations about the destruction of psychiatry and the support its destruction would give to revolutionary movements, a position popular in post-1968 France, had not materialized. Much less had conditions for the mass of mental patients notably improved.

The very patient organizations, always few in number, established to empower, house, and treat patients have themselves not been free of the internal struggles over goals, means, and power so common to all other organizations. The utopian view that ex-patients and patients would avoid forming hierarchical structures in the institutions they controlled is not being borne out, and ex-patient leaders have become connected with the "establishment" through funding arrangements and consultation with various mental health agencies, private and public. The American genius for absorbing at least the leadership among dissidents is under way.

Radical Left anti-psychiatry in a sense shared the views of psychiatrist-reformers of the early and midtwentieth century in seeing the problems surrounding the treatment of mental illness as the fault of the mental hospital as an institution. The break came when the anti-psychiatry critics attributed the failure of the mental hospital to the psychiatric profession and went farther in questioning the existence of mental illness. Another wing of recent anti-psychiatry, the radical Right, never made common cause with psychiatrists but instead categorically opposed psychiatry as a liberal, left-wing, subversive, anti-American plot. Unaffected by the anti-psychiatry among avant-garde intellectuals and unconventional psychiatrists, these activists incorporated their hatred and fear of psychiatry into a predominantly anti-Communist, nationalist world view.

In 1965 writer Donald Robison published in *Look Magazine* "The Far Right's Fight Against Mental Health,"[30] in which he captured the hostility toward psychiatry among those in the political far Right. A member of the John Birch Society is quoted as saying, "Mental health is alien and Communist-inspired," and a Wyoming chapter of the Daughters of the American Revolution "passed a resolution in 1960 charging that some psychiatrists use 'drugs, shock and lobotomy' on persons with 'certain ideological beliefs.' " Rightist Matt Cvetic charged that there was a " 'phony' concern about our so-called declining 'mental health' " planted by "Communist agents, fronters and sympathizers for the purpose of demoralizing the American people and spreading defeatism." Another rightist charged that "a substantial percentage" of mental patients are kidnapped sane people: "Will YOU sit idly by and allow them to be TORTURED and

MURDERED?'' The chief target of such extremists was the highly respectable National Association for Mental Health, successor to Beers's National Committee for Mental Hygiene, a supposed part of a Russian-run apparatus to brainwash the United States, an "ultimate instrument of communism for taking over the free world." Racism, anti-Semitism, anti-Catholicism, and anti-internationalism were significant components of this attack: The nefarious plot was not only Communist but was run by Jews, Catholics, and Negroes. In the Southwest and California the extremists, who besides the DAR and Birchers included members of neo-Nazi groups and White Citizens Councils, intimidated and smeared supporters of mental health associations and vehemently opposed, often successfully, the establishment of mental health clinics.[31]

Although there were obvious differences between the anti-psychiatry radical Right of the 1950s and 1960s and the anti-psychiatry radical Left of the 1960s and 1970s, some common tendencies deserve mention. Both groups saw psychiatry as part of a conspiracy to subvert the rights and well-being of the mass of the people in the interests of the few. The leftists believed that the "few" were the capitalists; the rightists, that the "few" were the advocates of Godless communism, the tool of Satan. Both rejected compromise or reform and argued for the destruction of psychiatry in order to insure the happiness of the masses or at least the God-fearing among them. The radical leftists, or at least some of them, were interested in the plight of the mental patient, though, and they were not ethnic or religious hatemongers. The radical rightists, among whom it is not always possible to distinguish between those concerned with politics or with religion, showed little concern with the actual mental patients or ex-patients. Interest was centered mainly on mental health advocates, who were the agents of the Communists or the devil or both.[32]

Among the rightist anti-psychiatry crusaders could be found fundamentalist Christian believers, who added anti-communism to the traditional anti-modernism that had distinguished them from mainstream, modernist Protestants earlier in the twentieth century. In the 1960s fundamentalism began to make significant inroads into the broader society beyond the Southern "Bible Belt," to the point where it was no longer a fringe movement. By the late 1970s and 1980s, with the rise of fundamentalism to national importance and to political influence in the Republican party, in part through the popularity of the televangelists, newly respectable fundamentalist leaders were softening their views of the medical profession in general and psychiatry in particular. Some of the "new" fundamentalists tended to ignore in their preaching the phenomenon of demonic possession, and some of the new charismatic religious groups were becoming involved in treating all sorts of mental disorders, sometimes in their own hospitals, and in cooperation with psychiatrists. The focus of these groups was on Christ as healer and their inheritance of his supernatural healing powers. Psychiatrists were also revising their approach to the charismatic, self-help programs of the religious sects and cults that had traditionally opposed psychiatry for spiritual reasons: Zealous groups such as the Unification Church and the Divine Light Mission, writes one psychiatrist, could "serve as adjuncts, even collaborators, in psychiatric care" and could "yield relief in psychopathology."[33]

From the early 1960s to the late 1970s, and with consequences still with us, psychiatry also became the focus of discontent among Americans who were not extremists. Much of this discontent revolved around legal issues, especially as the courts became more activist in implementing social policy. The scenario drawn by some midnineteenth-century jurists about the effect on American society if psychiatrists' claims to be the judges of human mentality were accepted were, in the opinion of some Americans, being realized a hundred years later. A number of books, some written by liberal psychiatrists, discussed the threat to individual rights and society posed by the growing powers of psychiatry, by psychiatrists' assertion of unjustified authority in many areas of American life. The courts, for example, sought the opinion of psychiatrists about the dangerousness of convicted criminals in order to guide judges and juries in sentencing, although psychiatrists were notoriously unsuccessful in making such predictions. Psychiatrists also played an increasingly important role in the disposition of cases involving juveniles in trouble with the law. Similarly psychiatrists were given, it was said, an unwarranted role in custody fights over children and in divorce cases, in settlements of claims for injury, and, during the Vietnam War, in determining who should be exempted from the draft or who might break down in military combat.

There was evidence supporting at least some of these criticisms. Some psychiatrists did, and still do, argue that criminality was an example of mental disorder. In the twentieth century psychoanalysts added their voices to those who thought punishment ineffective in controlling undesirable human behavior.[34] Psychoanalysis, moreover, found the origin of much behavior outside of consciousness: People did not know why they acted as they did and often could not control their actions. Then some psychiatrists expanded the concept of who could legitimately be considered mentally ill far beyond the limits of schizophrenia, manic-depressive disorders, and other chronic mental illnesses or psychoses to include virtually all troubled people, all driven by unconscious forces. These ideas inspired anxiety that no one could be held responsible for anything. Courts would be abandoned in favor of hospitals and doctors. And, indeed, in the twentieth century all sorts of people were withdrawn from the criminal justice system, especially youthful offenders. Traditional beliefs about good and evil or right and wrong were converted into medical questions: Society, it was feared, was abandoning religious morality and tradition.[35] A further issue surfaced in the Hinckley case, where the psychiatrist treating the troubled young man who shot President Reagan came under scrutiny for allegedly not preventing Hinckley from acting out his fantasies. As in the past, finding a defendant not guilty by reason of insanity still creates strong public distrust of psychiatry.

Another area of dispute arose when members of the legal profession inspired by the civil rights movement joined the anti-psychiatry "movement" to insist, as never before and with success, that the courts must protect and expand the individual rights of hospitalized mental patients. Allowing patients' rights not heretofore recognized—for example, the right to obtain appropriate treatment, the right to refuse treatment, and the abolition of involuntary commitment (except in cases of demonstrated dangerousness)—seriously diminished the authority of psychiatrists in mental hospitals. By the new rules, individual rights superseded the right of society to force upon adults unwanted hospitalization or treatment, except in a medical emergency or imminent danger posed by a supposedly deranged person. Although in practice the standard of dangerousness turned out to be elastic, it did significantly reduce the numbers of patients admitted to mental hospitals, and state courts held that hospitals must provide treatment or else discharge involuntary patients; some judges tried to insure improved care by mandating minimum standards of treatment.[36]

There is no doubt that the legal challenges of the 1960s and thereafter to the authority of psychiatry were in part stimulated by the perceived failure of psychiatry to provide humane and effective therapy in mental hospitals. The new legal rights granted to mental patients could be seen as reforms or outright anti-psychiatry. Psychiatrists tended to see them as anti-psychiatry in effect and sometimes in intent: The effect was certainly to deny to psychiatrists in mental hospitals the traditional authority that they claimed was essential to successful treatment and management of patients. Another effect was the discharge of many patients because the legal mandate to offer adequate therapy and decent living conditions was too costly to be carried out; whether such persons lived under better conditions "freed" from the control of psychiatrists, in the streets or in old-age homes, is debatable. The state legislatures' protection of the personal liberty of prospective patients by requiring a finding of dangerousness as a condition for admission to the mental hospital also effectively denied hospitalization to some who could get no treatment elsewhere. By the 1970s and especially the 1980s, hospitals, with the approval of most state legislatures, sought to admit as few patients as possible in an effort to cut costs. The result was a reduced hospital population and shorter duration of average residence of patients within the hospital. That this new system was an improvement over the old is not clear. No doubt some former hospitalized patients benefited, but others were harmed by the new activism of the courts. The problem was that the courts were not an effective means of forcing psychiatrists, mental hospitals, or state legislatures to do the right thing. The almost exclusive emphasis in many court decisions on the adversarial relationship between psychiatrists and patients protected patients' rights on the apparent assumption that the primary obstacles to their recovery were the hospital and the psychiatrists, and, as usual, no one thought much about the fate of the chronic, aging inmate. As one psychiatrist put it in 1974, patients were as a consequence "dying with [their] rights on."[37] By 1992, in the majority of American communities the new legal regime had broken down: A survey sponsored by the Public Citizen Health Research Group and the National Alliance for the Mentally Ill, supported by the American Psychiatric Association and the American Jail Association, found that, through lack of treatment programs, local jails have become, the Jail Association said, "the substitute institution of our neglect."[38]

Although psychiatrists' power was reduced, the public still viewed the psychiatric profession as a major player in the care of mentally disturbed patients, and the legal profession by the 1980s increasingly recognized that the basic assumptions of some of the legal critics of psychiatry were wanting. That mental disorders were the product of psychiatric mismanagement or venality, that the "insane" would disappear with the destruction of the psychiatric profession or mental hospitals, or that mental patients would be able to take advantage of their newly recognized rights seemed increasingly open to question.

The courts, moreover, still needed psychiatrists. After over a hundred years of complaints by lawyers that psychiatrists erroneously claimed to have knowledge about mental patients, in the late twentieth century the Supreme Court refused to accept psychiatrists' disclaimer of their ability reliably to predict dangerousness. The Court insisted that psychiatrists predict whether a particular defendant will be dangerous in the future and thus enable the judge to dispose of the defendant accordingly. Admittedly the newfound modesty of psychiatrists derives from their fear of being sued in cases where they did not warn of the danger that a patient under treatment posed.[39]

Jurists continue to dispute with psychiatrists over the nature of crime, over the legal responsibility of those found suffering from mental illness, and over the legitimate authority of psychiatry in the criminal justice system. Nor is it likely that these issues will have a definitive resolution, for they are ultimately not scientific questions. Science and medicine have influenced the way society decides these issues, but so do moral, religious, and social values and economic conditions, all of which are in constant change and which have often figured more significantly in anti-psychiatry attitudes and crusades than the condition and plight of the mentally ill.

Psychiatry itself has been reoriented, although how much is due to anti-psychiatry and economic stringency and how much to medical developments is difficult to say. Hospital psychiatry has become an endangered profession, and psychiatry has lost some of its previous status and power. Although probably many individual psychiatric practitioners had little awareness of the anti-psychiatry activism, the organized psychiatric profession, in the form of the American Psychiatric Association, did acknowledge the existence of the organized ex-patients and tried to work with them to redress their complaints. Psychoanalysis has declined; psychotherapy in general has given way to drug therapy, or combinations of both; and research into the biochemistry of behavior and the biology of the brain has come to the fore in the investigation of the etiology and treatment of mental disorder. Such research is leading to new support for psychiatry. As psychiatrist Melvin Sabshin noted in 1990, "Decision makers on Senate and House appropriation committees have commented frequently that they are now more willing to support the . . . Mental Health Administration because they can understand the palpable outcomes of the new generation of research."[40] Even Szasz's confidence that mental illness has no significant biological component has been shaken, as revealed in his 1987 book *Insanity: The Idea and Its Consequences.*[41]

In response to the new trends we have two recent books by American psychiatrists, from two opposing viewpoints, both critical of psychiatry, with arguments hotly propounded but not always substantiated or well thought out. Psychiatrist E. Fuller Torrey, a longtime critic of psychotherapy and of the medical model of psychiatry, who had written in 1974 on *The Death of Psychiatry,*[42] has become a strong advocate of the somatic approach to mental illness. In *Freudian Fraud,* published in 1992, he attributes the failures of post–World War II psychiatry to the influence of psychoanalysis.[43] Those psychoanalysts, he says, who designed the legislation creating the National Institute of Mental Health—Karl Menninger, Francis Braceland, and Robert Felix—were all Freudian and therefore imperialist in their thinking. They assumed that psychiatry or rather Freud had given them the means to solve social problems, not just those related to mental illness.[44] Torrey does not seem to be aware that an all-embracing view of the relevance of psychiatry to all human social problems did not originate with Freud and his followers but was apparent when mental hospitals and the profession of psychiatry appeared in the late eighteenth century. Freud developed a particular way of understanding human nature, which was used by some psychiatrists to comment on all manner of human activity, but the tendency of psychiatrists to do so long predated the twentieth century. And, of course, Freud the physician and scientist never abandoned somaticism; his interest and emphasis lay elsewhere.

Peter Breggin, in *Toxic Psychiatry,* which appeared in 1991, argues against the new "biopsychiatry," wherein "the brain-disabling principle applies to all of the most potent psychiatric treatments—neuroleptics, antidepressants, lithium, electroshock and psychosurgery. The principle states that all of the major psychiatric treatments exert their primary or intended effect by disabling normal brain function.'' Only in psychiatry did the physician damage the brain in order to gain control over the patient. ''If psychosurgery, electroshock or the more potent psychiatric drugs were refined to the point of harmlessness, they would approach uselessness. In biopsychiatry, unfortunately, it's the damage that does the trick.'' (That there might be a similar ''principle'' operating in the potent chemotherapy applied to various cancers Breggin does not acknowledge.) Even if some mental patients are discovered to have brain disease, he says, it would not ''change the fact'' that current psychiatric treatments further damage the brain.[45] Only a ''psychosocial'' approach could prove helpful to the mental patient, who is suffering primarily from pernicious family relations and a self-serving and misguided psychiatry. But once Breggin concedes the possibility that brain dysfunction may be the origin of some psychoses, then he cannot logically deny the possibility of successful treatment by biological means.

Breggin's argument against somatically oriented psychiatry is actually less theoretical than practical. Psychiatry, he contends, is more than an academic or a therapeutic discipline. ''Psychiatry is the political center of a multibillion-dollar psycho-pharmaceutical complex that pushes biological and genetic theories, as well as drugs, on the society. It is a political institution licensed by the state, financed by government, and empowered by the courts.'' Like others disturbed by the power of psychiatry, Breggin supports denying psychiatry the legal right to enforce hospitalization and treatment. He wants a free market, with no legal licensing requirements, where psychiatry would compete with psychotherapy and psychosocial alternatives and the right of people to practice mental healing with no let or hindrance.[46] Under such conditions many clients would not, he believes, choose the harmful psychosurgery, electroshock, or chemicals that are the present mainstay of psychiatry.

The perennial mind-body arguments continue. In recent years general systems theory has been most influential, and of late there have appeared a number of writings by philosophers, neurologists, psychiatrists, and psychologists arguing for a mind-brain identity approach.[47] Also by the 1980s, the revisionist history and sociology of mental illness that had helped to fuel contemporary anti-psychiatry had itself come under attack. Such criticism encompassed self-criticism among some revisionists themselves, who now recognized the inadequacy of social control theory in explaining the complexities and problems of psychiatry.[48]

Mental disorder, whatever its origins, is still with us; American society is still dealing with the consequences of deinstitutionalization; psychiatry, though changed, is not endangered; and chronically ill patients are still neglected. To some observers the clock has been turned back to preasylum days two centuries ago. Many Americans have abandoned the belief that it is possible, or economically feasible, to eliminate poverty and to provide for the needs of the disadvantaged, be they physically or mentally ill. This loss of nerve defeats not only the optimism attending the birth of modern psychiatry but also that form of anti-psychiatry that sought to force psychiatry to live up to its best and most hopeful ideals.

Anti-psychiatry is in a sense both a return to the past and a perverse ''fulfillment'' of psychiatry. Initially, psychiatry sought to treat and cure, and ultimately, ideally, to eradicate conditions today called psychoses. Much of anti-psychiatry has sought to negate mental illness altogether. And psychiatrists themselves in effect adopted this approach. Those who spearheaded deinstitutionalization and the community mental health movement, along with the radical critics within psychiatry, often ignored and thereby virtually denied the presence of psychosis. The problem that brought psychiatry as a profession into existence, insanity, is "solved" by disregarding it or by defining it away. But the sufferers do not go away.

Notes

1. A somewhat more detailed discussion of American Protestant attitudes toward insanity, plus a bibliography, appears in my "Madness and the Stigma of Sin in American Christianity" in Paul Jay Fink and Allan Tasman (eds.), *Stigma and Mental Illness* (Washington, D. C.: American Psychiatric Press, 1992), 73–84.

2. Attributing melancholy to sin was not confined to clergymen but was rather a commonly held view in Colonial New England. See, for example, Mary Ann Jimenez, *Early American Attitudes and Treatment of the Insane* (Hanover, New Hampshire: Published for Brandeis University Press by University Press of New England, 1987), 15; and Nancy Tomes, "Historical Perspectives on Women and Mental Illness" in Rima D. Apple (ed.), *Women, Health, and Medicine in America* (New Brunswick, New Jersey: Rutgers University Press, 1990), 154–156.

3. Otho T. Beall, Jr. and Richard H. Shryock, *Cotton Mather, First Significant Figure in American Medicine* (Baltimore: Johns Hopkins University Press, 1954); Kenneth Silverman, *The Life and Times of Cotton Mather* (New York: Columbia University Press, 1985), 309; Cotton Mather, *The Angel of Bethesda*, edited by Gordon W. Jones (Barre, Massachusetts: American Antiquarian Society and Barre Publishers, 1972); Jonathan Edwards (ed.), *An Account of the Life of the Late Reverend Mr. Brainerd* (Boston: 1749); Jonathan Edwards, *The Life of David Brainerd*, edited by Norman Pettit (New Haven: Yale University Press, 1985). Edwards, like Mather before him, considered "melancholy as a bodily disease which lowered men's resistance to secondary infections of satanic origin" (Gail Thain Parker, "Jonathan Edwards and Melancholy," *New England Quarterly*, xli [1968], 202).

4. For a history of healing and Christianity see Morton T. Kelsey, *Healing and Christianity in Ancient Thought and Modern Times* (New York: Harper & Row, 1976), 223ff; Leslie D. Weatherhead, *Psychology, Religion and Healing* (London: Hodder and Stoughton, 1951); on religious healing see also J. A. C. Murray, *An Introduction to a Christian Psycho-Therapy* (New York: Scribner, 1938).

5. See A. M. Bellwald, *Christian Science and the Catholic Faith, Including a Brief Account of New Thought and Other Modern Mental Healing Movements* (New York: Macmillan, 1922); Charles S. Braden, *Spirits in Rebellion: The Rise and Development of New Thought* (Dallas: Southern Methodist University Press, 1963); Sarah Elizabeth Titcomb, *Mind-Cure on a Material Basis* (Boston: Cupples, Upham, 1885).

6. The literature on Christian Science is very extensive; the following titles were most useful to me: Mary Baker G. Eddy, *Science and Health, with Key to the Scriptures* (Boston: Published by the Trustees under the Will of Mary Baker G. Eddy, 1934); Mary Baker Eddy, *Miscellaneous Writings, 1883–1896* (Boston: Christian Science Publishing Society, 1918); Mary Baker Eddy, *The First Church of Christ Scientist and Miscellany* (Boston: Published by the Trustees under the Will of Mary Baker G. Eddy, 1913); *A Century of Christian Science Healing* (Boston: Christian Science Publishing Society, 1966); Bellwald, *Christian Science and the Catholic Faith*; Charles S. Braden, *Christian Science Today: Power, Policy, Practice* (Dallas: Southern Methodist University Press, 1958); Horatio W. Dresser (ed.), *The Quimby Manuscripts* (New York: Julian Press, 1961); Edwin Franden Dakin, *Mrs. Eddy*, (New York: Grosset & Dunlap, 1929); Stephen Gottschalk, *The Emergence of Christian Science in American Religious Life* (Berkeley: Univer-

sity of California Press, 1973); Donald Meyer, *The Positive Thinkers' Religion as Pop Psychology, from Mary Baker Eddy to Oral Roberts* (New York; Pantheon, 1965); Frank Podmore, *Mesmerism and Christian Science: A Short History of Mental Healing* (Philadelphia: George W. Jacobs, 1909?); Julius Silberger, Jr., *Mary Baker Eddy: An Interpretive Biography of the Founder of Christian Science* (Boston: Little, Brown, 1980); Mark Twain, *Christian Science, with Notes Containing Corrections to Date* (New York: Harper, 1907); Sibyl Wilbur, *The Life of Mary Baker Eddy* (Boston: Christian Science Publishing Society, 1938); Irving C. Tomlinson, *Twelve Years with Mary Baker Eddy: Recollections and Experiences* (Boston: Christian Science Publishing Society, 1954); Stefan Zweig, *Mental Healers: Franz Anton Mesmer, Mary Baker Eddy, Sigmund Freud* (New York: Frederick Ungar, 1932); Robert Peel, *Mary Baker Eddy: The Years of Discovery* (New York: Holt, Rinehart and Winston, 1966).

7. Evans's views are expressed in the following books: W. F. Evans, *Soul and Body; or, The Spiritual Science of Health and Disease* (Boston: H. H. Carter, 1876); W. F. Evans, *Mental Medicine: A Theoretical and Practical Treatise on Medical Psychology*, 4th ed. (Boston: Carter & Pettee, 1872); W. F. Evans, *The Divine Law of Cure* (Boston: H. H. Carter, 1881); W. F. Evans, *The Mental-Cure, Illustrating the Influence of the Mind on the Body, Both in Health and Disease, and the Psychological Method of Treatment*, 6th ed. (Boston: Colby and Rich, 1884); W. F. Evans, *The Primitive Mind-Cure: The Nature and Power of Faith; or, Elementary Lessons in Christian Philosophy and Transcendental Medicine* (Boston: H. H. Carter, 1885).

8. For a historical treatment of dangerous and criminal insanity see Janet Colaizzi, *Homicidal Insanity, 1800–1985* (Tuscaloosa, Alabama: University of Alabama Press, 1989). On the history of early American psychiatry and the law, see also James C. Mohr, *Doctors and the Law: Medical Jurisprudence in Nineteenth-Century America* (New York: Oxford University Press, 1993); Janet Ann Tighe, "A Question of Responsibility: The Development of American Forensic Psychiatry, 1838–1930" (Ph.D. Diss., University of Pennsylvania, 1983); Norman Dain, *Concepts of Insanity in the United States, 1789–1965* (New Brunswick, New Jersey: Rutgers University Press, 1964).

9. See Norman Dain, *Clifford W. Beers, Advocate for the Insane* (Pittsburgh: University of Pittsburgh Press, 1981).

10. On the discussion about the Gheel system see Norman Dain, *Disordered Minds: The First Century of Eastern State Hospital in Williamsburg, Virginia, 1766–1866* (Williamsburg, Virginia: The Colonial Williamsburg Foundation, 1971), 128–134; and Gerald N. Grob, *The State and the Mentally Ill: A History of Worcester State Hospital in Massachusetts, 1830–1920* (Chapel Hill: University of North Carolina Press, 1966), 94–97.

11. Pliny Earle, *Memoirs of Pliny Earle, M.D., with Extracts from His Diary and Letters (1830–1892) and Selections from His Professional Writings (1839–1891)*, edited by F. B. Sanborn (Boston: Damrell & Upham, 1898), 273; Pliny Earle, "The Curability of Insanity," Read before the New England Psychological Society, on Retiring from Office as Its President, December 14, 1876; and Published by That Society (Utica, New York: Ellis H. Roberts & Co., Printers, 1877); see also Pliny Earle, "The Curability of Insanity," *American Journal of Insanity*, xlii (1885), 179–209 and Pliny Earle, *The Curability of Insanity: A Series of Studies* (1887; reprint, New York: Arno Press, 1972).

12. In the late eighteenth century, for example, Dr. Benjamin Rush, the so-called father of American psychiatry, advanced his political views by criticizing his opponents' actions as harmful to mental health. A Jeffersonian, Rush warned of the dangers to mental health in Federalist Alexander Hamilton's financial program: "The funding system, and speculation in bank script, and new lands have been fruitful sources of madness in our country." (Benjamin Rush, *Medical Inquiries and Observations upon the Diseases of the Mind*, 4th ed. [Philadelphia: John Grigg, 1830], 64.)

13. Letter from Mitchell to Clifford W. Beers, 2 April 1908 (copy), quoted in Dain, *Clifford W. Beers*, 98.

14. I do not suggest that in fact Freud or his followers were not initially committed to viewing

themselves as scientists, and indeed many Viennese psychoanalysts were neurologists who "shared with biologists a common interest in the biological foundation of mental and psychic processes," as historian Alfred Springer observes. "Because of this their interpretation of the impact of somatic structures and functions on the psychic and mental processes differed from that of early biological psychiatrists solely in the assumption that the relationship of brain structure and 'the soul' is not unidirectional but should be understood as a complex interrelation." (Alfred Springer, "Historiography and History of Psychiatry in Austria," *History of Psychiatry*, ii [1991], 257–258.)

15. The idea that insanity as well as emotional disorder was the price for civilization was a common view of many midnineteenth-century psychiatrists. See, for example, Edward Jarvis, *Cause of Insanity, An Address Delivered before the Norfolk, Massachusetts, District Medical Society* (Norfolk: 1851), 17. This view differed from Freud's in that those early American physicians and their successors assumed that one could reform society and thereby preserve civilization while eliminating insanity. Conversely, anti-psychiatry advocates who also believed that society was capable of being perfected sought a world free of insanity by eliminating psychiatry and its institutions.

16. On the relationship between the Roman Catholic church and psychiatry see Francis J. Braceland (ed.), *Faith, Reason and Modern Psychiatry: Sources for a Synthesis* (New York: P. J. Kenedy, 1955).

17. See David Musto, "What Happened to 'Community Mental Health,' " *Public Interest*, (Spring 1975), 59–60; Gerald N. Grob, *From Asylum to Community: Mental Health Policy in Modern America* (Princeton: Princeton University Press, 1991); Murray Levine, *The History and Politics of Community Mental Health* (New York: Oxford University Press, 1981).

18. Erving Goffman, *Asylums: Essays on the Social Situation of Mental Patients and Other Inmates* (Garden City, New York: Anchor Books, 1961).

19. For a somewhat more extensive discussion and bibliography of recent anti-psychiatry, especially among ex-patients, see my "Critics and Dissenters: Reflections on 'Anti-Psychiatry' in the United States," *Journal of the History of the Behavioral Sciences*, xxv (1989), 3–25. Among the most important and influential examples of the ex-patient literature are Judi Chamberlin, *On Our Own: Patient-Controlled Alternatives to the Mental Health System* (New York: Hawthorn Books, 1978); Lenny Lapon, *Mass Murderers in White Coats: Psychiatric Genocide in Nazi Germany and the United States* (Springfield, Massachusetts: Psychiatric Genocide Research Institute, 1986); Sherry Hirsch et al. (eds.), *Madness Network News Reader* (San Francisco: Glide Publications, 1974); David Hill, *The Politics of Schizophrenia: Psychiatric Oppression in the United States* (Lanham, Maryland: University Press of America, 1983). A compilation of anti-psychiatry writings by psychiatrists, psychologists, philosophers, legal scholars, and political scientists is Rem B. Edwards (ed.), *Psychiatry and Ethics: Insanity, Rational Autonomy, and Mental Health Care* (Buffalo, New York: Prometheus Books, 1982).

20. Szasz's most influential works are *The Myth of Mental Illness: Foundations of a Theory of Personal Conduct* (New York: Hoeber-Harper, 1964); *Law, Liberty, and Psychiatry: An Inquiry into the Social Uses of Mental Health Practices* (New York: Macmillan, 1963); and a collection of articles by various authors, *The Age of Madness: The History of Involuntary Mental Hospitalization Presented in Selected Texts*, edited with preface, introduction, and epilogue by Thomas S. Ssasz (New York: Jason Aronson, 1974).

21. See R. D. Laing, *The Politics of Experience* (New York: Ballantine Books, 1967).

22. See Thomas Scheff, *Being Mentally Ill: A Sociological Theory* (London: Weidenfeld & Nicolson, 1966) and *Labeling Madness* (New York: Prentice-Hall, 1975).

23. See, for example, David J. Rothman, *The Discovery of the Asylum: Social Order and Disorder in the New Republic* (Boston: Little, Brown, 1971), and Andrew T. Scull, *Museums of Madness: The Social Organization of Insanity in Nineteenth-Century England* (New York: St.

Martin's Press, 1979). Michel Foucault's major work on the subject is *Madness and Civilization: A History of Insanity in the Age of Reason* (New York: Pantheon Books, 1965).

24. Hans Eysenck, *The Future of Psychiatry* (London: Methuen, 1975), 16.

25. Hans Eysenck, *You and Neurosis* (Glasgow: Fontana, 1978), 17; see also Lawrie Reznek, *The Philosophical Defence of Psychiatry* (New York: Routledge, 1991), ch. 3.

26. Peter Sedgwick, *Psycho Politics* (London: Pluto Press, 1982), 30 (Sedgwick's italics).

27. James. S. Gordon, "Alternative Mental Health Services and Psychiatry," *American Journal of Psychiatry*, cxxxix (1982), 653–656.

28. An excellent study of the effects of deinstitutionalization is Ann Braden Johnson, *Out of Bedlam: The Truth about Deinstitutionalization* (New York: Basic Books, 1990). On the role of the law in the process see Rael Jean Isaac and Virginia C. Armat, *Madness in the Streets: How Psychiatry and the Law Abandoned the Mentally Ill* (New York: Free Press, 1990).

29. The National Alliance for the Mentally Ill has grown rapidly in size and power. Psychiatrist Melvin Sabshin notes that the "families of severely ill mental patients . . . felt attacked by psychotherapeutic and sociotherapeutic concepts in psychiatry" and find a somatic approach much more acceptable. The alliance's "passionate espousal of biological psychiatry" has been, moreover, of great help to psychiatry. (Melvin Sabshin, "Turning Points in Twentieth-Century American Psychiatry," *American Journal of Psychiatry*, cxlvii [1990], 1271.)

30. *Look Magazine*, 26 January, 1965, 28–32.

31. Ibid., 30–32. See also *The Doctors Speak Up: An Answer to Irresponsible Attacks on the Mental Health Program*, Prepared as a Public Service by the San Fernando Valley Doctors Committee on Mental Health, in collaboration with the San Fernando Valley Mental Health Association (n.p.: 1961?); and *The Facts . . . a Reply to the Anti-Mental Health Critics* (New York: National Association for Mental Health, 1962).

32. Important historical studies of the Right are Gary K. Clabaugh, *Thunder on the Right: The Protestant Fundamentalists* (Chicago: Nelson-Hall, 1974); George M. Marsden, *Fundamentalism and American Culture: The Shaping of Twentieth-Century Evangelicalism, 1870–1925*, (Oxford, New York: Oxford University Press, 1980); Richard Hofstadter, *The Paranoid Style in American Politics* (New York: Random House, 1965); Richard Hofstadter, *Anti-Intellectualism in American Life* (New York: Knopf, 1963); Daniel Bell (ed.), *The New American Right* (New York: Criterion Books, 1955). A brief overview of recent studies of the Right is Michael Kazin, "The Grass-Roots Right: New Histories of U.S. Conservatism in the Twentieth Century," *American Historical Review*, xcvii (1992), 136–155.

33. Marc Galanter, "Cults and Zealous Self-Help Movements: A Psychiatric Perspective," *American Journal of Psychiatry*, cxlvii (1990), 543–551, quotations from pp. 547, 545; Wade Clark Roof, *American Mainline Religion: Its Changing Shape and Future* (New Brunswick, New Jersey: Rutgers University Press, 1987); Richard John Neuhaus, *The Naked Public Square: Religion and Democracy in America*, 2d ed. (Grand Rapids, Michigan: Eerdmans Pub. Co., 1986).

34. See, for example, Karl Menninger, *The Crime of Punishment* (New York: Viking, 1969).

35. See Alexander D. Brooks, *Law, Psychiatry and the Mental Health System* (Boston: Little, Brown, 1974), 145–149; Bruce J. Ennis, *Prisoners of Psychiatry: Mental Patients, Psychiatrists, and the Law* (New York: Harcourt Brace Jovanovich, 1972); Jonas Robitscher, *The Powers of Psychiatry* (Boston: Houghton Mifflin, 1980); Lee Coleman, *The Reign of Terror: Psychiatry, Authority, and the Law* (Boston: Beacon Press, 1984); David Ingleby (ed.), *Critical Psychiatry: The Politics of Mental Health* (New York: Pantheon Books, 1980); Martin L. Gross, *The Psychological Society: A Critical Analysis of Psychiatry, Psychotherapy, Psychoanalysis and the Psychological Revolution* (New York: Random House, 1978). See also Reznek, *The Philosophical Defence of Psychiatry*, on the social origins of the determination of what is mental illness or disorder.

36. For brief discussions of these issues see Louis McGarry and Paul Chodoff, "The Ethics

of Involuntary Hospitalization'' in Sidney Bloch and Paul Chodoff (eds.), *Psychiatric Ethics* (Oxford, New York: Oxford University Press, 1984), 203–219; Bick Wanck, ''Two Decades of Involuntary Hospitalization Legislation,'' *American Journal of Psychiatry*, cxli (1985), 33–37; and Paul S. Appelbaum and Loren H. Roth, ''Involuntary Treatment in Medicine and Psychiatry,'' *American Journal of Psychiatry*, cxli (1985), 202–205.

37. D. A. Treffert, ''Dying with Your Rights On,'' Presented at the 12th Annual Meeting of the American Psychiatric Association, Detroit, Michigan, *American Journal of Psychiatry*, cxli (1974), 6–10; see also Morton Birnbaum, ''The Right to Treatment: Some Comments on Its Development'' in F. J. Ayd (ed.), *Medical, Moral and Legal Issues in Mental Health Care* (Baltimore: Williams & Wilkins, 1974), 97–141. For a graphic example of the ruinous effect on one person and his neighborhood of the failures of the recent policies regarding mental illness see *New York Times*, 3 Sept. 1992, A1, B4.

38. *New York Times*, 10 Sept. 1992, A18.

39. This was the well-known Tarasoff case, decided by the Supreme Court in 1974, and upon rehearing, again in 1976. See Loren H. Roth and Alan Meisel, ''Dangerousness, Confidentiality, and the Duty to Warn,'' *American Journal of Psychiatry*, cxxxiv (1977), 508–511. See also Colaizzi, *Homicidal Insanity*, ch. 9.

40. Sabshin, ''Turning Points in Twentieth-Century American Psychiatry,'' 1271.

41. Thomas Szasz, *Insanity: The Idea and Its Consequences* (New York: Wiley, 1987), 346ff.

42. E. Fuller Torrey, *The Death of Psychiatry* (Radnor, Pennsylvania: Chilton Book Co., 1974). See also his *The Mind Game: Witchdoctors and Psychiatrists* (New York: Emerson Hall Publishers, 1972).

43. E. Fuller Torrey, *Freudian Fraud: The Malignant Effect of Freud's Theory on American Thought and Culture* (New York: HarperCollins, 1992).

44. Ibid., 191.

45. Peter Breggin, *Toxic Psychiatry* (New York: St. Martin's Press, 1991), 58, 59, 60. A very different perspective is offered in, for example, Frank Ervin, ''Biological Intervention Technologies and Social Control,'' *American Behavioral Scientist*, xviii (1975), 617–635, and C. R. Jeffery and Ina A. Jeffrey, ''Psychosurgery and Behavior Modification: Legal Control Techniques Versus Behavior Control Techniques,'' *American Behavioral Scientist*, xviii (1975), 685–721.

46. Breggin, 408–409.

47. For the latter view see Reznek, *The Philosophical Defence of Psychiatry*; Aviel Goodman, ''Organic Unity Theory: The Mind-Body Problem Revisited,'' *American Journal of Psychiatry*, cxlviii (1991), 553–653; Jerome C. Wakefield, ''The Concept of Mental Disorder: On the Boundary Between Biological Facts and Social Values,'' *American Psychologist*, xlvii (1992), 373–388; Patricia Smith Churchland, *Neurophilosophy: Toward a Unified Science of the Mind-Brain* (Cambridge: MIT Press, 1986); Stephen Priest, *Theories of the Mind* (Boston: Houghton Mifflin, 1991), 113.

48. A recent critique and review of social control theorists is Abraham S. Luchins, ''Social Control Doctrines of Mental Illness and the Medical Profession in Nineteenth-Century America,'' *Journal of the History of the Behavioral Sciences*, xxix (1993), 29–47. The work of Michel Foucault has spawned a prolific literature, including of late critiques as well as explications; see a recent biography, James Miller, *The Passion of Michel Foucault* (New York: Simon & Schuster, 1993).

Index

CPSIA information can be obtained
at www.ICGtesting.com
Printed in the USA
LVHW080022170520
655837LV00003B/25